The M. D. Anderson Surgical Oncology Handbook

Second Edition

W9-CXQ-123

The M. D. Anderson Surgical Oncology Handbook

Second Edition

M. D. Anderson Cancer Center
Department of Surgical Oncology
Houston, Texas

Barry W. Feig, M.D.

David H. Berger, M.D.

George M. Fuhrman, M.D.

Editors

LIPPINCOTT WILLIAMS & WILKINS
A **Wolters Kluwer** Company
Philadelphia · Baltimore · New York · London
Buenos Aires · Hong Kong · Sydney · Tokyo

Acquisitions Editor: Lisa McAllister
Developmental Editor: Rebecca Irwin Diehl
Manufacturing Manager: Tim Reynolds
Production Manager: Cassie Moore
Production Editor: Aureliano Vázquez, Jr.
Cover Illustrator: Kevin Kall
Indexer: Victoria Boyle
Compositor: Circle Graphics
Printer: R. R. Donnelly, Crawfordsville

© 1999 by M. D. Anderson Cancer Center
Department of Surgical Oncology
Published by Lippincott Williams & Wilkins

Second Edition

Library of Congress Cataloging-in-Publication Data

The M. D. Anderson surgical oncology handbook / Barry W. Feig,
    David H. Berger, George M. Fuhrman, editors: M. D. Anderson
    Cancer Center, Department of Surgical Oncology. — 2nd ed.
        p.   cm.
    Includes bibliographical references and index.
    ISBN 0-7817-1581-4
    1. Cancer—Surgery—Handbooks, manuals, etc.   I. Feig,
Barry W. 1959–   .   II. Berger, David H., 1959–   .
III. Fuhrman, George M   IV. University of Texas M. D.
Anderson Cancer Center. Dept. of Surgical Oncology.
    [DNLM: 1. Neoplasms—surgery handbooks.   QZ 39M111
1999]
    RD651.M17   1999
    616.99'4059—dc21
    DNLM/DLC
    for Library of Congress   98-37038
                                                                    CIP

Printed in the United States of America

9 8 7 6 5 4 3 2 1

To our wives (Barbara, Adrianne, and Laura) and families, for their support, enthusiasm, and patience through our many years of training and continued long hours spent in the care of patients with cancer.

Contents

Foreword

Surgical oncology is a rapidly changing medical specialty that reflects our advancing understanding of cancer biology and treatment. The surgeon's role in cancer care has greatly expanded and diversified because of developments in the natural history of cancer, earlier detection of many cancers, and the increased availability of effective systematic therapy regimens. Thus, the surgeon today must posses up-to-date information and a broad set of clinical skills to participate as an effective partner in a multidisciplinary cancer care team and to ensure that the full range of diagnostic and treatment options are considered in the management of each patient's cancer.

The *M. D. Anderson Surgical Oncology Handbook, Second Edition*, helps equip the surgeon, experienced and in training, with current knowledge in the oncology field. Extensively revised, the second edition was written by surgical oncology fellows for an audience of students, residents and fellows, as well as members in allied medical fields. Each chapter outlines the essential elements of diagnosis, staging, and clinical management of solid tumors treated in surgical practice. It emphasizes the importance of multidisciplinary treatment planning, which is essential to the surgeon in counseling cancer patients.

Cancer therapy has evolved to the point that a multidisciplinary approach has become standard in treating most cancer patients, even those with early-stage disease. If the surgeon is to retain the primary coordinating role in cancer management, he or she must fully understand all modalities of oncology therapy and know how to deploy them. This role as coordinator of therapy demands knowledge about indications, risks, and the benefits of adjuvant chemotherapy, hormonal therapy, and radiation therapy.

Determining the most appropriate treatment plan for a surgical patient with cancer is one of the most difficult decisions in clinical medicine: the biological presentations of many cancers are varied, the treatment options and sequences are numerous, and patients' differing perceptions of quality of life are diverse. All these considerations have to be incorporated into an organized treatment plan. The surgical oncology handbook will help readers formulate these plans for their cancer patients.

The surgical oncology fellows (past and present) at the M. D. Anderson Cancer Center join me in dedicating this book to the cancer patients we serve. We hope it will be a valuable companion to the reader's daily rounds and study.

Charles M. Balch, M.D.
Professor of Surgery
President and CEO
City of Hope National Medical Center
Duarte, California 91010-3000

Preface

The *M. D. Anderson Surgical Oncology Handbook* was written in an attempt to document the philosophies and practices of the Department of Surgical Oncology at the M. D. Anderson Cancer Center. The purpose of the book is to outline basic management approaches based on our experience with surgical oncology problems at M. D. Anderson. The book is intended to serve as a practical guide to the established surgical oncology principles for treating cancer as it involves each organ system in the body. This second edition has included new chapters on basic science and the treatment of tumors of unknown primary origin. In addition, updated information has been added on new treatments and procedures including lymphatic mapping for breast cancer and melanoma, hyperthermic isolated limb perfusion for extremity melanoma and sarcoma, cryosurgery for liver tumors, as well as many other new advances in treatment.

This book is written by current and former surgical oncology fellows at M. D. Anderson. Although the target audience for the first edition was the surgical house staff and surgical oncology trainees, we found that there was a significantly wider appeal for the book across multiple disciplines and at various levels of training and experience. We have, therefore, widened the scope of the second edition to reach this broader group. The authors represent various training programs, and they have spent at least two years at the M. D. Anderson Cancer Center studying only surgical oncology. The diversity of authors allows us to present the current opinions and practices of the M. D. Anderson Department of Surgical Oncology, along with other opinions and treatment options practiced in our far-ranging surgical training. Although there is no "senior" well-known name associated with the book, the authors represent 160 years of surgical training; we have not, however, become dogmatic and unyielding in our medical practices.

This handbook is not meant to encompass all aspects of oncology in minute detail. Rather, it is an attempt to address commonly encountered as well as controversial issues in surgical oncology. While other authors present their opinions and approaches as firmly established, we have tried to point out controversies and show alternative approaches to these problems besides our own.

We would like to thank the surgical staff at the M. D. Anderson Cancer Center for their assistance with the content of this book and for their devoted teaching in the hospital clinics, wards, and operating rooms. In addition, we would particularly like to thank the patients seen and treated at M. D. Anderson for their warmth and appreciation of our care, as well as for their patience and understanding of the learning process.

B.W.F.
D.H.B.
G.M.F.

Contributing Authors

Paul M. Ahearne, M.D. *Junior Faculty Associate, Department of Surgical Oncology, University of Texas, M. D. Anderson Cancer Center, 1515 Holcombe Boulevard, Houston, Texas, 77030-4095*

David H. Berger, M.D. *Associate Professor, Department of Surgery, Medical College of Pennsylvania / , Hahnemann School of Medicine, 3300 Henry Avenue, Philadelphia, Pennsylvania 19129*

Diane C. Bodurka Bevers, M.D. *Assistant Professor, Department of Gynecologic Oncology, University of Texas, M. D. Anderson Cancer Center, 1515 Holcombe Boulevard, Box 67, Houston, Texas, 77030-4095*

Michael W. Bevers, M.D. *Assistant Professor, Department of Gynecologic Oncology, University of Texas, M. D. Anderson Cancer Center, 1515 Holcombe Boulevard, Box 67, Houston, Texas, 77030-4095*

Richard J. Bold, M.D. *Junior Faculty Associate, Department of Surgical Oncology, University of Texas, M. D. Anderson Cancer Center, 1515 Holcombe Boulevard, Houston, Texas, 77030-4095*

Michael Bouvet, M.D. *Assistant Professor, Department of Surgery, University of California, San Diego, 200 West Arbor Drive, San Diego, California, 92103*

James C. Cusack, Jr., M.D. *Assistant Professor, Department of Surgery, CB #7210, University of North Carolina School of Medicine, Chapel Hill, North Carolina, 27599-7210*

Mark G. Delworth, M.D. *Fellow, Department of Urology, University of Texas, M. D. Anderson Cancer Center, 1515 Holcombe Boulevard, Houston, Texas, 77030-4095*

Colin P.N. Dinney, M.D. *Assistant Professor, Department of Urology, University of Texas Medical School, Assistant Urologist, Department of Urology, University of Texas, M. D. Anderson Cancer Center, 1515 Holcombe Boulevard, Houston, Texas, 77030-4095*

Barry W. Feig, M.D. *Assistant Professor of Surgery, Department of Surgical Oncology, University of Texas, M. D. Anderson Cancer Center, 1515 Holcombe Boulevard, Box 106, Houston, Texas, 77030-4095*

George M. Fuhrman, M.D. *Program Director, Department of Surgery, Ochsner Clinic, 1514 Jefferson Highway, New Orleans, Louisiana, 70121*

Jeffrey E. Gershenwald, M.D. *Assistant Professor, Department of Surgical Oncology, University of Texas, M. D. Anderson Cancer Center, 1515 Holcombe Boulevard, Box 106, Houston, Texas, 77030-4095*

Ana M. Grau, M.D. *Research Fellow, Department of Surgical Oncology, University of Texas, M. D. Anderson Cancer Center, 1515 Holcombe Boulevard, Houston, Texas, 77030-4095*

Keith M. Heaton, M.D. *Junior Faculty Associate, Department of Surgical Oncology, University of Texas, M. D. Anderson Cancer Center, 1515 Holcombe Boulevard, Houston, Texas, 77030-4095*

Kelly K. Hunt, M.D. *Assistant Professor of Surgery, Department of Surgical Oncology, University of Texas, M. D. Anderson Cancer Center, Box 106, 1515 Holcombe Boulevard, Houston, Texas, 77030-4095*

Steven D. Leach, M.D. *Assistant Professor of Surgery, Vanderbilt University Medical School, T-2104 Medical Center North, 21st and Garland Streets, Nashville, Tennessee, 37232*

Jeffrey E. Lee, M.D. *Associate Professor, Department of Surgical Oncology, University of Texas, M. D. Anderson Cancer Center, 1515 Holcombe Boulevard, Box 106, Houston, Texas, 77030-4095*

Phillip B. Ley, M.D. *Clinical Assistant Professor, Department of Surgery, University of Mississippi Medical Center, 2500 N. State Street, Jackson, Mississippi, 39216; Attending Surgical Oncologist, Department of Surgery, Mississipi Baptist Medical Center, 1225 N. State Street, Jackson, Mississippi, 39202*

Sarkis H. Meterissian, M.D., F.R.C.S., F.A.C.S. *Assistant Professor, Department of Surgery, McGill University, McIntyre Medical Sciences Building, 3655 Drummond Street, Montreal, Quebec, H3G 1Y6, Canada; Assistant Surgeon, Department of Surgery, Royal Victoria Hospital, 687 Pine Avenue West, Montreal, Quebec, H3A 1A1, Canada*

Gregory P. Midis, M.D. *Assistant Professor, Department of Surgery, University of Tennessee Medical Center at Knoxville, 1924 Alcoa Highway, Knoxville, Tennessee, 37920*

Mira Milas, M.D. *General Surgery Resident, Department of Surgery, Emory University, 1364 Clifton Road NE, Altanta, Georgia 30322*

Alexander R. Miller, M.D. *Junior Faculty Associate, Department of Surgical Oncology, University of Texas, M. D. Anderson Cancer Center, 1515 Holcombe Boulevard, Houston, Texas, 77030-4095*

David B. Pearlstone, M.D.   *Junior Faculty Associate, Department of Surgical Oncology, University of Texas, M. D. Anderson Cancer Center, 1515 Holcombe Boulevard, Houston, Texas, 77030-4095*

A. Scott Pearson, M.D.   *Junior Faculty Associate, Department of Surgical Oncology, University of Texas, M. D. Anderson Cancer Center, 1515 Holcombe Boulevard, Box 106, Houston, Texas, 77030-4095*

George E. Peoples, M.D.   *Junior Faculty Associate, Department of Surgical Oncology, University of Texas, M. D. Anderson Cancer Center, 1515 Holcombe Boulevard, Houston, Texas, 77030-4095*

James A. Reilly, Jr., M.D.   *Clinical Assistant Professor, Department of Surgery, University of Nebraska, 600 S. 42nd Street, Omaha, Nebraska, 68198; Staff Surgeon, Department of Surgery, Nebraska Methodist Hospital, 8303 Dodge Street, Omaha, Nebraska, 68114*

Emily K. Robinson, M.D.   *Research Fellow, Department of Surgical Oncology, University of Texas, M. D. Anderson Cancer Center, 1515 Holcombe Boulevard, Box 106, Houston, Texas, 77030-4095*

Barry J. Roseman, M.D.   *Surgical Oncologist, Blount Memorial Hospital, 907 East Lamar Alexander Parkway, Maryville, Tennessee, 37804*

Francis R. Spitz, M.D.   *Assistant Professor, Department of Surgery, University of Pennsylvania, 3400 Spruce Street, Philadelphia, Pennsylvania, 19107*

Charles A. Staley, M.D.   *Assistant Professor of Surgery, Emory University Medical School, 1365 Clifton Road, NE, Atlanta, Georgia, 30322*

Jeffrey J. Sussman, M.D.   *Assistant Professor of Surgery, Department of Surgery, Division of Surgical Oncology, University of Cincinnati, Barrett Cancer Center, 234 Goodman Street, Cincinnati, Ohio, 45267-0772*

Stephen G. Swisher, M.D.   *Professor of Surgery, Department of Thoracic and Cardiovascular Surgery, University of Texas, M. D. Anderson Cancer Center, 1515 Holcombe Boulevard, Box 109, Houston, Texas, 77030-4095*

Kenneth K. Tanabe, M.D.   *Assistant Professor, Department of Surgery, Harvard Medical School, Assistant Surgeon, Massachusetts General Hospital, 100 Blossom Street, Boston, Massachusetts, 02114*

Paula M. Termuhlen, M.D.   *Assistant Professor, Department of Surgery, University of Nebraska Medical Center, 600 South 42nd Street, Omaha, Nebraska, 68198*

Douglas S. Tyler, M.D.   *Assistant Professor of Surgery, Duke University Medical Center, Box 3118, Durham, North Carolina, 27710*

Ara A. Vaporciyan, M.D.   *Assistant Professor of Surgery, Department of Thoracic and Cardiovascular Surgery, University of Texas, M. D. Anderson Cancer Center, 1515 Holcombe Boulevard, Box 109, Houston, Texas, 77030-4095*

Judith K. Wolf, M.D.   *Assistant Professor of Gynecology, Department of Gynecologic Oncology, University of Texas, M. D. Anderson Cancer Center, 1515 Holcombe Boulevard, Box 67, Houston, Texas, 77030-4095*

Alan M. Yahanda, M.D.   *Assistant Professor of Surgery, Division of Surgical Oncology, University of Michigan Medical Center, CGC 3304, 1500 East Medical Center Drive, Ann Arbor, Michigan, 48109-0932*

The M. D. Anderson Surgical Oncology Handbook

Second Edition

NOTICE

Care has been taken to confirm the accuracy of the information presented and to describe generally accepted practices. However, the authors, editors, and publisher are not responsible for errors or omissions or for any consequences from application of the information in this book and make no warranty, expressed or implied, with respect to the contents of the publication.

The indications and dosages of all drugs in this book have been recommended in the medical literature and conform to the practices of the general medical community. The medications prescribed do not necessarily have specific approval by the Food and Drug Administration for use in the diseases and dosages for which they are recommended. The package insert for each drug should be consulted for use and dosage as approved by the FDA. Because standards for usage change, it is advisable to keep abreast of revised recommendations, particularly those concerning new drugs.

Noninvasive Breast Cancer

Emily K. Robinson and Kelly K. Hunt

Noninvasive breast cancer comprises two separate entities: ductal carcinoma *in situ* (DCIS) and lobular carcinoma *in situ* (LCIS). DCIS and LCIS are defined as a proliferation of neoplastic epithelial cells confined to the mammary ducts or lobules, respectively, without demonstrable evidence of invasion through the basement membrane. Because they are noninvasive, DCIS and LCIS offer no risk of metastatic spread. The term *minimal breast cancer*, once used to encompass *in situ* lesions and invasive cancers less than 5 mm in diameter, has been abandoned because the prognosis and treatment strategies for each are entirely different.

Ductal Carcinoma *in Situ*

EPIDEMIOLOGY

Since the introduction of routine screening with mammography, the incidence of DCIS has increased threefold from that observed in older series, when DCIS remained undetected until it was palpable. In the United States, the incidence is now 10–20 per 100,000 woman-years, with the ratio of DCIS to LCIS being 6:1. The prevalence of DCIS has risen as the quality and sensitivity of mammography have improved, and DCIS currently accounts for 20–44% of all new screen-detected breast neoplasms.

The median age reported for patients with DCIS is 47–63 years, which is not different from that reported for patients with invasive carcinoma. Some studies have noted a trend toward a lower median age in patients with DCIS detected in screening examinations. The frequency of a family history of breast cancer among first-degree relatives of patients with DCIS (10–35%) is not different from that reported for women with invasive breast malignancies.

PATHOLOGY

Histologic Subtypes

DCIS is thought to arise from duct epithelium in the region of the terminal lobular-ductal unit and probably represents one stage in a continuum between atypical ductal hyperplasia and invasive carcinoma. DCIS comprises a heterogeneous group of lesions with variable histologic architecture, cellular characteristics, and clinical behavior. Malignant cells proliferate to obliterate the ductal lumen, and there may be an associated inflammatory reaction, stromal response, or lymphoid infiltration surrounding the duct.

DCIS is generally classified as one of five subtypes based on differences in the architectural pattern and nuclear features:

comedo, solid, cribriform, micropapillary, and papillary. Cribriform, comedo, and micropapillary are the most common subtypes, although two or more patterns coexist in up to 50% of cases.

As factors indicative of aggressive biology have been identified, classification systems of noninvasive breast cancer have undergone a fundamental change, from a strictly descriptive histologic nomenclature to a system that incorporates these prognostic factors and stratifies lesions based on their likelihood of recurrence. Lagios et al. identified high nuclear grade and comedo necrosis to be predictive of local recurrence. At 8 years, patients with high nuclear grade and comedo necrosis had a 20% local failure rate after breast conservation surgery and irradiation, compared with a 5% local failure rate for patients without necrosis and with a lower nuclear grade. Subsequently, Silverstein et al. (1996) developed the Van Nuys classification system in which patients with DCIS were assigned to one of three groups based on the presence or absence of high nuclear grade and comedo necrosis: group 1 had non-high-grade DCIS without comedo necrosis, group 2 had non-high-grade DCIS with comedo necrosis, and group 3 had high-grade DCIS with or without comedo necrosis. Two hundred thirty-eight patients treated with breast preservation surgery for DCIS were retrospectively stratified into these three groups. There was a statistically significant difference in disease-free survival between group 1 and groups 2 and 3. Intragroup disease-free survival was also analyzed according to treatment types, and there was no significant difference in disease-free survival for patients in groups 1 and 2 when they were treated with excision alone versus excision plus radiation therapy. In contrast, there was a statistically significant improvement in disease-free survival for those patients in group 3 (high-grade DCIS) who received adjuvant radiation therapy following tumor excision ($p = .001$).

Silverstein and colleagues subsequently proposed a treatment schema based on tumor characteristics that have been demonstrated by multivariate analysis to predict local recurrence. The Van Nuys Prognostic Index (VNPI) stratifies DCIS patients according to three significant predictors of local recurrence: tumor size, width of surgical excision margins, and pathologic classification (based on the Van Nuys classification system discussed earlier). Numerical values ranging from 1 (best) to 3 (worst) are assigned for each of the three predictors, the sum of which results in the VNPI score, which ranges from the lowest possible score of 3 to the highest possible score of 9. Based on the resultant VNPI score, either local excision, local excision plus radiotherapy, or mastectomy is recommended as treatment. Three hundred thirty-three DCIS patients treated with breast conservation therapy were retrospectively assigned a VNPI score and studied with local recurrence as the end point. Patients with VNPI scores of 3 or 4 did not appear to derive any extra benefit from the addition of radiation therapy over excision alone when evaluated for local recurrence-free survival. In contrast, local recurrence-free survival was increased by 17% ($p = .017$) by the addition of radiation therapy for patients with VNPI scores of 5, 6, or 7. Although patients with VNPI scores of 8 or 9 showed the greatest benefit with the addition of radiation therapy, local recurrence rates exceeded 60% in 8 years, regardless of irradiation. Therefore the authors recommended that these subgroups should be considered for mastectomy. The VNPI may become a useful adjunct in therapeutic decision making; however, its validity has yet to be tested prospectively.

MULTIFOCALITY

Multifocality is generally considered to be present when separate foci of DCIS occur more than 5 mm apart in the same breast quadrant. However, some investigators believe that multifocal disease may in fact represent intraductal spread from a single focus of DCIS. By careful serial subsectioning, Holland et al. demonstrated that multifocal lesions that appeared separate by traditional pathologic techniques were actually originating from the same focus in 81 of 82 mastectomy specimens.

MULTICENTRICITY

Multicentricity is defined as a separate focus of DCIS outside the index quadrant. The reported incidence of multicentricity may well depend on the extent of the pathologic review and therefore varies from 18% to 60% but is more likely around 30–40%. Mammary lobules are not constrained by the artificially imposed quadrant segregations; therefore contiguous intraductal spread may be interpreted as multicentricity on cursory pathologic examination. The biologic significance of multicentricity has been questioned, for close to 96% of all local recurrences after treatment for DCIS occur in the same quadrant as the index lesion, implicating residual untreated disease rather than multicentricity. Autopsy studies have reported a higher incidence of detection of DCIS than is evident in the general population, suggesting that not all DCIS lesions become clinically significant.

MICROINVASION

DCIS with microinvasion is generally defined as a predominantly noninvasive lesion with foci of invasive cancer, each measuring less than 1 mm. The incidence of microinvasion varies according to the size and extent of the ductal carcinoma *in situ*. Lagios et al. reported a 2% incidence of microinvasion in patients with DCIS measuring less than 25 mm, compared with a 29% incidence of microinvasion in index lesions larger than 26 mm. More recently, investigators have questioned the significance of distinguishing pure DCIS from DCIS with microinvasion. In a series by Wong et al., 41 patients presenting with DCIS and microinvasion had axillary nodal dissection as part of their treatment. There were no cases of nodal metastases, and none of the patients had recurrence of their disease with a median follow-up of 37 months. Silverstein et al. (1993) retrospectively compared patients with DCIS and those with DCIS with microinvasion. They found no difference in axillary node positivity, disease-free survival, or overall survival, and concluded that treatment for both forms of DCIS should be based on tumor size, margin status, ability to follow the patient mammographically, and the patient's desires and needs.

DIAGNOSIS

Clinical Presentation

In the past, patients with DCIS presented with a palpable mass, nipple discharge, or Paget's disease of the nipple. Occasionally, DCIS was an incidental finding in an otherwise benign biopsy specimen. The palpable lesions were large, and up to 25% demonstrated associated foci of invasive disease. The presence of occult invasion in these lesions as well as a 10% incidence of axillary metastasis led to the same treatment recommendations for patients with DCIS as for those with invasive breast cancer. Now that screening mammography is more prevalent, palpable or symptomatic DCIS with occult invasion and lymph node metastasis is rarely encountered, leading to a reassessment of treatment strategies.

Mammographic Features

Microcalcifications are the most common mammographic manifestation of DCIS and account for 80% of all carcinomas presenting with calcifications. Any interval change in a mammogram is associated with malignancy in 15–20% of cases and most often indicates *in situ* disease. Holland et al. described two different classes of microcalcifications: (1) those that are of the linear branching type and are associated with high nuclear-grade comedo-type lesions, and (2) fine, granular calcifications, which are associated with micropapillary or cribriform lesions (lower nuclear grade and no necrosis). These investigators demonstrated a significant difference in the mammographic versus pathologic extent of disease. The difference varied according to the histologic subtype of DCIS: In 44% of micropapillary tumors, the lesions were more than 2 cm larger by histologic examination than by mammographic estimate, compared with only 12% of the pure comedo subtype. However, with the addition of magnification views to the mammographic examination the extent of disease was underestimated in only 14% of micropapillary tumors.

Diagnostic Biopsy

Because most cases of DCIS are now detected as mammographic abnormalities, confirmational diagnosis by biopsy is critical. At the University of Texas M. D. Anderson Cancer Center, microcalcifications that are suspicious for malignancy are excised with the aid of mammographic needle localization. Nonpalpable mammographic masses that are visualized by ultrasound undergo ultrasound-guided fine-needle aspiration biopsy as a first step. Ultrasound can also be used in the operating room to guide excisional biopsy of these masses, alleviating the need for a prior needle localization procedure in the mammography suite. Stereotactic core needle biopsy can also be utilized in the diagnosis of mammographically detected lesions. This diagnostic modality should be used judiciously, and care should be taken not to completely excise all microcalcifications without placing a metallic marker to guide future surgical excision. In addition, calcifications that appear faintly or are deep in the breast and close to the chest wall may be difficult to target with stereotactic core biopsy.

The goal at the time of excisional biopsy should be to perform a margin-negative resection that can serve as a definitive segmental mastectomy. The margins should be at least 1 cm, with 2 cm being preferable. These specifications are based on the data by Holland et al., who demonstrated that up to 44% of lesions were found to extend more than 2 cm further on histologic examination than was estimated by mammography. Specimen radiography is essential to confirm the removal of all microcalcifications. After whole-specimen radiography, the specimen should be inked and then serially sectioned for repeat radiographic examination and pathologic examination to evaluate margin status and extent of disease.

Treatment

Traditionally, the treatment of DCIS has been mastectomy with or without low axillary lymph node dissection. Local-regional recurrence following mastectomy is reported to range from 0 to 4%, with from none to 4% of patients dying from the disease. As breast conservation techniques for invasive disease have been shown to be effective local therapy, the rationale for treating a premalignant (or noninvasive) condition with more radical surgery than its invasive counterpart has been questioned.

Mastectomy versus Breast Conservation Therapy

The rationale for total mastectomy to treat patients with DCIS is based on the incidence of multifocality and multicentricity as well as the possibility of occult invasion associated with the DCIS. Mastectomy remains the standard with which other proposed therapeutic modalities should be compared. A retrospective review by Balch et al. documented a local relapse rate of 3.1% and a mortality rate of 2.3% after mastectomy for DCIS. The cancer-related mortality following mastectomy for DCIS was calculated to be 1.7% in a series reported by Fowble and ranged from 0 to 8% in a review by Vezeridis and Bland.

The largest study comparing breast conservation therapy to mastectomy is Silverstein and colleagues' nonrandomized study of 277 cases of DCIS without microinvasion. Patients with tumors smaller than 4 cm with microscopically clear margins were treated with wide local excision and radiation therapy. Patients with tumors larger than 4 cm or positive margins were treated with mastectomy. The disease-free survival (freedom from local recurrence) at seven years was 98% in the mastectomy group versus 84% in the breast conservation therapy group ($p = .038$) with no difference in overall survival. Retrospective comparison of breast conservation surgery to mastectomy is difficult because of differences in tumor size, presentation, and follow-up. Crude local recurrences are higher after breast conservation surgery for DCIS (5–25%); however, with close follow-up the results of salvage surgery are excellent, and an increase in local recurrences has not affected overall survival. Solin et al. reviewed the records of 172 patients who underwent breast conservation therapy to evaluate pathologic characteristics of the primary tumor relative to local control, disease-free and overall survival, and freedom from distant metastasis. The only pathologic variable that correlated with the rate of local recurrence was the presence of comedo necrosis in tumors with nuclear grade 3 (8-year actuarial rate of local recurrence of 20% versus 5% in patients without necrosis). None of the pathologic variables examined correlated with overall survival, disease-specific survival, or freedom from distant metastasis. Patients with close or involved margins have a high rate of local recurrence, and large foci of DCIS (larger than 3 cm) may not only harbor occult invasive disease but are difficult to completely excise with cosmetically acceptable results. Therefore it is currently recommended that mastectomy be performed for large lesions (larger than 3 cm), lesions with a high nuclear grade, or pathologic evidence of close or involved margins when repeat local excision would not be cosmetically acceptable.

Wide Local Excision Alone

Data that support the use of wide local excision alone in the treatment of DCIS come from Lagios et al. In a report published in 1989, Lagios et al. noted that in 115 mastectomy specimens occult invasive cancer was identified only in breasts in which DCIS exceeded 45 mm and occurred in nearly 50% of breasts with DCIS larger than 55 mm in diameter. Subsequently, 79 patients with mammographically detected DCIS were treated by margin-negative wide local excision alone. The overall recurrence rate at 44 months was 10%, with 92% of the recurrences found in the same quadrant as the primary lesion and in the vicinity of the biopsy site. Fifty percent of the recurrences were invasive, but all were identified early by routine screening. Three patients had invasive recurrences that were stage I (T1a) at the time of excision, whereas a fourth patient, who developed a palpable recurrence and then initially refused treatment, had a 13-mm invasive lobular cancer with a single micrometastasis in a level 1 node. After a longer follow-up (124 months) of the same cohort of patients, local recurrence was 16% overall—33% for the subgroup of patients with high-grade lesions and comedo necrosis versus only 2% for patients with low- or intermediate-grade lesions.

Schwartz et al. reported on 70 patients with mammographically detected or incidentally discovered DCIS who were treated with wide local excision alone. The local recurrence rate at 49 months was 15%, with a 27% incidence of invasive recurrence. It should be noted that the follow-up on these patients was relatively short and that local recurrence following the diagnosis of DCIS without definitive treatment can occur 15–25 years later. These data taken together suggest that wide local excision alone may be appropriate therapy for a select subgroup of patients who have small, low-grade foci of DCIS excised with adequate margins and who can be followed diligently for recurrence.

Radiotherapy

The NSABP B-17 trial was designed to evaluate the role of radiotherapy in breast-conserving therapy for patients with DCIS. The 5-year event-free survival rate was 84.4% for the excision plus radiation therapy group and 73.8% for the lumpectomy-alone (wide local excision) cohort (p = .0001). The improvement in event-free survival was due to a decrease in local recurrence in the lumpectomy plus radiotherapy group: 7% versus 16.4% in the lumpectomy-alone group. Radiotherapy appears to decrease the incidence of local recurrence and the percentage of invasive recurrence. At 5 years, invasive recurrences decreased from 50% of the total recurrences after wide local excision alone to about 27% of those treated with radiotherapy. Difficulties with the B-17 trial included the following: (1) 45% of the lesions were smaller than 0.1 cm, (2) no reference was made to nuclear grade or comedo necrosis, and (3) in the subset of patients who developed local recurrences, invasive recurrences occurred relatively early (within 5 months), suggesting that some invasive tumors may have been misclassified as noninvasive. The ongoing EORTC-10853 trial was also designed to evaluate the role of adjuvant radiotherapy in the treatment of DCIS, but no preliminary statistical analysis has yet been performed. In a recent review by Silverstein et al. in which lesions were stratified according to the Van Nuys classification scheme, radiotherapy was of benefit (decreased local relapse) only in those patients with high nuclear-grade lesions. Clearly, future studies evaluating the role of radiotherapy should analyze subgroups based on pathologic indices (nuclear grade, comedo necrosis, margin status) in an attempt to identify the patients who will most likely benefit from adjuvant radiation. The current M. D. Anderson treatment algorithm is shown in Figure 1-1. Patients who would be considered for excision without radiotherapy have low nuclear grade, small tumor volume (<1 cm), and clear margins of resection (5–10 mm).

Tamoxifen

Two studies are now in progress to evaluate the effectiveness of tamoxifen in reducing recurrence in patients with DCIS. The NSABP B-24 trial and the United Kingdom Coordinating Committee for Cancer Research DCIS trial are both evaluating the role of tamoxifen in preventing subsequent invasive and *in situ* breast cancer in both the ipsilateral and contralateral breasts. At present, tamoxifen should be used as adjuvant treatment for patients with DCIS only in the context of a clinical trial.

Predictors of Local Relapse

There are no absolute indicators on which to base treatment strategies; however, multiple features of DCIS have been identified that are associated with a less favorable clinical course. Traditional pathologic variables such as large tumor size (>3 cm), high nuclear grade, comedo necrosis, and involved margins of excision are associated with a greater risk of local recurrence, as has been previously discussed. Involved margins of resection have been identified as the most important independent prognostic variable for predicting local relapse. As previously described, the VNPI developed by Silverstein combines three significant predictors of local recurrence: tumor size, margin width, and pathologic classification. In other studies, overexpression of multiple molecular markers such as HER-2/*neu*, nm23, heat shock protein, and metallothionein as well as DNA aneuploidy have also been associated with comedo lesions, but their independent prognostic significance has not been clarified.

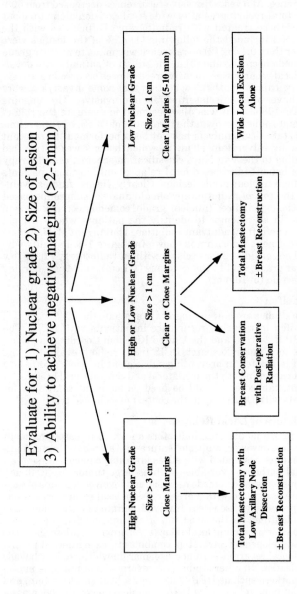

Fig. 1-1.   Guidelines for management of ductal carcinoma *in situ*.

SURVEILLANCE

Following breast conservation surgery, a postsurgical mammogram should be obtained to evaluate for residual microcalcifications. In addition, a mammogram should be obtained 3–4 months after the completion of radiation therapy to establish a new baseline. Follow-up of patients after conservative surgery with or without radiotherapy involves a twice-yearly physical examination and annual mammography for 5 years, with an annual physical examination and mammogram thereafter. Both patients treated with conservative therapy and patients treated with mastectomy should be monitored closely for new primary cancers in the contralateral breast. The risk that a new primary cancer will appear in the contralateral breast after treatment for DCIS approaches two to five times the risk of a first primary breast cancer and is approximately the same as the risk for a contralateral new primary cancer after invasive cancer.

Lobular Carcinoma *in Situ*

LCIS was first described as a distinct pathologic entity in 1941. During the era that followed, the treatment for LCIS was the same as that for invasive carcinoma—radical mastectomy. Haagensen is credited with altering the treatment philosophy for LCIS. In his review of 211 cases, he noted a 17% incidence of subsequent invasive carcinoma in women whose disease was diagnosed as LCIS and who were followed by observation only without undergoing surgery. The risk of developing a subsequent carcinoma was equal for both breasts, and only six women died of breast cancer. Haagensen concluded that close observation for LCIS allowed for early detection of subsequent malignancy, with associated high cure rates. Haagensen's rationale for observation as a treatment philosophy for LCIS was based on his view that patients with LCIS were at increased risk for developing invasive breast cancer but that LCIS itself did not differentiate into a malignancy.

EPIDEMIOLOGY

The true incidence and prevalence of LCIS are difficult to estimate because the diagnosis is most often a purely incidental finding. LCIS is not detectable by palpation, gross pathologic examination, or mammography. The incidence of LCIS has risen dramatically in recent years as a result of the increased use of screening mammography and therefore increased numbers of biopsies of mammographically detected non-LCIS breast abnormalities.

LCIS occurs most commonly in premenopausal women. Ninety percent of the women in Haagensen's series were premenopausal, and most studies have reported mean ages between 45 and 50 years. Estrogens are hypothesized to play an important role in the pathogenesis of LCIS. Postmenopausal regression of LCIS has been noted and may explain the decreased incidence in the elderly. The theory that LCIS represents a marker of increased risk for invasive breast carcinoma is supported by the fact that the mean age at diagnosis precedes that for invasive cancer by 10–15 years.

When the diagnosis of LCIS is established, there is a 0–6% chance that the patient has a synchronous invasive breast lesion. The risk of developing a subsequent invasive lesion has been estimated to be 0.5% per year of follow-up. The invasive malignancies seen in women with LCIS are ductal carcinomas in 60–70% of cases. This provides further evidence supporting the theory that LCIS does not differentiate into invasive carcinoma; if this were the case, a larger percentage of patients should develop invasive lobular carcinoma. The tumors that develop in women with LCIS are no more aggressive than invasive breast carcinomas not associated with LCIS.

PATHOLOGY

LCIS is characterized by an intraepithelial proliferation of the terminal lobular-ductal unit. The cells are slightly larger and paler than those normally lining the acini, but the lobular architecture is maintained. The cells have a homogeneous morphology and do not display prominent chromatin. The cytoplasm-to-nucleus ratio is normal, with infrequent mitoses and no necrosis. The basement membrane is not penetrated by the proliferating cells.

The diagnosis of LCIS involves the differentiation of LCIS from other forms of benign disease and from invasive lesions. In the absence of complete replacement of the lobular unit, atypical lobular hyperplasia becomes the designated pathologic term. Papillomatosis in the terminal ducts may have the appearance of LCIS but lacks the characteristic involvement of the acini. DCIS may extend retrograde into the acini but has a more characteristic anaplastic cell morphology. The LCIS is contained within the basement membrane, which distinguishes it from invasive lobular carcinoma.

Numerous studies have documented the multifocal and multicentric nature of LCIS. If diligently searched for, foci can be located elsewhere in the breast in almost all cases. In addition, LCIS is identified in the contralateral breast in 50–90% of cases. Thus the presence of LCIS reflects a phenotypic manifestation of a generalized abnormality present throughout both breasts. As a result, the treatment of LCIS should be directed not only at the index lesion but at both breasts.

DIAGNOSIS

Clinical Presentation

Because LCIS is not detectable by physical examination or mammography, it is most commonly diagnosed as an incidental finding in a breast biopsy specimen. Therefore the clinical presentation of patients with LCIS is similar to that of patients requiring breast biopsy for fibroadenoma, benign duct disease, DCIS, and invasive breast cancer.

Treatment

There are two treatment options for women with LCIS. The first is close clinical observation, as recommended by Haagensen.

The second is a surgical procedure that removes all tissue at risk for developing subsequent invasive disease. Because there is no risk of regional metastasis, axillary dissection is not required. Immediate breast reconstruction should be offered to patients at the time of mastectomy. Contralateral mirror-image breast biopsy, a procedure often advocated for LCIS, has fallen out of favor because an ipsilateral mastectomy and a negative mirror-image biopsy do not eliminate the need for close observation of the residual breast tissue.

Adjuvant therapy for LCIS is not indicated. However, because LCIS is a marker for patients at high risk of developing invasive breast cancer, patients with LCIS may be included in the NSABP chemoprevention trial (NSABP P-1). This trial is designed to evaluate the ability of tamoxifen to reduce the incidence of breast carcinoma in high-risk patients over placebo.

Selected References

Balch CM, Singletary SE, Bland KI. Clinical decision-making in early breast cancer. *Ann Surg* 217:207, 1993.

Fisher B, Costantino J, Redmond C, et al. Lumpectomy compared with lumpectomy and radiation therapy for the treatment of intraductal breast carcinoma. *N Engl J Med* 328:1581, 1993.

Fisher ER, Costantino J, Fisher B, et al. Pathological findings from the National Surgical Adjuvant Breast Project (NSABP) Protocol B-17. *Cancer* 75:1310, 1995.

Fowble B. Intraductal noninvasive breast cancer: a comparison of three local treatments. *Oncology* 3:51, 1989.

Frykberg ER, Bland KI. Overview of the biology and management of ductal carcinoma *in situ* of the breast. *Cancer* 74(1):350, 1994.

Goedde TA, Frykberg ER, Crump JM, et al. The impact of mammography on breast biopsy. *Am Surg* 58:661, 1992.

Haagensen CA, Lome N, Lattes R, et al. Lobular neoplasia (so-called lobular carcinoma *in situ*) of the breast. *Cancer* 42:757, 1978.

Holland R, Hendricks JH, Verbeek AL, et al. Extent, distribution, and mammographic/histological correlations of breast ductal carcinoma *in situ*. *Lancet* 335:519, 1990.

Lagios MD, Margolin FR, Westdahl PR, et al. Mammographically detected duct carcinoma *in situ*. *Cancer* 63:618, 1989.

Nielson M, Thomsen JL, Primdahl U, et al. Breast cancer and atypia among young and middle-aged women: A study of 110 medicolegal autopsies. *Br J Cancer* 56:814, 1987.

Page DL, Dupont WD, Rogers LW, et al. Continued local recurrence of carcinoma 15–25 years after a diagnosis of low grade ductal carcinoma *in situ* of the breast treated only by biopsy. *Cancer* 76:1197, 1995.

Schwartz GF, Finkel GC, Garcia JC, et al. Subclinical ductal carcinoma *in situ* of the breast. *Cancer* 70:2468, 1992.

Silverstein MJ, Waisman JR, Gierson ED, et al. Intraductal breast carcinoma (DCIS) with and without microinvasion: Is there a difference in outcome? *Proceedings of the American Society of Clinical Oncology,* abstract 24, p. 53, 1993.

Silverstein MJ, Cohlan BF, Gierson ED, et al. Ductal carcinoma *in situ*: 227 cases without microinvasion. *Eur J Cancer* 28:630, 1992.

Silverstein ML, Lagios MD, Craig PH, et al. A progonsotic index for ductal carcinoma *in situ* of the breast. *Cancer* 77:2267, 1996.

Silverstein MJ, Poller DN, Waisman JR, et al. Prognostic classification of breast ductal carcinoma *in situ*. *Lancet* 345:1154, 1995.

Solin LJ, Yeh IT, Kurtz J, et al. Ductal carcinoma *in situ* (intraductal carcinoma) of the breast treated with breast-conserving surgery and definitive irradiation. *Cancer* 71:2532, 1993.

Vezeridis MP, Bland KI. Management of ductal carcinoma *in situ*. *Surg Oncol* 3:309, 1994.

Wong JH, Kopald KH, Morton DL. The impact of microinvasion on axillary node metastases and survival in patients with intraductal breast cancer. *Arch Surg* 125:1298, 1990.

Invasive Breast Cancer

Paul M. Ahearne, Steven D. Leach,
and Barry W. Feig

Epidemiology

Breast cancer has become a leading health concern in the United States: 12% of American women will be diagnosed with breast cancer during their lifetimes, and more than 40,000 women will die of the disease each year. Breast cancer incidence rates have been increasing steadily since the start of data collection in the 1930s. In Connecticut, which has one of the oldest cancer registries in the country, the incidence of breast cancer rose by 1.2% per year from 1940 to 1982. According to the National Cancer Institute Surveillance, Epidemiology, and End Results Program (SEER), the incidence of breast cancer increased by 33% from 1973 to 1988. Because the breast cancer incidence rate increased by only 3% from 1973 to 1980, the majority of the increase occurred during the 1980s, indicating that this dramatic rise may be related to the increased use of mammographic screening during that time. If screening, and therefore increased detection, is responsible for the dramatic rise in incidence, a plateau should occur over the next few years.

Breast cancer is the leading cause of malignancy-related death among American women 15–54 years of age. The incidence of breast cancer increases rapidly during the fourth decade of life and becomes substantial before age 50. After menopause, the incidence continues to rise but at a much slower rate. Despite an increasing incidence, the mortality from breast cancer has remained relatively stable over the past several decades. This may be due to earlier detection of disease or advances in treatment. Among women younger than 50 years of age, breast cancer mortality has declined by 12%, whereas it has increased by 5% among women 50 years of age and older.

Risk Factors

The most important risk factor for the development of breast cancer is sex. The female-to-male ratio for breast cancer is 100:1. We therefore focus on risk factors related to the development of breast cancer in women.

Age is another important risk factor for the development of breast cancer. The risk that breast cancer will develop in a white American woman in a single year increases from 1:5,900 at age 30 to 1:290 at age 80.

Any family history of breast cancer increases a woman's risk of developing breast cancer. A more important increase in risk is associated with the presence of breast cancer in a first-degree relative. For a 30-year-old woman with a sister who had bilateral breast cancer before age 50, the cumulative probability of developing breast cancer by age 70 is 55%. This cumulative probability decreases to 8% for a woman whose sister developed unilateral breast cancer after age 50. The overall risk depends on the number of relatives with cancer, their ages at diagnosis, and whether the disease was unilateral or bilateral.

Genetic alterations predisposing individuals to breast cancer have received much attention recently. Although these gene mutations are inherited, only 5–10% of all breast cancer is thought to result from inheritance of a mutated gene. Autosomal dominant conditions include Li-Fraumeni syndrome, BRCA-1 and BRCA-2 mutations, Muir-Torre syndrome, Cowden's disease, and Peutz-Jeghers syndrome. Though autosomal dominant, these conditions do not always exhibit 100% penetrance. Other inherited conditions include the autosomal recessive disorder ataxia-telangiectasia.

The most recently publicized disorders have been the hereditary mutations with BRCA-1 or BRCA-2 genes. The BRCA-1 gene is found on the long arm of chromosome 17q. Risks of developing breast or ovarian cancer differ with site of mutation but are in the range of 37–87% by age 70 for breast cancer and 11–42% for ovarian cancer by age 60. The BRCA-2 gene is found on chromosome 13. In contrast to BRCA-1, BRCA-2 mutations are thought to be associated with breast cancer but not with ovarian cancer.

Prior breast cancer is a significant risk factor for the development of cancer in the contralateral breast, with an incidence of 0.5–1.0% per year of follow-up.

Pathologic findings that indicate increased risk of breast cancer can be divided into proliferative and nonproliferative breast disease. Nonproliferative breast diseases include adenosis, fibroadenomas, apocrine changes, duct ectasia, and mild hyperplasia. These histologic findings carry no increased risk of breast cancer. Histologic findings of proliferative breast disease can be divided into slightly increased, moderately increased, and high risk. Findings of moderate or florid hyperplasia without atypia, papillomas, or sclerosing adenosis carry a slightly increased risk (one and a half to two times that of the general population). Atypical ductal or lobular hyperplasia constitutes findings consistent with a moderately increased risk of developing breast cancer (four to five times). Histologic findings of LCIS represent a high-risk category (eight to 10 times). These findings represent a risk that applies equally to both breasts.

A number of endogenous endocrine factors have been implicated as risk factors in breast cancer, including age at menarche, age at menopause, parity, and age at first full-term pregnancy. The cumulative duration of menstruation also may be important. Women who menstruate for more than 30 years are at greater risk than those who menstruate for fewer than 30 years. The risk of breast cancer for women who experience menopause after age 55 is twice that of women who experience menopause prior to age 44. Although age at menarche is important, age at onset of regular menses may be even more critical. Women who have regular ovulatory cycles before age 13 have a fourfold greater risk than those whose menarche occurred after age 13 and who had a

5-year delay to the development of regular cycles. Age at first birth has a greater impact on risk than the number of pregnancies, with a woman who had her first child before age 19 having half the risk of a nulliparous woman. Interestingly, women who have their first child between 30 and 34 years of age have the same risk as nulliparous women, whereas women who have their first child after age 35 have a greater risk than nulliparous women. These observations indicate that the hormonal milieu at different times in a woman's life may affect her risk of breast cancer.

The potential of exogenous hormones to increase a woman's risk of breast cancer remains controversial. Recent evidence suggests that the benefits of hormone replacement therapy in postmenopausal women outweigh the risks. The benefits include decreased risk of coronary artery disease and stroke, as well as increased bone density. The longevity benefits extend especially to women in high-risk groups for coronary artery disease. However, after long-term use of hormone replacement therapy, the risk of breast cancer increases to a point at which continued use becomes of questionable benefit. No such benefits are proven for premenopausal women. Other studies suggest that prolonged use of oral contraceptives (greater than 10 years) may be associated with an increased risk of breast cancer.

Exposure to ionizing radiation for the treatment of Hodgkin's disease has been associated with an increased risk of cancer if the exposure was before age 30. The risk for the first 15 years after treatment is less than the risk after 15 years.

Both obesity and alcohol consumption have been implicated as potential risk factors for breast cancer. In general, obesity has not been identified as an important risk factor for breast cancer. Among premenopausal women, obesity is associated with a decreased incidence of breast cancer. In postmenopausal women, there is a clinically unimportant association of obesity with breast cancer. Despite the fact that a high-fat diet promotes mammary tumors in animals, only weak or nonexistent associations have been observed in human studies. No conclusive evidence has been published to link alcohol consumption with an increased risk of breast cancer.

Pathology

Invasive carcinomas of the breast tend to be histologically heterogeneous tumors. Overwhelmingly, these tumors are adenocarcinomas that arise from the terminal ducts. There are five common histologic variants of mammary adenocarcinoma.

1. Infiltrating ductal carcinoma accounts for 75% of all breast cancers. This lesion is characterized by the absence of special histologic features. It is hard when palpated and gritty when transected. It is associated with various degrees of fibrotic response. Often there is associated ductal carcinoma *in situ* (DCIS) within the specimen. Infiltrating ductal carcinomas commonly metastasize to axillary lymph nodes. The progno-

sis for patients with these tumors is poorer than that for patients with some of the other histologic subtypes. Distant metastases are found most often in the bones, lungs, liver, and brain.

2. Infiltrating lobular carcinoma is seen in 5–10% of breast cancer cases. Clinically, this lesion often presents as an area of ill-defined thickening within the breast. Microscopically, small cells in a single-file arrangement are seen. Infiltrating lobular cancers have a tendency to grow around ducts and lobules. Multicentricity is observed more frequently in infiltrating lobular carcinoma than in infiltrating ductal carcinoma. The prognosis for lobular carcinoma is similar to that of infiltrating ductal carcinoma. In addition to axillary lymph node metastasis, lobular carcinoma is known to metastasize to unusual sites, such as meninges and serosal surfaces, more often than do other forms of breast cancer.

3. Tubular carcinoma accounts for only 2% of all breast carcinomas. The diagnosis of tubular carcinoma is made only when more than 75% of the tumor demonstrates tubule formation. Axillary nodal metastases are uncommon with this type of tumor. The prognosis for patients with tubular carcinoma is considerably better than that for patients with other types of breast cancer.

4. Medullary carcinoma accounts for 5–7% of tumors. Grossly, medullary carcinomas are well circumscribed. Histologically, they are characterized by poorly differentiated nuclei, syncytial growth pattern, a well-circumscribed border, intense infiltration with small lymphocytes and plasma cells, and little or no DCIS. The prognosis for patients with medullary carcinoma is favorable only if all these characteristics are present.

5. Mucinous or colloid carcinoma constitutes approximately 3% of all breast cancers. It is characterized by an abundant accumulation of extracellular mucin surrounding clusters of tumor cells. Colloid carcinoma is slow-growing and tends to be bulky. If a breast carcinoma is predominantly mucinous, the prognosis is favorable. The mortality rate compared with that of invasive ductal carcinoma is 0.38.

There are several rarer special histologic types of breast malignancy, including papillary, apocrine, secretory, squamous cell, spindle cell, cystosarcoma phyllodes, and carcinosarcoma. Infiltrating ductal carcinomas occasionally have small areas containing one or more of these special histologic types. Tumors with these mixed histologies behave similarly to pure infiltrating ductal cancers.

Staging

Typically, breast cancer is staged using the American Joint Committee on Cancer (AJCC) guidelines. The TNM classifications and stage groupings for breast cancer are summarized in Table 2-1.

Table 2-1. Current AJCC TNM classification and stage grouping for breast carcinoma

TNM classification		Stage grouping			
Primary tumor (T)					
TX	Primary tumor cannot be assessed	Stage 0	Tis	N0	M0
T0	No evidence of primary tumor	Stage I	T1	N0	M0
Tis	Carcinoma in situ	Stage IIa	T0	N1	M0
T1	Tumor ≤2 cm in greatest dimension		T1	N1	M0
			T2	N0	M0
T2	Tumor >2 cm but ≤5 cm	Stage IIb	T2	N1	M0
T3	Tumor >5 cm		T3	N0	M0
T4	Tumor of any size with direct extension to chest wall or skin; includes inflammatory carcinoma	Stage IIIa	T0	N2	M0
			T1	N2	M0
			T2	N2	M0
			T3	N1,2	M0
Regional lymph nodes (N)					
NX	Regional lymph nodes cannot be assessed	Stage IIIb	T4	Any N	M0
N0	No regional lymph node metastases		Any T	N3	M0
N1	Metastasis to movable ipsilateral axillary lymph node(s)	Stage IV	Any T	Any N	M1
N2	Metastases to ipsilateral axillary lymph nodes fixed to one another or to other structures				
N3	Metastasis to ipsilateral internal mammary lymph nodes				
Distant metastasis (M)					
MX	Presence of distant metastasis cannot be assessed				
M0	No distant metastasis				
M1	Distant metastasis (includes ipsilateral supraclavicular node(s)				

Diagnosis

HISTORY AND PHYSICAL EXAMINATION

Diagnosis of breast cancer has undergone a dramatic evolution since the mid-1980s. Traditionally, 50–75% of all breast cancers were detected by self-examination. Subsequent to the widespread availability of mammographic screening programs, there has been a shift toward the diagnosis of clinically occult, nonpalpable lesions. Despite this trend, evaluation of the woman with potential breast cancer continues to be based on a careful history and physical examination.

The history is directed at assessing cancer risk as well as establishing the presence or absence of symptoms potentially related to breast disease. It should include the age of menarche, menopausal status, previous pregnancy, and use of oral contraceptives or postmenopausal replacement estrogens. A prior personal history of breast cancer is of obvious importance. In addition, careful documentation of a family history of breast cancer in first-degree relatives (i.e., mother or sister) should be sought.

In addition to determining cancer risk, the history should establish the presence or absence of specific symptoms potentially referable to breast cancer. It is worthwhile to inquire about breast pain and nipple discharge, although these symptoms are more commonly associated with nonmalignant processes, including fibrocystic disease and intraductal papilloma. Malaise, bony pain, and weight loss are rare but may indicate metastatic disease.

Physical examination of patients with potential breast cancer must constantly take into consideration the comfort and emotional well-being of the patient. Adequate privacy measures and good lighting are mandatory. Examination is initiated by careful visual inspection with the patient sitting upright. Nipple changes, gross asymmetry, and obvious masses are all noted. The skin must be carefully inspected for subtle changes; these can range from slight dimpling to the more dramatic *peau d'orange* appearance associated with locally advanced or inflammatory breast cancer.

Following careful inspection and with the patient remaining in the sitting position, the periclavicular regions are examined for potential nodal disease. Both axillae are then carefully palpated. If palpable, nodes should be characterized as to their number, size, and whether they are mobile or fixed. Examination of the axilla always includes palpation of the axillary tail of the breast; assessment of this area is often overlooked once the patient is placed in a supine position.

Palpation of the breast parenchyma itself is accomplished with the patient in a supine position and the ipsilateral arm placed over the head. The subareolar tissues and each quadrant of both breasts are systematically palpated. Dominant masses are noted with respect to their size, shape, location, consistency, and mobility. With experience, the examiner can begin to predict that the spherical, rubbery, movable mass occurring in a 25-year-old woman will prove to be a fibroadenoma and that the less circumscribed, firm, fixed lesion in a 50-year-old patient will likely prove malignant.

When subjected to critical analysis, however, physical examination often proves to be inadequate in differentiating benign from malignant breast masses. Various series have identified a 20–40% error rate, even among experienced examiners. Given this rate of inaccuracy, any persistent dominant breast mass occurring in a patient older than age 30 requires additional evaluation.

EVALUATION OF THE PALPABLE BREAST MASS

The choice of initial evaluation following the detection of a dominant breast mass should be individualized for each patient according to age, perceived cancer risk, and characteristics of the lesion in question. For most patients, mammographic evaluation is an important initial step. Mammography in this setting serves two purposes: (1) the risk of malignancy for the palpable lesion is further assessed, and (2) both breasts are screened for nonpalpable lesions. Bilateral synchronous cancers occur in about 3% of all cases; at least half of these lesions are nonpalpable.

For a palpable lesion, mammography may demonstrate the stellate or spiculated appearance typical of malignancy. Calcifications, nipple changes, and axillary adenopathy may also be visualized. Together, the presence or absence of these mammographic findings can predict malignancy with an overall accuracy of 70–80%. Mammography is least accurate in younger patients with dense breasts; it is rarely applied in patients under the age of 30.

Following mammographic evaluation, palpable masses suspected to be malignant should undergo fine-needle aspiration or needle-core biopsy. Some clinicians advocate needle aspiration at the time of initial evaluation, prior to mammography. For most patients, we defer biopsy until after mammographic examination is completed, as a needle-puncture hematoma will occasionally confuse future radiographic evaluation. For young patients with dense breasts in whom mammography is not contemplated, needle aspiration remains an ideal primary mode of evaluation.

Fine-needle aspiration with a 22-gauge needle allows for accurate differentiation between cystic and solid masses, and provides material for cytologic examination. Cystic lesions are not well visualized by mammography but are very well characterized by ultrasound. Benign breast cysts typically yield nonbloody fluid and become nonpalpable after aspiration. Bloody fluid should be submitted for cytologic analysis. In several large series, the incidence of malignancy among breast cysts is typically 1%; this is limited almost exclusively to those cysts that yield bloody fluid or have a residual mass following aspiration. Aspiration is often curative; only one in five breast cysts will recur following aspiration, and most of these are obliterated with a second drainage.

For solid lesions, several passes through the lesion with the syringe under constant negative pressure will typically yield ample material for cytologic evaluation. The material is evacuated onto a microscopic slide and immediately fixed in 95% ethanol. Multiple reports have demonstrated this technique to be simple, safe, and accurate in evaluating benign and malignant breast masses. For lesions interpreted as malignant, cytologic evaluation is unable to differentiate between *in situ* and invasive carcinoma. Needle-core biopsy allows the pathologist to distinguish invasive from *in situ* carcinoma by providing a core of tissue for histopathology. Nondiagnostic findings require open biopsy.

Although physical examination, mammography, and needle biopsy all carry error rates when used as single modalities, the combination of these three investigations has proven extremely accurate in predicting whether a palpable lesion is benign or malignant. For lesions with equivocal or contradictory results, open biopsy remains the definitive test.

EVALUATION OF NONPALPABLE LESIONS

Because of the increasing availability of mammographic screening programs, there has been a rapid increase in the diagnosis of nonpalpable breast cancer in the United States. Analysis of SEER data demonstrated a 213% increase in the age-adjusted incidence of DCIS among white women between the years 1983 and 1989, and a 140% increase in the incidence of node-negative invasive lesions smaller than 1 cm in diameter. During this same period, cancers larger than 2 cm in diameter and those associated with distant metastases have undergone a substantial decrease in incidence. Although these changes in the relative incidence of early and late lesions have not yet translated into changes in SEER breast cancer mortality, other studies have demonstrated the efficacy of screening mammography in preventing deaths from breast cancer. Among screened populations, breast cancer mortality appears to be reduced by approximately 30–40%, although the benefit of screening patients younger than age 50 remains controversial. Currently, the American Cancer Society recommends yearly screening mammography and clinical breast examination for all women 50 years and older. It is generally recommended that women between the ages of 40 and 50 be screened at least every other year.

Mammographic signs of malignancy can be divided into two main categories: microcalcifications and density changes. Microcalcifications can be either clustered or scattered; density changes include discrete masses, architectural distortions, and asymmetries. Mammographic findings most predictive of malignancy include spiculated masses with associated architectural distortion, clustered microcalcifications in a linear or branching array, or microcalcifications with a mass. The American College of Radiology (ACR) has published suggestions for reporting mammographic results. ACR categories range from I to V: I = negative (no findings), II = benign appearance, III = probably benign appearance, IV = findings suspicious for breast cancer, and V = highly suspicious for breast cancer.

Once screening mammography demonstrates a suspicious lesion, further evaluation is necessary. For lesions interpreted as "probably benign" (well-defined, solitary masses), careful counseling and repeat mammography in 6 months may be undertaken in low-risk patients. For appropriate lesions, additional examination using ultrasonography may identify a subset of cystic lesions that will not require biopsy. Ultrasound may also be used to guide fine-needle or needle-core biopsy. For suspicious lesions, some form of biopsy is required. Ultrasound-guided biopsy is not useful in the evaluation of microcalcifications; these are typically not sonographically visible. Mammography-guided stereotactic breast biopsy has emerged as a useful technique for nonpalpable lesions and microcalcifications.

BREAST BIOPSY TECHNIQUE

For either palpable or nonpalpable lesions, planning an optimal biopsy mandates careful consideration of at least three issues. First, the biopsy site may require future re-excision, even under a strategy of breast conservation. Second, the biopsy site must be incorporated into a future mastectomy incision should this form of treatment be chosen. Third, the biopsy must be constructed in a cosmetically optimal manner. All breast biopsies should be performed with the assumption that the target lesion is malignant.

Biopsies are typically performed in an outpatient setting using local anesthesia. In general, incisions must be planned carefully so that they can be incorporated into a mastectomy if that becomes necessary. Curvilinear incisions are often used to take advantage of decreased lines of tension along Langer's lines. Radial scars are generally avoided, except in the extreme medial aspect of the breast, where mastectomy incisions become radially oriented; lesions in the inner-lower quadrant are often best approached through a radial incision. Circumareolar incisions have obvious cosmetic advantage but carry the potential disadvantage of leading to sacrifice of areolar tissue should re-excision be required. Although a modest amount of peripheral "tunneling" is acceptable to maintain an incision within a potential mastectomy scar, extreme tunneling to the periphery of the breast from a central periareolar incision not only makes it virtually impossible to identify the tumor bed should re-excision be required, but also exposes an inordinate amount of breast tissue to potential contamination by tumor cells. In patients in whom breast conservation with axillary dissection is contemplated, the biopsy site should not be contiguous with the axillary incision. Separating these incisions provides a better cosmetic outcome (as the axillary drain will cause the biopsy cavity to become distorted if they are not separated) and may prevent tumor seeding of a previously negative axilla, thus avoiding the need to irradiate a dissected axilla.

The excisional breast biopsy has the potential to serve both diagnostic and local treatment purposes. It is reserved as a diagnostic tool when needle biopsy is impossible or inappropriate. The entire mass and a surrounding 1-cm rim of normal tissue should be excised. An excisional biopsy such as this will fulfill the requirements for "lumpectomy" and avoid subsequent re-excision.

For nonpalpable lesions, preoperative needle localization with a self-retaining hookwire is required. This procedure requires careful communication between radiologist and surgeon. For most lesions, the localizing needle is placed under mammographic guidance into the breast via the shortest direct path to the lesion. The self-retaining wire is placed through the needle, and the needle is removed. Postlocalization mammograms are then reviewed. Biopsy is undertaken with excision of a core of target breast tissue surrounding the wire tip. For superficial lesions, an ellipse of skin at the point of wire insertion may be removed en bloc with the underlying breast tissue. Postexcision specimen radiographs are essential to confirm successful biopsy.

Once the biopsy specimen has been excised, careful handling is critical. The surgeon should meticulously note the orientation of the excised breast tissue and hand-deliver the specimen to the pathology department. The lateral, medial, superior, inferior, superficial, and deep margins should be inked in a color-coded manner. For palpable lesions, material should be processed for receptor analysis and flow cytometry. Tissue to be assayed for steroid hormones should be rapidly frozen, because both estrogen and progesterone receptor concentrations have been shown to decline rapidly with warm ischemic time.

Closure of the biopsy incision must involve meticulous hemostasis. Deep parenchymal sutures often cause cosmetically unpleasing distortion of the residual breast and should be avoided. Drains are not used in the breast. The skin is closed with a subcuticular suture, and a light dressing is placed.

Pretreatment Evaluation

Once the diagnosis of breast cancer has been made, appropriate treatment planning involves some evaluation for the possibility of metastatic disease. For patients with stage I or stage II breast cancer, this is typically limited to complete history and physical examination, a chest radiograph, and evaluation of serum liver chemistries. The routine use of bone scans in asymptomatic patients with early-stage breast cancer carries an extremely low yield; several series have demonstrated only a 2% incidence of positive scans in this setting. In contrast, up to 25% of asymptomatic patients with apparent stage III cancer demonstrate positive bone scans; routine scanning in this population appears worthwhile. In the absence of elevated serum liver chemistries or palpable hepatomegaly, liver imaging is also not applied routinely in the preoperative evaluation of patients with early-stage disease. Supraclavicular ultrasound may be useful to rule out metastatic disease in patients with clinical N2 disease.

Treatment

Many of the current recommendations regarding therapy for invasive breast cancer have been influenced by the results of randomized, prospective clinical trials performed by the National Surgical Adjuvant Breast and Bowel Project (NSABP). A selected summary of these trials is presented in Table 2-2.

MICROINVASIVE BREAST CANCER

The diagnosis of microinvasive breast cancer has increased with the use of routine screening mammography. The incidence

Table 2-2. Selected summary of NSABP therapeutic trials for invasive breast cancer

Trial	Treatments	Outcome
NSABP B-04	Total mastectomy vs. total mastectomy with XRT vs. radical mastectomy	No difference in disease-free or overall survival
NSABP B-06	Total mastectomy vs. lumpectomy vs. lumpectomy with XRT	No difference in disease-free or overall survival; addition of XRT to lumpectomy reduced local recurrence rate from 39% to 10%
NSABP B-13	Surgery alone vs. surgery plus adjuvant chemotherapy in node-negative patients with ER-negative tumors	Improved disease-free survival for adjuvant chemotherapy group
NSABP B-14	Surgery alone vs. surgery plus adjuvant tamoxifen in node-negative patients with ER-positive tumors	Improved disease-free survival for adjuvant tamoxifen group
NSABP B-21	Lumpectomy plus tamoxifen vs. lumpectomy plus tamoxifen plus XRT vs. lumpectomy plus XRT for node-negative tumors <1 cm	Ongoing

ER = estrogen receptor; XRT = radiotherapy.

of this disease is difficult to determine because of overlap in the pathologic definition of microinvasion. The most accurate description is that of DCIS with limited microscopic stromal invasion below the basement membrane in one or several ducts, but not invading more than 10% of the surface of the histologic sections examined. Five to ten percent of patients with noninvasive breast cancer will be noted to have an area of microinvasion present on careful pathologic examination. The significance of the finding of a microscopic focal area of invasion is uncertain. The presence of lymph node metastasis associated with this diagnosis has been documented in 0–10% of all cases. Not surprisingly, those authors finding a low incidence of microinvasion deem an axillary lymph node dissection unnecessary for these patients. Most authors would agree that an axillary dissection is warranted in patients with an anticipated risk of lymph node metastasis of 10% or more, in order to accurately stage these patients.

At the University of Texas M. D. Anderson Cancer Center, we do not base the decision to perform an axillary dissection solely on the finding of a focal area of microinvasion. Other prognostic factors that need to be assessed are age, histology, hormone receptor status, and family history. An informed decision based on the risks and benefits of an axillary dissection is then made by the patient and physician. In most cases, patients with a single focus of microinvasion are adequately treated by simple excision with postoperative breast irradiation.

EARLY-STAGE BREAST CANCER (T1–T2, N0–N1)

About 75% of patients with breast cancer present with tumors less than 5 cm in diameter and no evidence of fixed or matted nodes. These patients with early-stage breast cancer are generally treated by one of three surgical options: (1) breast conservation surgery with irradiation, (2) modified radical mastectomy, or (3) modified radical mastectomy with either immediate or delayed reconstruction. With careful patient selection, the goal of maintaining either a conserved or reconstructed breast can be achieved in most cases.

BREAST CONSERVATION VERSUS MASTECTOMY

It is now clear that many patients with breast cancer can be effectively treated with breast conservation. Since 1970, seven different prospective randomized trials comparing breast conservation strategies with radical or modified radical mastectomy have failed to demonstrate any survival benefit to the more aggressive approach. Among these trials, the two most widely known were conducted by Veronesi et al. at the National Cancer Institute in Milan, Italy, and by Fisher et al. in conjunction with the NSABP in the United States. The Milan trial was limited to patients with stage I breast cancer (tumor <2 cm, negative axillary nodes) and compared radical mastectomy with a breast conservation strategy involving quadrantectomy, axillary dissection, and radiotherapy. No differences in local control, disease-free survival, or overall survival have been noted.

NSABP trial B-06 examined an expanded patient population that included women with primary tumors up to 4 cm in diameter and either N0 or N1 nodal status. Patients were randomized to one of three treatment strategies: modified radical mastectomy, lumpectomy with axillary dissection and radiotherapy, or lumpectomy and axillary dissection alone. Histologically negative margins were required in the breast conservation groups. Again, there were no differences in disease-free survival or overall survival among the three groups. Local recurrence, however, was markedly reduced by the addition of radiotherapy to lumpectomy and axillary dissection (12% versus 53% at 10 years). These results upheld breast conservation as appropriate treatment for patients with stage I or stage II breast cancer and made it clear that radiotherapy is required as an integral part of any breast conservation strategy. At the M. D. Anderson Cancer Center, we typically initiate radiotherapy 2–3 weeks following surgery or at the completion of postoperative adjuvant chemotherapy. A dose of 50 Gy is given through tangential ports using computerized dosimetry.

Although it is clear that breast conservation is equal to mastectomy for patients with stage I or II disease, the decision to embark on a treatment strategy involving breast conservation must be individualized for each patient. Numerous factors contribute to this decision. The patient's motivation and commitment to breast conservation must be strong, as daily outpatient radiation treatments over 5–6 weeks are required. The patient also must be willing to accept the risk of a 10–12% local recurrence rate within the conserved breast.

Other factors contributing to the choice between mastectomy and breast conservation surgery include the size of the breast, tumor size, tumor histology, tumor multicentricity, and patient age. For extremely small breasts, the cosmetic result may be unacceptable following local excision, especially for larger lesions. For large, pendulous breasts, lack of uniformity in radiation dosing may result in unattractive fibrosis and retraction. Patients with either extreme may benefit from a strategy of mastectomy and reconstruction, occasionally coupled with surgical augmentation or reduction of the contralateral breast. Patients with larger tumors also might be best served by mastectomy. At this point, there are no data to suggest that T3 lesions are adequately treated by breast conservation. From a purely practical point of view, local excision of such lesions rarely results in a cosmetically acceptable result. The ability of preoperative chemotherapy to downstage these tumors to the point where breast conservation may be undertaken provides an intriguing approach.

A number of attempts have been made to identify patients with a high rate of local recurrence following breast conservation based on the histology of the primary tumor. To date, there have been no documented differences in local recurrence among the various histologic subtypes. The risk of local recurrence has been shown to be higher for women less than 35 years old and for women whose tumors are greater than 2 cm in diameter regardless of lymph node status. For patients with positive lymph nodes, nuclear grade was also significantly correlated with recurrence.

AXILLARY DISSECTION

A substantial portion of patients with breast cancer present with axillary nodal metastases. In one series, 17% of patients with clinically T1N0 disease had histologically positive nodes; this figure rose to 27% for patients with clinically T2N0 disease. Other series have reported that 10% of patients with tumors less than 0.5 cm have positive axillary lymph nodes. Tumors 0.5–1.0 cm are associated with positive axillary lymph nodes in 13–22% of the patients. Tumors 1.0–2.0 cm in size were associated with up to 30% lymph node metastases. For either breast conservation surgery or modified radical mastectomy, axillary dissection remains an important component and a source of significant potential morbidity. It is clear that axillary dissection contributes little to overall survival but remains important for staging and local control.

The contribution of axillary dissection to local control is small but measurable. In the NSABP B-04 trial comparing radical mastectomy with simple mastectomy with and without radiation, 40% of patients with clinically negative axillae were found to have positive nodes at the time of radical mastectomy, and 1% of these patients eventually failed in the axilla. In patients with unoperated axillae, 18% (65 out of 365) eventually developed clinical adenopathy requiring delayed axillary dissection. Four of these patients eventually failed in the axilla in spite of delayed dissection. No survival disadvantage was seen for patients undergoing delayed versus immediate axillary dissection. Radiation was less effective than axillary dissection in preventing eventual failure in the axilla; this was especially true for patients with clinically positive nodes.

In addition to contributing to local control, axillary dissection provides important staging and prognostic information. As noted earlier, clinical staging of the axilla remains relatively inaccurate. However, nodal status remains a major predictor of outcome. For all patients with node-negative cancer, at least a 70% 10-year survival rate may be anticipated. This drops to 40% for patients with one to three positive nodes, and less than 20% for patients with four to 10 positive nodes. Micrometastatic disease (<2 mm in diameter) carries a better prognosis than macrometastatic disease. Independent of its contribution to subsequent treatment decisions, axillary dissection thus provides important prognostic information for the woman with breast cancer. As discussed later with regard to adjuvant chemotherapy, the contribution of axillary dissection to subsequent treatment planning is currently in flux.

We currently recommend an anatomic level I/II axillary lymph node dissection for all patients with stage I–II breast cancer. For patients with invasive breast cancer undergoing breast conservation therapy, axillary dissection should be performed via a separate axillary incision that does not extend anterior to the pectoralis fold. Axillary dissection should be directed toward en bloc removal of level I and level II nodal tissue. The addition of level III nodes to the dissection often requires division or resection of the pectoralis minor muscle and is of little benefit with respect to staging; only 1% of all patients show level III involvement in the absence of level I or II disease. On the other hand, level III dissections carry a substantially higher risk of subsequent lymphedema, especially if radiotherapy is used. The level I and II axillary dissection should preserve the long thoracic and thoracodorsal nerves and avoid stripping of the axillary vein. A closed-suction drain is placed and removed after the drainage has sufficiently decreased.

Whether axillary node dissection is necessary for all patients with invasive carcinoma remains controversial. Patients with early-stage disease with low risk of axillary node involvement may not require dissection. However, before such a treatment regimen can be recommended there must be (1) identification of the subgroup who is truly at low risk and (2) a randomized prospective trial to evaluate the issue. Another group of patients who may not benefit from axillary dissection consists of those who are receiving chemotherapy regardless of the nodal findings (i.e., premenopausal women with tumors >2 cm). These patients may be equally treated by axillary radiation at the time of their breast radiation. This issue also needs to be prospectively examined.

Another intriguing prospect regarding axillary dissection is that of lymphatic mapping and sentinel lymph node biopsy. Patients may not be good candidates if they have had previous excisional biopsies in the breast or axilla. The success rate of finding axillary sentinel nodes for breast cancer has been reported to be 65–98%. In one study, the sentinel nodes tested positive in 100% of the patients with positive axillary lymphatic disease. The sentinel lymph node was the only site of metastases in two-thirds of the patients. This is an interesting concept that warrants further investigation in large trials to determine the accuracy and predictive value of both positive and negative sentinel nodes.

BREAST RECONSTRUCTION

For patients not undergoing breast conservation, breast reconstruction should be considered a standard component of cancer therapy. Reconstruction may involve autologous tissue, synthetic implants, or a combination of both. Although satisfactory results can be obtained with either immediate or delayed reconstruction, we favor immediate reconstruction for most patients. Immediate reconstruction carries a substantial psychologic benefit for many women and often allows for a better cosmetic result. The initiation of adjuvant chemotherapy is not significantly delayed, and concerns that local recurrence may go undetected in a reconstructed breast are not well founded, especially for T1 and T2 lesions.

In our institution, 50% of all patients treated with mastectomy undergo immediate reconstruction. Although the method of reconstruction is individualized for each patient, either pedicled or free transverse rectus abdominus myocutaneous (TRAM) flaps are most commonly used. Contralateral augmentation or reduction may be performed to maximize symmetry. For premenopausal women with a perceived high risk for a contralateral second primary lesion, simultaneous contralateral mastectomy with bilateral free TRAM flap reconstruction is available. We typically perform a skin-sparing mastectomy in patients undergoing immediate breast reconstruction; the preservation of breast skin allows for a more natural contour to the reconstructed breast. To date, no increased risk of local recurrence has been observed for patients treated with skin-sparing techniques.

Although breast mound reconstruction may be undertaken immediately following mastectomy, nipple reconstruction is typically delayed 6–12 weeks to allow time for the reconstructed breast to remodel and attain its final shape and position. Only then can appropriate nipple position be determined. The nipple is formed by raising local skin flaps using local anesthesia; pigment is provided using tattooing techniques.

ADJUVANT CHEMOTHERAPY: NODE-POSITIVE PATIENTS

For both node-positive and node-negative patients, decisions regarding adjuvant chemotherapy must be individualized. Multiple factors must be considered, including patient age, overall health status, tumor size, estrogen receptor status, nodal status, and various other prognostic features, including ploidy, S-phase fraction, c-erbB-2 oncogene amplification, and cathepsin D expression. General guidelines regarding the use of adjuvant chemotherapy are presented in Table 2-3.

The first clear demonstrations that adjuvant chemotherapy was beneficial in a subset of women with breast cancer were provided by the NSABP in the United States and by the National Cancer Institute in Italy during the mid-1970s. In the Milan trial, surgery plus postoperative cyclophosphamide, methotrexate, and 5-fluorouracil (CMF) delivered over 12 monthly cycles was demonstrated to be superior to surgical therapy alone in a population of node-positive patients. Examination of the 15-year results from this trial shows a 10% improvement in both relapse-free survival and overall survival among treated patients. Subsequent trials have demonstrated a benefit for both pre- and postmenopausal patients and have shown that six treatment cycles are as effective as 12. Additional studies evaluating doxorubicin-based therapy in the adjuvant setting have not consistently demonstrated an advantage over CMF. The sequential administration of four cycles of doxorubicin followed by eight courses of CMF may provide some additional benefit, especially in patients with four or more positive nodes.

Initially applied to patients with metastatic, advanced, or recurrent disease, high-dose chemotherapy with autologous bone marrow transplantation is now also being applied in the adjuvant

Table 2-3.   Adjuvant chemotherapy recommendations for patients with invasive breast carcinoma based on tumor size, estrogen receptor (ER) expression, and nodal status

Tumor size	ER status	Nodal status	Recommended adjuvant therapy
≤1 cm	+/−	−	No adjuvant therapy required, especially for tumors with other favorable prognostic features (i.e., ploidy, S-phase, c-erb B-2, cathepsin D expression)
>1 cm	+	−	For women ≥50 yr, tamoxifen 10 mg bid; for women <50 yr, either cytotoxic chemotherapy (i.e., CMF vs. FAC) or tamoxifen as above
	−	−	Cytotoxic chemotherapy
Any size	+	+	For women ≥50 yr tamoxifen 10 mg bid × 5 yr +/− cytotoxic chemotherapy; for women <50 yr, cytotoxic chemotherapy +/− tamoxifen
	−	+	Cytotoxic chemotherapy

CMF = cyclophosphamide, methotrexate, and 5-fluorouracil;
FAC = 5-fluorouracil, doxorubicin, and cyclophosphamide.

setting. Early disease-free survival rates are encouraging; long-term results are lacking. These regimens are usually reserved for patients with an anticipated high rate of recurrence (i.e., ≥10 positive lymph nodes).

For patients with estrogen receptor–positive tumors, adjuvant therapy with tamoxifen may be considered. Among women with positive lymph nodes, the use of tamoxifen as a single adjuvant agent is typically limited to postmenopausal patients. The efficacy of antiestrogen therapy in the adjuvant setting has been demonstrated by several clinical trials, with the largest study published in 1987 from the Scottish Cancer Trials Office. In this study, 1,323 patients were randomized to receive either adjuvant tamoxifen (20 mg/day for 5 years) or observation alone following primary surgical treatment by mastectomy. Both pre- and post-menopausal patients were enrolled, and estrogen receptor positivity was not required. When patients in the observation group developed a recurrence, tamoxifen therapy was initiated; this feature allowed comparison of the benefit of adjuvant tamoxifen versus tamoxifen initiated at the time of clinical relapse. Overall, there was a 24% incidence of disease recurrence in the tamoxifen group compared with 38% in the observation group. An improvement in total survival was also noted among patients receiving adjuvant tamoxifen. Subgroup analysis according to menopausal, nodal, and estrogen receptor status demonstrated a benefit for each group examined, although the beneficial effect of adjuvant tamoxifen was most pronounced for postmenopausal node-positive patients with estrogen receptor levels exceeding 100 fmol/mg protein. This trial confirmed the efficacy of adjuvant tamoxifen and further identified this strategy as superior to a strategy of delayed tamoxifen initiated at the time of clinical relapse. Subsequent meta-analysis examining 28 different trials involving adjuvant tamoxifen confirmed a 16% reduction in the risk of death for women treated with tamoxifen. This benefit was limited to women older than the age of 50.

ADJUVANT CHEMOTHERAPY: NODE-NEGATIVE PATIENTS

During the 1980s, attention turned toward the possibility that adjuvant chemotherapy might benefit node-negative patients. In 1989, four reports were published in a single issue of the *New England Journal of Medicine* that addressed the potential benefit of adjuvant therapy in node-negative patients. Among these, NSABP trial B-13 reported on 679 node-negative patients with estrogen receptor–negative tumors who were randomized to receive either surgery alone or surgery followed by adjuvant therapy involving methotrexate, 5-fluorouracil, and leucovorin. The group receiving adjuvant therapy demonstrated an improvement in disease-free survival compared with the group treated with surgery alone (76% versus 62% at 7 years). Overall survival was increased in women over 49 (77% versus 91%, $p = .01$).

Controversy persists regarding the necessity of adjuvant therapy for patients with node-negative disease. Clearly, most patients do not require additional therapy, and recent work has been directed at identifying the subgroup of node-negative patients most likely to benefit. Toward this end, tumor size, nuclear grade, steroid receptor status, DNA ploidy, S-phase fraction, c-erbB-2 oncogene amplification, and cathepsin D expression have all been identified as prognostic variables that may assist in stratifying node-negative patients regarding the necessity of adjuvant therapy. Patients with diploid tumors that are smaller than 1 cm in diameter, have a low nuclear grade, and have a low S-phase fraction as determined by flow cytometry can expect a disease-free survival rate approaching 90% even without additional therapy. We currently do not recommend adjuvant cytotoxic therapy for this select, low-risk group of patients.

For node-negative patients whose tumors express estrogen receptors, adjuvant treatment with tamoxifen remains an attractive alternative. NSABP protocol B-14 examined the effectiveness of tamoxifen in both premenopausal and postmenopausal node-negative patients. Overall, 5-year disease-free survival was 82% in the tamoxifen-treated group and 73% for the placebo group ($p < .0001$). Overall survival was 93% in the treated and 90% in the untreated group ($p = 0.01$). Tamoxifen significantly reduced the rate of both local and distant failure as well as local recurrence following lumpectomy and radiotherapy. Of note, there was a 45% reduction in the incidence of contralateral breast cancer for tamoxifen-treated women; this finding has stimulated interest in the possibility that tamoxifen may be effective in the primary chemoprevention of breast cancer. The NSABP has embarked on a randomized trial of tamoxifen chemoprevention in women 60 years of age and older, as well as in women 35–59 years of age with a perceived high risk for breast cancer based on family history and other factors. Preliminary results from this trial, which randomized over 13,000 women, demonstrated a 45% reduction in the development of breast cancer.

Tamoxifen therapy is generally well tolerated; treatment-limiting adverse effects develop in less than 5% of all patients. Concerns regarding an increased incidence of endometrial cancer and thromboembolic events in women taking tamoxifen may be offset by beneficial effects on bone density and serum cholesterol, as well as an overall reduction in cardiovascular mortality. For these reasons, many practitioners recommend adjuvant tamoxifen therapy even for low-risk node-negative patients.

The merits of combining cytotoxic and hormonal therapies remain to be established. Although several trials have suggested a potential benefit to combination therapy, data remain inconclusive. NSABP protocol B-20 randomized patients with node-negative invasive breast cancer to receive either adjuvant tamoxifen alone or tamoxifen combined with one of two cytotoxic chemotherapy regimens. The results of this trial await long-term follow-up.

The 1992 St. Gallen Conference of a group of international breast experts made the following recommendations based on the available data regarding node-negative breast cancer:

1. Low-risk group (defined as DCIS tumors ≤1 cm or tumors of tubular, colloid, or papillary types <2 cm): No chemotherapy is necessary.
2. Good-risk group (defined as tumors >1 cm but ≤2 cm and ER positive): Tamoxifen is recommended for all age groups.

3. High-risk group (defined as any ER negative tumor >1 cm or any ER-positive tumor >2 cm or any tumor with nuclear grade III [poorly differentiated]): Standard chemotherapy is recommended (i.e., FAC vs CMF).

LOCALLY ADVANCED BREAST CANCER

Locally advanced breast cancer encompasses tumors with a broad range of biologic behavior. It is generally thought to include tumors that are large and/or have extensive regional lymph node involvement without evidence of distant metastatic disease on initial presentation. These patients are classified as having stage III disease according to the AJCC system. Approximately 10–20% of all breast cancer patients have stage III disease, which includes T3 tumors with N1, N2, or N3 disease; T4 tumors with any N stage; or any T stage with N2 or N3 regional lymph node involvement. Stage III disease is further subdivided into stage IIIa and stage IIIb (see Table 2-1). Approximately 25–30% of stage III breast cancers are inoperable at the time of diagnosis.

Because of the advanced stage of disease at diagnosis, many locally advanced breast cancers are discovered by the patient or her spouse. The rest are discovered during routine physical examination. On occasion, a discrete mass may not be present; rather, there is a diffuse infiltration of the breast tissue. These patients present with a breast that is asymmetric, immobile, and different in consistency from the contralateral breast. Seventy-five percent of stage III patients will have clinically palpable axillary or supraclavicular lymph nodes at the time of diagnosis. This clinical finding is confirmed on pathologic examination in 66–90% of patients. Of those patients with positive nodes, 50% will have more than four nodes involved by tumor. When appropriate staging is performed, 20% of stage III patients will have distant metastases at presentation. Distant metastases are also the most frequent form of treatment failure, usually appearing within 2 years of the initial diagnosis.

Both fine-needle aspiration and core-needle biopsy can be used to confirm the suspicion of breast cancer in these patients. These procedures usually are easily performed because of the large tumor size at presentation.

The Halsted radical mastectomy was initially thought to be the treatment of choice for locally advanced breast cancer; however, it proved to be inadequate in terms of both local control and long-term survival. In 1942, Haagensen reported a 53% local failure rate and no 5-year survival in a group of 1,135 stage III breast cancer patients.

The failure of surgery alone to control stage III breast cancer led to the use of radiotherapy as a single-agent treatment modality in this group of patients. However, the results with radiation therapy were in some cases inferior to those seen with surgery alone. The 5-year survival and local recurrence rates seen with radiation therapy alone were 10–30% and 25–70%, respectively.

The subsequent combination of surgery and radiotherapy for locally advanced breast cancer also resulted in poor overall results. The lack of efficacy in using a combination of two local treatment modalities confirmed the fact that stage III breast cancer is a systemic disease. Although there was a slight improvement in local control, 5-year survival was unchanged, as patients continued to succumb to distant metastases.

In the early 1970s, systemic combination chemotherapy was added to the local treatments for advanced breast cancer. Initial protocols were designed to administer the chemotherapy following local treatment. However, this sequence of treatment does not allow for any assessment of the efficacy of the chemotherapy, as all measurable disease is removed prior to administration of the drugs. This has led to the current practice of administering induction chemotherapy prior to any local treatment. This affords several advantages, including reduction of the initial tumor burden before surgery, ability to treat the potential systemic disease without delay, and ability to assess the response of the tumor to the treatment being rendered.

Several centers have reported experience with combined modality therapy for locally advanced disease. Although the protocols differ among institutions with respect to the specific chemotherapy regimens and the type of local treatment, all the studies have used induction chemotherapy followed by local treatment (surgery and/or radiotherapy) with a subsequent period of adjuvant chemotherapy. Based on these reports, it has now become the standard of care to treat patients with locally advanced breast cancer using this "sandwich" approach. Chemotherapy should consist of a doxorubicin-based regimen for four to six cycles, followed by surgery. Following surgery, adjuvant chemotherapy should precede radiotherapy to avoid interrupting the treatment of systemic disease because distant metastases are the most frequent form of treatment failure. The role of adjuvant hormonal therapy in this group of patients is still under investigation.

INFLAMMATORY BREAST CANCER

Inflammatory breast cancer is a rare, virulent form of locally advanced breast cancer. It represents 1–6% of all breast cancers and presents as erythema, warmth, and edema of the breast. Rapid onset of symptoms (within 3 months) is necessary to make the diagnosis of inflammatory carcinoma. The time course distinguishes this from locally advanced breast cancer with secondary lymphatic invasion, which usually progresses slowly over more than 3 months. Pain is also present in approximately one-half of these patients. These physical findings are often confused with an infectious process, resulting in frequent delays in diagnosis and treatment. Tumor emboli are seen in the subdermal lymphatics on microscopic examination. Biopsy for diagnosis should include a segment of involved skin because there is usually no dominant mass palpable on physical examination.

Inflammatory carcinoma, like other forms of locally advanced breast cancer, is a systemic disease. This was manifest in the poor outcome seen when local therapy was used as the only treatment modality. Median survival was less than 2 years, with 5-year survival rates around 5%.

The use of multimodality therapy in these patients has improved local control and survival compared with local therapy alone. Current therapy for inflammatory breast carcinoma at M. D. Anderson begins with chemotherapy. Patients with a complete or partial response proceed to surgery, which is followed by adjuvant chemotherapy and radiation therapy. Patients with progression of disease while on chemotherapy proceed to preoperative radiation therapy. Patients with less than partial response but no progression receive a second alternative chemotherapeutic regimen, followed by surgery for partial or complete response or radiation therapy for progression.

FOLLOW-UP AFTER PRIMARY TREATMENT OF INVASIVE BREAST CANCER

Following primary therapy for invasive breast cancer, patients must be made aware of the long-term risk for recurrent or metastatic disease. Although most series report most recurrences within the first 5 years of primary therapy, recurrences more than 20 years after primary therapy have been reported.

For each patient with breast cancer, follow-up evaluation should be individualized based on the treatments applied, the perceived risk of disease recurrence, and specific patient needs. Despite the availability of multiple biochemical and radiographic tests, periodic history taking and physical examination remain the most effective modalities for detecting recurrent disease. Numerous studies have demonstrated that 65–85% of all breast cancer recurrences may be detected by history and physical examination alone.

For patients who have undergone breast conservation therapy, follow-up examination should be undertaken every 4 months for the first 2 years, every 6 months for the third through fifth years, then yearly thereafter. Monthly self breast examination is also required. Mammography is obtained 6 months following the completion of breast conservation therapy to allow surgical and radiation changes to stabilize, and then on a yearly basis. For patients who have undergone mastectomy, a contralateral mammogram is obtained yearly. For both groups, further evaluation should be limited to yearly serum biochemical evaluation in patients who receive chemotherapy and a chest radiograph. The routine use of bone scans, skeletal surveys, and computed tomography scans of the abdomen and brain yields an extremely low rate of occult metastases in otherwise asymptomatic patients and is not cost-effective for patients with early-stage breast cancer.

LOCALLY RECURRENT BREAST CANCER

The time course, significance, and prognosis of locally recurrent breast cancer vary dramatically for patients undergoing breast conservation versus those undergoing mastectomy. Local recurrence rates of 5–10% at 8–10 years are reported in the conserved breast. This typically occurs over a protracted time period and is associated with systemic metastases in less than 10% of the patients. Local recurrence following lumpectomy remains curable in most cases; 50–63% of patients suffering local recurrence will remain disease-free 5 years after salvage mastectomy.

In contrast, local chest wall recurrence following mastectomy typically occurs within the first 2–3 years after surgery. It is associated with distant metastases in as many as two-thirds of the patients and predicts eventual death from breast cancer for many of the patients. One-third of patients with chest wall recurrence will have distant metastatic disease concurrent with their local recurrence; within 1 year, half will demonstrate distant disease. The median survival in this setting is 2–3 years.

Patients with apparently isolated local recurrence can often be treated without systemic cytotoxic chemotherapy. These patients should undergo complete restaging following the detection of recurrence; for patients with purely local recurrence, treatment with surgical excision combined with radiotherapy provides better local control than either modality used alone.

METASTATIC BREAST CANCER

Metastatic breast cancer generally cannot be cured; the median survival following the detection of metastases is 2 years. Treatment in this setting is purely palliative, although significant prolongation of survival can be obtained with appropriate therapy. For patients with overt metastases, the decision to treat with either systemic chemotherapy or hormonal therapy rests on several issues: patient age, physiologic status, disease-free interval, estrogen receptor status of the primary tumor, rapidity of metastatic growth, and whether the metastatic disease is skeletal or visceral. In selected patients who have isolated skeletal, pericardial, or pleural disease following a substantial disease-free interval (i.e., >2 years), radiotherapy with or without hormonal manipulation is often the most attractive strategy. In patients with a shorter disease-free interval and rapidly growing visceral (i.e., liver, lung, central nervous system) metastases, cytotoxic chemotherapy is usually required. Although doxorubicin remains the single agent with the highest response rate for advanced breast cancer, an actual benefit in terms of overall survival compared with nondoxorubicin-containing regimens remains difficult to establish. Most patients are initially treated with CMF, with doxorubicin reserved for disease progression. In selected patients with good performance status, high-dose chemotherapy with autologous stem cell rescue using hematologic growth factor support represents a potential treatment strategy. Response rates exceed 50%, and 1-year survival rates of 60% are reported. Long-term data are unavailable. At present, it remains unclear which chemotherapeutic agents are best used under such a strategy as well as which subsets of patients are most likely to benefit.

BREAST CANCER AND PREGNANCY

The incidence of breast cancer detected during pregnancy is 2 per 10,000 gestations, accounting for 2.8% of all breast malignancies. The diagnosis of breast cancer is typically more difficult in the gravid female because of several factors, including a low level of suspicion based on generally young patient age, the relative frequency of nodular changes in the breast during pregnancy, and the fact that increased breast density during pregnancy renders mammographic imaging less accurate. For these reasons the diagnosis of breast cancer during pregnancy is frequently delayed.

This feature, rather than specific differences in the biology of breast cancer among gravid and nongravid females, likely explains the relatively poor prognosis for women with breast cancer detected during pregnancy. When matched for tumor stage, pregnant women with breast cancer appear to have a prognosis no worse than nonpregnant patients.

Because of the inaccuracy of mammography in this setting, all persistent, suspicious breast masses discovered during pregnancy should undergo evaluation either by fine-needle aspiration, needle-core biopsy, or excisional biopsy. Excisional biopsy under local anesthesia represents a safe procedure at any time during pregnancy. Once a diagnosis of malignancy is established, subsequent treatment decisions are influenced by their timing with respect to the specific trimester of pregnancy. For women who want to complete their pregnancies, the goal should be curative treatment of the breast cancer without injury to the fetus. It is important to note that numerous studies have demonstrated that termination of pregnancy in hopes of minimizing hormonal stimulation of the tumor has no benefit to maternal survival.

Surgical treatment of gestational breast cancer is generally conducted in a manner identical to nongestational breast cancer. There is no evidence that extra-abdominal surgical procedures are associated with premature labor or that the typically used anesthetic agents are teratogenic. For women desiring modified radical mastectomy as primary therapy, this can be undertaken at any point during pregnancy without undue risk to mother or fetus. For cancer detected during the third trimester, delays in primary treatment of up to 4 weeks to allow for delivery prior to surgery appear to be acceptable. If modified radical mastectomy is undertaken during pregnancy, breast reconstruction should not be performed simultaneously; a symmetric result is impossible until the postpartum appearance of the contralateral breast is known.

For women desiring breast conservation, treatment is complicated by the fact that radiotherapy is contraindicated during pregnancy. For cancers detected during the third trimester, lumpectomy and axillary dissection can safely be performed using general anesthesia, with radiotherapy delayed until after delivery. Longer delays may be detrimental to maternal outcome, although the time limit within which radiotherapy must be carried out to minimize the risk of local recurrence is unknown.

It may be necessary to administer cytotoxic adjuvant chemotherapy during pregnancy, raising fears of congenital malformations. Most series have demonstrated no increased risk of fetal malformation for chemotherapy administered during the second and third trimesters. In contrast, chemotherapy administration during the first trimester is associated with an increased incidence of spontaneous abortion and congenital malformation, especially when methotrexate is used.

CYSTOSARCOMA PHYLLODES

Cystosarcoma phyllodes represents an uncommon group of neoplasms, accounting for only 0.3–0.9% of all breast tumors. The term *cystosarcoma* is antiquated nomenclature that has generated great confusion regarding this diagnosis. Phyllodes tumors may actually be either benign or malignant and exhibit a wide spectrum of metastatic potential. Features suggesting malignancy include large tumor size, stromal atypia, an infiltrating margin, and frequent mitoses. Nevertheless, the clinical course is often difficult to predict based on histologic appearance alone. When metastases do occur, common sites include the lung, bone, and mediastinum.

Women with phyllodes tumors present at a median age of 50 years. These tumors are typically quite large, with a mean diameter of 4–5 cm. Given the fact that phyllodes tumors are mammographically indistinguishable from fibroadenomas, the decision to perform excisional biopsy is usually based on large tumor size, a history of rapid growth, and the age of the patient.

Appropriate treatment for phyllodes tumors remains complete surgical excision. The decision to perform wide local excision versus total mastectomy has traditionally been based on the size of the lesion and the potential for malignancy based on histologic appearance. Depending on the series, the incidence of subsequent recurrence ranges from 4% to 20% for histologically benign lesions, and from 8% to 37% for tumors considered histologically malignant. Local recurrences are typically salvageable with total mastectomy and have no impact on overall survival. Because these tumors are almost always unifocal, breast conservation should be considered, especially for patients with T1–T2 lesions. For all phyllodes tumors, the incidence of axillary nodal metastases is less than 1%, obviating the need for lymphadenectomy. To date, no role for radiotherapy, chemotherapy, or hormonal therapy has been established for this disease.

Selected References

Abner AL, Recht A, Eberlein T, et al. Prognosis following salvage mastectomy for recurrence in the breast after conservative surgery and radiation therapy for early-stage breast cancer. *J Clin Oncol* 11:44, 1993.

Balch CM, Singletary SE, Bland KI. Clinical decision-making in early breast cancer. *Ann Surg* 217:207, 1993.

Barnovon Y, Wallack MK. Management of the pregnant patient with carcinoma of the breast. *Surg Gynecol Obstet* 171:347, 1990.

Deckers PJ. Axillary dissection in breast cancer: When, why, how much, and for how long? *J Surg Oncol* 48:217, 1991.

Early Breast Cancer Trialists' Collaborative Group. Effects of adjuvant tamoxifen and of cytotoxic therapy on mortality in early breast cancer: An overview of 61 randomized trials among 28,896 women. *N Engl J Med* 319:1681, 1988.

Fisher B, Constantino J, Redmond C, et al. A randomized clinical trial evaluating tamoxifen in the treatment of patients with node-negative breast cancer who have estrogen-receptor-positive tumors. *N Engl J Med* 320:479, 1989.

Fisher B, Redmond C, Dimitrov NV, et al. A randomized clinical trial evaluating sequential methotrexate and fluorouracil in the treatment of patients with node-negative breast cancer who have estrogen-receptor-negative tumors. *N Engl J Med* 320:473, 1989.

Fisher B, Redmond C, Fisher ER, et al. Ten-year results of a randomized clinical trial comparing radical mastectomy and total mastectomy with or without radiation. *N Engl J Med* 312:674, 1985.

Fisher B, Redmond C, Poisson R, et al. Eight-year results of a randomized clinical trial comparing total mastectomy and lumpectomy with or without irradiation in the treatment of breast cancer. *N Engl J Med* 320:822, 1989.

Grodstein F, Meir S, Graham C, et al. Postmenopausal hormone therapy and mortality. *N Engl J Med* 336:1769, 1997.

Harris JR, Lippman ME, Veronesi U, et al. Breast cancer. *N Engl J Med* 327:319, 390, 473, 1992.

Henderson IC. Risk factors for breast cancer development. *Cancer* 71(6)(Supp):2128, 1993.

Hortobagyi GN, Buzdar AU. Locally advanced breast cancer: A review including the M. D. Anderson experience. In J Ragaz, IM Ariel (eds.), *High Risk Breast Cancer*. Berlin: Springer-Verlag, 1991.

Margolese R, Poisson R, Shibata H, et al. The technique of segmental mastectomy (lumpectomy) and axillary dissection: A syllabus from the NSABP workshops. *Surgery* 102:828, 1987.

McGuire WL, Clark GM. Prognostic factors and treatment decisions in axillary node-negative breast cancer. *N Engl J Med* 326:1756, 1992.

Salvadori B, Cusumano F, Del Bo R, et al. Surgical treatment of phylloides tumors of the breast. *Cancer* 63:2532, 1989.

Veronesi U, Saccozz R, Del Vecchio M, et al. Comparing radical masectomy with quadrantectomy, axillary dissection, and radiotherapy in patients with small cancers of the breast. *N Engl J Med* 305:6–11, 1981.

Melanoma

Jeffrey E. Gershenwald, Jeffrey J. Sussman, and Jeffrey E. Lee

Epidemiology

Although melanoma is a relatively uncommon malignancy worldwide, its incidence is increasing dramatically. It is estimated that 40,300 new cases were diagnosed in the United States in 1997, an 18% increase in the incidence from 1995. Overall, the incidence rate for melanoma is now increasing faster than that for any other cancer. Melanoma is the most common cancer in American women 25–29 years of age and the second most common in American women 30–34 years old (second only to breast cancer). Incidence varies from 4 to 30 per 100,000 persons, increasing at lower latitudes. Melanoma incidence is similar in men and women and increases from the age of 10 years to the fifth decade. Approximately 1 in 87 Americans alive today will develop melanoma in their lifetime; lifetime risk is expected to be 1 in 75 by the year 2000. Melanoma occurs primarily in whites, although other races are also affected. There have been changes in the distribution and stage of melanoma at diagnosis over the past 30 years, with an increase in thinner lesions. Most melanomas seen at many institutions now measure less than 1 mm thick.

Risk Factors

1. *Previous melanoma:* The risk of developing a second melanoma in a patient who has had a melanoma is 3–7%; this represents a 900-fold higher risk than that of the general population.
2. *Fair complexion*: Fair or red hair, light skin, blue eyes, and a propensity to sunburn are associated with an increased risk of melanoma.
3. *Sunlight exposure*: Occasional or recreational exposure to sunlight, especially a history of severe blistering sunburn, has been associated with an increased risk of melanoma. The effects of sunlight have been attributed to exposure to ultraviolet B radiation.
4. *Benign nevi*: Though a benign nevus is most likely not a precursor of melanoma, the presence of large numbers of nevi has been consistently associated with an increased risk of melanoma.
5. *Family history*: See the next item, "genetic predisposition."
6. *Genetic predisposition*: Specific genetic alterations have been implicated in the pathogenesis of melanoma. At least four distinct genes—located on chromosomes 1p, 6q, 7, and 9—may play a role in melanoma. A tumor suppressor gene located on

chromosome 9p21 is probably involved in familial and sporadic cutaneous melanoma. Deletions or rearrangements of chromosomes 10 and 11 are also well documented in cutaneous melanoma.

7. *Atypical mole and melanoma syndrome* (AMS): Previously known as dysplastic nevus syndrome, AMS is characterized by the presence of large numbers of atypical moles (dysplastic nevi) that represent a distinct clinicopathologic type of melanocytic lesion. They can be precursors of melanoma as well as markers of increased melanoma risk. The actual frequency of an atypical mole progressing to melanoma is small. After identification of AMS, patients should be followed closely and family members should be screened.

Pathology

There are four major melanoma growth patterns:

1. *Superficial spreading melanoma* constitutes the majority of melanomas (about 70%) and generally arises in a preexisting nevus.
2. *Nodular melanoma* is the second most common growth pattern (15–30%). Nodular melanomas are more aggressive tumors and usually develop more rapidly than superficial spreading melanomas.
3. *Lentigo maligna melanoma* does not have the same propensity to metastasize as do other histologies. Lentigo maligna melanomas constitute a small percentage of melanomas (4–10%) and are typically located on the face in older Caucasian women. They are usually large (>3 cm at diagnosis), flat lesions and are uncommon before age 50.
4. *Acral lentiginous melanoma* occurs on the palms (palmar) or soles (plantar) or beneath the nail beds (subungual), although not all palmar, plantar, and subungual melanomas are acral lentiginous melanomas. These melanomas account for only 2–8% of melanomas in Caucasian patients but for a substantially higher proportion of melanomas (35–60%) in darker-skinned patients. Acral lentiginous melanomas are the most aggressive histologic type. They are generally large, with an average diameter of approximately 3 cm.

Clinical Presentation

Clinical features of melanoma include (1) variegated color, (2) irregular raised surface, (3) irregular perimeter, and (4) surface ulceration. Any pigmented lesion that undergoes a change in size, configuration, or color should be biopsied. The **ABCD**s of early diagnosis provide an easy way by which physicians and individuals may become familiar with the early signs of malignant melanoma. *A* denotes lesion asymmetry; *B*, border irregularity; *C*, color variegation; and *D*, diameter greater than 6 mm.

When a patient presents with a lesion suspicious for melanoma, a thorough physical examination must be performed, with particular emphasis on the skin, all nodal basins, and subcutaneous tissues. Chest radiograph and liver function studies should be obtained. Further evaluation is based on pathologic findings. We discourage routine extensive evaluation with computed tomography or bone scan because their yield in the absence of symptoms, abnormal laboratory findings, or an abnormal chest radiograph is very low in patients with primary melanoma.

Staging

Collaboration between the American Joint Committee on Cancer (AJCC) and the Union Internationale Contre le Cancer has resulted in the current clinical staging system for melanoma (Table 3-1).

Two methods have been used to microstage primary melanoma. Breslow's microstaging determines the thickness of the lesion using an ocular micrometer to measure the total vertical height of the melanoma from the granular layer to the area of deepest penetration. Clark's microstaging defines levels of invasion reflecting increasing depth of penetration into the dermis. Discrepancies between the Clark's level and the Breslow's thickness occur frequently. For localized primary melanoma, the Breslow's thickness is the single most significant prognostic factor.

Significant prognostic factors for patients with primary melanoma not included in the AJCC staging system include ulceration, sex, and the anatomic location of the primary lesion. Ulceration, male sex, and location on the trunk or head are all associated with a worse prognosis. (The reader is also referred to Buzaid et al. for an excellent critical review of the current staging system for melanoma.)

Biopsy

The choice of biopsy technique varies according to the anatomic site, size, and shape of the lesion. Definitive therapy must be considered in choosing a biopsy technique. Either an excisional biopsy or an incisional biopsy using a scalpel or punch is acceptable. An excisional biopsy allows the pathologist to more accurately determine the thickness of the lesion. For excisional biopsies, a narrow margin of normal-appearing skin (1–3 mm) is taken with the specimen. An elliptical incision is used to facilitate closure. The biopsy incision should be oriented to facilitate later wide local excision (e.g., longitudinally on extremities) and minimize the need for a skin graft to provide wound closure. We reserve punch biopsy for lesions that are large, are located on anatomic areas where maximum preservation of surrounding skin is important, or can be completely excised with a 6-mm punch. Punch biopsies should be performed at the most raised or darkest area of the lesion. Full-thickness biopsy into the subcutaneous tissue must be performed to properly microstage the lesion.

Table 3-1. AJCC melanoma staging system*

TNM Classification

Primary tumor (pT)

pTX	Primary tumor cannot be assessed
pT0	No evidence of primary tumor
pTis	Melanoma *in situ* (Clark's level I)
pT1	Primary tumor ≤0.75 mm thick and/or invades papillary dermis (Clark's level II)
pT2	Primary tumor 0.76–1.50 mm thick and/or invades to papillary-reticular dermal interface (Clark's level III)
pT3	Primary tumor 1.51–4.00 mm thick and/or invades the reticular dermis (Clark's level IV)
pT4	Primary tumor >4.00 mm thick and/or invades the subcutaneous tissue (Clark's level V) and/or satellite(s) within 2 cm of the primary tumor

Regional lymph nodes (N)

NX	Regional lymph nodes cannot be assessed
N0	No regional lymph node metastasis
N1	Metastasis ≤3 cm in greatest dimension in any regional lymph node
N2	Metastasis >3 cm in greatest dimension in any regional lymph node(s) and/or in-transit metastasis

Distant metastasis (M)

MX	Distant metastasis cannot be assessed
M0	No distant metastasis
M1	Distant metastasis

Stage grouping

Stage 0	pTis	N0	M0
Stage I	pT1	N0	M0
	pT2	N0	M0
Stage II	pT3	N0	M0
	pT4	N0	M0
Stage III	Any pT	N1	M0
	Any pT	N2	M0
Stage IV	Any pT	Any N	M1

*The AJCC Melanoma Committee recommends that when there is a discrepancy between tumor thickness and Clark's level, the pT category be based on the less favorable finding.
(Adapted from ID Fleming, JS Cooper, DE Henson, et al. (eds). *AJCC Cancer Staging Manual* (5th ed). Philadelphia: Lippincott, 1997.)

Shave biopsies are contraindicated if a diagnosis of melanoma is being considered. Fine-needle aspiration biopsy may be used to document nodal and extranodal melanoma metastases but should not be used to diagnose primary melanomas. We send all pigmented lesions for permanent-section examination only and perform definitive surgery at a later time.

Markers of melanocytic cells can be useful in confirming the diagnosis of melanoma. Two widely used antibodies employed in immunohistochemical evaluations are S-100 and HMB-45. S-100 is expressed by more than 90% of melanomas but also by several other tumors and some normal tissues, including dendritic cells. Although the monoclonal antibody HMB-45 is relatively specific for proliferative melanocytic cells and melanoma, it is not as sensitive as S-100.

Management of Local Disease

Local control of a primary melanoma requires wide excision of the tumor or biopsy site down to the deep fascia with a margin of normal-appearing skin. Risk of local recurrence correlates more with tumor thickness than with margins of surgical excision. It is rational to excise melanomas using surgical margins that vary according to tumor thickness.

MARGINS

The first randomized study involving surgical margins for melanomas less than 2 mm thick was reported by the World Health Organization (WHO) Melanoma Group. In an update of the study of 612 evaluable patients randomly assigned to receive a 1-cm or 3-cm margin of excision, there were no local recurrences among patients with melanomas thinner than 1 mm. There were four local recurrences in the 100 patients with melanomas 1–2 mm thick, and all four patients had received 1-cm margin excisions. There was no statistically significant difference in survival between the 1-cm and the 3-cm surgical margin groups. These results demonstrate that a narrow excision margin for thin (<1 mm) melanomas is safe.

A multi-institutional prospective randomized trial from France compared a 5-cm margin with a 2-cm margin in 319 patients with melanomas ≤2 mm thick. There were no differences in local recurrence rate or survival.

A randomized prospective study conducted by the Intergroup Melanoma Committee evaluated 2-cm versus 4-cm radial margins of excision for intermediate-thickness melanomas (1–4 mm). There was no difference in local recurrence rate between the 2-cm and the 4-cm margin groups. Of note is that 46% of the 4-cm group required skin grafts, whereas only 11% of the 2-cm group did ($p < .001$). These data strongly support the use of a 2-cm margin for intermediate-thickness lesions.

Although these randomized prospective trials demonstrated the efficacy of 1-cm and 2-cm excision margins for thin and intermediate-thickness melanomas, respectively, the optimal management of thick melanomas (>4 mm thick) is still unknown. A retrospective review of 278 patients with thick primary melanomas demonstrated that the width of the excision margin (≤2 cm versus >2 cm) did not significantly affect local recurrence, disease-free survival, or overall survival after a median follow-up of 27 months.

General recommendations for margins are as follows:

1. *Thin melanomas* (<1 mm thick) have a minimal risk of local recurrence. Wide excision with a 1-cm margin of normal-appearing skin is recommended.
2. *Intermediate-thickness melanomas* (1–4 mm thick) have an increased risk of local recurrence. A 2-cm margin can be safely used.
3. *Thick melanomas* (>4 mm thick) have a risk of local recurrence that may exceed 10–20%. A 2-cm margin is probably safe, although no prospective randomized trials have specifically addressed this thickness group.

CLOSURE

If there is any question about the ability to achieve suitable wound closure, a plastic or reconstructive surgeon should be consulted. Options for closure include primary closure, skin grafting, and local and distant flaps.

Primary closure is the method of choice for most lesions, but it should be avoided when it will distort the appearance of a mobile facial feature or interfere with function. Many defects can be closed using an advancement flap, undermining the skin and subcutaneous tissues to permit primary closure. Primary closure usually requires that the longitudinal axis of an elliptical incision be at least three times the short axis. Closure of the wound edges is usually performed in two layers. This may consist of a dermal layer of 3–0 or 4–0 undyed absorbable sutures, and either interrupted skin closure using 3–0 or 4–0 nonabsorbable sutures or a running subcuticular skin closure using 4–0 monofilament absorbable sutures.

Application of a *skin graft* is one of the simplest reconstructive methods. Split-thickness skin grafts are the most commonly used. For lower-extremity primary lesions, split-thickness grafts should be harvested from the extremity opposite the melanoma. A full-thickness skin graft can provide a result that is both durable and of high aesthetic quality. The most common use of the full-thickness graft has been on the face, where aesthetic considerations are most significant. Donor sites for full-thickness skin graft to the face should be chosen from locations that are likely to match the color of the face, such as the postauricular or preauricular skin or the supraclavicular portion of the neck.

Local flaps offer a number of advantages for reconstruction of defects that cannot be closed primarily, especially on the distal extremities and on the head and neck. Color match is excellent, durability of the skin is essentially normal, and normal sensation is usually preserved. Transposition flaps and rotation flaps of many varieties have been successfully used.

Distant flaps should be used when sufficient tissue for a local flap is not available and when a skin graft would not provide adequate wound coverage. Myocutaneous flaps and free flaps can be used. Discussion of such complex methods is beyond the scope of this chapter, but these techniques are familiar to plastic and reconstructive surgeons.

SPECIAL ANATOMIC SITES

Fingers and Toes

More than three-fourths of subungual melanomas involve either the great toe or the thumb. A melanoma located on the skin of a digit or beneath the fingernail should be removed by a digital amputation, saving as much of the digit as possible. In general, amputations are performed at the middle interphalangeal joint of the fingers or proximal to the distal joint of the thumb. More proximal amputations are not associated with a prolongation of survival. For a melanoma located on a toe, an amputation of the entire digit at the metatarsal-phalangeal joint is indicated. Lesions arising between two toes often require the amputation of both surrounding toes.

Sole of the Foot

Excision of a melanoma on the plantar surface often produces a sizable defect in a weight-bearing area. If possible, a portion of the heel or ball of the plantar surface should be retained to bear the greatest burden of pressure. Where possible, deep fascia over the extensor tendons should be preserved as a base for skin coverage. Rotation flaps or myocutaneous free flaps are recommended for coverage of weight-bearing areas.

Face

Facial lesions usually cannot be excised with more than a 1-cm margin because of adjacent vital structures. The tumor diameter, thickness of the melanoma, and its exact location on the face must all be considered when determining margin width.

Breast

Wide local excision with primary closure is the treatment of choice for melanoma on the skin of the breast; mastectomy is not generally recommended. As with any trunk lesion, lymphoscintigraphy should be done before selective lymphadenectomy (see later) or prophylactic lymph node dissection.

SPECIAL CLINICAL SITUATIONS

Giant Congenital Nevi

Decisions about the management of giant congenital nevi are difficult because such lesions are often so extensive that prophylactic surgical excision is impossible. When the location and size of a lesion permit prophylactic excision, excision should be done before the age of 2 years.

Mucosal Melanoma

Patients with true mucosal melanoma—including melanoma of the mucosa of the head and neck, vagina, and anal canal—have a poor prognosis regardless of surgical therapy. We generally do not recommend an aggressive surgical approach to patients with clinically localized disease. We reserve extended resection for bulky or recurrent tumors and favor therapeutic over elective lymph node dissection (see later). In particular, we recommend local excision of anal melanomas over abdominoperineal resection. Abdominoperineal resection is associated with a much higher morbidity, leaves the patient with a permanent colostomy, offers no survival advantage, and does not treat at-risk inguinal nodes unless combined with groin dissection. Adjuvant radiotherapy may be considered for patients with mucosal melanoma in an attempt to decrease locoregional recurrence.

Desmoplastic Melanoma

Desmoplastic or neurotropic melanoma is a rare variant of melanoma. Desmoplastic melanomas have a propensity for perineural invasion and infiltration of the blood vessel adventitia. These tumors often recur locally. Frozen-section examination must be performed to ensure that excision margins are free of tumor. Adjuvant radiotherapy may decrease the risk of local recurrence.

Pregnancy

The precise influence of pregnancy or hormonal manipulation on the clinical course of malignant melanoma has not been defined. There is no conclusive evidence that concurrent pregnancy has an adverse effect on the disease course. Several large studies report no difference in outcome between gravid and non-gravid patients with primary melanoma. Surgery is the treatment of choice in pregnant patients with early-stage melanoma. There is no proof that abortion of the pregnancy protects the mother from subsequent development of metastases. Although there are differing opinions on planning a pregnancy after a diagnosis of melanoma, the weight of evidence does not demonstrate an increased risk for developing metastatic disease with pregnancy. Furthermore, several studies have found no association between oral contraceptive use and survival in melanoma.

General recommendations for managing melanoma during pregnancy are as follows:

1. The ultimate decision about continuing or terminating a pregnancy should be left to the patient and family.
2. A patient who presents with a primary melanoma during pregnancy should be evaluated with the minimum number of diagnostic tests.
3. The primary melanoma should be excised under appropriate anesthesia. Elective lymph node dissection should not be performed. However, therapeutic dissection of regional lymph nodes should be considered, if warranted.
4. In pregnant patients with systemic metastases, the decision to abort or continue the pregnancy must be made on a case-by-case basis. Systemic chemotherapy during the second and third trimesters does not usually cause abnormalities in fetal development, unless alkylating agents are used.
5. If the mother had melanoma during pregnancy, the placenta should be examined histologically for evidence of metastasis

at the time of delivery. Additionally, the child should be monitored carefully for metastatic disease during the first 6–12 months of life.

6. Women of child-bearing age who have melanoma should probably not become pregnant or take oral contraceptives for 2 years after their treatment. Those 2 years represent the period of greatest risk for relapse with metastases. Conversely, however, should pregnancy occur during this time, abortion of the pregnancy is not necessary.

Management of Local Recurrence and In-Transit Disease

The overall risk of local recurrence is low—3% in a collected series of 3,520 patients. Local recurrence usually develops within 5 years after primary melanoma excision. Local recurrence implies a poor prognosis and often portends distant metastases. In a study of 95 patients with local recurrences, the median survival was 3 years, with a 10-year survival rate of only 20%.

In-transit metastases are located between the primary melanoma and the first major regional nodal basin. The incidence of in-transit metastases is 2–3%. Regional nodal metastases occur in about two-thirds of patients with in-transit metastases and, if present, are associated with lower survival rates. Patients with few in-transit metastases have better prognoses than those with multiple lesions.

Comparison studies of treatment alternatives for local recurrences and in-transit disease have not been performed. Options include surgical excision, regional chemotherapy using isolated limb perfusion, and radiotherapy.

A single local recurrence in a patient whose primary melanoma had favorable prognostic features can be excised and no further treatment given. Alternatively, adjuvant treatment can be considered, for example, in the form of high-dose interferon-alpha. Patients with multiple local recurrences, with local recurrence and poor prognostic features of the primary melanoma, or with in-transit metastases may be considered for regional treatment. Regional treatment options include isolated limb perfusion and radiotherapy using a high-dose-per-fraction technique. Rarely, amputation may be necessary for extensive or deeply infiltrative lesions involving the foot, hand, arm, or leg.

Melphalan is the most active single agent for use in hyperthermic isolated limb perfusion. Complete response rates average 40% in patients with measurable disease. Recent nonrandomized studies of hyperthermic limb perfusion by Leinard et al. have reported a high complete response rate (90%) using a combination of melphalan, tumor necrosis factor-alpha (TNF-alpha), and interferon-gamma, compared with melphalan alone (52%). The durability of these responses has not yet been reported. Fraker et al. reported a 100% response rate in patients treated with melphalan alone and a 90% response rate in patients perfused with melphalan, interferon-gamma, and TNF-alpha. This latter combination resulted in a higher complete response rate (80% versus 61%). A multicenter randomized trial is currently under way comparing perfusion using melphalan alone with perfusion using the combination of melphalan, TNF-alpha, and interferon-gamma. Significant palliation of regional symptoms (pain, edema, bleeding, and ulceration) has also been achieved at the National Institutes of Health using multiagent perfusion regimens in patients with locally advanced extremity melanoma.

Hyperthermic isolated limb perfusion continues to be associated with significant regional toxicity, including myonecrosis, nerve injury, and arterial thrombosis, sometimes requiring major amputation. Systemic toxicity, including hypotension and adult respiratory distress syndrome, is sometimes seen with the addition of TNF-alpha to the regimen. The treatment requires a high degree of technical expertise and carries a significant risk of major complications, including limb loss. The procedure should therefore be performed only in centers that have experience with the technique, preferably in the setting of a clinical trial. At present, there is little evidence to justify the use of prophylactic perfusion except as part of a clinical trial.

Management of Regional Disease

Regional lymph nodes are the most common site of metastatic melanoma. Effective palliation and sometimes cure can be achieved in patients with regional metastases. Fine-needle aspiration can often yield a diagnosis in patients who develop clinically enlarged regional nodes. Open biopsy is sometimes warranted. If, by clinical examination, the index of suspicion for metastases is high, definitive surgical treatment can be performed without open biopsy.

Surgical excision of nodal metastases is the only effective treatment to achieve local disease control and cure. In patients with clinical stage III disease, a biopsy or partial lymphadenectomy results in lower survival rates compared with a complete lymphadenectomy. Incomplete lymph node dissection is unacceptable. Some surgeons prefer to perform lymphadenectomy only for clinically demonstrable nodal metastases. This type of excision has been termed *delayed or therapeutic lymph node dissection* (TLND). Other surgeons choose to excise the nodes even when they appear normal in patients who are at increased risk of developing nodal metastases. This excision has been termed *immediate, prophylactic, or elective lymph node dissection* (ELND). More recently, many surgeons have adopted a selective approach to regional lymphadenectomy based on the technique of intraoperative lymphatic mapping and sentinel lymph node identification developed by Morton.

ELND has the theoretic advantage of treating melanoma nodal metastases at a relatively early stage in the natural history of the disease. Its disadvantage is that some patients undergo surgery when they do not have nodal metastases. Thus an advantage of TLND is that only patients with demonstrable metastases undergo major operations; this reduces the number of potentially unnecessary lymphadenectomies while not necessarily reducing the chance for cure. The disadvantage of TLND is that delaying treatment until lymph node metastases are clinically palpable may result in many patients having distant micrometastases at the time of lymphadenectomy. Chances for cure may therefore be diminished. The technique of lymphatic mapping and sentinel lymph node biopsy offers a selective approach to ELND that satisfies many proponents both of ELND and of TLND.

ELECTIVE LYMPH NODE DISSECTION

The role of ELND in the management of clinically localized (stage I and II) primary melanoma has been the focus of great debates. Although ELND does not offer a survival benefit to all patients, recently completed prospective randomized trials suggest that some subsets of patients benefit from ELND.

Tumor thickness is the primary tumor feature that best predicts regional and distant metastases and is therefore the most important (but not sole) guide in selecting who might benefit from an ELND. Thin melanomas (<1 mm) are generally localized and are associated with a 95% or greater cure rate following wide local excision alone. ELND does not benefit these patients. Intermediate-thickness melanomas (1–4 mm) confer an increased risk (up to 60%) of occult regional metastases but a relatively low risk (<20%) of distant metastases. Patients with these lesions might benefit from ELND. Thick melanomas (>4 mm) carry a high risk for regional nodal micrometastases (>60%) as well as a high risk (>70%) of occult distant disease at the time of initial presentation. In fact, the risk of distant microscopic metastases is so high in these patients that it may negate any potentially curative benefit of a regional operation. Therefore regional lymph node dissection in patients with thick primary melanomas has generally been deferred until nodal metastases become clinically evident.

Several nonrandomized studies involving melanomas from all anatomic sites showed significantly improved survival with ELND for a subgroup of patients with intermediate-thickness melanomas. In studies at at least two institutions, however, longer follow-up eliminated the previously reported survival benefit attributed to ELND. Nevertheless, these investigations did provide evidence that patients with intermediate-thickness primaries could benefit from ELND and identified appropriate subsets of patients to include in prospective randomized trials.

The first two prospective trials to evaluate ELND in the treatment of stage I and II melanoma were an international cooperative study conducted by the WHO Melanoma Group and a study at the Mayo Clinic. These studies clearly demonstrated that not all patients benefit from ELND. Both studies included melanomas of all thicknesses and did not specifically address the potential benefit of ELND for the subgroup of patients with intermediate-thickness melanomas.

Two contemporary prospective randomized trials of ELND have been completed. Their design was influenced by identification of the limitations of earlier prospective trials (preponderance of women with thin extremity lesions) and by findings supporting ELND in patients with intermediate-thickness melanomas in retrospective studies. The WHO Trunk Trial evaluated the role of ELND in patients with truncal melanomas thicker than 1.5 mm and stratified patients according to tumor thickness and gender. Long-term results of this trial have not been reported. More recently, the Intergroup Melanoma Committee studied patients with melanomas 1–4 mm thick at any anatomic site; patients were stratified by tumor thickness, presence or absence of ulceration, and anatomic subsite. The first analysis, which was recently reported, noted no overall survival benefit in patients who underwent ELND compared with those who had wide local excision alone. However, two subsets of patients were identified who received a significant benefit from ELND: (1) patients ≤60 years of age and (2) patients whose tumors were 1.1–2.0 mm thick. These subsets represent combinations of prospectively and retrospectively defined criteria. The early results of this trial can be incorporated at the surgeon's discretion into surgical strategies for patients ≤60 years of age, especially when the primary tumor is 1.1–2.0 mm thick.

INTRAOPERATIVE LYMPHATIC MAPPING AND SENTINEL LYMPH NODE BIOPSY

A rational alternative to ELND has emerged that has already significantly altered the surgical approach to primary melanoma in several large cancer centers, including M. D. Anderson. This new approach, termed *selective lymphadenectomy*, includes lymphatic mapping and sentinel lymph node (SLN) biopsy and relies on the concept that finite regions of the skin drain first to specific lymph nodes—sentinel lymph nodes—within the regional basin via an organized system of afferent lymphatic channels. At the time of wide excision a vital blue dye (patent blue V or isosulfan blue) is injected intradermally at the primary melanoma or biopsy site. Exploration of the draining nodal basin (identified by prior lymphoscintigraphy) allows the lymphatic channels and the first draining (i.e., sentinel) lymph node to be identified by their uptake of the blue dye. Using this technique, Morton proved that (1) the SLN is the first node to which a cutaneous primary melanoma is likely to metastasize, and (2) the histologic status of the SLN reflects the histologic status of the remainder of the regional nodal basin. This approach spares patients with a histologically negative SLN the morbidity and expense of an unnecessary procedure, since ELND is offered only to patients in whom metastatic melanoma is identified in the SLN. Two subsequent series have confirmed the results of the original trial: the SLN was identified in ≥85% of patients, and in ≤8% of patients metastatic melanoma was identified elsewhere in the regional nodal basins (by concomitant lymphadenectomy at the time of SLN biopsy) when the SLN was histopathologically free of tumor.

It is imperative that the surgeon contemplating the use of these techniques in his or her practice have adequate pathology and nuclear medicine support; close collaboration is essential to perform these procedures accurately.

Technique

To improve SLN localization, two techniques—preoperative lymphoscintigraphy and intraoperative radiolymphoscintigraphy accompanied by use of a hand-held gamma probe—have been incorporated into our treatment strategy for patients with clinically node-negative primary melanoma.

Lymphoscintigraphy is an essential adjunct to determine which regional basins are at risk in patients with primary melanomas located in ambiguous drainage sites (e.g., trunk, head, and neck), since historical lymphatic drainage guidelines are often inaccurate. The test involves the intradermal injection of a radiocolloid such as technetium 99m-labeled human serum albumin around the primary tumor site and subsequent nuclear scanning of regional nodal basins. This technique can also be used to localize potential SLNs, *prior* to surgical exploration, within epitrochlear or popliteal nodal regions in patients with primary tumors distal to the elbow or knee, respectively. This technique may occasionally identify a SLN present outside typical lymphatic drainage basins, especially in patients with truncal primaries. It is not uncommon for two or more nodal basins to be identified by these scans.

Following the intradermal injection of 0.5–1.0 mCi of unfiltered technetium 99mTc sulfur colloid 1–4 hours before surgery, lymphatic mapping is subsequently performed with the aid of a hand-held gamma probe. This device, designed for intraoperative use, permits the surgeon to identify the region or regions of greatest radiotracer uptake, which correspond to the sites of the SLNs. This technology is based on the principle that the radiolabeled colloid is actively incorporated into the draining SLN. Accurate localization can therefore be obtained before incision, resulting in better-directed and smaller incisions as well as rapid intraoperative identification of the node. Although some groups rely on only one of these techniques (vital blue dye or intraoperative lymphoscintigraphy with use of a hand-held gamma probe), we believe that these two techniques are complementary and have incorporated both into our current practice. Our experience with the combination demonstrates an SLN identification rate of >99%.

Prognostic Value of SLN Status

Following the demonstration that the histologic status of the SLN accurately reflects the histologic status of the nodal basin, several major centers incorporated selective lymphadenectomy into their approach for primary melanoma patients with clinically negative regional nodal basins. The experience at M. D. Anderson Cancer Center and Moffitt Cancer Center has been presented. Lymphatic mapping and SLN biopsy were successful in 580 of 612 patients (95%) who underwent the procedure. SLN status was the most significant prognostic factor with respect to disease-free, distant disease-free, and disease-specific survival by univariate and multivariate analyses (Fig. 3-1).

A National Cancer Institute–sponsored international, multicenter prospective randomized trial of SLN biopsy is currently accruing stage I and II patients with melanomas thicker than 1 mm. Patients are randomized (2:1) to receive either wide local excision and SLN biopsy or wide local excision alone. This trial will address the following issues: (1) What is the long-term false-negative rate for SLN biopsy? (2) What, if any, survival benefit is achieved with selective node dissection in patients with micrometastatic regional nodal involvement? (3) What is the therapeutic benefit, if any, of removing a histologically negative SLN that actually harbors submicroscopic disease?

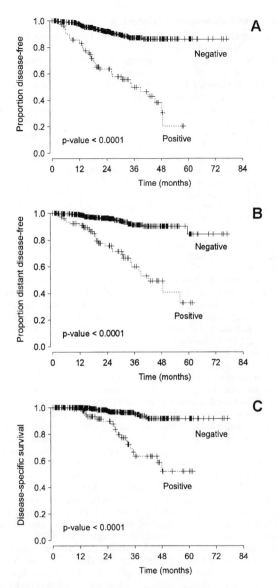

Fig. 3-1. Kaplan-Meier survival curves for patients undergoing successful lymphatic mapping and sentinel lymph node (SLN) biopsy stratified by positive or negative SLN status. (A) Disease-free survival. (B) Distant disease-free survival. (C) Disease-specific survival. Disease-free, distant disease-free, and disease-specific survivals were significantly better for patients with a negative SLN biopsy (each $p < .0001$).

Pathologic Evaluation of the SLN

The recently reported survival benefit for patients with nodal metastases treated systemically with high-dose interferon-alpha-2b provides an important impetus for accurate assessment of nodal status in patients with clinically negative nodal basins. Several investigators have demonstrated that SLN biopsy is an accurate way to detect disease in the nodal basin without complete lymphadenectomy. However, conventional histologic techniques for evaluating lymph nodes (i.e., bisection of lymph nodes followed by hematoxylin and eosin [H&E] staining) may underestimate disease, primarily because of sampling error. The combination of serial sectioning and immunostaining improves the detection of microscopic metastases in examined nodes.

We recently reported on patterns of failure in a consecutive cohort of 243 M. D. Anderson patients who underwent lymphatic mapping, had a negative SLN biopsy, and were then followed expectantly with the remaining lymph nodes intact. Eleven percent developed local recurrences, in-transit metastases, regional nodal metastases, and/or distant metastases during the follow-up period (median follow-up, 3 years). Although failure in the regional nodal basin was rare, the regional nodes represented the most common site of first recurrence in this population: 4% of patients developed a nodal metastasis in the previously mapped basin, alone or at the same time as recurrence elsewhere. Three potential mechanisms can be offered to explain these false-negative findings: (1) technical failure—the true SLN was not identified; (2) pathologic failure—the appropriate lymph node was removed but routine histologic evaluation failed to identify microscopic disease; and (3) biologic failure—recurrence occurred in a nodal basin as a result of residual microscopic satellite or in-transit disease that persisted after wide excision of the primary tumor. Therefore, paraffin blocks of the SLN specimens from patients who developed recurrent melanoma were re-evaluated using a combination of serial sectioning and immunohistochemical staining (S-100 and HMB-45). The SLNs demonstrated evidence of occult disease in 80% of the patients who developed nodal metastasis. In contrast, no evidence of micrometastatic nodal disease was demonstrated by any of these techniques in patients who had only local, in-transit, and/or distant recurrence.

Recently, the molecular biologic technique of reverse transcriptase-polymerase chain reaction (RT-PCR) to detect tyrosinase mRNA has been reported to increase detection of occult disease. The obvious potential advantage of RT-PCR is that the entire node can be evaluated, minimizing sampling error. A potential drawback of this technique is that "disease" found at this submicroscopic level may not be clinically relevant in patients whose SLNs are negative by other pathologic techniques. Although recent data suggest that PCR-based prognostic evaluations may be clinically relevant, longer follow-up is required before such evaluations become a standard of care. The recently initiated Sunbelt Melanoma Trial will prospectively evaluate the relative clinical importance of conventional histology, serial sectioning, and molecular staging in patients undergoing lymphatic mapping and SLN biopsy.

Current Practice Guidelines

In general, we have adopted the technique of selective lymph-adenectomy (lymphatic mapping and SLN biopsy) into the treatment of patients with stage I and II melanoma. All patients diagnosed with primary cutaneous melanoma are offered the procedure if the primary melanoma is at least 1.0 mm thick or, if less than 1.0 mm, is at least Clark's level IV, is ulcerated, or demonstrates evidence of regression and if there is no evidence of metastatic melanoma in regional lymph nodes and distant sites by physical examination and staging evaluation (chest x-ray and measurement of lactic dehydrogenase levels).

Patients in whom the primary tumor arises in areas of potentially ambiguous drainage (for example, the trunk) undergo preoperative lymphoscintigraphy. Technetium 99m-labeled human serum albumin is intradermally administered to establish lymphatic drainage patterns and identify those basins at risk for metastatic melanoma. Patients receive an intradermal injection of 0.5–1.0 mCi of unfiltered technetium 99m-labeled sulfur colloid 1–4 hours before surgery. In addition, 1–3 ml of isosulfan blue dye is injected intradermally around the intact tumor or biopsy site immediately prior to surgery. Lymphatic mapping is subsequently performed with the aid of a hand-held gamma probe. In patients undergoing mapping of more than one basin, the basin with predominant drainage by preoperative lymphoscintigraphy is explored first. An SLN is defined as one that localizes blue dye and/or concentrates radiolabeled colloid and is located within or, more recently, near a regional nodal basin. All patients also have wide local excision of the primary melanoma with margins appropriate for tumor thickness.

Excised SLNs are analyzed by conventional histologic staining (hematoxylin and eosin [H&E]) of grossly sectioned specimens. Histologic serial sectioning is performed on all nonpositive SLNs. Immunohistochemical staining using antisera to the S-100 protein and/or the melanoma antigen HMB-45 is generally performed only if suspicious cells are seen to clarify equivocal H&E findings. Frozen-section analysis is utilized only to confirm the presence of metastatic melanoma in SLNs that are grossly suspicious.

When the SLN is negative no further surgery is done; the remaining regional nodes are left intact. For those patients in whom the SLN or SLNs contain evidence of metastatic melanoma, TLND of the affected basins is recommended.

Postoperative follow-up consists of physical examination, chest x-ray, and determinations of lactic dehydrogenase levels. Further investigations, including computed tomography and/or magnetic resonance imaging, are also performed selectively to confirm abnormal findings suggestive of metastatic melanoma. A routine program of postoperative surveillance can be based on tumor thickness and results of SLN biopsy; one standard follow-up schedule for patients treated at M. D. Anderson Cancer Center consists of evaluation every 3–4 months for the first 2 years, every 6 months in years 3–5, and annually thereafter.

In centers where a selective approach to ELND is not feasible, the results of the Intergroup Melanoma Committee trial can be incorporated into surgical strategies for patients ≤60 years, especially when the primary tumor is 1.1–2.0 mm thick.

TECHNICAL CONSIDERATIONS

Axillary Lymph Node Dissection

General

Axillary dissection must be complete and include the level III lymph nodes (Fig. 3-2). The arm, shoulder, and chest are prepared and included in the surgical field.

Incision

We use a horizontal, slightly S-shaped incision beginning anteriorly along the superior portion of the pectoralis major muscle, traversing the axilla over the fourth rib, and extending inferiorly along the anterior border of the latissimus dorsi muscle.

Skin Flaps

Skin flaps are raised anteriorly to the midclavicular line, inferiorly to the sixth rib, posteriorly to the anterior border of the latissimus dorsi muscle, and superiorly to just below the pectoralis major insertion. The medial side of the latissimus dorsi muscle is dissected free from the specimen, exposing the thoracodorsal vessels and nerve. The lateral edge of the dissection then proceeds cephalad beneath the axillary vein. These maneuvers allow the remainder of the dissection to proceed from medial to lateral. The fatty and lymphatic tissue over the pectoralis major muscle is dissected free around to its undersurface, where the pectoralis minor muscle is encountered. The interpectoral groove is exposed.

Lymph Node Dissection

The medial pectoral nerve is preserved. The interpectoral nodes are dissected free. Exposure of the upper axilla is obtained by bringing the patient's arm over the chest by adduction and internal rotation. If nodes are bulky, the pectoralis minor muscle may need to be divided. Dissection proceeds from the apex of the axilla inferolaterally. The upper axillary lymph node dissection should be sufficiently complete that the thoracic outlet beneath the clavicle, Halsted's ligament, and the subclavius muscle can be visualized (Fig. 3-3). Fatty and lymphatic tissues are dissected downward over the brachial plexus and axillary artery until the axillary vein is exposed. The apex of the dissected specimen is tagged. Dissection then continues until the thoracodorsal vessels and the long thoracic and thoracodorsal nerves are identified. The fatty tissue between the two nerves is separated from the subscapularis muscle. The specimen is removed from the lateral chest wall. Intercostobrachial nerves traversing the specimen are sacrificed. The specimen is swept off the latissimus dorsi and the serratus anterior muscles.

Wound Closure

One 10-mm closed-suction catheter is placed percutaneously through the inferior flap into the axilla. An additional catheter may be inserted through the inferior flap and placed over the pectoralis major muscle. The skin is closed with interrupted 3–0 undyed absorbable sutures and running 4–0 subcuticular undyed absorbable sutures.

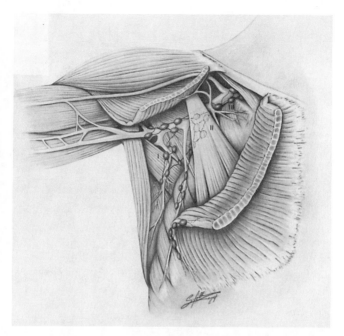

Fig. 3-2. Lymphatic anatomy of the axilla demonstrating the three groups of axillary lymph nodes defined by their relationship to the pectoralis minor muscle. The highest axillary nodes (level III) medial to the pectoralis minor muscle should be included in an axillary lymph node dissection for melanoma. (From CM Balch, GW Milton, HM Shaw, S-J Soong [eds.]. *Cutaneous Melanoma*. Philadelphia: Lippincott, 1985.)

Postoperative Management

Suction drainage is continued until output is less than 30 ml per day. By approximately the tenth day, the suction catheters are removed, regardless of the amount of drainage, to avoid infection. Any subsequent collections of serum are treated by needle aspiration. Mobilization of the arm is discouraged during the first 7–10 days after surgery. Over the ensuing 4 weeks, gradual mobilization of the arm is encouraged. The complication rate for axillary lymph node dissection is low. The most frequent complication is wound seroma.

Groin Dissection

For groin dissection, the patient is placed in a slight frog-leg position.

Incision

A reverse lazy "S" incision is made from superomedial to the anterior superior iliac spine, vertically down to the inguinal

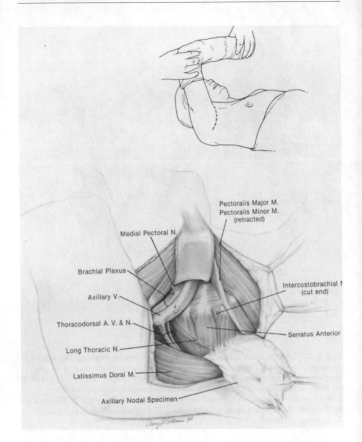

Fig. 3-3. Access to the upper axilla. The arm is draped so that it can be brought over the chest wall during the operation. This facilitates retraction of the pectoralis muscles upward to reveal level III axillary lymph nodes. (From CM Balch, GW Milton, HM Shaw, S-J Soong [eds.]. *Cutaneous Melanoma*. Philadelphia: Lippincott, 1985.)

crease, obliquely across the crease, and then vertically down to the apex of the femoral triangle.

Skin Flaps

The limits of the skin flaps are medially to the pubic tubercle and the midbody of the adductor magnus muscle, laterally to the lateral edge of the sartorius muscle, superiorly to above the inguinal ligament, and inferiorly to the apex of the femoral triangle. We sometimes incorporate an ellipse of skin with the specimen.

Lymph Node Dissection

Dissection is carried down to the muscular fascia superiorly (Fig. 3-4). All fatty, node-bearing tissue is swept down to the inguinal ligament and off the external oblique fascia. Medially, the

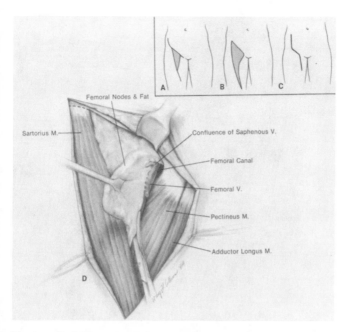

Fig. 3-4. Technique of inguinal lymph node dissection. (From CM Balch, GW Milton, HM Shaw, S-J Soong [eds.]. *Cutaneous Melanoma.* Philadelphia: Lippincott, 1985.)

spermatic cord or round ligament is exposed and nodal tissue is swept laterally. Nodal tissue is swept off the adductor fascia to the femoral vein. At the apex of the femoral triangle, the saphenous vein is divided. Laterally, nodal tissue is dissected off the sartorius muscle and the femoral nerve. With dissection in the plane of the femoral vessels, the nodal tissue is elevated up to the level of the fossa ovalis, where the saphenous vein is suture ligated at its junction with the femoral vein. The specimen is dissected to beneath the inguinal ligament, where it is divided. Cloquet's node (the lowest iliac node) is sent as a separate specimen for frozen-section examination (Fig. 3-5).

Sartorius Muscle Transposition

The sartorius muscle is divided at its insertion on the anterior superior iliac spine (Fig. 3-6). The lateral femoral cutaneous nerve is preserved. The proximal two or three neurovascular bundles going to the sartorius muscle are divided to facilitate transposition. The muscle is placed over the femoral vessels and tacked to the inguinal ligament, fascia of the adductor, and vastus muscle groups.

Wound Closure

The skin edges are examined for viability and trimmed back to healthy skin, if necessary. Two closed-suction drains are placed

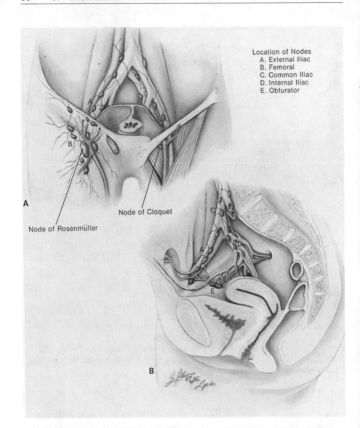

Fig. 3-5. (A) Lymphatic anatomy of the inguinal area demonstrating the superficial and deep lymphatic chains. The node of Cloquet lies at the transition between the superficial and deep inguinal nodes. It is located beneath the inguinal ligament in the femoral canal. (B) The iliac nodes include those on the common and superficial iliac vessels and the obturator nodes. Obturator nodes should be excised as part of an iliac nodal dissection. (From CM Balch, GW Milton, HM Shaw, S-J Soong [eds.]. *Cutaneous Melanoma.* Philadelphia: Lippincott, 1985.)

through separate stab wounds inferiorly. One is laid medially and the other is laid laterally within the operative wound. The wound is closed with interrupted 3–0 undyed absorbable sutures and skin staples.

Postoperative Management
    The patient begins ambulating the day following surgery and is measured for a custom-fit elastic stocking to be used during the day for 6 months. After this period, the stocking may be discontinued if no leg swelling occurs. We use a mild diuretic, such as hydrochlorothiazide, on an individual basis.

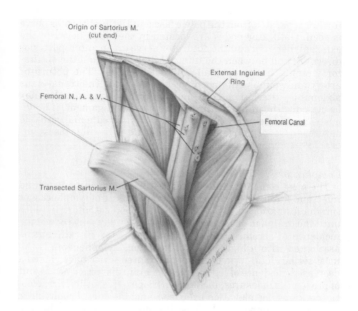

Origin of Sartorius M.
(cut end)

External Inguinal
Ring

Femoral N., A. & V.

Femoral Canal

Transected Sartorius M.

Fig. 3-6.   Transection of the sartorius muscle at its origin on the anterior superior iliac spine in preparation for transposition over the femoral vessels and nerves. (From CM Balch, GW Milton, HM Shaw, S-J Soong [eds.]. *Cutaneous Melanoma.* **Philadelphia: Lippincott, 1985.)**

Dissection of the Iliac and Obturator Nodes

We perform deep (iliac) dissection for the following indications: (1) known involvement (revealed by preoperative mapping studies), (2) more than three grossly positive nodes in the superficial specimen, or (3) frozen-section examination of Cloquet's node that reveals metastatic tumor. To gain access to the deep nodes, we extend the skin incision superiorly. The external oblique muscle is split from a point about 8–10 cm superomedial to the anterior superior iliac spine to the lateral border of the rectus sheath. The internal oblique and transversus abdominis muscles are divided, and the peritoneum is retracted superiorly. An alternative approach is to split the inguinal ligament vertically, medial to the femoral vein. The ureter is exposed as it courses over the iliac artery. Dissection continues in front of the external iliac artery to separate the external iliac nodes. The inferior epigastric artery and vein are divided if necessary. Dissection of the lymph nodes continues to the common iliac artery. Nodes in front of the external iliac vein are dissected to the point at which the latter proceeds under the internal iliac artery. The plane of the peritoneum is traced along the wall of the bladder, and the fatty tissues and lymph nodes are dissected off the perivesical fat starting at the internal iliac artery. Dissection is completed on the medial wall of the external iliac vein, and the nodal chain is further separated from the pelvic fascia until the obturator nerve is seen. Obturator nodes are located in the space between the external iliac vein and the obturator nerve (in an anteroposterior direction) and between the internal iliac artery and the obturator foramen (in a cephalad–caudad direction). The obturator artery and vein usually need not be disturbed. The transversus abdominis, internal oblique, and external oblique muscles may be closed with running sutures. The inguinal ligament, if previously divided, is approximated with interrupted nonabsorbable sutures to Cooper's ligament medially and to the iliac fascia lateral to the femoral vessels.

Complications

The most common acute postoperative complication is wound infection. Rates range from 5% to 19%. The rate of lymphocele or seroma formation is 3–23%. Leaving suction catheters in place until the drainage decreases to 40–50 ml per day may reduce the incidence of seroma. However, prolonged stay of catheters is associated with a higher rate of infection. Lymphedema is the most serious long-term complication. Three series have shown a decreased incidence of leg edema after groin dissection as a result of preventive measures, including perioperative antibiotics, elastic stockings, leg elevation exercises, and diuretics. Prophylactic measures are important because it is difficult to reverse the progression of edema. Skin flap problems occur with some frequency. Expectant management of ischemic edges often results in full-thickness necrosis and prolonged hospitalization. Therefore if edges are of questionable viability, the patient is returned to the operating room early for flap revision. Clinically detectable deep vein thrombosis is uncommon.

Neck Dissection

Metastases to lymph nodes from primary melanomas in the head and neck were previously believed to follow a predictable pattern. However, lymphatic drainage from primary melanomas of the head and neck can be multidirectional and unpredictable; preoperative lymphoscintigraphy is needed to identify the basins at risk for metastases. ELND or sentinel lymph node biopsy (see later) may be misdirected in up to 59% of patients if the operation is based on classic anatomic studies without such preoperative evaluation. These findings strongly support the use of lymphoscintigraphy in these patients.

Radical neck dissection is generally recommended when nodal metastases are clinically evident. Otherwise, modified neck dissection that spares the spinal accessory nerve, the sternomastoid muscle, and the internal jugular vein is generally preferred.

Melanomas arising on the scalp or face anterior to the pinna of the ear and superior to the commissure of the lip are at risk of metastasizing to parotid lymph nodes. This parotid chain of nodes is contiguous with the cervical nodes. It is advisable to combine neck dissection with parotid lymph node dissection when parotid nodes are clinically involved or at risk.

ADJUVANT THERAPY

Biologic Therapy

High-dose interferon-alpha-2b has recently been approved by the U.S. Food and Drug Administration as adjuvant treatment for high-risk melanoma patients. Approval was based on the results of the Eastern Cooperative Oncology Group (EST 1684) prospective randomized trial for melanoma patients at high risk of recurrence. The majority (75%) of patients had clinically palpable nodal disease. A regimen of adjuvant high-dose interferon-alpha-2b (20 million units/m^2/day intravenously for 4 weeks followed by 10 million units/m^2 subcutaneously thrice weekly for the next 48 weeks) resulted in improved relapse-free and overall survival in high-risk (especially stage III) patients compared with patients who did not receive this therapy (Fig. 3-7). For the overall trial, the median relapse-free survival was improved from 1.0 to 1.7 years (26% versus 37% at 5 years) and overall survival from 2.8 to 3.8 years (37% versus 46% at 5 years). Although the absolute improvement in overall survival was low (9%) and the toxicity was high (two deaths; 67% of patients experienced grade 3 toxicity; 50% of patients either stopped treatment early or required dose reduction), interferon-alpha-2b currently represents the only adjuvant therapy with efficacy.

Further trials are needed to clarify dosing schedules, compare interferon with other therapies, and evaluate interferon's efficacy in patients with minimal nodal disease (i.e., SLN microscopically positive and/or PCR positive). Some of these questions will be addressed in the multicenter Sunbelt Melanoma Trial.

Current candidates for adjuvant interferon include patients with locally recurrent, nodal, in-transit, or satellite disease. Optimally, eligible patients should be entered into available trials.

Radiotherapy

The role of radiotherapy as adjuvant treatment after TLND or as an alternative to ELND in the regional treatment of patients with intermediate to thick melanomas has not been clearly defined. Adjuvant radiotherapy, either alone in clinically node-negative patients or in conjunction with surgery in pathologically node-positive patients, has resulted in a locoregional control rate in excess of 85%. Proof of a therapeutic benefit from adjuvant radiotherapy can be obtained only from a prospective randomized trial. Such a trial has been initiated by the Radiation Therapy Oncology Group. Patients with head and neck primary tumors, with multiple involved regional nodes, or with extracapsular extension of regional lymphatic metastases should be considered for adjuvant radiotherapy.

Chemotherapy

No confirmed studies have demonstrated a benefit of adjuvant chemotherapy in melanoma patients at high risk for relapse. On the contrary, a randomized trial of adjuvant dacarbazine versus no adjuvant treatment resulted in a statistically significant decrease in survival in the adjuvant treatment arm. Adjuvant systemic therapy should be considered only in the context of a clinical trial.

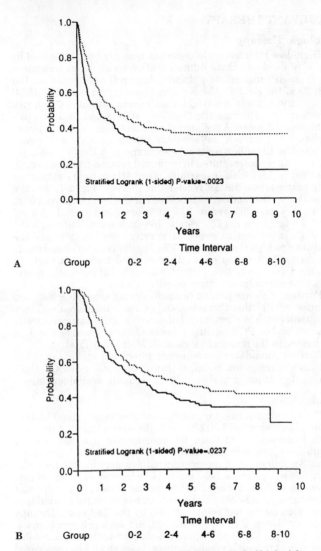

Fig. 3-7.   Relapse-free (A) and overall (B) survival of high-risk stage III patients participating in EST 1684. (From JM Kirkwood, MH Strawderman, MS Ernstoff, et al. Interferon-alpha-2b adjuvant therapy of high risk resected cutaneous melanoma: the Eastern Cooperative Oncology Group trial EST 1684. *J Clin Oncol* 14:7, 1996.)

melanoma: The Eastern Cooperative Oncology Group trial EST 1684. *J Clin Oncol* 14:7, 1996.

Krag DN, Meijer SJ, Weaver DL, et al. Minimal-access surgery for staging of melanoma. *Arch Surg* 130:654, 1995.

Leinard D, Ewalenko P, Delmotte JJ, et al. High dose recombinant tumor necrosis factor alpha in combination with interferon gamma and melphalan in isolation perfusion of the limbs for melanoma and sarcoma. *J Clin Oncol* 10:52, 1992.

Livingston PO, Wong GYC, Adluri S, et al. Improved survival in stage III melanoma patients with GM2 antibodies: A randomized trial of adjuvant vaccination with GM2 ganglioside. *J Clin Oncol* 12:1036, 1994.

Mansfield PF, Lee JE, Balch CM. Melanoma: Surgical controversies and current practice. *Curr Probl Surg* 31:253, 1994.

McCarthy WH, Shaw HM, Milton GW. Efficacy of elective lymph node dissection in 2,347 patients with clinical stage I malignant melanoma. *Surg Gynecol Obstet* 161:575, 1985.

Milton GW, Shaw HM, McCarthy WH, et al. Prophylactic lymph node dissection in clinical stage I cutaneous malignant melanoma: Results of surgical treatment in 1319 patients. *Br J Surg* 69:108, 1982.

Morton DL, Foshag LJ, Hoon DSB, et al. Prolongation of survival in metastatic melanoma after active specific immunotherapy with a new polyvalent melanoma vaccine. *Ann Surg* 216:463, 1992.

Morton DL, Wen DR, Wong JH, et al. Technical details of intraoperative lymphatic mapping for early stage melanoma. *Arch Surg* 127:392, 1992.

Norman J, Cruse CW, Espinoza C, et al. Redefinition of cutaneous lymphatic drainage with the use of lymphoscintigraphy for malignant melanoma. *Am J Surg* 162:432, 1991.

Reintgen DS, Balch CM, Kirkwood J, et al. Recent advances in the care of the patient with malignant melanoma. *Ann Surg* 225:1, 1997.

Reintgen D, Cruse CW, Berman C, et al. The orderly progression of melanoma nodal metastases. *Ann Surg* 220:759, 1994.

Reintgen DS, Cox EB, McCarty KM Jr, et al. Efficacy of elective lymph node dissection in patients with intermediate thickness primary melanoma. *Ann Surg* 198:379, 1983.

Rosenberg SA, Yannelli JR, Yang JC, et al. Treatment of patients with metastatic melanoma with autologous tumor infiltrating lymphocytes and interleukin-2. *J Natl Cancer Inst* 86:1159, 1994.

Ross MI. Surgical management of stage I and II melanoma patients: Approach to the regional lymph node basin. *Semin Surg Oncol* 12:394, 1996.

Ross M, Reintgen DS, Balch C. Selective lymphadenectomy: Emerging role of lymphatic mapping and sentinel node biopsy in the management of early stage melanoma. *Semin Surg Oncol* 9:219, 1993.

Sim FH, Taylor WF, Pritchard DJ, et al. Lymphadenectomy in the management of stage I malignant melanoma: A prospective randomized study. *Mayo Clin Proc* 61:697, 1986.

Thompson JF, McCarthy WH, Bosch CMJ, et al. Sentinel lymph node status as an indicator of the presence of metastatic melanoma in regional lymph nodes. *Melanoma Res* 5:255, 1995.

Travis J. Closing in on melanoma susceptibility gene(s). *Science* 258:1080, 1992.

Veronesi U, Adamus J, Bandiera DC, et al. Delayed regional lymph node dissection in stage I melanoma of the skin of the lower extremities. *Cancer* 49:2420, 1982.

Veronesi U, Adamus J, Bandiera DC, et al. Inefficacy of immediate node dissection in stage I melanoma of the limbs. *N Engl J Med* 297:627, 1977.

Veronesi U, Cascinelli N, Adamus J, et al. Primary cutaneous melanoma 2 mm or less in thickness: Results of a randomized study comparing wide with narrow surgical excision: A preliminary report. *N Engl J Med* 318:1159, 1988.

Wang X, Heller R, Van Voorhis N, et al. Detection of submicroscopic metastases with polymerase chain reaction in patients with malignant melanoma. *Ann Surg* 220:768, 1994.

Nonmelanoma Skin Cancer

Keith M. Heaton

Epidemiology and Etiology

Basal cell carcinoma (BCC) and squamous cell carcinoma (SCC) of the skin are the most common malignancies in the Caucasian population. They account for almost one-third of all cancers in the United States, with more than 600,000 new cases and 2,000 deaths from nonmelanoma skin cancer reported in 1992. These figures most likely underestimate the true prevalence of BCC and SCC because most cases are diagnosed and treated in an out-patient setting and therefore are not recorded in a tumor registry.

Exposure to sunlight is the principal cause of BCC and SCC, although each can occur in sites protected from the sun, such as the genitals and lower extremities. Other known causes of nonmelanoma skin cancer include exposure to ultraviolet (UV) light, chemical carcinogens such as arsenic and hydrocarbons, human papillomavirus, ionizing radiation, cigarette smoking, and chronic irritation or ulceration (e.g., decubitus ulcers). In addition, patients who are immunocompromised have a much higher incidence of skin cancer.

Differential Diagnosis

A variety of benign skin lesions either are precursor lesions of malignant tumors or are difficult to distinguish from malignant tumors.

Keratoacanthoma is a benign tumor that usually presents in elderly people as a single, raised 1- to 2-cm lesion with a characteristic horn-filled crater. Although there is a characteristic phase of rapid growth, spontaneous involution occurs within a few months and is usually complete by 6 months. This lesion can be difficult to distinguish from SCC and therefore requires a biopsy that includes a segment of adjoining normal skin to confirm the diagnosis.

Actinic keratosis also may be confused with early SCC. This benign tumor most commonly presents as multiple lesions on sun-exposed areas in middle-aged individuals with fair complexions, although single lesions can occur. Actinic keratosis is characterized by hyperkeratosis and is usually less than 1 cm in diameter. Cryotherapy or topical fluorouracil are the standard treatments. Persistent lesions require excisional biopsy because the incidence of SCC arising from actinic keratoses approaches 20%.

Bowen's disease represents a benign lesion that has malignant potential. It is frequently solitary and manifests as a slowly enlarging erythematous patch of skin with a sharp but irregular outline. Crusting is commonly noted in the center. Bowen's disease is thought to result from prolonged sun exposure. Histologically, the lesion is an intraepithelial SCC. Complete excision is required because the incidence of SCC developing in patients with Bowen's disease is as high as 11%. Lesions that occur in unexposed areas are frequently due to arsenic ingestion and are associated with an increased incidence of visceral cancer.

There is no known precursor lesion for BCC.

Squamous Cell Carcinoma

Approximately 80% of UV light–induced SCCs develop on the arms, head, and neck. Patients with SCC often have actinic keratoses. SCC associated with exposure to ionizing radiation occurs at sites affected by chronic radiation dermatitis. SCC arises from basal keratinocytes of the skin and typically presents as a firm nodule on an erythematous base with elevated borders and indistinct margins. Central ulceration or crusting may be present. Histologically, SCC is characterized by irregular nests of epidermal cells invading the dermis in varying degrees. Grading is based on the degree of cell differentiation. The greater the differentiation, the less the invasive tendency and the better the prognosis. The more poorly differentiated neoplasms show no evidence of keratinization and exhibit marked cellular atypia, making them difficult to distinguish from anaplastic melanoma, lymphoma, or mesenchymal tumors.

SCC may metastasize to regional lymph nodes and eventually to distant sites, including bone, brain, and lungs. The rate of metastases with SCC varies according to prognostic factors such as anatomic site, depth of invasion, and degree of differentiation. For example, SCC arising from actinic keratosis has a low propensity to metastasize (0.5%), whereas SCC arising from a chronic sinus tract or from a previously irradiated area metastasizes much more frequently (20–30%). The overall rate of metastasis for SCC of the skin is 2%.

Basal Cell Carcinoma

BCC is a malignant neoplasm that arises from the basal cell layers of the epidermis and adnexal structures. Ninety-five percent occur in patients more than 40 years of age. BCC develops on hair-bearing skin, most commonly on sun-exposed areas, and approximately 85% of lesions are found on the head and neck. Pruritus and bleeding are common symptoms, and patients frequently complain of a bleeding sore that heals partially and then ulcerates again.

Histologically, most BCCs are well differentiated. Tumors consist of palisading basal cells with uniform, elongated nuclei and very little cytoplasm.

There are five common forms of BCC:

1. *Noduloulcerative*, which is characterized by a waxy, nodular lesion with an ulcerated center.

2. *Pigmented*, which is similar in gross appearance to nodulo-ulcerative BCC but has pigmentation. This lesion can be difficult to distinguish from seborrheic keratosis and nodular melanoma.
3. *Sclerosing or morphea-form*, which appears as a single, flat, indurated, off-white, ill-defined macule. Histologic sections show a dense, fibrous connective-tissue stroma in which small groups and narrow strands of basaloid cells are embedded. It is very similar to the microscopic appearance of metastatic breast carcinoma and desmoplastic epithelioma.
4. *Superficial*, which occurs commonly on the trunk as an ill-defined, red, scaly macule.
5. *Fibroepithelial*, which also usually occurs on the trunk and manifests as a flesh-colored papule without surrounding inflammatory changes.

The natural history of BCC depends on the histologic subtype. Fibroepithelial and superficial BCC remain stable and grow slowly. The noduloulcerative and pigmented types also grow slowly but invade locally by peripheral and deep extension. This invasion can, in rare instances, lead to destruction of vital organs and eventually death. Sclerosing BCC is biologically more aggressive and difficult to treat because of indistinct margins and deep infiltration.

Metastases from BCC are very rare (0.0028% in one large study). Lesions at increased risk for metastasis are typically located on the head or neck, are large and locally invasive, and persist despite repeated surgery and radiotherapy. Most metastases are found in the regional lymph nodes, but distant organs may be involved.

Kaposi's Sarcoma

Kaposi's sarcoma (KS), a neoplasm of vascular endothelial cells, is characterized by the presence of bluish-red nodules, edema, and hemosiderin deposition. Prior to 1981, about 100 new cases of this disease were diagnosed in the United States each year. The incidence has since risen dramatically, particularly in immunosuppressed or human immunodeficiency virus (HIV)–positive patients. Prior to 1981 and the HIV disease epidemic, KS most commonly occurred on the feet of men of Jewish or Italian descent in the sixth to eighth decade of life. Typical KS patients today are immunocompromised. These people develop a much more virulent, systemic form of the disease, with occasional lymph node and/or gastrointestinal involvement.

Sebaceous Carcinoma

Sebaceous carcinoma accounts for only 0.2–4.6% of all cutaneous neoplasms. It usually presents as a slow-growing, hard, yellow nodule arising from the sebaceous glands of the face and eyelids. Apocrine and eccrine sweat gland carcinomas are even rarer, with fewer than 100 cases reported annually.

Syndromes Associated with Skin Cancers

Xeroderma pigmentosum is a rare (1 in 250,000 persons) autosomal-recessive disease characterized by severe sun sensitivity, photophobia, cutaneous pigmentary changes, advanced sun damage, and development of malignant cutaneous neoplasms, especially BCC, SCC, and melanoma.

Sebaceous nevus of Jadassohn usually manifests as a single, oval, alopecic, orange-yellow plaque on the scalp of a child. At puberty, the lesion becomes verrucous. In adult life, both benign and malignant skin tumors (particularly BCC) may develop.

Basal cell nevus syndrome is a genetic form of BCC inherited by an autosomal-dominant gene. The lesions appear on the skin between puberty and 35 years of age and can range in number from a few to several hundred. Most lesions remain quiescent, but some may become locally aggressive.

Biopsy Techniques

Four principal biopsy techniques are used for cutaneous malignancies. A *shave biopsy* is obtained by slicing a superficial portion of the tumor with a scalpel. A *punch biopsy* obtains a deeper specimen by introducing a sharp, cylindrical instrument into the reticular dermis or subcutaneous tissue. An *incisional biopsy* removes only a portion of the tumor, whereas the entire lesion is removed with an *excisional biopsy*. To facilitate accurate diagnosis, the technique selected should be the one that yields the optimal pathologic specimen. For example, the diagnosis of SCC can be missed with a shave biopsy. Therefore a deep punch biopsy, incisional biopsy, or excisional biopsy is indicated when SCC is suspected. These more definitive techniques are also indicated in suspected cases of pigmented or sclerosing BCC or to confirm the diagnosis of benign keratoacanthoma. Shave biopsy may be used in cases of noduloulcerative or superficial BCC.

Staging

The current American Joint Committee on Cancer (AJCC) staging system for BCC and SCC of the skin is shown in Table 4-1.

Treatment

Once the histologic diagnosis has been made, numerous factors must be considered in determining the appropriate therapy. These factors include the histopathologic type, location, and size of the tumor; the age and general medical condition of the patient; patient preference; and cost. Commonly used treatments for nonmelanoma skin cancers are excisional surgery, Mohs' surgery, cryosurgery, curettage and electrodesiccation, and radiotherapy.

Table 4-1.   TNM staging for squamous cell carcinoma and basal cell carcinoma of the skin

Primary tumor (T)

Tx	Not assessable
Tis	Carcinoma *in situ*
T0	No primary tumor present
T1	Tumor ≤2 cm, strictly superficial, or
T2	Tumor >2 cm but <5 cm or with minimal dermal infiltration
T3	Tumor >5 cm or with deep infiltration of dermis
T4	Tumor involving other structures such as muscle, bone, or cartilage

Nodal involvement (N)

Nx	Not assessable
N0	No evidence of regional lymph node involvement
N1	Evidence of mobile ipsilateral regional lymph nodes
N2	Evidence of contralateral mobile lymph nodes
N3	Fixed regional lymph nodes

Distant metastasis (M)

Mx	Not assessable
M0	No known distant metastasis
M1	Distant metastasis present

Staging

Stage I	Any T	N0	M0
Stage II	Any T	N1–3	M0
Stage III	Any T	Any N	M1

Source: Adapted from AK Patterson, RG Geronemu. Cancers of the Skin. In VT DeVita Jr, S Hellman, SA Rosenberg (eds): *Cancer: Principles and Practice of Oncology* (3rd ed). Philadelphia: Lippincott, 1989.

SURGICAL EXCISION

Excisional surgery is effective for all types of nonmelanoma skin cancer and is a mainstay of therapy. Complete excision of a tumor has the advantage of allowing evaluation of the tumor margins. Most excisions are performed in an elliptical fashion along Langer's cleavage lines (the lines of skin tension) to achieve a good cosmetic result. Elliptical excisions are easily performed on the trunk, extremities, cheeks, forehead, chin, and scalp; however, special consideration must be given to excision of lesions from the lip, eyelids, alar rim of the nose, and ears. In these locations, a wedge-shaped excision may be preferable to minimize distortion. There is no uniform recommendation regarding the size of surgical margins, but many surgeons use margins of 3–5 mm for small, well-defined lesions and margins of at least 1 cm for large lesions or more aggressive subtypes. Simple primary closure, a local flap, a skin graft, or healing by second intention can be used to repair the defect.

For a neoplasm with the potential to metastasize, clinical evaluation of the regional lymph nodes is mandatory. However, lymph node dissection should be performed only if there is clinically palpable lymphadenopathy and a biopsy of an enlarged node has demonstrated metastatic disease.

MOHS' MICROGRAPHIC SURGERY

Mohs' surgery is a specialized technique in which serial horizontal sections of excised tissue are systematically mapped and microscopically evaluated by frozen-section examination. Because margins are checked thoroughly at the time of surgery, this technique is a major improvement in the treatment of difficult and recurrent skin cancers, allowing complete removal of tumor with minimal loss of normal tissue. However, Mohs' surgery is both time-consuming and expensive. The choices for repair after Mohs' surgery are similar to those with excisional surgery.

CRYOSURGERY

Cryosurgery uses liquid nitrogen delivered by a spray apparatus or a cryoprobe under local anesthesia. It is effective in the treatment of premalignant tumors. However, the local failure rate is high even for experienced cryosurgeons. Favorable anatomic sites for cryosurgery include the eyelids, ears, face, neck, and trunk. Particular care must be taken when treating tumors of the nasolabial fold, inner canthi of the eyes, and periauricular areas. These sites usually require a wider margin of freezing to help prevent recurrence because there is often deep infiltration. Cryosurgery should not be the first-choice therapy for malignant tumors.

CURETTAGE AND ELECTRODESICCATION

Dermatologists commonly use curettage and electrodesiccation to treat BCC and superficial SCC. A curette is first used to debulk and delineate the tumor from the surrounding normal skin based on differences in tissue consistency. The remaining lesion is then electrodesiccated or obliterated with a carbon dioxide laser. Usually two or three office visits are required to completely remove the tumor, depending on its size. This method is appropriate for small superficial or noduloulcerative BCCs and for SCCs with clearly defined borders. It should not be used for tumors larger than 2 cm. Because of wound contracture, distortion is especially likely to occur around the eyes and mouth. Curettage and electrodesiccation are particularly useful for lower-extremity tumors or when optimal cosmetic results are not essential.

RADIOTHERAPY

Prior to initiation of radiotherapy, a biopsy should always be performed to confirm the diagnosis and document the type of neoplasm. Radiotherapy is most appropriate for primary SCC and

BCC, although recurrences (of tumors previously treated by other means) can also be treated. However, treatment is costly and the cure rate is low. Radiotherapy is particularly advantageous in elderly or debilitated patients and in patients at high risk for surgical complications.

CHEMOTHERAPY

Topical fluorouracil may be used to treat premalignant lesions. Available as creams and solutions, fluorouracil is applied twice daily for 4–6 weeks. Treatment causes oozing, crusting, and ulceration of the lesion, with healing taking 3–6 weeks after treatment stops. The recurrence rate after treatment with topical fluorouracil may be higher than that with other therapies.

Intralesional interferon-alpha is currently being evaluated as a treatment for noduloulcerative and superficial BCC and for SCC. Although it offers good cosmetic results, studies have found recurrence rates to be higher and cure rates lower than with other treatment modalities. The use of interferon is classified as investigational at this time.

PHOTODYNAMIC THERAPY

Photodynamic therapy, another investigational treatment, involves the intravenous administration of a systemic photosensitizer followed by nonionizing radiation to preferentially destroy neoplastic tissue. The photosensitizer is cleared from most organs by 48–72 hours but is retained by the tumor, skin, and reticuloendothelial system. Exposure to light at 630 nm produces oxygen free radicals and selectively kills the tumor cells. Preliminary results show success rates of 85–100% for BCC. Patients must be shielded from sunlight for the duration of therapy.

Screening and Prevention

The key to preventing nonmelanoma skin cancer is reducing one's exposure to sunlight. People of all ages should protect their skin by staying out of the sun, particularly during the middle of the day; by wearing protective clothing; and by applying sunscreens with a sun protection factor of 15 or higher to all exposed areas. Although most chemical sunscreens (p-aminobenzoic acid [PABA], benzophenones, cinnamates, salicylates, and anthranilates) absorb and filter out UVB radiation, only the benzophenones and anthranilates absorb UVA radiation.

Because there are no completely satisfactory topical sunscreens, other strategies have been attempted. However, chemoprophylaxis with beta-carotene or isotretinoin has failed to show any significant reduction in the risk of developing nonmelanoma skin cancer.

The rising incidence of skin cancers underscores the need for effective measures to control them. Because of its ease, screening for skin cancer is theoretically promising, but few data demonstrate its effectiveness. Nevertheless, monthly at-home examination using full-length and hand-held mirrors of all areas of the body is useful for detecting skin changes. Any change in an existing lesion or the appearance of a new lesion should be brought to the attention of a physician.

Selected References

Arnold HL, Odom RB, James WD (eds.). *Andrew's Diseases of the Skin* (8th ed). Philadelphia: Saunders, 1990.

Koh HK, Geller AC, Miller DR, et al. Can screening for melanoma and skin cancer save lives? *Dermatol Clin* 9:795, 1991.

Kuflik EG, Gage AA. The five-year cure rate achieved by cryosurgery for skin cancer. *J Am Acad Dermatol* 24:1002, 1991.

Miller PK, Roenigk RK, Brodland DG, et al. Cutaneous micrographic surgery: Mohs' procedure. *Mayo Clin Proc* 67:971, 1992.

O'Donoghue MN. Sunscreen: One weapon against melanoma. *Dermatol Clin* 9:789, 1991.

Patterson AK, Geronemu RG. Cancers of the skin. In VT DeVita, Jr, S Hellman, SA Rosenberg (eds.), *Cancer: Principles and Practice of Oncology* (3rd ed). Philadelphia: Lippincott, 1989.

Preston DS, Stern RS. Nonmelanoma cancers of the skin. *N Engl J Med* 327:1649, 1992.

Robinson JK. Advances in the treatment of nonmelanoma skin cancer. *Dermatol Clin* 9:757, 1991.

Silverman CK, Kopf AW, Grin JM, et al. Recurrence rates of treated basal cell carcinomas. *J Dermatol Surg* 17:713, 1991.

Urbach F. Incidence of nonmelanoma skin cancer. *Dermatol Clin* 9:751, 1991.

Wick MR. Kaposi's sarcoma unrelated to the acquired immunodeficiency syndrome. *Curr Opin Oncol* 3:377, 1991.

Bone and Soft-Tissue Sarcoma

A. Scott Pearson, Sarkis H. Meterissian,
and Kenneth K. Tanabe

Soft-Tissue Sarcomas

EPIDEMIOLOGY AND RISK FACTORS

Approximately 6,000 people are diagnosed in the United States each year as having soft-tissue sarcomas, rare tumors that account for less than 1% of all newly diagnosed adult cancers in the United States annually. More common in children, soft-tissue sarcomas represent 7% of all malignancies diagnosed in the pediatric population. Because of the ubiquity of connective tissue, soft-tissue sarcomas are found throughout the body, including the extremities, head and neck, abdominal wall, and retroperitoneum. Approximately 50% of sarcomas occur in the extremities, 15% in the trunk, and 15% in the retroperitoneum. Lower-extremity lesions are 3.5 times more common than upper-extremity lesions. The thigh is the most common area affected by this tumor. The incidence of sarcomas is equivalent in men and women. Risk factors for soft-tissue sarcoma include the following:

1. *Environmental factors.* Exposure to herbicides has been linked in some studies to an increased risk for the development of soft-tissue sarcoma. Exposure to asbestos has been associated with the development of mesotheliomas. Hepatic angiosarcoma is associated with thorotrast, vinyl chloride, and arsenic exposure. Although patients with sarcoma frequently report a history of trauma in the tumor area, a causal relationship has not been established.

2. *Previous radiation exposure.* Rarely, sarcomas may develop in areas exposed to radiotherapy, such as the chest wall of women who have received radiotherapy for breast cancer. The risk of postradiotherapy sarcomas increases with increasing dosage. The interval between irradiation and the development of sarcoma is usually at least 10 years. Sarcomas occurring after radiation exposure are most commonly malignant fibrous histiocytomas.

3. *Chronic lymphedema.* Chronic lymphedema such as that experienced after axillary dissection has been associated with lymphangiosarcoma (Stewart-Treves syndrome).

4. *Genetic predisposition.* Specific inherited genetic alterations have been associated with an increased risk of bone and soft-tissue sarcomas. For example, patients with Gardner's syndrome (familial polyposis) have a higher than normal incidence of desmoids; patients with germ line mutations in the tumor suppressor gene P53 (Li-Fraumeni syndrome) have a high incidence of sarcomas; and patients with von Recklinghausen's disease who have abnormalities in the neurofibromatosis type 1

gene (NF1) tend to develop neurofibrosarcomas. Soft-tissue sarcomas can occur in patients with hereditary retinoblastoma as a second primary malignancy. Cytogenetic aberrations such as chromosome translocations have been characterized in sarcomas.

5. *Oncogene changes.* Germ line defects in P53 have been identified in families studied who are affected by Li-Fraumeni syndrome, suggesting that inactivation of P53 by mutation may play an etiologic role in the development of soft-tissue sarcomas. Amplification of the MDM2 gene, whose protein product binds to the P53 protein, has been detected in sarcoma specimens. Alterations in the retinoblastoma gene (Rb) have been implicated in sarcoma pathogenesis. Future studies will undoubtedly uncover more information on the genetic alterations that result in sarcoma formation.

PATHOLOGY

The term *sarcoma* is Greek for "fish flesh," referring to the tumor's tendency to feel fleshy when palpated, unlike the more common scirrhous variants of many carcinomas. Mesodermal cells give rise to the connective tissues distributed throughout the body, including pericardium, pleura, blood vessel endothelium, smooth and striated muscle, bone, cartilage, and synovium, and are the cells from which nearly all sarcomas originate. Consequently, sarcomas develop in a wide variety of anatomic sites. Although schwannomas (peripheral nerve sheath tumors) arise from Schwann's cells, which are derived from neuroectoderm rather than mesodermal cells, schwannomas are still commonly considered sarcomas. Several histologic types of sarcomas have been characterized. This characterization can be difficult and is aided by electron microscopy. Desmin, vimentin, S-100, and keratin are proteins identified by immunohistochemistry that can further delineate the cell of origin. The relative frequencies of soft-tissue sarcomas (Table 5-1) differ among institutions, depending on referral patterns, study exclusion criteria, and time period examined. For example, malignant fibrous histiocytoma was rarely reported before 1972; however, since that time it has gained increasing recognition and is now the most common histologic diagnosis in many published series. Approximately 15% of all soft-tissue sarcomas occur in the retroperitoneum. Of tumors that occur in the retroperitoneum, approximately 80% are malignant, with liposarcoma, fibrosarcoma, leiomyosarcoma, and malignant fibrous histiocytoma accounting for the vast majority of histologic types identified. It is not uncommon for a patient's tumor to be classified differently by different pathologists. The concordance rate among competent pathologists in assigning a sarcoma to a histologic subtype is approximately 65%. Few pathologists have the opportunity to study many of these rare tumors during their careers, and this lack of experience may contribute to the relatively low concordance rate. However, when different histologic types are grouped together according to histologic grade, it becomes apparent that tumors of different histologic type but of common histologic grade behave similarly with respect to distant metastasis and effect on patient survival. There are several different sarcoma grading schemes in use. Knowledge

Table 5-1. The relative incidence of the most common histologic types of soft-tissue sarcoma treated at M. D. Anderson Cancer Center, 1963–1977

Histologic classification	Incidence (%)
Malignant fibrous histiocytoma	20
Neurofibrosarcoma	20
Fibrosarcoma	14
Liposarcoma	14
Synovial sarcoma	8
Unclassified sarcoma	6
Rhabdomyosarcoma	6
Leiomyosarcoma	5
Epithelioid sarcoma	2
Angiosarcoma	1
Other	4

Source: Adapted from RD Lindberg, RG Martin, MM Romsdahl, et al. Conservative surgery and postoperative radiotherapy in 300 adults with soft-tissue sarcomas. *Cancer* 47:2391, 1981.

of the histologic grade is critical in the formulation of treatment plans. The criteria used to determine grade include differentiation, cellularity, amount of stroma, vascularity, degree of necrosis, and mitoses per high-power field. Metastases are uncommon in patients with low-grade sarcomas, in contrast to patients with intermediate- or high-grade sarcomas. Lymph node metastases from sarcoma are rare, occurring in less than 3% of adult patients. Only three histologic types of sarcoma metastasize to regional lymph nodes: Epithelioid sarcomas metastasize to regional nodes in approximately 20% of cases, with rhabdomyosarcomas and malignant fibrous histiocytomas metastasizing to regional nodes significantly less frequently (10% and 5%, respectively).

STAGING

The American Joint Committee for Cancer Staging (AJCC) system for staging soft-tissue sarcomas relies on histologic grade, tumor size, nodal status, and presence or absence of distant metastases (Table 5-2). An alternate system for extremity soft-tissue sarcoma staging has been proposed by Enneking and colleagues and relies on histologic grade (low versus high), anatomic location (intracompartmental versus extracompartmental), and presence or absence of metastases. In this staging scheme, anatomic location may be a pseudonym for tumor size because large tumors are generally not confined to a single compartment. In nearly all published reports, histologic grade is a statistically significant prognostic factor for disease-free and overall survival. Tumor size at presentation is also an important determinant of outcome. Tumors larger than 5 cm have a higher incidence of both distant metastasis and local recurrence and are associated with a worse overall survival rate than tumors that are smaller than

Table 5-2.   The AJCC staging system for sarcoma of soft tissues

Histologic grade of malignancy (G)

GX	Grade cannot be assessed
G1	Well differentiated
G2	Moderately differentiated
G3	Poorly differentiated
G4	Undifferentiated

Primary tumor (T)

TX	Primary tumor cannot be assessed
T0	No evidence of primary tumor
T1	Tumor 5 cm or smaller in greatest dimension
T2	Tumor larger than 5 cm in greatest dimension

Regional lymph nodes

NX	Regional lymph nodes cannot be assessed
N0	No regional lymph node metastases
N1	Regional lymph node metastases

Distant metastases (M)

MX	Presence of distant metastases cannot be assessed
M0	No distant metastases
M1	Distant metastases

Stage grouping

Stage IA	G1	T1	N0	M0
Stage IB	G1	T2	N0	M0
Stage IIA	G2	T1	N0	M0
Stage IIB	G2	T2	N0	M0
Stage IIIA	G3,4	T1	N0	M0
Stage IIIB	G3,4	T2	N0	M0
Stage IVA	Any G	Any T	N1	M0
Stage IVB	Any G	Any T	Any N	M1

Source: Adapted from OH Beahrs, DE Henson, RVP Hutter, et al (eds). *Manual for Staging of Cancer* (4th ed). Philadelphia: Lippincott, 1992.

5 cm at presentation. Local recurrence is an independent adverse prognostic factor in many published series.

CLINICAL PRESENTATION

Most extremity soft-tissue sarcomas present as an asymptomatic mass, and therefore the size at presentation usually depends on the anatomic site of the tumor. For example, although a 2- to 3-cm tumor may become readily apparent on the back of the hand, a tumor in the thigh may grow to 10–15 cm in diameter before it becomes apparent. Frequently, a traumatic event to the affected area will call attention to the pre-existing lesion. Some patients present with pain; however, there appear to be no signs or symptoms that reliably distinguish between benign and malignant soft-tissue tumors. Small lesions that by clinical history have been unchanged for several years may be closely observed without biopsy. However, a biopsy should be performed for all other tumors. Retroperitoneal soft-tissue sarcomas nearly always present as asymptomatic masses and generally grow to large sizes (median approximately 15 cm) because of the abdomen's ability to accommodate slow-growing tumors with few symptoms. Patients may present with neurologic symptoms from compression of lumbar or pelvic nerves. On occasion, patients may present with obstructive gastrointestinal symptoms related to displacement or direct tumor involvement of an intestinal organ.

EXTREMITY SOFT-TISSUE SARCOMAS

Biopsy

Appropriate biopsy of an extremity lesion suspected of being a soft-tissue sarcoma requires avoidance of several potential pitfalls. Core-needle biopsies and fine-needle aspirations have been demonstrated to be accurate diagnostic tools at large centers with extensive experience in the management of these tumors. However, tissue samples larger than those provided by needle biopsy may be necessary to obtain sections of viable tissue adequate for determination of grade and histologic type. Excisional biopsy is indicated for lesions smaller than 3 cm. Soft-tissue tumors larger than 3 cm in diameter should be assessed by incisional biopsy, regardless of whether malignancy is suspected. This technique provides adequate tissue for analysis without disturbing the tissue planes that surround the tumor, and it leaves the bulk of the tumor intact to aid in performing a subsequent wide local excision. The biopsy incision should be oriented so that a subsequent wide local excision can easily encompass the biopsy site and scar. Biopsy incisions should generally be oriented along the long axis of an extremity or parallel to the dominant underlying muscle group on the trunk. An improperly oriented biopsy incision may result in a much larger surgical defect than would otherwise be necessary to appropriately excise the biopsy cavity. This in turn may result in significantly larger postoperative radiotherapy fields to encompass all tissues at risk. The need for adequate hemostasis after a biopsy cannot be overemphasized. Extravasation of blood allows dissemination of tumor cells along the planes of blood extravasation and therefore increases the volume of tissue requiring treatment by radiotherapy or surgical excision.

Work-up

After establishing a diagnosis of an extremity soft-tissue sarcoma, it is important to assess the extent of local disease and search for distant metastases. Magnetic resonance imaging (MRI) provides a more accurate delineation of muscle groups affected by the primary tumor than does computed tomography (CT). MRI also provides sagittal and coronal views and better distinction between bone, vascular structures, and tumor than does CT. However, both techniques provide the information essential for planning a surgical resection. The possibility of bone invasion by tumor should be addressed by either MRI or plain bone radiography. Radionuclide bone scans cannot distinguish between bone invasion by tumor and increased periosteal blood flow in reaction to an adjacent tumor. High-quality cross-sectional images usually obviate the need for arteriography, especially for extremity and trunk tumors. Soft-tissue sarcomas very rarely metastasize to lymph nodes, so lymphangiography is never indicated. Positron emission tomography (PET) scanning measures metabolic activity of the tumor and may become an additional imaging technique to correlate with tumor grade. The most common site for the distant spread of extremity sarcomas is the lungs. CT is more sensitive than conventional tomography in the detection of lung, pleural, and mediastinal metastases. However, because it also detects many more lesions that on subsequent evaluation prove to be unrelated benign conditions, CT is less specific than conventional tomography. Chest CT is used most often in patients with high-grade lesions. Searches for bone and brain metastases are rarely indicated, unless symptoms of metastases to these sites are present.

Management of Local Disease

The success of local tumor control depends on several tumor-related and treatment-related prognostic factors. Patients with sarcomas that are recurrent, large (>5 cm), and/or high grade have a higher risk of recurrence. Older patients (>50 years of age) may have a higher risk of local recurrence than do younger patients. Local control rates based on stage are shown in Table 5-3.

Surgery

Elective regional lymphadenectomy is rarely indicated in patients with soft-tissue sarcoma and should be considered only in patients with epithelioid sarcomas. Because the pseudocapsule that forms around a sarcoma always contains malignant cells, shelling a sarcoma out of its pseudocapsule is inadequate treatment and nearly always leads to a local recurrence. The concept of radical resection with wide surgical margins and entire muscle group excision was a major breakthrough in extremity sarcoma management, with a reduction in the local recurrence rate to 20%. However, although radical resection was a step forward, several problems remained. First, in patients with large lesions, these resections were extremely morbid, often requiring amputation or causing other significant functional and/or cosmetic deficits. Second, many patients who underwent radical resection for large, high-grade lesions developed distant disease despite adequate local control. Finally, some sarcomas arise in areas where anatomic constraints limit the surgical margins obtainable. Although the need

Table 5-3. Local control and disease-free survival rates by AJCC stage in 220 patients with soft-tissue sarcomas treated with surgery and radiotherapy at the Massachusetts General Hospital, 1971–1985

| | | 5-year actuarial rates (%) | |
AJCC stage*	Number of patients	Local control	Disease-free survival
IA	15	100	100
IB	25	91	96
IIA	32	86	88
IIB	53	85	53
IIIA	31	92	89
IIIB	61	73	44
IVA	3	100	100
Total	220	86	70

* AJCC staging according to 1988 guidelines, which used three categories for histopathologic grade rather than the current four-grade system.
Source: Adapted from HD Suit, HJ Mankin, WC Wood, et al. Treatment of the patient with stage M0 soft tissue sarcoma. *J Clin Oncol* 6:854, 1988.

for radical excision may be unavoidable in some instances, the modern approach to extremity soft-tissue sarcoma entails an aggressive effort to achieve limb salvage. Small (<5 cm), low-grade tumors are usually amenable to therapy by wide local excision only, with margins of 2 cm. The resection should include skin when applicable, in addition to soft tissue around the tumor. Biopsy sites including the biopsy tract should be included en bloc with the specimen.

Radiotherapy

With larger, higher-grade lesions, adjuvant radiotherapy has been demonstrated to be effective in reducing local recurrence. A randomized, prospective study from the NCI established that the addition of radiotherapy to limb-sparing surgery results in local control rates and survival equal to those associated with amputation. Radiotherapy may be delivered preoperatively, postoperatively, intraoperatively, or by brachytherapy; no randomized studies have been performed to compare these methods. At the University of Texas M. D. Anderson Cancer Center radiotherapy is preferentially used preoperatively rather than postoperatively. The radiotherapy fields can be smaller preoperatively because they do not need to encompass all tissue areas and planes exposed during surgical resection. Additionally, radiotherapy doses of 50 Gy given preoperatively yield results comparable to those with higher doses given postoperatively because of relative tissue hypoxia in surgical wounds. More recently, the use of brachytherapy techniques has resulted in tumor control that is comparable to that achieved with external beam radiotherapy. This technique involves placement of catheters in the bed of the resected tumor. Radioactive seeds are then loaded into the catheters on the fifth postoperative day. An additional benefit of brachytherapy is that only 5 days of treatment are required rather than 5–6 weeks needed for external beam radiotherapy. Moreover, there is no delay in resection as with preoperative radiotherapy, which requires 1 week of healing for each 10 Gy of radiation delivered. The frequency of wound complications with brachytherapy is similar to that seen with postoperative radiotherapy (approximately 10%), as compared with the 30% frequency seen with preoperative irradiation. Finally, because there is less radiation scatter, brachytherapy is the radiotherapy technique of choice for sarcomas near joints, immature epiphyses, or gonads. Ongoing prospective trials may better define the indications of the various radiotherapeutic approaches. The overall 5-year survival rates are dependent on stage at presentation and are shown in Table 5-3.

Adjuvant Chemotherapy

The role of adjuvant chemotherapy in the treatment of extremity soft-tissue sarcoma remains controversial. Because of the high incidence of distant metastases with high-grade lesions, several prospective studies have been initiated in an attempt to improve outcome. However, prospective randomized adjuvant chemotherapy trials have failed to demonstrate an improvement in disease-free and overall survival for treated patients. A recent meta-analysis was performed on all randomized trials to evaluate the effect of adjuvant chemotherapy on localized, resectable soft-tissue sarcomas. This study showed that doxorubicin-based chemotherapy significantly improved the time to local and distant recurrence and overall recurrence-free survival. Most regimens use combinations of drugs, with doxorubicin and ifosfamide being the most active. Clinical response rates have been 40–50% at best, and the regimens used have been associated with significant toxicities. Because of the poor response and severe side effects associated with adjuvant chemotherapy, it is used in the neoadjuvant (preoperative) setting at M. D. An-derson. Patients with high-grade lesions who respond with primary tumor shrinkage after two or three courses of multi-agent chemotherapy are continued on this treatment regimen after tumor resection. Patients whose tumors do not respond are offered other systemic treatments, thereby avoiding the toxicity of a chemotherapy regimen to which they have demonstrated insensitivity. In a retrospective review of this approach at M. D. Anderson, marked improvement in overall, disease-free, and distant disease-free survival rates was seen in patients who responded to neoadjuvant therapy. To facilitate limb-sparing in those patients with extremity tumors that may require amputation, a trial utilizing limb perfusion is now being evaluated. The technique is similar to that used for melanoma. Melphalan and tumor necrosis factor-alpha are used in the perfusate. Agents commonly used in the treatment of sarcoma, such as adriamycin, are being investigated for use in limb perfusion.

Management of Local Recurrence

Up to one-third of patients with extremity sarcoma will have recurrent disease. It remains unclear whether a local recurrence contributes to distant metastases and diminished survival. Although patients with local recurrences have a worse overall survival rate than those who maintain local disease control, a local recurrence may be a marker rather than a source of distant metastases. Microscopically positive surgical margins increase the risk for local recurrence but do not adversely influence overall survival. Studies have shown that patients with isolated local recurrences may be successfully re-treated with additional surgery and adjuvant radiotherapy. In a retrospective analysis of 39 patients with locally recurrent soft-tissue sarcomas, Singer et al. found that of the 21 patients with an isolated local recurrence, 14 (67%) were successfully retreated by an aggressive reexcision. An isolated local recurrence should be aggressively treated with a negative-margin re-resection (amputation if necessary), with the addition of radiotherapy. Patients previously treated with external beam radiotherapy can still receive radiotherapy by either a brachytherapy or intraoperative radiotherapy technique.

Management of Distant Disease

Distant metastases are the most common cause of death from soft-tissue sarcomas, and most treatment failures at distant sites occur within 2 years. The incidence of metastases is 40% in patients with intermediate- and high-grade extremity sarcomas, compared with only 5% in patients with low-grade sarcomas. Within each histologic grade, the incidence of metastases increases with increasing primary tumor size. The most common site of metastases is the lungs, and 50% of first recurrences are isolated lung metastases. In the absence of extrapulmonary metastases, lung metastases should be resected if the patient is medically fit to withstand a thoracotomy and the lesions are amenable to resection. A complete resection can result in a 15–30% 5-year survival rate. Disease-free interval and number of metastases have an impact on prognosis. Patients with a disease-free interval of more than 12 months and fewer than four lung nodules have a better prognosis after lung metastases resection. With the advent of thoracoscopic techniques, an aggressive approach to isolated pulmonary metastases should be encouraged.

General Recommendations

General recommendations for management of extremity soft-tissue sarcomas are as follows:

1. Soft-tissue tumors (benign or malignant) smaller than 3 cm should be evaluated by excisional biopsy with 1- to 2-cm margins.
2. Larger soft-tissue tumors should be evaluated by incisional biopsy.
3. Wide local excision with 2-cm margins is adequate therapy for low-grade lesions smaller than 5 cm.
4. Radiotherapy plays a critical role in the management of larger lesions.
5. Patients with high-grade sarcomas should be offered adjuvant chemotherapy.
6. An aggressive surgical approach should be taken in the management of patients with an isolated local recurrence or isolated resectable distant metastases.

RETROPERITONEAL SARCOMAS

Although significant advances in the understanding of extremity soft-tissue sarcomas have resulted in improved treatments and outcomes, similar progress has not been achieved in the understanding and treatment of retroperitoneal soft-tissue sarcomas. Patients with retroperitoneal soft-tissue sarcomas generally have a worse prognosis than those with extremity sarcomas. Retroperitoneal soft-tissue sarcomas grow to larger sizes before they become clinically apparent, and they often involve important vital structures that preclude surgical resection. Furthermore, the surgical margins that can be obtained around these sarcomas are often inadequate because of anatomic constraints. The most common histologies include liposarcoma and leiomyosarcoma.

Biopsy

In patients with retroperitoneal tumors, it is important to distinguish a sarcoma from lymphoma or a germ-cell tumor. A testicular exam should be performed on all male patients and beta-HCG and AFP obtained as indicated. Therefore, unlike extremity lesions, CT-directed fine-needle aspiration is indicated. If fine-needle aspiration is nondiagnostic, a CT-directed core-needle biopsy can be performed. These techniques will spare most patients an open laparotomy for diagnosis.

Work-up

The single most informative study in the work-up of a retroperitoneal sarcoma is a CT scan, which can identify the mass and adjacent organs that may be involved as well as the presence of liver metastases. Because retroperitoneal soft-tissue sarcomas may metastasize to the lungs, a thoracic CT scan is indicated. MRI will reveal the same information as well as provide coronal and sagittal views and better delineation of the retroperitoneal mass from vessels and bone. Angiography is indicated when CT or MRI suggests the presence of visceral artery encasement. Bilateral renal function must be assessed preoperatively because nephrectomy is frequently required (33%), although renal preservation is becoming more common.

Management of Local Disease

The best chance for long-term survival in patients with retroperitoneal sarcoma is offered by a resection with tumor-free margins. Patients with clear radiographic evidence of unresectability should be operated on only for specific symptoms amenable to surgical treatment, such as intestinal obstruction or bleeding. Patients with partially resected tumors have the same overall survival rate as patients who undergo laparotomy with only a biopsy for unresectable disease. However, patients with well-differentiated liposarcomas may benefit symptomatically from repeated debulking. The first step of an operation for a retroperitoneal sarcoma is determination of resectability based on the absence of liver metastases, sarcomatosis, and tumor invasion of unresectable structures. An organ or mesentery attached to a retroperitoneal sarcoma may be invaded by tumor and should be resected en bloc with the specimen. The tumor itself should not be violated, and a biopsy is rarely indicated, unless the tumor cannot be distinguished from a lymphoma preoperatively. Only 50% of patients who undergo surgical exploration have completely resectable tumors. For patients able to have complete resection, 5-year survival is approximately 50–60%.

Adjuvant Therapy

In patients whose initial or recurrent tumor is not resectable, it may be possible to downstage the lesion with neoadjuvant chemotherapy and radiotherapy. This approach is used only if surgery would be possible with tumor shrinkage; it is not used adjuvantly after resection. No studies have demonstrated a benefit from adjuvant chemotherapy, external beam radiotherapy, or intraoperative radiotherapy after complete resection of a retroperitoneal sarcoma; these modalities remain investigational. At M. D. Anderson, patients selected for neoadjuvant therapy receive ifosfamide with hypofractionated (short-course) external beam radiotherapy (36 Gy over 10 days). This is done in an attempt to avoid radiation enteritis in long-term survivors. After treatment, patients are restudied radiographically to assess resectability. An additional trial, studying the use of intraoperative radiation to the tumor bed in an attempt to decrease local recurrence, is being evaluated. Brachytherapy can be used, depending on the status of margins on frozen-section examinations.

Management of Recurrent Disease

Retroperitoneal sarcomas will recur in two-thirds of patients. In addition to recurring locally in the tumor bed and metastasizing to the lungs, retroperitoneal leiomyosarcoma and malignant fibrous histiocytoma readily spread to the liver. Also, retroperitoneal sarcomas can recur diffusely throughout the peritoneal cavity (sarcomatosis). The approach to resectable recurrent disease after treatment of a retroperitoneal sarcoma is similar to the approach taken after the recurrence of an extremity sarcoma. Isolated liver metastases, if stable over several months, may be amenable to resection.

Well-differentiated liposarcoma may recur in a poorly differentiated form. This dedifferentiated retroperitoneal liposarcoma is more aggressive with greater propensity for distant metastasis than its well-differentiated precursor.

FOLLOW-UP

Follow-up of patients with extremity and retroperitoneal soft-tissue sarcomas must be extremely stringent in the first 2 years after therapy because approximately 80% of all recurrences become evident during this period. Patients should have a complete history and physical examination every 3 months and a chest radiograph every 6 months for the first 2 years. If the chest radiograph reveals a suspicious nodule, a CT scan of the chest should be obtained for confirmation. A CT scan or, if available, an MRI of the tumor site should be performed every 6 months during the initial 2 years, particularly if the primary tumor was deeply situated and the site is therefore not amenable to simple clinical examination. Ultrasound is becoming increasingly used to follow extremity sites of resection. Thereafter, patients should be seen every 6 months for the next 3 years, with a chest radiograph and appropriate imaging of the original tumor site done yearly. After 5 years, patients should be seen and a chest radiograph should be taken on a yearly basis.

OTHER SOFT-TISSUE LESIONS

Sarcoma of the Breast

Sarcomas in the breast are rare tumors. These include angiosarcoma, stromal sarcoma, fibrosarcoma, and malignant fibrous histiocytoma. Cystosarcoma phyllodes is generally excluded from this group. Size of the tumor is an important prognostic indicator. As in extremity sarcoma, patients with tumors less than 5 cm have better overall survival than those with tumors greater than 5 cm. Complete excision with negative margins is the primary therapy. Mastectomy carries no additional benefit if complete excision can be accomplished by wide local excision. Because of low rates of regional lymphatic spread, axillary dissection is not routinely indicated. Neoadjuvant chemotherapy or radiation may be considered for patients with large, higher-risk tumors.

Desmoids

Desmoid tumors do not metastasize and are best considered low-grade sarcomas. Approximately half of these tumors arise in the extremity, with the remaining lesions located on the trunk or in the retroperitoneal position. Abdominal wall desmoids are associated with pregnancy and are thought to be under hormonal influence. Patients with Gardner's syndrome may have retroperitoneal desmoids as an extracolonic manifestation of the disease. Surgical resection with wide local excision should be the primary therapy of desmoid tumors. Local recurrence may occur in up to one-third of patients. Adjuvant radiation therapy has been associated with reduced local recurrence.

Dermatofibrosarcoma Protuberans

Dermatofibrosarcoma protuberans (DFSP) is a neoplasm arising in the dermis that may occur anywhere in the body. Approximately 40% arise on the trunk, with most of the remaining tumors distributed between the head and neck and extremities. The lesion presents as a nodular, cutaneous mass with slow and persistent growth. Satellite lesions may be found with larger tumors. Wide local excision is recommended, although recurrence rates are as high as 30–50%.

Bone Sarcomas

EPIDEMIOLOGY

Malignant tumors arising from the skeletal system are rare, representing only 0.2% of primary cancers. Osteosarcoma and Ewing's sarcoma are the two most common bone tumors. They occur mainly during childhood and adolescence. Chondrosarcoma is the most common bone sarcoma that develops after skeletal maturity. Osteosarcoma most commonly involves the distal femur, proximal tibia, or humerus. Rarely are the bones of the hands or feet involved. The most common sites of involvement by

Ewing's sarcoma are the femur, pelvis, tibia, and fibula. Unlike osteosarcoma, Ewing's sarcoma may involve the flat bones and the axial skeleton. Chondrosarcoma occurs most commonly in the pelvis, proximal femur, and shoulder girdle.

STAGING

As with soft-tissue sarcomas, histologic grade is a crucial component of staging bone sarcomas. The staging system proposed by Enneking is shown in Table 5-4.

DIAGNOSIS

Plain radiography in conjunction with a thorough history and physical examination is essential to make an accurate diagnosis. Malignant bone tumors have irregular, poorly defined borders. In addition, there is evidence of bone destruction and periosteal reaction. Soft-tissue extension is a common finding. Plain radiographs may differentiate Ewing's sarcoma from osteosarcoma based on the characteristic diaphyseal involvement, "moth-eaten" appearance, and classic "onion skin" appearance of the periosteum in Ewing's sarcoma. Once a malignant bone tumor is suspected, bone scintigraphy, MRI, CT, and angiography are required prior to biopsy to delineate the local tumor extent, vascular displacement, and compartmental localization. The serum alkaline phosphatase level is elevated in approximately 50% of osteosarcoma cases. If elevated at initial presentation, the alkaline phosphatase level is an excellent marker of treatment response and disease recurrence.

Table 5-4. Staging system for sarcoma of bone

Primary tumor (T)			
T1		Intracompartmental lesion	
T2		Extracompartmental lesion	
Tumor grade (G)			
G1		Low grade	
G2		High grade	
Distant metastases (M)			
M0		No distant metastases	
M1		Distant metastases	
Stage grouping			
Stage IA	G1	T1	M0
Stage IB	G1	T2	M0
Stage IIA	G2	T1	M0
Stage IIB	G2	T2	M0
Stage IIIA	G1, 2	T1	M1
Stage IIIB	G1, 2	T2	M1

Source: Adapted from WF Enneking, SS Spanier, MA Goodman. A system for the surgical staging of musculoskeletal sarcoma. *Clin Orthop* 153:106, 1980.

BIOPSY

The first step in treatment is a carefully planned and meticulously executed biopsy. If the biopsy incision is poorly placed, the chance for a limb-sparing procedure may be lost. Unlike extremity soft-tissue sarcomas, for which an incisional biopsy is favored, a trephine or core-needle biopsy is optimal for bone sarcomas and is best done under radiographic guidance. Precautions should be taken to avoid contamination of uninvolved soft tissue. Adequate hemostasis is critical.

TREATMENT

Surgery

During the 1950s and 1960s, amputation was the standard surgical approach to bone sarcomas. Currently, treatment involves limb salvage whenever feasible. Management of localized sarcoma requires coordination of staging studies, biopsy, surgery, and adjuvant therapy. Successful limb-sparing surgery consists of three phases: tumor resection, bone reconstruction, and soft-tissue coverage. The contraindications for limb-sparing surgery include major neurovascular involvement, pathologic fractures, inappropriately placed biopsy incision, and extensive soft-tissue involvement. Surgical resection is usually the only modality indicated for the management of chondrosarcomas. The indications for primary resection of Ewing's sarcoma are a lesion in an expendable bone, a lesion in the pelvic region (after chemotherapy), a tumor that arises at or below the knee in a child younger than 6 years of age, or the expectation that a major uncorrectable functional deformity will result from radiotherapy.

Chemotherapy

Chemotherapy has revolutionized the approach to most bone sarcomas and is considered standard care for osteosarcoma and Ewing's sarcoma. The bleak 15–20% survival rate with surgery alone during the 1960s has improved to 55–80% with the addition of combination chemotherapy to surgical resection. The timing of chemotherapy, the mode of delivery, and the drug combinations continue to be studied in multi-institutional trials. Adjuvant preoperative chemotherapy is an attractive option because of its potential to downstage tumors, thus allowing for the maximal application of limb-sparing surgery.

Radiotherapy

Because osteosarcomas are generally radioresistant, the major role for radiotherapy is in the palliation of large, unresectable tumors. Acceptable palliation can be achieved in up to 75% of patients with large, unresectable primary tumors. Adjuvant external beam radiotherapy may improve 5-year survival rates for osteosarcomas of the maxilla and mandible by enhancing local control. For most localized Ewing's sarcomas, radiotherapy is the primary mode of therapy. In conjunction with chemotherapy, doses of 50–60 Gy achieve local tumor control in up to 85% of cases without surgery.

RECURRENT DISEASE

Bone tumors disseminate almost exclusively through the bloodstream. Lymphatic metastases are rare and a poor prognostic sign. The lungs are the most common site of distant disease, followed by the bony skeleton. With the use of adjuvant chemotherapy, bony metastases are becoming a more common form of initial distant relapse. It is important to note that patients with Ewing's sarcoma may present with distant disease as long as 15 years after initial diagnosis. Tumor nodules located within the same bone as the initial tumor (skip metastases) are a feature of high-grade lesions. An aggressive approach to recurrent disease, similar to that for soft-tissue sarcomas, should be used.

Sacrococcygeal Chordoma

The notochordal remnant is the origin of this rare tumor. Chordomas are locally aggressive tumors with high recurrence rates. Vague symptoms often result in delayed presentation. Surgical resection should involve a multidisciplinary approach of surgical oncologist, neurosurgeon, and reconstructive plastic surgeon. A two-part procedure is used at our institution. The first portion involves an anterior approach during which blood supply to the tumor, arising from the iliac vessels, is controlled. Several days later, a posterior approach is used to resect the tumor. Radiation therapy should be considered because of high rates of local recurrence.

Selected References

Barkley HT, Martin R G, Romsdahl MM, et al. Treatment of soft tissue sarcomas by preoperative irradiation and conservative surgical resection. *Int J Radiat Oncol Biol Phys* 14:693, 1988.

Brennan MF, Casper E S, Harrison LB, et al. The role of multimodality therapy in soft-tissue sarcoma. *Ann Surg* 214:328, 1991.

Casson AG, Putnam JB, Natarajan G, et al. Five year survival after pulmonary metastasectomy for adult soft tissue sarcoma. *Cancer* 69:662, 1992.

Chang AE, Kinsella T, Glatstein E, et al. Adjuvant chemotherapy for patients with high-grade soft-tissue sarcomas of the extremity. *J Clin Oncol* 6:1491, 1988.

Chang AE, Matory YL, Dwyer AJ, et al. Magnetic resonance imaging versus computed tomography in the evaluation of soft tissue tumors of the extremities. *Ann Surg* 205:340, 1987.

Glenn J, Sindelar WF, Kinsella T, et al. Results of multimodality therapy of resectable soft-tissue sarcomas of the retroperitoneum. *Surgery* 97:316, 1985.

Gutman H, Pollock RE, Benjamin RS, et al. Sarcoma of the breast: Implications for extent of therapy. The M. D. Anderson experience. *Surgery* 116:505, 1994.

Huth J F, Eilber FR. Patterns of metastatic spread following resection of extremity soft-tissue sarcomas and strategies for treatment. *Semin Surg Oncol* 4:20, 1988.

Jaques DP, Coit DG, Hajdu SI, et al. Management of primary and recurrent soft-tissue sarcoma of the retroperitoneum. *Ann Surg* 212:51, 1990.

Lienard D, Ewalenko P, Delmotte JJ, et al. High-dose recombinant tumor necrosis factor alpha in combination with interferon gamma and melphalan in isolation perfusion of the limbs for melanoma and sarcoma. *J Clin Oncol* 10:52, 1992.

Lindberg RD, Martin RG, Romsdahl MM, et al. Conservative surgery and postoperative radiotherapy in 300 adults with soft-tissue sarcomas. *Cancer* 47:2391, 1981.

Localio AS, Eng K, Ranson JHC. Abdominosacral approach for retrorectal tumors. *Am Surg* 179:555, 1980.

Mazanet R, Antman KH. Adjuvant therapy for sarcomas. *Semin Oncol* 18:603, 1991.

Pezzi CM, Pollock RE, Evans HL, et al. Preoperative chemotherapy for soft tissue sarcoma of the extremities. *Ann Surg* 211:476, 1990.

Pisters PWT, Harrison LB, Woodruff JM, et al. A prospective randomized trial of adjuvant brachytherapy in the management of low grade soft tissue sarcomas of the extremity and superficial trunk. *J Clin Oncol* 12:1150, 1994.

Potter DA, Kinsella T, Glatstein E, et al. High-grade soft tissue sarcomas of the extremities. *Cancer* 58:190, 1986.

Razek A, Perez C, Tefft M, et al. Intergroup Ewing's sarcoma study: Local control related to radiation dose, volume and site of primary lesion in Ewing's sarcoma. *Cancer* 46:516, 1980.

Rosenberg SA. Adjuvant chemotherapy of adult patients with soft tissue sarcomas. *Important Adv Oncol* 273, 1985.

Rosenberg SA, Tepper J, Glatstein E, et al. The treatment of soft-tissue sarcomas of the extremities: Prospective randomized evaluations of (1) limb-sparing surgery plus radiation therapy compared with amputation and (2) the role of adjuvant chemotherapy. *Ann Surg* 196:305, 1982.

Sarcoma Meta-analysis Collaboration. Adjuvant chemotherapy for localised resectable soft-tissue sarcoma of adults: Meta-analysis of individual data. *Lancet* 350:1647, 1997.

Storm FK, Mahvi D M. Diagnosis and management of retroperitoneal soft-tissue sarcoma. *Ann Surg* 214:2, 1991.

Suit HD, Mankin HJ, Wood WC, et al. Treatment of the patient with stage M0 soft tissue sarcoma. *J Clin Oncol* 6:854, 1988.

Verweij A, van Oosterom A, Somers R, et al. Chemotherapy in the multidisciplinary approach to soft tissue sarcomas: EORTC soft tissue and bone sarcoma group studies in perspective. *Ann Oncol* 3(Suppl 2):75, 1992.

Carcinoma of the Head and Neck

Mira Milas

Epidemiology

This chapter focuses on squamous cell carcinomas (SCCs) of the head and neck and on salivary gland tumors; thyroid and parathyroid tumors are discussed in Chapter 16.

Approximately 67,000 cancers of the head and neck are diagnosed in the United States each year, accounting for 2–3% of all cancers. The relative frequencies of primary head and neck tumors by site are 40% in the oral cavity, 25% in the larynx, 15% in the oropharynx, 7% in the major salivary glands, and 13% at other sites. The male-to-female ratio is 3:1, and the average age at onset is approximately 50 years.

There is an increased incidence of SCC in patients with heavy tobacco and alcohol exposure. Some studies have shown an association between SCC and syphilis, viruses (Epstein-Barr virus, herpes simplex virus, human papillomavirus), occupational exposure (sawdust, metal dust), ultraviolet light exposure, and neglect of oral hygiene.

Pathology

SCC is by far the most common tumor encountered, comprising >90% of all head and neck cancers. The cancer may be intraepithelial (*in situ*) or invasive, in which case it is classified as well differentiated, moderately differentiated, poorly differentiated, or undifferentiated based on decreasing amounts of keratinization. This histologic grading has not consistently predicted clinical behavior. There are four morphologic growth patterns: exophytic, ulcerative, infiltrative, and verrucous. The ulcerative type is most common and portends a poor prognosis. Premalignant lesions include leukoplakia (white plaque), hyperplasia (thickened mucosa), erythroplakia (velvety red area), and dysplasia; the last two have the highest propensity for malignant transformation. Regional metastasis to cervical lymph nodes is common and related to size and thickness of the primary tumor. The most frequent sites for distant metastases are the lungs, liver, and bone.

Clinical Presentation and Evaluation

SCC of the mucous membranes of the head and neck can arise from any of the premalignant lesions or an ulcer, spread in area and depth, and eventually invade adjacent structures. Signs and symptoms of SCC of the head and neck include a nonhealing ulcer, neck mass, bleeding, otalgia, unexplained facial pain, dysphagia, odynophagia, and hoarseness.

The presence of such symptoms necessitates a detailed clinical examination. Bimanual palpation of the neck, oral cavity, tonsils, and base of the tongue is required in every patient. In addition, the nasal cavity, nasopharynx, oropharynx, hypopharynx, and larynx should be examined; in skillful hands, these examinations can all be done with a mirror, but flexible endoscopy can also provide valuable clinical information. Approximately 5% of patients with head and neck cancer will have a second primary SCC of the head and neck, esophagus, or lung, which can best be evaluated by panendoscopy (direct laryngoscopy, esophagoscopy, and bronchoscopy with directed biopsy). A CT scan from the skull base to the clavicle is an extremely informative test and should be part of the clinical work-up prior to panendoscopy and biopsy. The CT scan is useful for identification of occult tumors, local tumor extension, and lymph node disease. In a patient with a clinically apparent primary tumor, a biopsy specimen can be obtained with a scalpel, punch forceps, or fine needle in an outpatient setting. A chest radiograph and liver function studies are adequate screening examinations for distant metastatic disease. An isolated pulmonary nodule seen on chest radiograph in a patient with a known SCC of the head and neck more likely represents a primary lung cancer (second primary) than metastatic disease from the head and neck primary tumor. A diagnostic biopsy of the lung lesion is necessary before treatment of the head and neck cancer is undertaken.

Two mistakes commonly made in the evaluation of patients with head and neck tumors can lead to treatment delays. First, an incomplete examination of the upper aerodigestive system can allow one to miss small lesions. It is imperative that patients who present with symptoms suggestive of head and neck cancer be evaluated by a physician experienced in performing a thorough head and neck examination. The second common mistake occurs when patients with a cervical mass experience delays in referral for biopsy while long courses of antibiotic therapy are tried. A patient with persistent adenopathy after a 2-week course of antibiotics should be evaluated with a fine-needle aspiration biopsy.

Staging

Head and neck cancers are staged according to the TNM system of the American Joint Committee on Cancer Staging (AJCC) (Table 6-1). The T staging is based on the location of the primary tumor and thus varies for each site in the head and neck. Prognosis correlates strongly with stage at diagnosis. For many head and neck cancer sites, survival exceeds 80% in patients with stage I disease. Most patients, however, have stage III or IV disease at diagnosis and a survival rate of less than 40%.

Table 6-1. AJCC staging system for head and neck cancers

Stage grouping

Stage I	T1, N0, M0
Stage II	T2, N0, M0
Stage III	T3, N0, M0
	T1-3, N1, M0
Stage IV	T4, N0 or N1, M0
	Any T, N2 or N3, M0
	Any T, any N, M1

Primary tumor (T) dependent on anatomic location

Regional lymph nodes (N)

N0	No regional lymph node metastasis
N2a	Metastasis in single ipsilateral lymph node >3 cm but <6 cm
N2b	Metastasis in multiple ipsilateral lymph nodes, none >6 cm
N2c	Metastasis in bilateral or contralateral lymph nodes, none >6 cm
N3	Metastasis in a lymph node >6 cm

Metastatic disease

M0	No evidence of distant metastasis
M1	Evidence of distant metastasis

Source: Adapted from OH Beahrs, DE Henson, RVP Hutter, et al (eds). *Manual for Staging of Cancer* (4th ed). Philadelphia: Lippincott, 1992.

General Principles of Treatment

Surgery, radiotherapy, or both are the conventional treatment modalities used in the management of head and neck tumors. In general, chemotherapy and immunotherapy are appropriate only as part of clinical protocols, as palliative measures in patients with incurable disease, or for tumors that persist after conventional therapy.

Surgical resection generally offers the best chance for complete tumor cure and provides a specimen that can be used to verify the adequacy of excision margins. Morbidity is minimal when the tumor is small and accessible, but significant cosmetic and functional deficits are not unusual after resection of large tumors; disabilities can be minimized with appropriate reconstructive techniques.

Radiotherapy is effective in the treatment of head and neck tumors. The advantage of radiotherapy is that anatomic structures can be preserved while local tumor control is achieved. However, irradiation of the head and neck produces acute mucositis and, over the long term, xerostomia, fibrosis of the skin and soft tissue, and altered pituitary and thyroid function.

Surgery and radiotherapy are often combined to achieve local control of head and neck cancer. Most surgeons prefer that radiation be administered postoperatively, where it seems to lead to better response rates than before surgery. The main indications for postoperative radiation are high risk of local and regional failure (stage III and IV disease), residual tumor at surgical margins, and histopathologic features that suggest unusual tumor aggressiveness (i.e., vessel invasion, perineural invasion, anaplastic appearance, multiple positive nodes, or extracapsular nodal spread).

Rehabilitation is important during and after treatment, and includes physical and occupational therapy, speech and swallowing rehabilitation, and nutritional support. A novel and still experimental strategy of chemoprevention is currently being evaluated in clinical trials, which administer retinoid-derived compounds to decrease the incidence of second primary tumors and to induce regression of premalignant lesions. Similarly, clinical trials are currently in place to evaluate the usefulness of gene therapy (e.g., restoration of the normal p53 gene) in the treatment of head and neck malignancies.

Neck Dissection

There are several approaches to the treatment of lymph node metastases in patients with head and neck cancer. Metastatic SCC to a single small neck node without extracapsular tumor spread can be controlled with either radiation alone or neck dissection. When disease in the neck is more extensive ($\geq$N2, extranodal spread), combined surgery and radiation therapy treatment is important because neither modality alone leads to successful tumor control.

Surgical treatment of the neck relies on three major types of neck dissection: radical neck dissection, modified radical neck dissection, or selective neck dissection. The classical *radical neck dissection* refers to removal of all ipsilateral cervical lymph nodes in levels I–V (Fig. 6-1). The dissection extends from the inferior border of the mandible to the clavicle, posteriorly to the anterior border of the trapezius muscle, and anteriorly to the lateral border of the sternohyoid muscle. The depth of dissection extends to the fascia overlying the anterior scalene and levator scapulae muscles. The spinal accessory nerve, internal jugular vein, and sternocleidomastoid muscle are removed.

Modified radical neck dissection was developed to reduce the morbidity of the classical operation. The modified dissection still removes all lymph nodes routinely excised in a radical neck dissection. However, at minimum the spinal accessory nerve is preserved, as are frequently also the internal jugular vein and sternocleidomastoid muscle.

Selective neck dissection is the term reserved for less extensive lymph node dissections. The most common selective dissection is the supraomohyoid neck dissection, in which submental, submandibular, and upper and middle jugular lymph nodes (levels I–III) are removed. Such procedures are used to remove lymph nodes corresponding to the most significant drainage basins of specific head and neck tumor sites, and are usually employed for

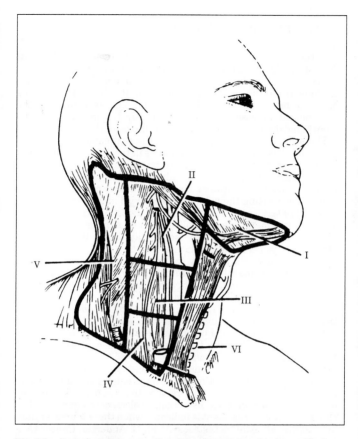

Fig. 6-1. Lymph node groups. Level I, submental and submandibular lymph node groups; level II, upper jugular group; level III, middle jugular groups; level IV, lower jugular group; level V, posterior triangle group; level VI, anterior compartment group.

staging a patient with nonpalpable neck nodes. Another common selective neck dissection, used to treat patients with posterior scalp melanoma, is the posterolateral neck dissection. In this procedure, the suboccipital, retroauricular, upper jugular, middle jugular, and lower jugular lymph nodes (levels II–V) are removed. Finding nodal disease may warrant progression to a more extensive neck dissection.

At the University of Texas M. D. Anderson Cancer Center, the neck dissection most commonly performed for a primary cancer of the head and neck is a modified radical neck dissection. It is employed to treat neck metastases when they are identified and electively for conclusive staging of cervical lymph node disease. The radical neck dissection is reserved for treatment of disease that has extended into the sternocleidomastoid muscle, jugular vein, or spinal accessory nerve.

Carcinoma of the Oral Cavity

In the United States, cancer of the oral cavity develops in about 30,000 people and causes about 10,000 deaths annually. The incidence is twice as high in males as in females. The oral cavity extends from the vermillion border of the lips to the plane between the junction of the hard and soft palates. It includes the lips, buccal mucosa, gingiva, retromolar trigone, floor of the mouth, hard palate, and anterior two-thirds of the tongue.

The staging system for tumors of the oral cavity is shown in Table 6-2. The treatment for carcinoma of the oral cavity is determined by location and stage of the primary tumor. For small stage T1 and some stage T2 tumors, radiation or surgery yield similar results. Surgical treatment for stage T1 oral cancer is accomplished by excising the primary tumor with an adequate margin (approximately 1 cm) and repairing the defect by primary closure, local advancement flaps, or split-thickness skin grafts. Stage T2 disease can be treated in the same way, but a flap closure is almost always necessary for larger defects.

Radiotherapy as a primary treatment modality for cancers of the oral cavity may involve interstitial radioactive implants, external beam therapy, or both. Small superficial cancers can be treated with interstitial implants: local control rates of 80–95% can be achieved for T1–T2 lesions of the oral tongue and floor of the mouth. Cancers arising at other sites are usually best treated with surgical excision. Postoperative adjuvant external beam radiotherapy is effective in improving local control rates for tumors likely to recur (T3 and T4).

Lymph nodes that are clinically involved with tumor are always treated with a neck dissection. However, treatment of the clinically uninvolved neck is still controversial, with three options available: observation, elective neck dissection, or elective irradiation. Most clinicians believe treatment is indicated when there is greater than 20% chance of nodal metastases. At M. D. Anderson Cancer Center, most, if not all, stage T1 and T2 oral cavity carcinomas are treated with primary surgical excision and a supraomohyoid neck dissection. If there is no nodal involvement or if only a single node is involved, without evidence of extracapsular extension, postoperative radiotherapy is not given. If there are multiple positive nodes

Table 6-2.   Staging system for oral cavity tumors

Tis	Carcinoma *in situ*
T1	Tumor ≤2 cm at greatest dimension
T2	Tumor >2 cm but not 4 cm at greatest dimension
T3	Tumor >4 cm at greatest dimension
T4	Tumor invades adjacent structures (e.g., cortical bone, deep extrinsic muscle of tongue, maxillary sinus, or skin)

Source: Adapted from OH Beahrs, DE Henson, RVP Hutter, et al. (eds). *Manual for Staging of Cancer* (4th ed). Philadelphia: Lippincott, 1992.

or extranodal extension, postoperative radiotherapy to the neck is used to lower the incidence of disease recurrence. Radiotherapy for clinically negative cervical nodes is reserved for patients whose primary tumor is to be treated by radiotherapy as well.

Early lesions have a reasonably good prognosis, but the 5-year disease-free survival rate for patients with advanced oral cavity cancers has remained about 30–40% over the past 20 years. Adverse prognostic factors include site of the lesion, depth of invasion, and presence of nodal metastases.

LIP

Small lesions of the lip can be cured with either radiation or surgical excision. Most T1 lesions are best treated by surgery alone, with a greater than 90% 5-year survival rate. However, T1 lesions of the commissure are best treated by radiotherapy. Lesions larger than 2 cm should be treated by surgical excision with immediate reconstruction and postoperative radiotherapy. Invasion of the mental nerve is associated with an 80% incidence of node involvement and only a 35% 5-year survival rate.

FLOOR OF THE MOUTH

Small lesions confined to the floor of the mouth can be treated by intraoral excision with tumor-free surgical margins or radiotherapy. Floor-of-the-mouth lesions frequently involve adjacent structures, such as the deep muscles of the tongue and mandible. In most cases, a cheek flap with marginal or segmental mandibulectomy is required to obtain adequate margins.

TONGUE

Carcinoma of the tongue is the most common intraoral malignancy. An intraoral glossectomy can be performed for patients with lesions limited to the anterior or middle third of the oral tongue. Tumor thickness is the most accurate predictor of lymph node involvement. Lesions thinner than 1 cm have a minimal incidence of lymph node involvement. Thicker lesions have a greater than 20% chance of lymph node positivity; therefore a supraomohyoid neck dissection should be included in the treatment of patients with a tongue carcinoma 1 cm or thicker and a clinically uninvolved neck. The lower jugular nodes are typically involved in patients with clinically positive cervical nodes; therefore a complete modified radical neck dissection is required. Tumors of the posterior oral tongue with extension into the base of the tongue are best treated by a transcervical excision combined with an en bloc neck dissection. Smaller surgical defects can be allowed to heal by primary intention, while larger ones may require split-thickness skin grafting; in some instances, the edge of the tongue can be approximated upon itself.

HARD PALATE

Most SCCs of the upper gum and hard palate begin on the gingiva and can be excised with negative margins. Large lesions of the palate that have invaded the bone will require a partial maxillectomy. Reconstruction for maxillary defects of the oral cavity is best achieved using a prosthetic dental appliance.

Carcinoma of the Larynx

The incidence of carcinoma of the larynx in the United States is approximately 13,000 cases per year, with a male-to-female ratio of 9:1. Most patients are middle-aged or older men who smoke tobacco and drink alcohol. There is also a risk associated with exposure to the human papillomavirus.

The larynx has three subsites: the glottis (true vocal cords), the supraglottis (false cords, epiglottis, aryepiglottic folds, arytenoids, and ventricles), and the subglottis (inferior border of vocal cords to inferior border of cricoid cartilage). The lymphatics of the larynx are numerous, except over the vocal cords, where the mucosa is thin, adheres tightly to the vocal ligament, and lacks lymphatic channels. Above the level of the ventricles, the efferent lymphatics of the superior portion of the larynx extend to the pyriform sinus upward to join the jugular chain. From the inferior larynx, the efferent lymphatics drain into the pretracheal, paratracheal, and deep cervical lymph nodes. The lymphatic drainage of the larynx is usually bilateral, and any laryngeal tumor, except a lesion of the true vocal cords, should be considered a midline cancer with the propensity to metastasize to bilateral neck nodes.

Glottic carcinomas are those that involve the upper surface of the vocal cords and continue down to 1 cm below this plane. Glottic cancers account for 65% of cancers of the larynx. They usually are well differentiated, grow slowly, and metastasize late. Metastasis occurs only after the disease has infiltrated muscle or has spread beyond the limits of the true vocal cords into the paraglottic space or from the anterior commissure into the pretracheal region.

Supraglottic cancers account for 35% of laryngeal tumors. They are usually aggressive tumors causing both local extension and lymph node metastasis. The lymphatic channels of the supraglottis drain to the jugulodigastric and middle and inferior internal jugular chains. Supraglottic tumors have a high risk of bilateral nodal involvement.

Subglottic cancers are rare. They commonly produce extension into the lymph nodes of the prelaryngeal area, inferior internal jugular chain, and thyroid gland, and have a high risk of bilateral cervical metastasis.

The staging system for tumors of the larynx is summarized in Table 6-3.

PATIENT EVALUATION

The initial presenting symptoms of cancer of the larynx depend on the site and stage of the disease. Only lesions of the true vocal cords produce early symptoms and give a chance for intervening at an early stage of disease. Supraglottic lesions are usually discovered at a much later stage upon development of dysphagia, odynophagia, hemoptysis, or referred otalgia. Often supraglottic

Table 6-3.   Staging system for cancers of the larynx

Supraglottis

T1	Tumor confined to site of origin
T2	Tumor involving adjacent supraglottic sites, without glottic fixation
T3	Tumor limited to the larynx, with fixation and/or extension to the postericoid medial wall of the pyriform sinus or pre-epiglottic space
T4	Massive tumor extending beyond the larynx to involve the oropharynx, soft tissues of the neck, or destruction of thyroid cartilage

Glottis

T1	Tumor confined to vocal folds, with normal vocal cord mobility
T2	Tumor extension to supraglottis and/or subglottis with normal or impaired vocal cord mobility
T3	Tumor confined to larynx, with fixation of the vocal cords
T4	Massive tumor, with thyroid cartilage destruction and/or extension beyond the confines of the larynx

Source: Adapted from OH Beahrs, DE Henson, RVP Hutter, et al. (eds). *Manual for Staging of Cancer* (4th ed). Philadelphia: Lippincott, 1992.

tumors produce a large lesion that can eventually impair motion of the vocal cord and cause hoarseness. Physical examination usually reveals either an exophytic or a submucosal lesion. CT is very useful for determining paraglottic, subglottic, pyriform sinus, and extralaryngeal involvement, and for revealing clinically occult lymph node disease.

TREATMENT

The goal of treatment for laryngeal carcinoma is tumor extirpation while preserving voice function if possible. Mucosal stripping of the cord can be effective treatment for patients with carcinoma *in situ*, but repeated attempts at stripping leave the cord difficult to examine for the development of a malignant lesion. Therefore radiotherapy is recommended for patients with recurrent premalignant vocal cord lesions. In general, radiotherapy can also satisfy treatment goals for patients with T1 and T2 lesions, although some surgeons still choose to operate on early laryngeal cancers. More advanced cancer usually requires removal of all or part of the larynx and postoperative irradiation.

The local control rate for T1 and T2 lesions treated by radiotherapy is 71–100%. Salvage laryngectomy improves the local control rate to 88–100%. The local control rate for patients with T3 laryngeal carcinomas treated by surgery and radiotherapy is 85%, with a 67% 5-year survival rate. Patients with T4 lesions treated by surgery and radiotherapy can anticipate a 30–50% 5-year survival rate.

Surgery

A vertical laryngectomy (hemilaryngectomy) is used for patients with T1 or T2 vocal cord tumors who are not candidates for radiotherapy (usually due to prior irradiation). Hemilaryngectomy can also be used in select patients with persistent or recurrent disease after radiotherapy. It preserves voice function with some hoarseness. A supraglottic laryngectomy is used for patients with early (T1 or T2) supraglottic cancers. It is often associated with aspiration and is contraindicated in patients with poor pulmonary function. Total laryngectomy is the procedure of choice for patients with stage T3 or T4 cancers of the larynx. This procedure is seldom performed when patients have normal vocal cord mobility. A wide-field laryngectomy includes the paralaryngeal soft tissue, which extends between the internal jugular veins and the lymph nodes in levels II–V (see Fig. 6-1). In some instances, portions of the hypopharynx will also need to be removed, in which case a 1-cm mucosal margin is desirable because of the risk of submucosal microscopic disease. An ipsilateral thyroid lobectomy is indicated when the tumor involves the subglottis, pyriform apex, or paratracheal nodes, or when the tumor extends through the thyroid cartilage on the same side as the lesion.

Radiotherapy

Early (stage T1 or T2) glottic and supraglottic cancers respond to external beam radiotherapy, and tumor control is usually achieved with a 65- to 70-Gy dose. Glottic tumors, which have a low incidence of lymph node involvement, can be treated through small portals that encompass only the larynx. With careful treatment, there is minimal damage to normal tissues, and the patient can retain a normal voice. Supraglottic tumors, because of their higher incidence of lymph node involvement, require larger fields that encompass the lymphatic drainage of the neck. Lymph nodes in the primary drainage basin, if clinically uninvolved, should be treated with a 50-Gy dose.

Postoperative radiotherapy to the primary site and/or the regional lymph nodes is indicated for patients who have undergone a total laryngectomy and who have multiple positive lymph nodes, extranodal disease, close or positive surgical margins, T4 disease, or subglottic extension of tumor. Patients who have undergone a tracheotomy to achieve airway control prior to laryngectomy also require postoperative radiotherapy to control disease at the tracheostoma.

Carcinoma of the Oropharynx, Nasopharynx, and Hypopharynx

The oropharynx begins at the ring bounded by the anterior tonsillar pillars, uvula, and base of tongue. Superiorly, the soft palate separates it from the nasopharynx, and inferiorly, the epiglottis divides it from the hypopharynx. Pain, dysphagia, and a neck mass are the most common presenting symptoms in patients with oropharyngeal cancer. External beam and/or interstitial radiation has been used for curative treatment and results in overall local control rates for all primary sites ranging from 90% (T1) to 55% (T4). Cancers of the tonsillar fossa respond best to radiotherapy. Surgical excision of all but the smallest palatal and tonsillar lesions is generally inadequate. Larger lesions most frequently involve the supraglottic pharynx and are treated as described earlier.

Nasopharyngeal carcinoma is uncommon in most of the world, with highest incidence in China and Africa, where it seems related to risk factors in the diet and viral agents (EBV). A neck mass is the presenting complaint in 90% of patients; other symptoms include nasal obstruction and abnormalities of hearing. One-fourth of patients have invasion of tumor into the base of skull and cranial nerve deficits. Treatment usually involves radiotherapy of the primary tumor and draining lymph nodes. Surgical resection, even of small tumors, is limited because of high associated morbidity. Overall 5-year survival is 50%.

The hypopharynx is the region of entrance to the esophagus and includes the pyriform sinuses, posterior pharyngeal wall, and postcricoid area. Seventy percent of cancers occur in the pyriform sinus and produce few symptoms until they are advanced. Diffuse local spread and lymph node metastases are common. Combined modality treatment is usually required, as is total laryngectomy in most patients. Hypopharyngeal cancer is difficult to control and has poor 5-year survival rates: 25% without nodal disease and 10% in presence of nodal metastases.

Cervical Lymph Node Metastasis from an Unknown Primary Tumor

Benign conditions, inflammatory and infectious diseases, and primary and metastatic cancer can lead to the development of an enlarged cervical lymph node. A complete history and physical examination, as well as fine-needle aspiration biopsy, are helpful in diagnosing the correct etiology. Among malignancies, SCC of the head and neck is by far the most common reason for enlarged cervical lymph nodes, followed by lymphoma and solid tumor metastases, including those from lung, breast, and thyroid cancer. Management of biopsy-proven malignancy in a cervical lymph node when no primary tumor is apparent can be very challenging.

A thorough search for a primary tumor is essential and should be the first priority of management. Knowledge of lymphatic drainage patterns and the metastatic propensity of various cancers can provide some clues. Metastatic SCC in a cervical node may have originated in many different sites. The location of the node can provide valuable diagnostic information as to the possible origin of the primary tumor. A valuable diagnostic strategy, however, is to consider whether the lymph node malignancy is of squamous or nonsquamous origin. The clinical management then becomes organized according to a very specific course in each case.

Most patients with metastatic SCC to lymph nodes in zones II or III have a primary in the nasopharynx, tonsil, or tongue base (Waldeyer's ring). They should undergo careful clinical examination with panendoscopy. In the absence of overt anomalies, a CT or MRI scan of the head and neck may be a useful next step. The patient should also be scheduled for an exam under anesthesia in the operating room for the purpose of obtaining biopsies. How to perform the biopsy is debatable. One approach advocates "blind" biopsies of the ipsilateral nasopharynx, tonsil, base of tongue, pyriform sinus, and even postcricoid area. Alternatively, only sites of mucosal abnormalities, however minor, are biopsied. If the primary tumor is identified, an appropriate treatment decision can be made that incorporates both the primary tumor and the cervical node. If the primary remains unidentified, the neck is treated with a modified or radical neck dissection, depending on the extent of lymph node disease, and radiation therapy is administered to Waldeyer's ring and both necks. An ipsilateral tonsillectomy is also recommended.

A patient with a cervical lymph node metastasis and a small tumor of the head and neck that is detected only by an examination under general anesthesia can usually be treated by radiotherapy alone. The cervical lymphatics can be adequately treated with radiotherapy if the involved lymph node is small (<3 cm) based on physical examination and CT scan, although some surgeons advocate a neck dissection in all patients to determine the extent of regional disease. A modified radical neck dissection should be performed if the enlarged lymph node is larger than 3 cm or if residual disease persists after radiotherapy.

For cervical lymph node metastases that are adenocarcinoma or other nonsquamous carcinomas, the strategy is completely different. These tumors most likely originate below the level of the clavicles. Extensive work-up consisting of CT of the chest and abdomen, imaging of the bowel, and bone scan to exclude other sites of distant metastasis should be made before the neck is treated. Again, if the primary is not identified, the neck is treated with surgery and radiotherapy as described for squamous metastases.

The finding of metastatic thyroid carcinoma in a cervical lymph node is sufficient information to proceed with neck exploration and thyroidectomy. Lymphoma can be diagnosed by fine-needle aspiration but cannot be subtyped; therefore an accessible lymph node should be removed. The diagnosis of adenocarcinoma requires an evaluation of the salivary glands if the node is cephalad in the neck. Needle biopsy evidence of adenocarcinoma in inferior neck nodes should prompt an evaluation of the lungs, breasts, pancreas, and colon.

Five-year survival rates of 50% have been reported for patients with cervical metastases from an unknown primary tumor. Close follow-up is mandatory, as the primary site will become evident in 15–20% of patients over 5 years. The 5-year survival rate for patients with metastatic adenocarcinoma to the cervical lymph nodes is less than 5%.

Carcinoma of the Salivary Glands

The parotid, submandibular, and submaxillary glands are the major salivary glands and together account for more than 95% of salivary gland tumors. The remaining tumors involve minor salivary glands, which are small foci of glandular tissue found in submucosa throughout the oral cavity with highest density on the palate. Salivary gland tumors appear sporadically (5–10% of all head and neck tumors) and are not associated with smoking, alcohol use, or other environmental factors.

Neoplasms of the parotid gland account for 90% of all tumors of the three major salivary glands. Submandibular gland tumors are less common (10%), and submaxillary ones are exceedingly rare (<1%). The smaller the size of a salivary gland, the greater the likelihood that a tumor will be malignant. Three-fourths of parotid tumors will be benign, whereas 50% of submandibular and virtually all sublingual tumors are malignant.

The most common benign tumors are pleomorphic adenomas and benign cystic lymphomatosum (Warthin's tumor, which is almost exclusive to the parotid). The most common malignant histologic types are mucoepidermoid, adenoid cystic carcinoma, and adenocarcinoma. The parotid may be the site of metastatic disease (cutaneous head tumors, bronchogenic, and breast cancer) or lymphoma.

The superficial portion of the parotid gland is the largest and rests lateral to the facial nerve. The deep lobe is medial to the facial nerve and extends to the retromandibular and parapharyngeal spaces. Drainage to the mouth is via Stensen's duct. There are numerous lymph nodes within the parotid gland itself; lymphatic drainage then goes to preauricular, infra-auricular, and deep upper jugular lymph nodes.

The submandibular glands are paired glands located medial to the body of the mandible and thus adjacent to all structures within the submandibular triangle: the facial vessels, the marginal mandibular branch of the facial nerve, the lingual vessels and nerve, and the hypoglossal nerve. Wharton's duct opens into the floor of the mouth. The submandibular gland is invested with the superficial layer of cervical fascia and has lymphatic drainage into the deep jugular chain.

The sublingual glands are located on the paramedian floor of the mouth just deep to the mucosa and superficial to the mylohyoid muscle.

PATIENT EVALUATION

Asymptomatic swelling is the initial complaint in the overwhelming majority of patients with salivary gland tumors.

Facial paralysis (especially if associated with a small mass), enlarged regional lymph nodes, and fixation to skin or adjacent tissues are very strong indications of malignancy. Episodic swelling associated with meals suggests an obstructive or inflammatory process. Diffuse submandibular gland enlargement is benign in 90% of patients, but duct obstruction by an underlying malignancy needs to be excluded in all cases. Other symptoms, like pain and rapid growth, do not distinguish infiltrative from inflammatory disease consistently well. Differentiation from collagen vascular diseases, such as Wegener's granulomatosis and Sjögren's syndrome, that affect the parotid is necessary. Any mass in the preauricular area or the angle of the mandible should be presumed to arise from the parotid gland.

Fine-needle aspiration (FNA), which has a sensitivity greater than 95%, is a useful biopsy technique. It is employed often to distinguish inflammatory and neoplastic enlargements of the submandibular gland. Use of FNA or open biopsy for diagnosing parotid lesions is more controversial. Most parotid neoplasms will require surgical removal. Therefore the usefulness of FNA must be weighed against whether the decision to proceed with surgery will be changed. FNA is rarely indicated for minor salivary glands; biopsy with cup forceps is performed instead.

The role of CT in the evaluation of salivary tumors is limited to patients with symptoms suspicious of malignancy or when distinction between inflammatory and neoplastic disease remains unclear. A CT scan is valuable to identify tumor extension into the deep parotid lobe and parapharyngeal space.

TREATMENT

Surgery is the treatment of choice for salivary gland neoplasms. Many surgeons rely on intraoperative frozen-section biopsy to determine the extent of surgical procedure.

Benign neoplasms can be cured if completely excised, which usually is accomplished by superficial parotidectomy or submandibular excision. The facial nerve can be "peeled off" benign tumors without risk of recurrence. Violating the capsule of pleomorphic adenomas predisposes to recurrence.

Current treatment of malignant salivary tumors mainly involves surgery and radiation. Extent of surgery is dictated by tumor size and degree of local extension, and should include a rim of normal tissue. In the case of the parotid gland, the minimum operation is a superficial parotidectomy. For lesions of the submandibular gland, adequate surgical excision includes removal of the gland and the associated investing fascia and lymph nodes. In some instances, resection of part or all of the mandible, floor of the mouth, lingual and hypoglossal nerves, and a supraomohyoid neck dissection will be necessary. No chemotherapy regimen has proved to be effective, and immunotherapy is in the clinical trial phase.

Every effort should be made to preserve facial nerve function, even when dealing with malignancy, unless the tumor has adhered to or directly invaded the nerve. If the facial nerve must be sacrificed, it should be immediately reconstructed with either a nerve graft or a cranial nerve XII–VII anastomosis. Postoperative radiotherapy should be planned. There is no evidence that this approach compromises local and regional control.

Only node-positive necks, where malignancy in lymph nodes was detected either before or during surgery, require neck dissection. Postoperative radiation to the neck is indicated in almost all cases of cervical metastatic disease.

Postoperative radiotherapy to the surgical area for malignant tumors is indicated in almost all cases except for small, low-grade tumors. Typically, radiotherapy is given for high-grade mucoepidermoid carcinoma, adenoid cystic carcinoma, adenocarcinoma, malignant mixed tumor, SCC, multicentric recurrent pleomorphic adenoma, and highly cellular acinic cell carcinoma. Radiotherapy is also beneficial for patients with perineural invasion, positive nodes, skin involvement, or microscopic residual disease.

Overall, 20% of patients will develop distant metastasis. The 5-year survival rates for patients with malignant salivary gland tumors vary from 95% for low-grade mucoepidermoid carcinoma to 75% for adenoid cystic carcinoma and 50% for high-grade mucoepidermoid carcinoma and malignant mixed tumors.

Surveillance

Following curative treatment of head and neck cancers, patients must be closely followed for the development of local as well as distant recurrences. Physical examination performed by someone skilled in examination of the head and neck is the most important part of the postoperative follow-up. At M. D. Anderson, follow-up of patients occurs every 3 months for the first 2 years postoperatively, then every 6 months for the next 3 years, and yearly thereafter. A chest radiograph and liver function studies are performed yearly.

Selected References

Byers RM. The role of a modified neck dissection. In C Jacobs (ed.), *Cancers of the Head and Neck*. Boston: Martinus Nijhoff, 1987.

Byers RM, Wolf PF, Ballantyne AJ. Rationale for elective modified neck dissection. *Head Neck* 10:160, 1988.

Clayman GL. Gene therapy for head and neck cancer. *Head Neck* 17:535, 1995.

Crissman JD, Gluckman J, Whiteley J, et al. Squamous cell carcinoma of the floor of mouth. *Head Neck* 3:2, 1980.

Eiband JD, Elias GE, Suter CM, et al. Prognostic factors in squamous cell carcinoma of the larynx. *Am J Surg* 158:314, 1989.

Frankenthaler RA, Luna MA, Lee SS, et al. Prognostic variables in parotid gland cancer. *Arch Otolaryngol Head Neck Surg* 117:1251, 1991.

Gluckman J, Gullane P, Johnson J. *Practical Approach to Head and Neck Tumors*. New York: Raven Press, 1994.

Khuri FR, Lippman SM, Spitz MR, et al. Molecular epidemiology and retinoid chemoprevention of head and neck cancer. *JNCI* 89:199, 1997.

Lefebvre JL, Degueant C, Castelain B, et al. Interstitial brachytherapy and early tongue squamous cell carcinoma management. *Head Neck* 12:232, 1990.

Mendenhall WM, Million RR, Sharkey DE, et al. Stage T3 squamous cell carcinoma of the glottic larynx treated with surgery and/or radiation therapy. *Int J Radiat Oncol Biol Phys* 10:357, 1984.

Mendenhall WM, Parsons JT, Stringer SP, et al. T1–T2 vocal cord carcinoma: A basis for comparing the results of irradiation and surgery. *Head Neck Surg* 10:373, 1988.

Myers EN, Suen JC (eds.). *Cancer of the Head and Neck*. Philadelphia: Saunders, 1996.

Rice DM, Spiro RH (eds.). *Current Concepts in Head and Neck Cancer*. Atlanta: American Cancer Society, 1989.

Ridge JA, Hooks MA, Lee R, Benner SE. Head and neck tumors. In R Pazdur, L Coia, W Hoskins, L Wagman (eds.), *Cancer Management: A Multidisciplinary Approach*. Huntington, New York: PRR, Inc., 1996.

Robbins KT, Medina JE, Wolfe GT, et al. Standardizing neck dissection terminology. Official report of the Academy's Committee for Head and Neck Surgery and Oncology. *Arch Otolaryngol Head Neck Surg* 117:601, 1991.

Wang RC, Goepfert H, Barber A, et al. Squamous cell carcinoma, metastatic to the neck from an unknown primary site. In DL Larson, AJ Ballantyne, OM Guillamondegui (eds.), *Cancer in the Neck*. New York: Macmillan, 1986.

Weber RS, Byers RM, Petit B, et al. Submandibular gland tumors. *Arch Otolaryngol Head Neck Surg* 116:1055, 1990.

Weber RS, Callender DL. Laryngeal conservation. *Semin Radiat Oncol* 2:149, 1992.

Thoracic Malignancies

Ara A. Vaporciyan and Stephen G. Swisher

Primary Neoplasms of the Lung

In 1997 lung cancer will account for an estimated 160,000 deaths and 170,000 new cases of cancer in the United States. Though less publicized than breast or prostate cancer, lung cancer is the most common cause of cancer-related death in both men and women. Approximately 25% of all cancer deaths are attributable to lung cancer. However, as seen in Fig. 7-1, the overall age-adjusted death rates for lung cancer have begun to level off (although they continue to rise in women). This leveling off is attributable to an overall decrease in the number of males who smoke. Unfortunately, this good news is countered by a disturbing increase in smoking among certain minority and adolescent age groups. The overall 5-year survival rate for lung cancer is only 14%, primarily because the disease is usually advanced at presentation. If the disease is found at an early stage, the 5-year survival rate approaches 60–70%.

EPIDEMIOLOGY

Smoking is the primary etiology in more than 80% of lung cancers, and secondhand smoke increases the risk of lung cancer by 30%. Despite the strong association of lung cancer with smoking, only 15% of heavy smokers develop such cancers. Giant bullous emphysema and airway obstructive disease can act synergistically with smoking to induce lung cancer, perhaps because of poor clearance and trapping of carcinogens. Industrial and environmental carcinogens have been implicated, including residential radon gas, asbestos, uranium, cadmium, arsenic, and terpenes.

PATHOLOGY

Lung cancer can be broadly separated into two groups: non–small cell lung cancers (NSCLC) and small cell lung cancers (SCLC). This is a popular division because, for the most part, NSCLC patients are often treated with surgery when the tumor is localized, whereas SCLC patients are almost always treated nonsurgically with chemotherapy and radiation therapy. The three major types of NSCLC are adenocarcinoma, squamous cell carcinoma, and large cell carcinoma (Table 7-1).

NSCLC

Adenocarcinoma has become the most common type of NSCLC and accounts for more than 40% of cases. It is the most common lung cancer found in nonsmokers and women. The lesions tend to be located in the periphery and to develop systemic metastases even in the face of small primary tumors.

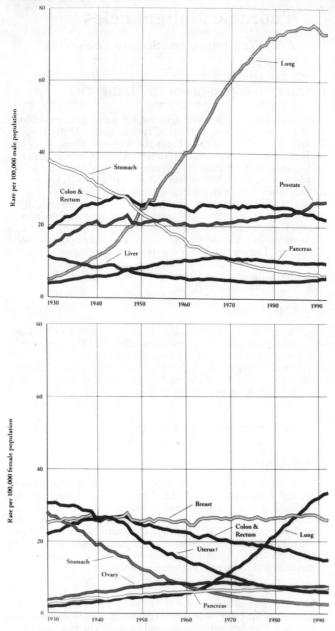

Fig. 7-1.   The age-adjusted cancer death rate continues to rise in females but appears to have leveled off in males.

Table 7-1. Frequency of histologic subtypes of primary lung cancer

Cell type	Estimated frequency (%)
Non–small cell lung cancer	
Adenocarcinoma	40
Bronchoalveolar	2
Squamous cell carcinoma	25
Large cell carcinoma	7
Small cell lung cancer	
Small cell carcinoma	20
Neuroendocrine, well differentiated	1
Carcinoids	5

Bronchoalveolar cell carcinoma is regarded as a subset of ade-nocarcinoma, whose incidence appears to be increasing with time. This tumor is also associated with women and nonsmokers and can present as a single mass, multiple nodules, or an infiltrate. The clinical course can vary from indolent progression to rapid diffuse dissemination.

Squamous cell carcinoma accounts for approximately 25% of all lung cancers. Most (66%) present as central lesions and are asso-ciated with cavitation in 7-10% of cases. Unlike adenocarcinoma, the tumor often remains localized, tending to spread initially to regional lymph nodes rather than systemically.

Large cell carcinoma accounts for approximately 7–10% of all lung cancers. Clinically, large cell carcinomas behave aggres-sively, with early metastases to the regional nodes in the medi-astinum and distant sites such as the brain.

SCLC

Small cell carcinoma is associated with neuroendocrine carci-noma because of ultrastructural and immunohistochemical simi-larities. Some pathologists feel small cell carcinomas represent a spectrum of disease beginning with the well-differentiated, benign carcinoid tumor (Kulchitsky I), including the less differ-entiated atypical carcinoids (Kulchitsky II) or neuroendocrine carcinomas, and ending with the undifferentiated small cell carcinomas (Kulchitsky III). Small cell carcinomas tend to pre-sent with metastatic and regional spread and are usually treated with chemotherapy with or without radiation therapy. Surgery is only used to remove the occasional localized peripheral nodule.

Carcinoids tend to arise from major bronchi and are central tumors. Metastasis is rare. Immunohistochemically, carcinoids express neuron-specific enolase (NSE), chromogranin, and synap-tophysin virtually without exception.

Neuroendocrine carcinomas or *atypical carcinoids* occur more peripherally than carcinoids and have a more aggressive course, although surgery should still be considered according to clinical stage. Without appropriate immunostaining, they may inadver-tently be classified as large cell carcinomas.

DIAGNOSIS

Signs and symptoms occur in 90–95% of patients at the time of diagnosis. Intraparenchymal tumors cause cough, hemoptysis, dyspnea, wheezing, and fever (often due to infection from proximal bronchial tumor obstruction). Regional spread of the tumor within the thorax can lead to pleural effusions or chest wall pain. Less common symptoms are superior vena cava syndrome, Pancoast's tumor, Horner's syndrome, and involvement of the recurrent laryngeal nerve, the phrenic nerve, the vagus nerve, or the esophagus. Paraneoplastic syndromes are found in 10% of lung cancer patients, most commonly those with SCLC. These syndromes are numerous and can affect endocrine, neurologic, skeletal, hematologic, and cutaneous systems.

A standard chest radiograph (CXR) is the initial diagnostic study for the evaluation of suspected lung cancer. The limit of detection of a lung mass is approximately 7 mm. Computed tomography (CT) can provide additional information and should include imaging of the liver and adrenals to rule out two common sites for intra-abdominal metastases. CT helps assess local extension to other thoracic structures as well as the presence of mediastinal adenopathy. Unfortunately, CT cannot definitively predict mediastinal nodal involvement because not all malignant lymph nodes are enlarged and many enlarged nodes are simply larger because of proximal infection. Lymph nodes larger than 1 cm have a 30% chance of being benign, whereas lymph nodes smaller than 1 cm still have a 15% chance of containing tumor. Because of this uncertainty, histologic confirmation is required to confirm the presence of mediastinal adenopathy. Histologic confirmation can be obtained by CT-guided fine-needle aspiration, bronchoscopy-directed Wang needle aspiration, or mediastinoscopy. At present, magnetic resonance imaging (MRI) adds little to the information gained by CT imaging, and other modalities such as PET scanning are still being evaluated. Because of their low yield, bone scans and MRI or CT of the brain should only be obtained when symptoms of metastatic disease are present (i.e., bone pain, headaches, or visual disturbances).

Histologic diagnosis of a lung tumor can be obtained by sputum cytology and bronchoscopy (central lesions) or by fluoroscopic fine-needle aspiration (FNA), or CT-guided biopsy (peripheral lesions). In certain patients whose probability of having cancer is high, the diagnosis can be obtained at the time of surgery (thoracotomy or video-assisted thoracic surgery [VATS]) with frozen-section analysis of a wedge resection.

STAGING

The primary goal of pretreatment staging is to determine the extent of disease so that prognosis and treatment can be determined. In SCLC, most patients present with metastatic or advanced locoregional disease. A simple two-stage system classifies the SCLC as limited or extensive disease. Limited disease is confined to one hemithorax, ipsilateral or contralateral hilar or mediastinal nodes, and ipsilateral supraclavicular lymph nodes. Extensive disease has spread to the contralateral supraclavicular nodes or distant sites such as the contralateral lung, liver, brain, or bone marrow. Staging for SCLC requires a bone scan, bone marrow biopsy, and CT scans of the abdomen, brain, and chest.

Staging of NSCLC has most recently involved a system proposed in 1985: the International Lung Cancer Staging System or International Staging System (ISS). This system is based on TNM classifications as shown in Tables 7-2. Survival rates for patients with NSCLC by stage of disease are shown in Fig. 7-2. Because of heterogeneity within groups, further modifications to the ISS have been proposed that involve splitting stage I into IA (T1N0) and IB (T2N0) and stage II into IIA (T1N0) and IIB (T2N0) and moving the good-prognosis T3N0 patients (chest wall involvement without nodal spread) into IIB. Staging of NSCLC involves a thorough history and physical examination, CXR, and CT scans of the chest and upper abdomen. Because of the low yield in asymptomatic patients, a bone scan or CT or MRI of the brain should only be obtained when suspected by history.

TREATMENT

Pretreatment Assessment

Once a patient has been staged clinically with noninvasive tests, a physiologic assessment should be performed to determine the patient's ability to tolerate different therapeutic modalities. In addition to a general evaluation of the patient's overall medical status, specific attention should be paid to the cardiovascular and respiratory systems. Cardiovascular screening should include a history and physical examination as well as a CXR and EKG. Patients with signs and symptoms of significant cardiac disease should undergo further noninvasive testing, including either exercise testing, echocardiography, or nuclear perfusion scans. Significant reversible cardiac problems should be addressed prior to therapy (i.e., chemotherapy, radiation therapy, or surgery).

The pulmonary reserve of lung cancer patients is commonly diminished as a result of tobacco abuse. Simple spirometry is an excellent initial screening test to quantify a patient's pulmonary reserve and ability to tolerate surgical resection. A postoperative forced expiratory volume in 1 second (FEV_1) of less than 0.8 liter or less than 35% of predicted is associated with an increased risk of perioperative complications, respiratory insufficiency, and death. The predicted postoperative FEV_1 is estimated by subtracting the contribution of the lung to be resected from the preoperative FEV_1. In certain instances, the lung to be resected does not contribute much to the preoperative FEV_1 because of tumor, atelectasis, or pneumonitis. Thus more accurate determination of predicted postoperative FEV_1 can be obtained by performing a ventilation perfusion scan and subtracting the exact contribution of the lung to be resected. In patients who fail spirometry criteria but are still felt to be operative candidates, oxygen consumption studies can be obtained that measure both respiratory and cardiac capacity. A maximum oxygen consumption (VO_2 max) of greater than 15 ml min^{-1} kg^{-1} indicates low risk, whereas a VO_2 max of less than 10 ml min^{-1} kg^{-1} is associated with high risk (a

Table 7-2. TNM descriptors

Primary tumor (T)

TX   Primary tumor cannot be assessed or tumor proven by the presence of malignant cells in sputum or bronchial washings but not visualized by imaging or bronchoscopy

T0   No evidence of primary tumor

Tis   Carcinoma *in situ*

T1   Tumor ≤3 cm in greatest dimension, surrounded by lung or visceral pleura, without bronchoscopic evidence of invasion more proximal than the lobar bronchus* (i.e., not in the main bronchus)

T2   Tumor with any of the following features of size or extent:
         >3 cm in greatest dimension
         Involving main bronchus, ≥2 cm distal to the carina
         Invading the visceral pleura
         Associated with atelectasis or obstructive pneumonitis that extends to the hilar region but does not involve the entire lung

T3   Tumor of any size that directly invades any of the following: chest wall (including superior sulcus tumors), diaphragm, mediastinal pleura, parietal pericardium; or tumor in the main bronchus <2 cm distal to the carina but without involvement of the carina; or associated atelectasis or obstructive pneumonitis of the entire lung

T4   Tumor of any size that invades any of the following: mediastinum, heart, great vessels, trachea, esophagus, vertebral body, carina; or tumor with a malignant pleural or pericardial effusion,† or with satellite tumor nodule(s) within the ipsilateral primary-tumor lobe of the lung

Regional lymph nodes (N)

NX   Regional lymph nodes cannot be assessed

N0   No regional lymph node metastasis

N1   Metastasis to ipsilateral peribronchial and/or ipsilateral hilar lymph nodes, and intrapulmonary nodes involved by direct extension of the primary tumor

N2   Metastasis to ipsilateral mediastinal and/or subcarinal lymph nodes(s)

N3   Metastasis to contralateral mediastinal, contralateral hilar, ipsilateral or contralateral scalene, or supraclavicular lymph node(s)

Distant metastasis (M)

MX   Presence of distant metastasis cannot be assessed

M0   No distant metastasis

M1   Distant metastasis present‡

---

* The uncommon superficial tumor of any size with its invasive component limited to the bronchial wall, which may extend proximal to the main bronchus, is also classified T1.

† Most pleural effusions associated with lung cancer are due to tumor. However, there are a few patients in whom multiple cytopathologic examinations of pleural fluid show no tumor. In these cases, the fluid is nonbloody and is not an exudate. When these elements and clinical judgment dictate that the effusion is not related to the tumor, the effusion should be excluded as a staging element and the patient's disease should be staged T1, T2, or T3. Pericardial effusion is classified according to the same rules.

‡ Separate metastatic tumor nodule(s) in the ipsilateral nonprimary-tumor lobe(s) of the lung also are classified M1.

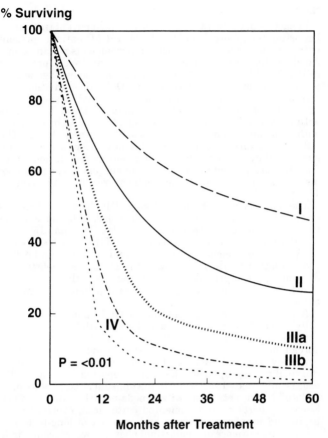

Fig. 7-2. Cumulative survival according to clinical stage of non–small cell lung cancer.

mortality rate of more than 30% in some series). Additional risk factors for lung resection include a predicted postoperative diffusing capacity (DLCO) or maximum ventilatory ventilation (MVV) of less than 40% and hypercarbia (>45 mm CO_2) or hypoxemia (<60 mm O_2) on preoperative arterial blood gases. In conjunction with clinical assessment, these tests can help identify those patients at high risk for complications during and after surgical resection.

Preoperative training with an incentive spirometer, initiation of bronchodilators, weight reduction, good nutrition, and cessation of smoking for at least 2 weeks prior to surgery can help minimize complications and improve performance on spirometry for patients with marginal pulmonary reserve.

NSCLC

In early-stage NSCLC, surgery is a critical part of treatment. Unfortunately, more than 50–70% of NSCLC patients present with advanced disease for which surgery alone is not an option. An algorithm for treatment based on clinical stage is presented in Fig. 7-3. Physiologically fit patients with early-stage lesions (stage I or II) are treated with surgery. Definitive radiation therapy is indicated if surgery cannot be tolerated. Five-year survival rates of 60–70% and 39–43% can be achieved for patients with stage I and II disease, respectively. Chest wall involvement without nodal spread (T3N0) was formally considered stage IIIa, but because survival rates of 33–60% have been achieved with surgery, they are now considered as early-stage lesion (stage IIa). If these patients cannot tolerate surgery because of poor medical status, definitive radiation can result in survivals of 15–35%.

The remainder of patients with stage IIIa disease (N2 disease or chest wall with nodal involvement) classically have a poor response to surgery, with 5-year survivals of less than 15%. The standard treatment for these patients and those with stage IIIb or IV includes chemotherapy (VP-16 and cisplatin) and definitive radiation therapy for local palliation. Some reports have demonstrated improved survival when chemotherapy is combined with radiation therapy as opposed to radiation therapy alone.

A small subset of stage IIIb tumors can be approached surgically. These tumors are considered stage IIIb because of local extension (T4N0) into adjacent structures rather than systemic spread (nodes, hematogenous metastases) and may benefit from aggressive surgical resection of the atrium, carina, or vertebrae. Survival rates of up to 30% have been reported. Metastatic disease is only treated surgically in the unusual circumstance of an isolated brain metastasis with a node-negative lung primary. Several reports have documented better local control (in the brain and lung) with surgery and a subset of long-term survivors. The presence of mediastinal nodes, however, contraindicates surgical resection and mandates radiation therapy for the lung primary.

Surgery

Pneumonectomy

The removal of the whole lung was previously the most commonly performed operation for NSCLC; it now accounts for only 20% of all resections. Although a more complete resection is accomplished using pneumonectomy versus parenchyma-conserving techniques (lobectomy), it comes at the cost of higher mortality (4–10%) and morbidity without clear survival benefits.

Lobectomy

The similar survival of patients treated by lobectomy versus pneumonectomy, along with the lower morbidity and mortality associated with lobectomy, make lobectomy the preferred method of resection. Sleeve lobectomies and bronchoplasty procedures in which portions of the main bronchus are removed without loss

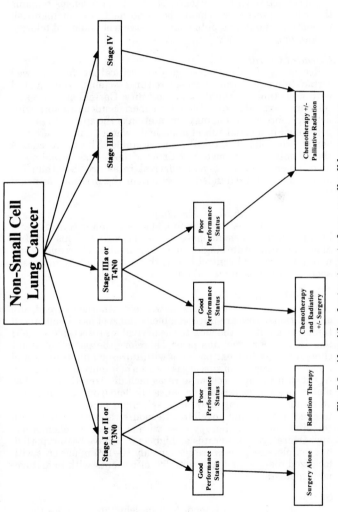

Fig. 7-3. Algorithm for treatment of non–small cell lung cancer.

of the distal lung have further decreased the need for pneumonectomies.

Lesser Resections

Segmentectomies and nonanatomic resections (wedge resection and lumpectomy) are associated with increased local recurrence when compared with lobectomy. The general consensus remains that these procedures should be performed only in high-risk patients with minimal pulmonary reserve who could not tolerate a lobectomy.

Extended Operations

Recent improvements in surgery and critical care have allowed certain tumors, previously considered unresectable, to be removed with acceptable morbidity and mortality. Carinal sleeve resections and extended resections for superior sulcus tumors with hemivertebrectomy and instrumentation of the spine can now be performed in a small subset of patients whose tumors were previously considered surgically unresectable. These procedures should only be performed in patients without mediastinal nodal involvement because 5-year survival rates are less than 5% for patients with extended resections in the presence of nodal involvement.

Mediastinal Lymph Node Dissection

Complete mediastinal lymph node dissection is controversial because survival benefits have not been clearly demonstrated. It allows more accurate staging and determination of prognosis and may improve local control but at the cost of slightly increased operative time (20 minutes) and morbidity.

Chemotherapy

Almost 50% of patients present with extrathoracic spread, and an additional 15% are unresectable because of locally advanced tumor. In addition, the long-term survival for resectable stage II and IIIa tumors remains poor. Therefore the use of adjuvant chemotherapy to treat patients with unresectable tumors and improve the results of surgery is an area of intense investigation. Agents with proven response rates include cisplatin and other platinum analogs, ifosfamide, vinca alkaloids, mitomycin C, and etoposide. Promising new agents include edatrexate, gemcitabine, taxanes, and navelbine. Response rates are higher with combination chemotherapy than with single-agent chemotherapy. Overall response rates as high as 80% have been reported, but complete responses are seen in only 10–15% of patients with localized disease and less than 5% of patients with hematogenous metastases.

SCLC

Unlike NSCLC, SCLC tends to be disseminated at presentation and is therefore not amenable to cure with surgery or thoracic radiation therapy alone. Without treatment, the disease is rapidly fatal, with few patients surviving more than 6 months. Fortunately, SCLC is very sensitive to chemotherapy, and more than two-thirds of patients achieve a partial response after systemic therapy with multidrug regimens. Treatment of SCLC therefore revolves around systemic chemotherapy. An algorithm based on the extent of disease is presented in Fig. 7-4. Complete response is seen in as many as 20–50% of patients with limited disease, but these responses are not durable, and the 5-year survival rate is still less than 10%.

Chemotherapeutic regimens for SCLC most commonly include combinations of cyclophosphamide, cisplatin, etoposide, doxorubicin, and vincristine. Thoracic radiotherapy has been shown to improve local control of the primary tumor and is often included as part of the treatment for limited SCLC. In addition, because brain metastases are noted in 80% of patients with SCLC during the course of their disease, patients who show no evidence of brain metastases on CT scans and who achieve a good response from therapy are usually treated with prophylactic brain irradiation to minimize the chances of developing this morbid site of treatment failure.

There does exist a small role for surgical resection of SCLC. Solitary peripheral pulmonary nodules with no evidence of metastatic disease after evaluation with bone scan, bone marrow biopsy, and CT of the abdomen, brain, and chest can be treated with lobectomy and postoperative chemotherapy if mediastinoscopy is negative. In these select patients, 5-year survival of 50% has been achieved for T1N0, T2N0, and completely resected N1 disease. Surgery for more central lesions, however, has not been demonstrated to improve survival over that achieved with chemotherapy and radiotherapy alone.

Surveillance

The few treatment options for tumor recurrence in NSLC have limited the cost-effectiveness of aggressive radiologic surveillance following surgical resection. Nevertheless, there is an increased incidence of second primary lung cancers (3% per year), and annual or semiannual CXR may help detect these lesions. Any patient who develops symptoms in the interim should also be evaluated aggressively for recurrence or a new primary.

Metastatic Neoplasms to the Lung

The lung and liver are the most common sites of metastases. Patients with isolated lung metastases can achieve survival rates of 25–40% if complete surgical resection is obtained. Because metastases can recur, resection involves nonanatomic wedge or laser resections to preserve the lung parenchyma.

PATHOLOGY

The biology of the underlying primary malignancy determines the behavior of its metastases. Metastases may occur via hematogenous, lymphatic, direct, or aerogenous routes. Thirty percent of lung cancer patients die with isolated pulmonary metastases.

DIAGNOSIS

Because of their predominantly peripheral localization, most pulmonary metastases remain asymptomatic, with fewer than

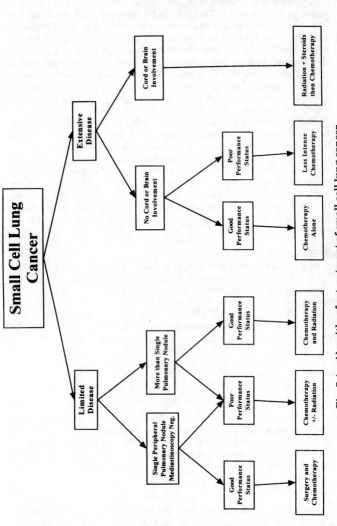

Fig. 7-4. Algorithm for treatment of small cell lung cancer.

5% showing symptoms at presentation. Diagnosis is commonly made during radiographic follow-up after treatment of the primary malignancy.

Routine CXR during surveillance after cancer treatment is an effective means of screening patients for pulmonary metastases. Indeed, several studies have demonstrated the increased sensitivity of CT over standard CXR. However, the cost-effectiveness of CT for screening remains low, and no data as yet suggest that early detection with CT leads to improved survival. Planning of surgical interventions, however, should be based on CT findings, even though CT scanning still misses approximately 30% of the nodules found at surgery.

When multiple pulmonary nodules are present in patients with a known previous malignancy, the likelihood of metastatic disease approaches 100%. New solitary lesions, however, often represent primary lung cancers because many of the risk factors are similar.

STAGING

No valid staging system exists for pulmonary metastases. The International Registry of Lung Metastases (IRLM) has identified three parameters of prognostic significance: resectability, disease-free interval, and number of metastases. The present criteria for resectability include resectable pulmonary nodules, control of the primary tumor, adequate predicted postoperative pulmonary reserve, and no extrathoracic metastases. Favorable histologies for long-term survival following resection include sarcoma, breast, colon, and genitourinary metastases. Unfavorable histologies include melanomas, esophageal, pancreatic, and gastric cancers.

TREATMENT

Surgery

Preoperative evaluation for resection of pulmonary metastases is similar to that for any other pulmonary resection. Because of the increased risk of recurrent metastases and need for future thoracotomies, parenchyma-conserving procedures are favored (wedge resection, laser or cautery excision). The various surgical approaches include the following:

Median sternotomy allows bilateral exploration with one incision. Lesions located near the hilum can be difficult to reach, and exposure of the left lower lobe—especially in patients with obesity, cardiomegaly, or an elevated left hemidiaphragm—is poor.

Bilateral anterothoracosternotomy (clamshell procedure) allows excellent exposure of both hemithoraces, including the left lower lobe, although some surgeons feel the incision increases postoperative pain.

Posterolateral thoracotomy is a more common incision for access to the lung. The limitation to one hemithorax, however, necessitates a second staged operation for removing bilateral metastases.

Thoracoscopic resection allows visualization of both hemithoraces during the same anesthetic. Pleural-based lesions are therefore easily visualized and excised. Unfortunately, the ability to carefully evaluate the parenchyma for deeper or smaller nonvisualized lesions is poor, and some reports suggest an increased risk of local recurrence with thoracoscopy.

At the time of surgery, wedge resections with a 1-cm margin are preferred. If multiple nodules within one segment, lobe, or lung preclude resection of multiple wedges, then laser resections can be performed.

Adjuvant Therapy

Radiotherapy's role in the treatment of pulmonary metastases is limited to the palliation of symptoms of advanced lesions with extensive pleural, bony, or neural involvement. The value of chemotherapy pre- or postoperatively remains controversial. There are many isolated reports of the benefit of chemotherapy, especially when the primary tumor is sensitive (e.g., osteosarcoma, teratoma, and other germ cell tumors). However, improvements in survival are more difficult to achieve when the primary is of other types.

Surveillance

The frequency and intensity of follow-up after resection are determined by the primary tumor but usually involve annual or biannual CXR. CT scans should be reserved for evaluations subsequent to abnormal CXR findings or evaluation of adjuvant therapies.

Neoplasms of the Mediastinum

The mediastinal compartment can harbor a number of lesions of congenital, infectious, developmental, traumatic, or neoplastic origin. Earlier recommendations advocated a direct surgical approach to all mediastinal tumors, with biopsy or debulking of unresectable lesions. However, recent advances in imaging and noninvasive diagnostic techniques, as well as improvements in chemotherapy and radiotherapy, have led to a more conservative approach, with management decisions based on better preoperative evaluation.

PATHOLOGY

A recent study combining nine previous series was performed to better approximate the true incidence of mediastinal lesions (Table 7-3). In adults, neurogenic and thymic tumors contribute 19% and 23%, respectively, to the overall incidence, whereas in children they contribute 39% and 3%, respectively. This section will not attempt to describe the myriad of cystic and other rare miscellaneous lesions but will concentrate on the more common diagnoses.

Neurogenic tumors include schwannoma, neurofibroma, ganglioneuroblastoma, neuroblastoma, pheochromocytoma, and paraganglioma. They are the most common tumors arising in the posterior compartment.

Thymoma arises from thymic epithelium, although its microscopic appearance is a mixture of lymphocytes and epithelial

Table 7-3. Overall incidence of mediastinal tumors

Thymic	19 (3)*
Neurogenic	23 (39)*
Lymphoma	12
Germ Cell	12
Cysts	18
Mesenchymal	8
Miscellaneous	8

* ( ) incidence in children

cells. Thymomas are classified as lymphocytic (30% of cases), epithelial (16%), mixed (30%), and spindle cell (24%). Histologic evidence of malignancy is difficult to obtain, as benign and malignant lesions can have similar histologic and cytologic features. Surgical evidence of invasion at the time of resection is the most reliable method of differentiating between malignant and benign thymomas.

Lymphomas make up approximately 50% of childhood and 20% of adult anterior mediastinal malignancies. They are treated nonsurgically but may require surgery to secure a diagnosis.

Germ cell tumors are comprised of teratomas, seminomas, and nonseminomatous germ cell tumors. Teratomas are the most common and are mostly benign. Malignant teratomas are very rare and often widely metastatic at the time of diagnosis. Seminomas progress in a locally aggressive fashion. Nonseminomatous malignant tumors include embryonal carcinoma and choriocarcinoma, both of which carry a poor prognosis, and the more favorable endodermal sinus tumor.

Miscellaneous cysts and mesenchymal tumors include thyroid goiters, thyroid malignancies, mediastinal parathyroid adenomas, bronchogenic cysts, pericardial cysts, duplications, diverticula, and aneurysms.

DIAGNOSIS

Mediastinal lesions are most commonly asymptomatic. When symptoms do occur, they result from compression of adjacent structures or systemic endocrine or autoimmune effects of the tumors. Children, with their smaller chest cavities, tend to have symptoms at presentation (two-thirds of children versus only one-third of adults) and more commonly have malignant lesions (greater than 50%). Symptoms can include cough, stridor, and dyspnea (more common in children) as well as symptoms of local invasion such as chest pain, pleural effusion, hoarseness, Horner's syndrome, upper-extremity and back pain, paraplegia, and diaphragmatic paralysis.

Chest radiography remains a mainstay of diagnosis. Fifty percent of lesions are diagnosed by CXR. The position of the tumor within the mediastinum on lateral projection can help tailor the differential diagnosis (Fig. 7-5, Table 7-4). The standard for further assessment of the lesion is CT scanning, specifically with contrast enhancement. Certain tumors and benign conditions can be diagnosed or strongly suggested by their appearance on CT

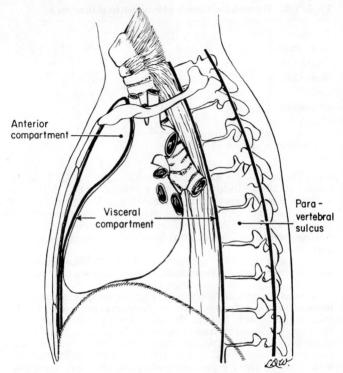

Anterior compartment

Visceral compartment

Para-vertebral sulcus

Fig. 7-5. Anatomic boundaries of mediastinal masses according to one commonly used classification.

scans. Angiography and/or MRI may be required if a major resective procedure is planned and vascular involvement suspected. Nuclear imaging—such as thyroid and parathyroid scanning, gallium scanning for lymphoma, and metaiodobenzylguanidine scanning for pheochromocytomas—may also be indicated.

The use of serum markers can be of some assistance in the diagnosis of some germ cell and neuroendocrine tumors. In addition, the association of myasthenia gravis with thymoma can also assist in the diagnosis.

Because many mediastinal tumors are treated without surgery, a determined effort should be made to achieve a tissue diagnosis noninvasively. FNA, with its reasonable sensitivity, is an excellent starting point, but the diagnosis of lymphoma can be difficult because only a limited number of cells are retrieved. Bronchoscopy and esophagoscopy can also be useful if symptoms and/or imaging studies suggest tumor involvement.

If these procedures cannot help make a diagnosis then a mediastinoscopy to access paratracheal lesions can be performed. Although the risk of vascular or tracheobronchial injury is present,

Table 7-4. Usual location of the common primary tumors and cysts of the mediastinum

Anterior compartment	Visceral compartment	Paravertebral sulci
Thymoma	Enterogenous cyst	Neurilemoma-schwannoma
Germ cell tumors	Lymphoma	Neurofibroma
Lymphoma	Pleuropericardial cyst	Malignant schwannoma
Lymphangioma	Mediastinal granuloma	Ganglioneuroma
Hemangioma	Lymphoid hamartoma	Ganglioneuro-blastoma
Lipoma	Mesothelial cyst	Neuroblastoma
Fibroma	Neuroenteric cyst	Paraganglioma
Fibrosarcoma	Paraganglioma	Pheochromocytoma
Thymic cyst	Pheochromocytoma	Fibrosarcoma
Parathyroid adenoma	Thoracic duct cyst	Lymphoma
Aberrant thyroid		

the incidence of complications is very low in experienced hands. If more invasive procedures are required to make the diagnosis, an anterior or parasternal mediastinotomy (Chamberlain procedure) or thoracoscopy can be performed. Rarely, a sternotomy or thoracotomy will be required to obtain a tissue diagnosis.

STAGING

Staging is determined by the specific histology identified and its extent at the time of diagnosis.

TREATMENT

Therapy, like staging, is determined by the type of tumor and its histology (see Table 7-5). The primary determination to be made is whether the lesion will require resection as part of its treatment or whether chemotherapy and/or radiotherapy is

Table 7-5. Frequency and treatment of malignant chest wall tumors

Cell type	Estimated frequency (%)	Standard therapy
Chondrosarcoma	35	Surgical resection
Plasmacytoma	25	Radiation + chemotherapy
Ewing's sarcoma	15	Surgery + chemotherapy
Osteosarcoma	15	Surgery + chemotherapy
Lymphoma	10	Chemotherapy ± radiation

sufficient. Thymomas should all be resected, with the possibility of postoperative radiotherapy. Benign neurogenic tumors are sometimes observed in older debilitated patients; however, if the patient is otherwise healthy or if malignant potential is suspected, then resection should be pursued. Germ cell tumors should be treated on the basis of their histology. In particular, benign teratomas should be resected, seminomas should be treated with radiation therapy, and nonseminomatous tumors should be treated initially with chemotherapy. In the subset of nonseminomatous tumors that have a residual mass but negative markers, surgical resection should be performed to rule out residual tumor. Lymphomas should not be resected and should be treated with radiation and/or chemotherapy on the basis of their stage and histology (i.e., Hodgkin's versus non-Hodgkin's).

SURVEILLANCE

The frequency and intensity of follow-up after resection are determined by the primary tumor. Chest radiography remains the mainstay of surveillance, with CT scanning reserved for evaluation subsequent to abnormal CXR findings.

Neoplasms of the Chest Wall

Primary chest wall malignancies account for less than 1% of all tumors and include a wide variety of bone and soft-tissue lesions. The absence of large series makes the prospective evaluation of treatment options difficult. As more patients with these tumors are treated at large referral institutions, the initiation of multi-institutional trials will help settle some of the more controversial aspects of therapy.

PATHOLOGY

Primary chest wall tumors include chondrosarcoma (20%), Ewing's sarcoma (8–22%), osteosarcoma (10%), plasmacytoma (10–30%), and infrequently, soft-tissue sarcoma. Chondrosarcomas arise from the ribs in 80% of cases and from the sternum in the remaining 20%. They are related to prior chest wall trauma in 12.5% of cases and are very radio- and chemoresistant. Ewing's sarcoma is part of a spectrum of disease having primitive neuroectodermal tumors at one end and Ewing's sarcoma at the other. Multimodality therapy, including both radiotherapy and chemotherapy, has been shown to be beneficial for this tumor. Osteosarcomas are best treated with neoadjuvant therapy, with prognosis being predicted by the tumor's response to chemotherapy. Plasmacytoma confined to the chest must be confirmed by evaluating the remaining skeletal system. Surgery can then be used to confirm the diagnosis. If radiotherapy is unable to achieve local control, then resection may be indicated. Soft-tissue sarcomas are rare and are primarily resected. Adjuvant therapy is based on tumor histology.

DIAGNOSIS

Chest wall tumors are asymptomatic in 20% of patients, whereas the remaining 80% have an enlarging mass. Fifty to sixty percent of these patients will have associated pain. Radiographic assessment usually includes CXR and CT; however, MRI is being used instead with increasing frequency because its ability to image in multiple planes with superior anatomic distinction can better reveal disease extent than CT or plain radiography. Pathologic diagnosis is made with FNA (64% accuracy) or core-cutting biopsy (96% accuracy).

STAGING

Chest wall lesions are staged according to the primary tumor identified. Most progress to pulmonary or hepatic metastases without lymphatic involvement.

TREATMENT

As outlined earlier, the treatment of chest wall lesions is determined by the diagnosis. Most, with few exceptions, require resection as part of the treatment. Posterior lesions reaching deep to the scapula or lesions that require resection of less than two ribs do not require reconstruction of the chest wall. However, all other lesions require some form of stable reconstructive technique. A simple mesh closure using Marlex or Proline mesh is acceptable as long as the material is secured in position under tension. Some surgeons feel there is a loss of tensile strength over time. A more rigid prosthesis is methyl methacrylate sandwiched between two layers of Marlex mesh. Long-term seroma formation plagues all types of repair, particularly this latter repair technique.

If the chest wall lesion involves the overlying muscle or the skin, a large defect may be present after resection. This may require a muscle flap for final reconstruction, especially if postoperative radiotherapy is considered. Though description of the techniques available is beyond the scope of this manual, let it be said that a combination of muscle flap with primary skin closure, muscle flap with skin grafting, or myocutaneous flap coverage can be used.

SURVEILLANCE

Once treated and in remission, chest wall tumors tend to recur locally or with pulmonary or hepatic metastases. Regular follow-up with careful examination and a CXR should suffice to detect all significant sites of recurrence.

Neoplasms of the Pleura

There are two main types of pleural neoplasms. Malignant pleural mesothelioma remains an uncommon and highly lethal tumor with no adequate method of treatment. It behaves primarily as a locally aggressive tumor with locally invasive failure after therapy and only metastasizes late in its course. Its relationship with asbestos exposure was suggested in the 1940s and 1950s, and clearly established in 1960. A more localized pleural tumor, known as localized fibrous tumor of the pleura, can also occur; when malignant, it is frequently classified as a localized mesothelioma.

PATHOLOGY

Localized mesotheliomas and malignant localized fibrous tumors of the pleura are very rare. There is some controversy as to whether these lesions are even mesothelial at all because no epithelial component may be identifiable. More commonly, a benign localized fibrous tumor of the pleura is found. On the other hand, diffuse pleural mesothelioma is always a malignant process. There is a 20-year latency for development of this disease after exposure to asbestos. A recent surge in the incidence of this disease reflects the widespread use of asbestos in the 1940s and 1950s, and this surge should continue because mechanisms for limiting occupational asbestos exposure were not instituted until the 1970s. Mesothelioma almost always exhibits an epithelial component, which can be combined with sarcomatoid features. Thus it can be hard to differentiate this lesion from metastatic adenocarcinoma. Immunohistochemistry and electron microscopy, however, have aided in establishing the diagnosis.

DIAGNOSIS

The presentation of mesothelioma is often vague and nonspecific, with dyspnea and pain common in 90% of patients. Radiographic diagnosis in the early stage is often difficult, with the findings limited to a pleural effusion in many cases. Even CT may fail to identify any other abnormalities at this stage. The classic finding of a thick, restrictive pleural rind is a late finding. Thoracentesis is diagnostic in 50% of patients, and pleural biopsy is positive in 33%. If the diagnosis remains elusive, a thoracoscopy is diagnostic in 80% of patients.

STAGING

A staging system for mesothelioma has been proposed by Butchart and is shown in Table 7-6.

TREATMENT

The treatment of mesothelioma is still evolving. Attempts at radical resections, such as extrapleural pneumonectomy, have led to some improvements in local control but only limited impact on survival at the cost of a significantly increased operative risk. Likewise, chemotherapy and radiotherapy have had only limited effects, with less impact on palliation. Institutional trials are under way to examine new methods of treatment, such as intrapleural instillation of new chemotherapeutic agents.

SURVEILLANCE

Mesotheliomas tend to recur locally. CT scans are required to detect recurrences or follow residual disease. Unfortunately, treatment options are limited, but they do include radiation therapy and chemotherapy.

Table 7-6. Staging of mesothelioma

Stage	Characteristic
I	Within the capsule of the parietal pleura: ipsilateral pleura, lung, pericardium, or diaphragm
II	Tumor involving the chest wall or mediastinum: esophagus, trachea, or great vessels
	Positive lymph nodes within the chest
III	Tumor penetrating the diaphragmatic muscle to involve the peritoneum or the retroperitoneal space; tumor penetrating the pericardium to involve its internal surface or the heart
	Involvement of the opposite pleura
	Positive lymph nodes outside the chest
IV	Distant blood-borne metastases

Selected References

Anderson BO, Burt ME. Chest wall neoplasms and their management. *Ann Thorac Surg* 58:1774, 1994.

Dartevelle PG. Extended operations for the treatment of lung cancer. *Ann Thorac Surg* 63:12, 1997.

Ginsberg RJ, Rubinstein LV. Randomized trial of lobectomy versus limited resection for T1 N0 non–small cell lung cancer: Lung cancer study group. *Ann Thorac Surg* 60:615, 1995.

Moreno de la Santa P, Butchart EG. Therapeutic options in malignant mesothelioma. *Curr Opin Oncol* 7:134, 1995.

Mountain CF. Revisions in the international system for staging lung cancer. *Chest* 111:1710, 1997.

Nesbitt JC, Putnam JB, Walsh GL, et al. Survival in early-stage non–small cell lung cancer. *Ann Thorac Surg* 60:466, 1995.

Parker SL, Tong T, Bolden S, et al. Cancer statistics, 1997. *CA Cancer J Clin* 47:5, 1997.

Pastorino U, Buyse M, Friedel G, et al. Long-term results of lung metastasectomy: Prognostic analyses based on 5206 cases. *J Thorac Cardiovasc Surg* 113:37, 1997.

Roth JA, Fossella F, Komaki R, et al. A randomized trial comparing perioperative chemotherapy and surgery with surgery alone in resectable stage III non-small cell lung cancer. *J Natl Cancer Inst* 86:673, 1994.

Shields TW. Primary mediastinal tumors and cysts and their diagnostic investigation. In Shields TW (eds.), *Mediastinal Surgery*. Philadelphia: Lea & Febiger, 1991.

Sugarbaker DJ, Jaklitsch MT, Liptay MJ. Mesothelioma and radical multimodality therapy: Who benefits? *Chest* 107:345S, 1995.

Walsh GL, Morice RC, Putnam JB, et al. Resection of lung cancer is justified in high-risk patients selected by exercise oxygen consumption. *Ann Thorac Surg* 58:704, 1994.

Walsh GL, O'Connor M, Willis KM, et al. Is follow-up of lung cancer patients after resection medically indicated and cost effective? *Ann Thorac Surg* 60:1563, 1995.

8

Esophageal Carcinoma

Ara A. Vaporciyan and Stephen G. Swisher

Carcinoma of the esophagus accounted for approximately 12,500 new cases and 11,500 deaths in the United States in 1997. In the last 30 years the overall 5-year survival rate for this cancer has improved from 3% to 15%. Even though esophageal cancer is curable at an early stage, overall survival is poor because the large majority of tumors are quite advanced at presentation. Recent treatment strategies have included multimodality approaches combining surgery, radiation therapy, and chemotherapy. These regimens have resulted in 5-year survival rates of 40–75% in the subset of patients who achieve a complete histologic response after preoperative chemotherapy and radiation therapy.

Etiology

The worldwide incidence of esophageal cancer varies more than that of any other cancer. In the United States, the rate of esophageal cancer is approximately seven cases per 100,000 people, whereas in high-risk areas of China, Iran, and Russia, the incidence is closer to 100 per 100,000 people. These geographic variations imply an etiologic role for local environmental or dietary carcinogens.

A number of compounds and clinical diagnoses are associated with an increased risk of squamous cell cancer (SCC) of the esophagus, including low socioeconomic status, race, and increased tobacco and alcohol use. Additional risk factors include N-nitrosamines, achalasia, tylosis, caustic strictures, celiac disease, and Plummer-Vinson syndrome.

The risk factors for esophageal adenocarcinoma differ markedly from those of esophageal SCC and include the presence of gastroesophageal reflux and Barrett's esophagus. High-risk patients include young white males with a history of gastroesophageal reflux.

Pathology

There are two histologic types of esophageal cancer: adenocarcinoma and SCC. Adenocarcinoma is uncommon worldwide but has shown a marked increase in the last decade in the United States. The percentage of adenocarcinomas increased from 17% to 31% from 1976 to 1984. Approximately 15% of all esophageal cancers occur in the upper third of the esophagus, 50% in the middle third, and 35% in the lower third. Adenocarcinomas usually occur in the distal third of the esophagus, often in association with Barrett's esophagus or a proximal gastric carcinoma extending into the esophagus.

Diagnosis

The initial symptoms of esophageal cancer in 90% of patients are dysphagia and weight loss. Dysphagia occurs when the diameter of the esophagus is narrowed to less than 13 mm. Occasionally, the onset of dysphagia is sudden; however, most patients present with vague symptoms of mild dysphagia that precede their presentation to their physicians by 3–6 months. In approximately 50% of patients, variable degrees of odynophagia (painful swallowing) are present. Less common symptoms include regurgitation of undigested food, retrosternal or epigastric pain, and aspiration pneumonia. Patients with locally advanced lesions may also present with hematemesis, melena, tracheo-esophageal fistula, hemoptysis, or hoarseness. Erosion into the aorta with exsanguinating hemorrhage has been reported. Although infrequent, bleeding from the tumor mass can occur in 4–7% of patients.

Findings at exam depend in large part upon the degree of weight loss. Enlarged cervical or supraclavicular lymph nodes can be biopsied with fine-needle aspiration (FNA), and bone pain should be evaluated with a bone scan to exclude distant metastases. All neurologic symptoms (e.g., headaches, visual disturbances) should also be assessed with a computed tomography (CT) or magnetic resonance imaging (MRI) scan of the brain.

Initial radiographic evaluation should include a chest x-ray (CXR) and barium swallow study. The barium study should include double contrast to completely evaluate the mucosa of the esophagus as well as to evaluate the stomach for evidence of disease or abnormalities that would preclude its use as a conduit. CT scans of the chest and abdomen should also be obtained to evaluate local invasion of mediastinal structures as well as significant adenopathy.

Endoscopic evaluation of the esophagus should be performed to obtain a histologic diagnosis and to identify any intramural metastases. Endoscopic dilation of tight strictures can be done to allow passage of the endoscope beyond the tumor. Involvement of the upper or middle third of the esophagus mandates bronchoscopy to rule out tracheobronchial involvement.

Staging

The TNM staging system for the cervical and thoracic esophagus is outlined in Table 8-1. Clinical evaluation, especially of nodal metastases, is difficult. CT scanning can provide some evidence of tumor extension and, to a lesser degree, nodal metastases with a reported accuracy of 88–100% and 78–85%, respectively. The addition of endoscopic ultrasound allows more subtle differentiation of the depth of tumor involvement and reportedly better results than CT, but it does not add significantly to the identification of nodal metastases. Evaluation of nodal metastases remains the role of the surgeon at exploration.

Table 8-1.   TNM staging for esophageal cancer

Primary tumor (T)

Tx	Primary tumor cannot be assessed
T0	No evidence of primary tumor
Tis	Carcinoma *in situ*
T1	Tumor invades lamina propria or submucosa
T2	Tumor invades muscularis propria
T3	Tumor invades adventitia
T4	Tumor invades adjacent structures

Regional lymph nodes (N)

Nx	Regional nodes cannot be assessed
N0	No regional node metastasis
N1	Regional node metastasis

Distant metastasis (M)

Mx	Presence of distant metastasis cannot be assessed
M0	No distant metastases
M1	Distant metastasis

Stage grouping

Stage 0	Tis	N0	M0
Stage I	T1	N0	M0
Stage IIA	T2	N0	M0
	T3	N0	M0
Stage IIB	T1	N1	M0
	T2	N1	M0
Stage III	T3	N1	M0
	T4	Any N	M0
Stage IV	Any T	Any N	M1

Treatment

Patients should be approached with the intent to perform a surgical resection since this affords the best chance for cure (Fig. 8-1). Even though the pathologic stage correlates well with prognosis, accurate clinical staging is difficult because of the inability to evaluate occult nodal involvement. All patients who can physiologically tolerate resection and are without clinically evident distant metastases should undergo surgery. If distant metastases or advanced locoregional disease are found at exploration, nonoperative palliation should be performed because of the high perioperative mortality associated with surgical bypass (approximately 20%).

Operative mortalities for transhiatal or transthoracic esophagectomies in recent series are less than 5%, with rates of morbidity ranging from 10% to 27%. Five-year survival rates range from 68% to 85% for stage I and II patients and from 15% to 28% for stage III disease (Fig. 8-2). Unfortunately, the vast majority (70%) of patients have stage III or IV disease at presentation.

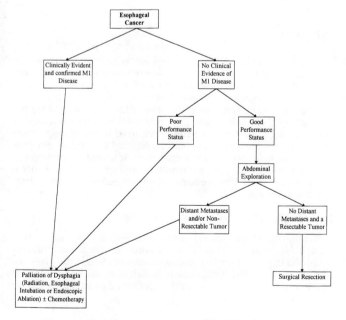

Fig. 8-1. Algorithm for treatment of esophageal cancer.

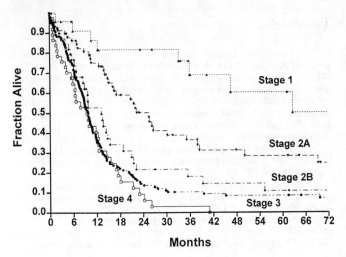

Fig. 8-2.   Survival curves of esophageal cancer.

Surgery

Surgical resection remains the best curative treatment for early-stage esophageal cancer. Five-year survival rates of 70% are reported for stage I disease (see Fig. 8-2). Advanced disease, however, is rarely cured by surgery but often provides the best long-term palliation of dysphagia. Because of the longitudinal spread of esophageal carcinoma via the submucosal lymphatics, a total or subtotal esophagectomy is usually required to completely excise the tumor. Segmental resections are plagued by positive margins and a high incidence of local recurrence. Adjuvant chemotherapy and radiation therapy may ultimately improve survival. At present, however, no definitive survival advantage for adjuvant therapy has been shown.

PREOPERATIVE EVALUATION

Evaluation of pulmonary reserve and cardiac status is warranted for most patients. Specific considerations that require attention in patients with esophageal cancer include the presence and severity of nutritional depletion, dehydration, and anemia. If present, these conditions should be corrected as expeditiously as possible.

INITIAL EVALUATION

All operations begin with a thorough abdominal exploration for evidence of metastases. The two most common sites of metastatic disease are the liver and the celiac nodes. If metastatic disease is identified, surgical resection should only be performed if nonsurgical palliation of dysphagia is not possible. After a complete abdominal exploration, the stomach is mobilized by dividing the gastrocolic ligament caudally and short gastric vessels with preservation of the right gastric and gastroepiploic arteries. The lesser omentum is divided close to the liver and the left gastric vessel is identified and ligated. A pyloroplasty or pyloromyotomy is performed to avoid gastric stasis, which can accompany division of the vagus nerves during esophageal transection.

SUBTOTAL ESOPHAGECTOMY

Distal esophageal tumors located at the gastroesophageal junction can be managed by subtotal esophagectomy with adequate local control. Known as an Ivor Lewis (or Tanner-Lewis modification) esophagectomy, this requires a right thoracotomy to complete the mobilization of the esophagus and create an intrathoracic esophagogastric anastomosis, usually at the level of the azygous vein. The proximal esophageal margin should be examined for the presence of cancer; if cancer is present, a total esophagectomy should be performed. A cervical anastomosis is preferred in this situation because of the increased risk of a high intrathoracic anastomosis.

TOTAL ESOPHAGECTOMY

Proximally located tumors (cervical or upper esophagus) require a total esophagectomy because of the difficulty of achieving negative margins with segmental resections (i.e., Ivor Lewis). Two popular methods differ by the presence or absence of thoracotomy for esophageal mobilization. The esophagus can be mobilized using a right thoracotomy with the conduit brought substernally or through the posterior mediastinum to the neck for anastomosis. Alternatively, a transhiatal esophagectomy can be performed with mobilization of the intrathoracic esophagus from the esophageal hiatus and the thoracic inlet without the need for a thoracotomy.

The advantage of the transhiatal technique is that it avoids a thoracotomy while achieving a complete removal of the esophagus. Potential disadvantages of the transhiatal technique include less complete periesophageal lymphadenectomy and risk of tracheobronchial or vascular injury during blunt dissection of the esophagus. In addition, a cervical anastomosis is associated with a higher anastomotic leak rate (12% vs. 5%) than is an intrathoracic anastomosis, although mortality is much less from a cervical leak than from a thoracic leak (2% vs. 50%). Multiple series have failed to show differences in morbidity, mortality, or cure following transhiatal or transthoracic esophageal resection. Either technique is acceptable, provided the surgeon performing the operation has adequate experience.

RECONSTRUCTION FOLLOWING RESECTION

The stomach, colon, and jejunum have all been successfully used as replacement conduits after esophagectomy. The stomach is the preferred conduit because of the ease of mobilization and excellent blood supply. Pyloroplasty or pyloromyotomy is required to avoid gastric stasis secondary to the division of the vagi during esophagectomy. No difference has been seen in leak rate or development of strictures following the closure of stapled or hand-sewn anastomoses.

The colon is the most common alternative when the stomach is not available. Either the right or left colon can be used, although the segment of left and transverse colon supplied by the left colic artery is generally longer. The colonic arterial anatomy should be evaluated preoperatively by arteriography, and the colonic mucosa should be evaluated preoperatively by colonoscopy to rule out any colonic pathology. Alternatives to gastric or colonic conduits include free jejunal grafts, which have been used successfully after resection of hypopharyngeal or upper cervical esophageal tumors. The mesenteric vessels are usually anastomosed to the external carotid artery and the internal jugular vein.

PALLIATION FOR UNRESECTABLE TUMORS

Methods of nonoperative palliation have improved dramatically. Patients with a large tracheal-esophageal fistula should now be treated with stenting rather than bypass. Endoscopic laser therapy, electrocoagulation, and most recently, photodynamic therapy are all effective methods of palliation, with reported success rates of 80–100%. If these treatment options fail, an endoscopic prosthesis can be placed. Good results are reported in many patients. However, ulceration, obstruction, dislocation, and aspiration have all been reported in association with these techniques.

Recently, improvements in definitive radiation therapy and chemotherapy have also provided excellent means for short-term palliation. Unfortunately, long-term local control is still poor with nonoperative treatment (40% locoregional failure).

Adjuvant Therapy

Radiotherapy alone, as a treatment for esophageal cancer, is associated with a 5-year survival of less than 10%. Prospective trials have demonstrated improved survival with chemoradiation. Therefore radiation should always be combined with chemotherapy for palliation of esophageal cancer unless chemotherapy is contraindicated. Preoperative radiation therapy has not been shown to improve resectability or survival. Postoperative radiation therapy may decrease the incidence of local recurrence following resection of certain high-risk tumors (those with positive margins or nodal involvement).

When examining results of single and multiagent chemotherapy trials, several principles must be recognized. SCCs are more responsive to chemotherapy than adenocarcinomas, and multiagent chemotherapy is more effective than single-agent chemotherapy for SCC. Single agents used for esophageal cancer include 5-fluorouracil, cisplatin, mitomycin C, and methotrexate, with reported response rates of from 0 to 42%. Multiagent regimens include some combination of 5-fluorouracil, cisplatin and, recently, taxol, with response rates of 30–70%. Unfortunately, when used alone, these agents produce short-lived responses that are not accompanied by significant improvements in survival.

The postoperative use of single or multiple chemotherapeutic agents with or without radiation therapy has not increased survival, although some studies suggest that postoperative radiation therapy may improve locoregional control. Encouraging results with phase II preoperative chemotherapy and radiation therapy trials await confirmation by larger randomized phase III studies. At present, however, no definitive evidence exists to mandate preoperative chemotherapy or radiation therapy.

Surveillance

A barium swallow study should be done in the first preoperative month as a baseline study. Asymptomatic patients can be followed with yearly physical exams and CXR. Any symptoms (e.g., pain, dysphagia, weight loss) should be aggressively evaluated by CT scan, barium studies, or endoscopy. Benign strictures at the anastomosis should be treated with dilation. Unfortunately, treatment options are limited for locoregional or distant recurrences. If radiotherapy was not given pre- or postoperatively, then it can be used along with the previously mentioned nonoperative methods of palliation (stenting, dilation, coring, or laser resection).

Selected References

DeMeester TR, Barlow AP. Surgery and current management for cancer of the esophagus. In SA Wells (ed.), *Current Problems in Surgery*. Chicago: Year Book Medical Publishers, 1988.

Forastiere AA, Orringer MB, Perez-Tamayo C, et al. Preoperative chemoradiation followed by transhiatal esophagectomy for carcinoma of the esophagus: final report. *J Clin Oncol* 11:1118, 1993.

Herskovic A, Martz K, Al-Sarraf M, et al. Combined chemotherapy and radiotherapy compared with radiotherapy alone in patients with cancer of the esophagus. *N Engl J Med* 326:1593, 1992.

Knyrim K, Wagner HJ, Bethge N, et al. A controlled trial of an expansile metal stent for palliation of esophageal obstruction due to inoperable cancer. *N Engl J Med* 329:1302, 1993.

Roth JA, Pass HI, Flanagan MM, et al. Randomized clinical trial of preoperative and postoperative adjuvant chemotherapy with cisplatin, vindesine and bleomycin for carcinoma of the esophagus. *J Thorac Cardiovasc Surg* 96:242, 1988.

Swisher SG, Holmes EC, Hunt KK, et al. The role of neoadjuvant therapy in surgically resectable esophageal cancer. *Arch Surg* 131: 819, 1996.

Swisher SG, Hunt KK, Holmes EC, et al. Changes in the surgical management of esophageal cancer from 1970 to 1993. *Am J Surg* 169:609, 1995.

Swisher SG, Mansfield P. Esophageal carcinoma management. In Meyers MA (ed.), *Neoplasms of the Digestive Tract: Imaging, Staging and Management*. Philadelphia: Lippincott-Raven 1997.

Gastric Carcinoma

David B. Pearlstone and Charles A. Staley

Epidemiology

Gastric cancer is the eighth most common cancer among males in the United States and is expected to account for 22,400 new cases and 14,000 deaths in 1997. In 1930 gastric cancer was the most commonly reported malignancy in the United States. The incidence of gastric cancer in the United States, however, declined steadily from 1930 to 1980, and from 1980 to 1990 the incidence has plateaued. The approximate incidence in the United States is 10 per 100,000 people, compared with 780 per 100,000 people in Japan. Survival of patients with gastric cancer remains poor, with the overall 5-year survival rate being 15%.

Risk Factors

Many factors have been associated with an increased risk of gastric cancer. Diet is thought to play a major role. Geographic regions with diets high in salt and smoked foods are associated with a high incidence of gastric carcinoma, whereas diets high in raw vegetables, vitamin C, and antioxidants may be protective. Animal studies have shown that polycyclic hydrocarbons and dimethylnitrosamines, substances produced after prolonged smoking of fish and meat, can induce malignant gastric tumors. In the United States, male gender, black race, and low socioeconomic class are associated with a higher risk of gastric carcinoma. A specific occupational hazard may exist for metal workers, miners, and rubber workers, and for workers exposed to dust from wood and asbestos. Cigarette smoking poses a clear risk, possibly as a result of decreased vitamin C levels, but alcohol consumption has not been as consistently correlated with the development of gastric cancer. An association of gastric carcinoma with blood group A patients was described in 1953, but the relative risk is only 1.2. Familial clusterings, though rare, have been reported.

Helicobacter pylori, a gram-negative microaerophilic bacterium, living within the mucous layer in the gastric pits, has been implicated in the genesis of gastric carcinoma. This association is based on the increased incidence of *H. pylori* infection in areas where there is a high rate of gastric cancer and an increased incidence of infection in patients with gastric cancer in the United States.

Gastric polyps are rarely precursors of gastric cancer. Hyperplastic polyps, the polyps most commonly found in the stomach, are benign lesions. Villous adenomas do have malignant potential, not only within the polyp itself, but elsewhere in the stomach. These adenomatous polyps, however, represent only 2% of all gastric polyps. Pernicious anemia is associated with a 10%

incidence of gastric cancer, a risk that is about 20 times that of the normal population. The risk of developing carcinoma in a chronic gastric ulcer is small; however, up to 10% of patients with gastric cancer will have been misdiagnosed as having a benign-appearing gastric ulcer when evaluated by upper GI contrast study only. Operations for benign peptic ulcers also appear to be associated with an increased risk of subsequent stomach cancer. Typically appearing 15 or more years after gastrectomy, so-called gastric stump cancer has been variously reported to occur anywhere from zero to five times as often as in individuals without previous gastric resection. Chronic atrophic gastritis and the often subsequent intestinal metaplasia are also risk factors for gastric carcinoma but may not be direct precursor conditions. Interestingly, however, no association has been seen between long-term H2 blockade and gastric cancer.

Most recently, a number of genetic alterations have been found to be associated with gastric cancer. A study of p53 expression in 418 patients with gastric cancer revealed that p53 expression was detectable in more than 55% of tumors; however, there was no correlation between p53 expression and depth of invasion, lymph node involvement, or survival.

Pathology

Ninety-five percent of gastric cancers are adenocarcinomas, arising almost exclusively from the mucus-producing rather than the acid-producing cells of the gastric mucosa. Lymphoma, carcinoid, leiomyosarcoma, and squamous cell carcinoma make up the remaining 5%. In the United States, gastric cancer is macroscopically divided into ulcerative (75%), polypoid (10%), scirrhous (10%), and superficial (5%). Adenocarcinoma of the stomach is an aggressive tumor, often metastasizing early via both lymphatic and venous routes and directly extending into adjacent structures. Extension through the serosal surface can lead to peritoneal tumor implantation and drop metastases to pelvic structures.

Two histologic types of gastric cancer are recognized: intestinal and diffuse. Each type has distinct clinical and pathologic features. The *intestinal* type is found in regions with a high incidence of gastric cancer and is characterized pathologically by the tendency of malignant cells to form glands. The tumors are usually well differentiated; consist of papillary, glandular, and tubular variants; and are associated with metaplasia or chronic gastritis. They occur more commonly in older patients and tend to spread hematologically to distant organs. The *diffuse* type is identified by the lack of organized gland formation, is usually poorly differentiated, and is composed of signet ring cells. This type of tumor is more common in younger patients with no history of gastritis and spreads by transmural extension as well as through lymphatic invasion. The incidence of diffuse-type tumors is relatively constant among many countries and appears to be increasing overall.

In the past, most gastric cancers were localized in the antrum (60–70%). However, from 1980 to 1990, there has been an increase in tumors of the cardia, which now account for up to 40% of all gastric carcinomas. Nine percent of patients have tumor involvement of the entire stomach, known as *linitis plastica*; this entity portends a dismal prognosis. In general, gastric tumors are more common on the lesser curve of the stomach than on the greater curve. In the United States, the incidence of synchronous lesions is 2.2%, compared with an incidence of up to 10% in Japanese patients with pernicious anemia.

Clinical Presentation

Gastric carcinoma usually lacks specific symptoms early in the course of the disease. The vague epigastric discomfort and indigestion are usually ignored by the patient. Patients are often treated presumptively for benign disease for 6–12 months without diagnostic studies even being performed. Rapid weight loss, anorexia, and vomiting occur more frequently in advanced disease. The most frequent presenting symptoms of 1,121 patients at Memorial Sloan-Kettering Cancer Center were weight loss, pain, vomiting, and anorexia. The epigastric pain is usually similar to benign ulcer pain, can mimic angina, and many times is relieved by eating food. Dysphagia is usually associated with tumors of the cardia or gastroesophageal junction. Antral tumors may cause symptoms of gastric outlet obstruction. Large tumors that directly invade the transverse colon may present with colonic obstruction. Physical examination will reveal a palpable mass in up to 30% of patients, and about 10% of patients will present with one or more signs of metastatic disease. The most common indications of metastasis include a palpable supraclavicular node (Virchow's node), a mass palpable on rectal exam (Blumer's shelf), a palpable periumbilical lymph node (Sister Mary Joseph node), ascites, jaundice, a liver mass, or a pelvic mass. The most common site of hematogenous spread is to the liver. Gastric tumors may be associated with chronic blood loss, detected as occult blood in the stool, but massive upper GI bleeding is rare.

Preoperative Evaluation

Early diagnosis remains the only hope for cure in gastric cancer. This implies the need for investigation of the vaguest of upper GI symptoms or realistic and appropriate screening programs. Historically, the barium upper GI x-ray series was the gold standard for the diagnosis of gastric cancer. However, this test has an accuracy of only 70–80% and a false-negative rate of 10–20%. Contrast radiologic studies have largely been replaced, however, by flexible fiberoptic endoscopy, which allows for not only more detailed real-time examination of the gastric mucosa, but the possibility of biopsy and a definitive tissue diagnosis. An accurate diagnosis can be made from four to six biopsies and cytologic brushings in more than 90% of patients.

Once the tissue diagnosis has been made, computed tomography (CT) evaluation allows visualization of the stomach, perigastric area, and distant sites such as the liver, nodal basins, and peritoneum. Overall, CT scans have an accuracy of 90% for liver disease, 60% for nodal disease, and 50% for peritoneal disease. Focal wall thickening may be an important but sometimes misleading CT finding. Early small tumors, peritoneal disease, and invasion of adjacent organs are often missed by CT. In Cook and colleagues' report on 37 patients who underwent laparotomy after preoperative CT scans, 61% of the patients were understaged by CT, most frequently because of missed nodal, liver, or peritoneal disease. In addition, not all adenopathy seen on CT scan represents metastasis. CT evaluation of regional lymph nodes has a sensitivity of 67% and a specificity of 61%. Komaki et al. found that massive adenopathy represented metastatic disease in 96% of cases but that a single enlarged node was metastatic only 48% of the time. Most authors agree that nodes larger than 6 mm are suspicious for cancer.

Endoscopic ultrasound (EUS) has become the gold standard for preoperative T and N staging of gastric cancer. EUS is more accurate than CT in staging the depth of primary tumor invasion (T) and regional lymph node metastases (N). EUS is not helpful, however, in evaluating distant metastatic disease.

Elevated levels of carcinoembryonic antigen (CEA) are seen in only 30% of patients with gastric carcinoma. Because the CEA level is usually normal in early cancer, it is not a useful screening marker. Serial determinations of CEA level may be helpful in evaluating tumor recurrence or tumor response to treatment in patients who present with an elevated level.

The limitations of CT and EUS in evaluating peritoneal disease have led many surgeons to use diagnostic laparoscopy to avoid an unnecessary laparotomy in patients with unsuspected metastatic disease. In a recent analysis by Lowy et al. of 71 patients who were deemed resectable by current-generation CT, staging laparoscopy revealed unappreciated distant metastatic disease in 16 patients (23%). Only one of these patients required palliative surgery. Utilizing combined CT and laparoscopic staging, resectability rate was 93% for patients operated on with curative intent. Diagnostic laparoscopy is an important part of the preoperative evaluation, unless a palliative resection for bleeding or obstruction is planned.

Staging

The current American Joint Committee on Cancer (AJCC) staging for gastric cancer is listed in Table 9-1. This system uses depth of penetration of the gastric wall as the guideline for T stage. Nodal involvement is classified as N0–N2 as described in Table 9-1. Nodes in the retropancreatic, para-aortic, hepatoduodenal, and mesenteric areas, as well as sites of distant organ metastasis, are considered M1 disease.

The Japanese staging system for gastric cancer is different from that used in Western countries, making it difficult to compare reports on the disease. The most confusing difference is in the staging classification of the lymph nodes. The Japanese system describes four major nodal groups (N1–N4) that encompass

Table 9-1. TNM staging system for gastric carcinoma

T1	Tumor invades lamina propria or submucosa
T2	Tumor invades muscularis propria or subserosa
T3	Tumor penetrates serosa
T4	Tumor invades adjacent organ structures
N0	No metastases in lymph nodes
N1	Metastasis in perigastric lymph node(s) within 3 cm of primary tumor
N2	Metastasis in perigastric lymph node(s) >3 cm from primary tumor, or in lymph nodes along left gastric, common hepatic, splenic, or celiac arteries
M0	No evidence of distant metastasis
M1	Evidence of distant metastasis

Staging				
	IA	T1	N0	M0
	IB	T1	N1	M0
		T2	N0	M0
	II	T1	N2	M0
		T2	N1	M0
		T3	N0	M0
	IIIA	T2	N2	M0
		T3	N1	M0
		T4	N0	M0
	IIIB	T3	N2	M0
		T4	N1	M0
	IV	T4	N2	M0
		Any T, N	M1	

Source: Adapted from OH Beahrs, DE Henson, RVP Hutter, et al. (eds).
AJCC Manual for Staging of Cancer (4th ed). Philadelphia: Lippincott, 1992.

16 separate locations of nodal tissue (Fig. 9-1). Nodes closest to the primary tumor and within the perigastric tissue of the lesser and greater curvatures constitute the N1 group. It is important to note that the specific nodal tissue included in the N1 nodal grouping varies, depending on the anatomic location of the tumor. Lymph nodes along the blood vessels from the celiac axis to the stomach, as well as lymph nodes >3 cm from the primary tumor, make up the N2 nodal group. N3 nodes are found in the hepato-duodenal ligament, retropancreatic tissue, and celiac axis (Table 9-2). N4 nodes are located in the para-aortic tissue. The N3 and N4 designations in the Japanese system would constitute distant metastatic disease (M1) in the AJCC system.

Older Japanese studies used a different coding system for the extent of lymph node resection (Table 9-3). In an R0 resection the N1 nodes are incompletely removed; R1 resections include only N1 nodes as well as omentectomy; R2 resections include N1 as well as N2 nodes; and so on.

Recent attempts have been made to adopt a uniform classification of the extent of resection and nodal dissection so that results

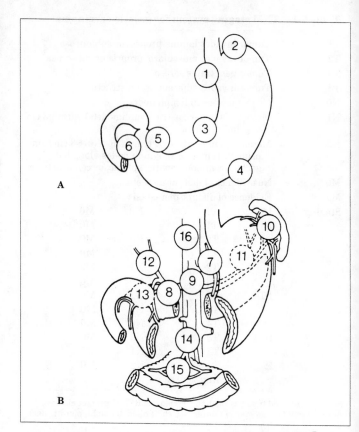

Fig. 9-1.   Japanese classification of regional gastric lymph nodes.
(A) Perigastric lymph nodes. 1: right pericardial; 2: left pericardial;
3: lesser curvature; 4: greater curvature; 5: suprapyloric; 6: infra-
pyloric. (B) Extraperigastric lymph nodes. 7: left gastric artery; 8:
common hepatic artery; 9: celiac artery; 10: splenic hilus; 11: splenic
artery; 12: hepatic pedicle; 13: retropancreatic; 14: mesenteric root;
15: middle colic artery; 16: para-aortic. (Adapted from Y Kodama,
K Sugimachi, K Soejima, et al. Evaluation of extensive lymph node
dissection for carcinoma of the stomach. *World J Surg* 5:242, 1981.)

can be appropriately compared. In the currently adopted system
R0 resection indicates removal of all tumor tissue; R1 resection
indicates microscopic residual disease left behind; and R2 resections leave macroscopic disease. Nodal dissections are classified
corresponding to TNM nodal staging: D1 nodal dissection entails
removal of all nodal tissue within 3 cm of the primary tumor,
whereas a D2 dissection includes removal of nodes more than
3 cm away from the primary, as well as along the common
hepatic, splenic, and left gastric arteries.

Table 9-2. Lymph node groupings according to site of tumor*

| | Location of primary tumor | | | |
Group	Entire stomach	Lower third	Middle third	Upper third
N1	1–6	3–6	1, 3–6	1–4
N2	7–11	1, 7–9	2, 7–11	5–11
N3	12–14	2, 10–14	12–14	12–14

* 1–14 correspond to the lymph nodes described in Fig. 9–1.
Source: Adapted from KE Behrns, RR Dalton, JA van Heerden, et al. Extended lymph node dissection for gastric cancer. Is it of value? *Surg Clin North Am* 72:433, 1992.

Table 9-3. Japanese classification of gastric resection

R0	Total gastrectomy with incomplete removal of N1 nodes
R1	Total gastrectomy with complete removal of N1 nodes
R2	Total gastrectomy with complete removal of N2 nodes
R3	Total gastrectomy with complete removal of N3 nodes
R4	Total gastrectomy with complete removal of N4 nodes

Surgical Treatment

SURGICAL OPTIONS

In the absence of documented metastatic disease, aggressive surgical resection of gastric tumors is justified. The appropriate surgical procedure for a given patient must take into account the location of the lesion and the known pattern of spread.

Proximal Tumors

The optimal surgical management of proximal gastric tumors is controversial. The options include total gastrectomy and proximal subtotal gastrectomy. In general, proximal tumors are more advanced at presentation and have a poorer long-term prognosis than distal cancers. Consequently, palliative, rather than curative, resections are more likely to be performed in patients with proximal tumors. Because of the advanced stage at diagnosis of most tumors of the cardia, some authors argue that any operation is realistically a palliative procedure and that therefore one should always perform the simpler proximal subtotal gastrectomy, especially because total gastrectomy does not improve prognosis for patients with stage III and IV disease. However, a survival benefit and lower recurrence rate have been shown for patients with stage I and II disease who undergo a total gastrectomy.

At M. D. Anderson, we perform a total gastrectomy with Roux-en-Y reconstruction for proximal gastric lesions. This procedure has the advantage of avoiding alkaline reflux gastritis associated with proximal subtotal gastrectomy. There is no significant increase in mortality or morbidity with total gastrectomy compared with proximal subtotal gastrectomy.

Mid-body Tumors

Mid-stomach tumors comprise 15–30% of all gastric cancers. Based on the same arguments discussed for proximal tumors, we recommend total gastrectomy for tumors located in the mid-body of the stomach.

Distal Tumors

Distal tumors account for about 35% of all gastric cancers. The standard operation for these lesions is a distal subtotal gastrectomy with or without a regional lymphadenectomy. This procedure entails resection of approximately three-fourths of the stomach, including the majority of the lesser curvature. Studies have shown that microscopic invasion beyond a distance of 6 cm from the gross tumor is virtually nonexistent. We therefore recommend a 5- to 6-cm resection margin when possible. Even if this distance is achieved, margins must still be checked by frozen-section analysis.

Splenectomy

Splenectomy is not performed unless there is tumor adherence or invasion of the spleen. Routine splenectomy does not improve survival but does increase the morbidity of gastrectomy. If a splenectomy is contemplated due to tumor adherence, pneumococcal vaccine should be given preoperatively.

Lymphadenectomy

Probably the single greatest current controversy in gastric surgery is the role of extended lymphadenectomy in gastric cancer. Radical lymphadenectomy was adopted based on an initial report in 1981 by Kodama et al. that showed a survival benefit for patients with serosal or regional lymph node involvement who underwent an R2 (in the older Japanese system) or R3 lymphadenectomy. Patients undergoing radical lymphadenectomy had a 39% 5-year survival rate, compared with 18% for an R1 lymphadenectomy. Figure 9-2 shows the site-specific extent of dissection for an R1 and R2 lymphadenectomy. Many other studies from Japan have shown a similarly significant survival benefit for patients undergoing radical lymphadenectomy. Unfortunately, most Western studies have not been able to repeat the Japanese results, which contributes to this already significant controversy.

The difference in survival between Japanese and Western studies appears to result from several causes. The significant differences in the staging systems between the two countries make it difficult to compare the survival rate stage for stage between studies. In addition, the Japanese nodal dissection and pathologic analysis is much more meticulous and extends out to the quaternary nodes (N4) in many cases. Western series, on the other hand,

Lower third lesions

R1

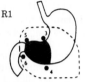

R2

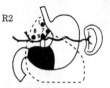

3 Lesser curvature	1 R Cardiac
4 Greater curvature	7 L Gastric artery
5 Suprapyloric	8 Hepatic
6 Infrapyloric	9 Celiac

Middle third lesions

R1

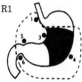

R2

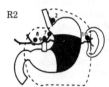

1 R cardiac	2	L cardiac*
3 Lesser curvature	7	L gastric artery
4 Greater curvature	8	Hepatic artery
5 Suprapyloric	9	Celiac
6 Infrapyloric	10	Splenic hilar
	11	Splenic artery

Upper third lesions (includes cardia)

R1

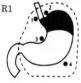

R2

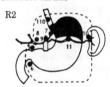

1 R cardiac	5	Suprapyloric*
2 L cardiac	6	Infrapyloric*
3 Lesser curvature	7	L gastric artery
4 Greater curvature	8	Hepatic artery
and short gastric	9	Celiac
	10	Splenic hilar
	11	Splenic artery
	110	Paraesophageal
		(cardia lesions)

Fig. 9-2. Extent of R1 and 2 lymphadenectomy by tumor location.
Dashed line indicates the scope of the lymphadenectomy. An R2
dissection must remove all the R-1-designated lymph nodes as
well as the majority of the R2 lymph nodes. The asterisk indicates
those nodes for which removal is optional. (From J Smith, MH Schiu,
L Kelsey, et al. Morbidity of radical lymphadenectomy in the
curative resection of gastric carcinoma. *Arch Surg* 126:1469, 1991.)

potentially understage patients because in many cases only peri-gastric nodes are dissected and the involvement of N2 and M1 nodes is not evaluated. Mass screening programs in Japan have increased the percentage of early-stage cancers (30% versus 5% in the United States). It is also postulated that there is an inherent difference in the biology of gastric cancer between the two countries, with the Japanese having a less aggressive form of tumor. Furthermore, most of the Japanese data compare results of radical lymphadenectomy to historical controls from previous decades rather than conducting prospective randomized trials. The higher percentage of early-stage gastric cancer being diagnosed currently in Japan could account in part for this increased survival over historical controls. At least one report from Japan was unable to show any benefit of R3 over R2 dissection.

Wanebo et al. reviewed the results of a prospectively gathered data base that included 18,346 cases of gastric cancer from 200 tumor registries in the United States. Patients undergoing D2 nodal dissections (including lymph nodes >3 cm from the primary tumor) had no increase in median survival time (19.7 months versus 24.8 months) or in 5-year survival rate (26.3% versus 30%), compared with patients undergoing D1 dissection. Similar results have been shown in a prospective randomized study from South Africa. In contrast, a 10-year study from Austria prospectively assigned 345 patients with potentially curable gastric cancer to extended lymphadenectomy; these patients had 5- and 10-year survivals similar to those of patients in Japanese studies, with no increase in morbidity or mortality. Shiu et al. (1987) retrospectively reviewed 210 patients with gastric cancer at Memorial Sloan-Kettering Cancer Center and found that a lymphadenectomy that failed to include the lymph nodes at least one echelon beyond the histologically involved nodes was predictive of a poor prognosis. They also showed that there was not a significant difference in morbidity between the R1 and R2 nodal dissections. In a recent study from Holland, Bonenkamp et al. reported on 711 patients prospectively randomized to D1 or D2 nodal dissections. Patients undergoing more extended lymphadenectomy had a significantly higher operative mortality and experienced significantly more complications. Survival data from these patients have yet to be reported.

SURGICAL TECHNIQUE

Total Gastrectomy

Once the preoperative work-up excludes the presence of distant metastases or an unresectable tumor, the patient should undergo diagnostic laparoscopy. If laparoscopy is negative, an open laparotomy, exploration, and gastrectomy are performed through a midline or bilateral subcostal incision. For a total gastrectomy, the dissection is begun by holding up the omentum and dissecting down the anterior leaf of the transverse mesocolon, thereby separating the omentum from the mesocolon. The right gastroepiploic vessels are ligated at their origin, and the subpyloric nodes are dissected with the specimen. The first portion of the duodenum is mobilized and divided 2 cm distal to the pylorus. The lesser omentum is then dissected free at the inferior edge of the liver. The left gastric artery is ligated at its origin. It is important to remember that an aberrant or accessory left hepatic artery may originate from the left gastric artery and reside in the lesser omentum. If an extended lymphadenectomy is done, the celiac, hepatic artery, and splenic artery nodes are dissected along with the specimen. The short gastric vessels are ligated up to the gastroesophageal junction (GEJ). Dissection around the GEJ will free 7–8 cm of distal esophagus, which facilitates transection of the esophagus with adequate proximal margins. After the esophagus is divided, the resection margins are checked by frozen-section examination. If the tumor is adherent to the spleen, pancreas, liver, diaphragm, or mesocolon, the involved organs are removed en bloc.

There are many types of reconstruction, but the most frequently used is a Roux-en-Y anastomosis. If a significant portion of the distal esophagus is resected, a left thoracoabdominal or right Ivor-Lewis approach may be used. Reconstruction with pouches and loops to act as reservoirs has no benefit over a straight Roux-en-Y reconstruction. Care is taken to ensure a Roux limb of at least 45 cm. A feeding jejunostomy tube is placed for postoperative nutritional support.

Subtotal Gastrectomy

A subtotal gastrectomy is approached in the same way as described earlier for a total gastrectomy except that only about 80% of the distal stomach is resected (Fig. 9-3). A small remnant of stomach remains and is supplied by the short gastric vessels. We prefer to perform a Roux-en-Y reconstruction, but a loop gastrojejunostomy can be done if there is no tension on the anastomosis.

Complications

Postoperative complications are listed in Table 9-4. The most devastating complication of a gastric resection is an anastomotic leak, which is seen in 3–12% of patients. We no longer routinely obtain a barium upper GI series before oral feeding is begun. Leaks can occur late, and an intact anastomosis early in the postoperative period does not guarantee an uncomplicated course. Feeding is begun if the patient is asymptomatic. Upper GI contrast studies are only performed based on clinical indications (i.e., fever, tachycardia, tachypnea). Because the food reservoir is gone, many patients must initially change their eating habits to six small meals per day. Many patients are discharged on supplemental jejunostomy feedings until their oral intake is adequate. Within several months, most patients will increase their intestinal capacitance and be able to eat larger meals less frequently (three or four meals per day).

SURGICAL RESULTS

The overall 5-year survival rate for gastric cancer is 10–21% in most Western series, a consequence of the advanced stage of disease at presentation in most patients. There is a slightly better prognosis in patients resected for cure (5-year survival rate of 24–57%). This is in contrast to the 50% 5-year survival reported in the Japanese literature. Overall 5-year survival rates for Japan and the United States are listed by TNM stage in Table 9-5.

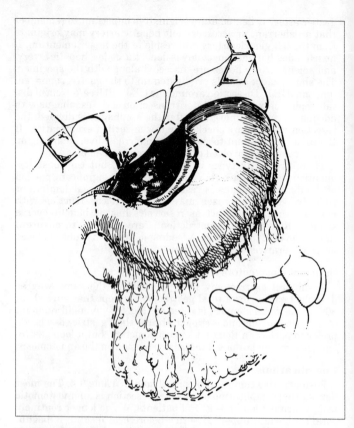

Fig. 9-3.   Resection margins of subtotal gastrectomy. Inset
shows placement of anastomosis. (From JS MacDonald, G Steele, LL
Gunderson. Cancer of the stomach. In VT DeVita, S Hellman,
SA Rosenberg (eds.), *Cancer: Principles and Practice of Oncology*
[4th ed]. Philadelphia: Lippincott, 1993.)

In 1989, Cady et al. reviewed their series of 211 gastric cancer
patients. Of these, 17% were not explored because of distant
metastatic disease or diffuse peritoneal spread identified preoperatively, whereas 83% underwent a laparotomy. Of those
patients undergoing laparotomy, 58% underwent resection; 34%
of the procedures were performed for cure and 24% for palliation.
These patients were treated before the more widespread availability of diagnostic laparoscopy. The overall 5-year survival rate
for all 211 patients was 21%, but those patients who underwent
surgical resection had a 5-year survival rate of 36%. This figure
increased to 58% for those patients resected with curative intent.
The percentage of patients with proximal cancers undergoing
curative resection was half that of patients with distal cancers.
Fifteen percent of the patients had linitis plastica; these patients

Table 9-4. Complications of gastric resection

Complication	Percentage of patients
Pulmonary	3–55
Infectious	3–22
Anastomotic	3–21
Cardiac	1–10
Renal	1–8
Bleeding	0.3–5
Pulmonary embolus	1–4

had a median survival of 12 months. Resection should be avoided in these patients unless palliation of an obstructing or bleeding tumor is necessary.

Multiple prognostic variables for gastric cancer were reviewed by Shiu et al. in 1989. The five independent variables found to correlate with a poor prognosis were high TNM stage, metastatic involvement of four or more lymph nodes, poorly differentiated tumors, splenectomy, and regional lymphadenectomy not extensive enough relative to the nodal stage. These variables all had a negative impact on survival.

Disease recurrence has been analyzed in autopsy, reoperative, and clinical series. Some component of disease failure can be found in up to 80% of patients following gastrectomy. In 1982, Gunderson and Sosin analyzed patterns of failure in a prospective study of 109 patients who had undergone a gastric resection and were then subjected to reoperation at the University of Minnesota. Of the 107 evaluable patients, 86 (80%) had recurrent disease. Locoregional failure alone occurred in only 22 (9%) of the patients, but peritoneal seeding was seen as a component of recurrence in 53.7% of those patients who failed. Isolated distant

Table 9-5. Five-year survival rates after gastrectomy (%)

Stage		Japan	United States
N0	T1	80	90
	T2	60	58
	T3	30	50
	T4	5	20
N1		53	20
N2		26	10
N3		10	—
N4		3	—
Overall		50	15

Source: Adapted from Y Noguchi Y, T Imada, A Matsumoto, et al. Radical surgery for gastric cancer: A review of the Japanese experience. *Cancer* 64:2053, 1989.

metastases were uncommon but occurred as some component of failure in 29% of the group.

In 1990, Landry et al. from Massachusetts General Hospital reviewed disease recurrence in 130 patients resected for cure. The overall locoregional failure rate was 38% (49/130): 21 patients (16%) had locoregional failure alone, 28 patients (22%) had locoregional failure and distant metastasis, and 39 patients (30%) had distant metastases alone. Locoregional recurrence increased with the degree of tumor penetration through the gastric wall. The most frequent sites of locoregional recurrence were the gastric remnant at the anastomosis, the gastric bed, or the regional nodes. The overall incidence of distant metastases was 52% (67 patients), and an increased incidence was seen with advancing stage of disease. The overall recurrence rate was 68% (88 patients).

Early Gastric Cancer

In the early 1960s, the Japanese defined early gastric cancer as carcinoma limited to the mucosa and submucosa regardless of the presence or absence of lymph node metastasis. This pathologic classification is based on the high cure rate in this group of patients. Although the incidence of early gastric cancer has increased in the United States (from approximately 5% to 15% of all gastric cancers), aggressive screening in Japan has resulted in an even greater increase in incidence in that country, from 5% to 30%, during the last 15 years. The mean age of patients at diagnosis in Western studies is 63, whereas in Japanese patients it is 55. Most patients present with GI symptoms similar to those of peptic ulcer disease, including epigastric pain and dyspepsia. In contrast to advanced gastric cancer, it is uncommon to see significant weight loss in these patients at the time of diagnosis.

The use of endoscopy and biopsy has been instrumental in the ability to diagnose early gastric cancer. In collected Western series, only 22% of cancers were diagnosed by a barium upper GI study, as compared with 80% by endoscopy. The Japanese have classified early gastric cancer pathologically based on its gross endoscopic appearance. They define three basic types of tumors: type I, protruded; type II, superficial; and type III, excavated. By the TNM classification, early gastric cancer would include all T1 tumors with any N stage of disease.

The surgical procedure performed in the patient with early gastric cancer is based on the location, extent of the lesion, and nodal disease. Most reports in the Western literature favor subtotal gastrectomy as the procedure of choice for early gastric cancer, with total gastrectomy reserved for proximal tumors or multifocal disease. This approach has resulted in a 5-year survival rate of approximately 85%, which compares favorably with the Japanese experience of a 5-year survival rate reportedly greater than 90%. The Japanese have been unable to show a survival benefit for radical lymphadenectomy in patients with histologically uninvolved lymph nodes. However, an improved survival rate has been noted in patients with lymph node metastases who undergo a radical lymphadenectomy compared with patients undergoing an R1 dissection. Despite a high potential cure rate, it must be remembered that 10–15% of these early tumors will have positive lymph nodes that may occasionally extend to the N2 nodal basin. Therefore several authors recommend that an extended lymphadenectomy (R2) be performed in these highly curable patients.

Adjuvant Therapy

POSTOPERATIVE CHEMOTHERAPY

Only a minority of patients who undergo resection for gastric cancer are actually cured, as 70–80% develop recurrences after gastric resection. Effective adjuvant therapy is needed to impact on survival; results, however, have been inconsistent at best. In general, no survival benefit has been reproduced consistently with adjuvant treatment of gastric cancer. Two early studies conducted by the Veterans Administration Surgical Adjuvant Group (VASAG) investigated the use of thiotepa and floxuridine (FUDR) following surgical resection. There was no survival benefit seen in either study, and the toxicity of thiotepa was substantial. A meta-analysis by Hermans et al. reviewed the results of 11 randomized trials of adjuvant chemotherapy involving 2,096 patients and concluded that postoperative chemotherapy offers no survival advantage compared with surgery alone.

Three trials have studied the use of 5-fluorouracil (5-FU) and semustine (methyl-CCNU) as adjuvant therapy. The Gastrointestinal Tumor Study Group (GITSG) evaluated patients who were randomly assigned to receive no additional therapy or 18 months of 5-FU and methyl-CCNU. A survival benefit was noted in patients receiving chemotherapy. However, an Eastern Cooperative Oncology Group (ECOG) trial using the same doses and schedule of chemotherapy failed to demonstrate any survival benefit. A third study by VASAG using the same agents but a different dosing schedule also found no survival benefit. Without a clear benefit in using 5-FU and methyl-CCNU and with a significant risk of treatment-induced acute nonlymphocytic leukemia, many investigators believe that this adjuvant regimen is inappropriate.

A single study from Spain by Estape et al. with a follow-up of 10 years has shown a survival benefit with the use of adjuvant mitomycin C. The chemotherapy schedule used in this study was 20 mg/m^2 given IV once every 6 weeks for four cycles. Of 37 patients in the control arm, 31 died of recurrent disease, compared with 16 of 33 patients in the treatment group. The most significant advantage was seen in patients with T3, N0, M0 tumors. The major criticism of this study is the relatively small sample size. Other studies have used mitomycin C in combination with 5-FU and either cyclophosphamide or cytosine arabinoside. These studies have been unable to show any survival benefit in the group of patients receiving adjuvant chemotherapy.

More recently, chemotherapy regimens that include doxorubicin have been studied. Several groups have reported no survival benefit in trials with 5-FU, doxorubicin, and mitomycin C (FAM) in an adjuvant setting.

Two studies have looked at patients randomly assigned to receive no additional therapy or radiotherapy with concurrent 5-FU. Dent studied 142 patients but found no benefit to this combined regimen. A second study by Moertel showed a benefit of chemotherapy plus radiotherapy, but the study results were skewed by 10 patients who were randomized to the experimental arm but refused treatment.

PREOPERATIVE CHEMOTHERAPY

Preoperative, or neoadjuvant, chemotherapy offers the potential to downstage disease and the ability to evaluate tumor sensitivity to a chemotherapeutic regimen. If the tumor responds to the neoadjuvant therapy, treatment can be continued postoperatively. Several trials have evaluated etoposide, cisplatin, and either 5-FU or doxorubicin in the neoadjuvant setting. Response rates have ranged from a clinical response of 21–31% to a complete pathologic response rate of from 0 to 15%. Currently, M. D. Anderson is evaluating a neoadjuvant regimen consisting of 5-FU, cisplatin, and leucovorin, followed postoperatively by continued chemotherapy and radiation. Until randomized trials are conclusive, neoadjuvant therapy should be reserved for a protocol setting.

INTRAOPERATIVE RADIOTHERAPY

Most of the data available on intraoperative radiotherapy (IORT) for gastric cancer are based on the reports of Abe and Takahashi from Japan. Their prospective nonrandomized trial looked at 110 patients who had surgery alone and 84 patients who had surgery plus IORT. The 5-year survival rates were similar in stage I patients; however, a suggestion of a survival benefit was seen in stage II, III, and IV patients receiving IORT. In contrast, a small (less than 40 patients) randomized IORT study done at the National Cancer Institute showed neither a disease-free nor an overall survival benefit with IORT, despite a marked decrease in locoregional recurrence.

Management of Advanced Disease

PALLIATIVE SURGERY

Because few patients present with early-stage disease, 70% of patients with gastric cancer will be treated for palliation alone. The procedures available for palliation are resection, bypass, intubation, or laser fulguration. The particular treatment rendered must be individualized for each patient. The symptoms that commonly require palliation are obstruction, bleeding, and intractable pain. Pyloric obstruction can be relieved by a gastroenterostomy or resection. Obstruction of the cardia is best treated by resection, but laser ablation may be used for patients at high operative risk with a reasonable degree of success. The best results with laser ablation are obtained with lesions smaller than 5 cm in diameter. Acute bleeding may be controlled by endoscopy and cautery, angiographic embolization, or resection. Chronic blood loss may be treated with cautery or radiotherapy. Good palliation is obtained with surgery 50% of the time. The operative mortality ranges from 6% to 22%. Mean survival after palliative treatment is 4.2 months and ranges from 0 to 13 months.

CHEMOTHERAPY

The effect of chemotherapy on advanced gastric carcinoma has been disappointing. Several single-agent drug regimens have been tested, including 5-FU, doxorubicin, and mitomycin C. The response rates have ranged from 17% to 30%; however, the responses have generally been brief and have not had a significant impact on survival.

Numerous attempts have been made to develop effective combination chemotherapy using known active agents. The combination of 5-FU, doxorubicin, and mitomycin C (FAM) was studied in the 1980s. Initially, it produced a response rate of 42% and a median response duration of 9 months, but there were no complete responses. Other reports on FAM have shown similar results. Etoposide has been used in combination with doxorubicin and cisplatin (EAP). Although a single report showed a 64% response rate, other investigators have not been able to achieve such high response rates and have documented significant morbidity and mortality due to myelosuppression. As a result, etoposide has been tried in combination with other chemotherapeutic agents, including leucovorin and 5-FU, with varying results. This regimen is well tolerated by older, high-risk patients. Methotrexate has been combined with doxorubicin and 5-FU in clinical trials to produce a regimen termed FAMTX. Response rates have ranged from 33% to 59% with complete response rates and median survival times reported as high as 21% and 9 months, respectively.

No regimen of combination chemotherapy has been shown to be decisively superior to single-agent therapy. However, many investigators are encouraged by the initial results with FAMTX.

RADIOTHERAPY

There are several isolated case reports of radiotherapy being beneficial when used as palliative treatment for advanced gastric carcinoma. However, no large prospective trial has been able to show any long-term benefit for radiotherapy in advanced disease.

INTRAPERITONEAL HYPERTHERMIC PERFUSION

The use of intraperitoneal (IP) chemotherapy has been investigated for several years, particularly in the treatment of ovarian and colorectal cancers. IP 5-FU was initially shown to decrease peritoneal recurrence in patients with colorectal cancer. Koga et al. reviewed their experience with a combination of hyperthermia and mitomycin C used in an adjuvant setting for gastric cancer. The authors showed that this procedure was technically feasible and safe. Patients who underwent perfusion did not have an increased incidence of postoperative complications. Yonemura et al. have reported that adjuvant hyperthermic IP chemotherapy with mitomycin C, etoposide, and cisplatin after gastric resection in patients with peritoneal seeding resulted in a complete response in eight of 43 patients (19%) and partial response in nine of 43 (21%). A randomized trial of gastric cancer patients with gross serosal invasion, but no evidence of peritoneal metastases showed hyperthermic IP chemotherapy with mitomycin C reduced the incidence of peritoneal recurrence but had no influence on 5-year survival. Fujimoto et al. evaluated 59 patients who underwent gastrectomy followed by randomization to no further therapy or IP hyperthermic perfusion therapy. The perfused patients survived longer than the controls (1-year survival rate 80.4% versus 34.2%, respectively). Patients with peritoneal seeding also had a significant survival benefit when perfused with hyperthermic mitomycin C. This technique is currently under investigation in several centers in the United States.

IMMUNOTHERAPY

A number of investigators have recently examined the use of immunologic agents in an adjuvant role for patients with gastric cancer both alone and in combination with chemotherapy. Maehara et al. reported that patients randomized to receive standard chemotherapy with intra-peritoneal injection of the streptococcal preparation OK-432 had significantly decreased rates of peritoneal recurrence and longer survival times compared with patients receiving chemotherapy alone. Studies are ongoing and the future role of immunomodulators in gastric cancer remains to be defined.

Figure 9-4 outlines the treatment approach to gastric cancer at M. D. Anderson Cancer Center.

Surveillance

Patients are examined every 3 months for the first 2 years following resection of a gastric adenocarcinoma. A careful history and physical examination are performed, along with laboratory studies (complete blood count and liver function tests). Chest x-rays are obtained every 6 months. Patients may have a CT scan performed 1 year after surgery and yearly thereafter. Those who undergo a subtotal gastrectomy should be considered for yearly endoscopy as well.

Gastric Lymphoma

In contrast to the decreasing incidence of gastric adenocarcinoma, the incidence of gastric lymphoma is steadily increasing. The stomach is the most common site for lymphoma in the gastrointestinal tract, accounting for two-thirds of GI lymphomas. Non-Hodgkin's lymphomas are the second most common malignancy of the stomach after adenocarcinoma. The average age of patients is 60 years. The most frequent symptoms at the time of presen-

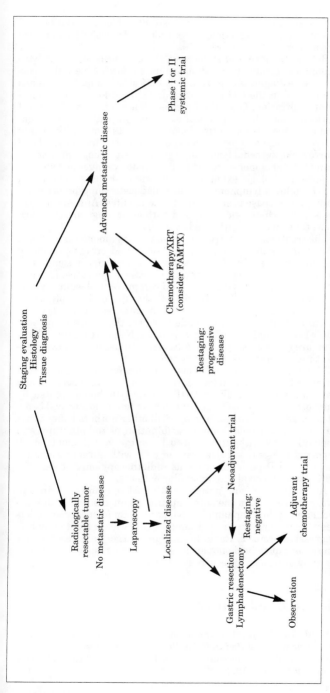

Fig. 9-4. M. D. Anderson outline for the evaluation and treatment of gastric adenocarcinoma.

tation are pain (68%), weight loss (28%), bleeding (28%), and fatigue (16%). Obstruction, perforation, and massive bleeding are uncommon.

Before the advent of endoscopy, the diagnosis of gastric lymphoma was usually made at operation. Endoscopy permits a correct tissue diagnosis approximately 80% of the time. Most lesions are located in the distal stomach and spread locally by submucosal infiltration. Once the diagnosis has been made, a careful work-up—including a physical examination (with special attention to adenopathy), routine laboratory tests along with lactate dehydrogenase and beta$_2$-microglobulin determinations, a bone marrow biopsy, pedal lymphangiogram, chest radiograph, and CT scan of the abdomen—should be done to fully stage the extent of disease. Pathologic examination shows most cases to be B-cell non-Hodgkin's lymphoma (diffuse histiocytic subtype predominant). The disease is staged using the modified Ann Arbor staging system. Histologic grade and pathologic stage are two variables that independently predict survival.

The treatment of gastric lymphoma varies among institutions, with some centers using surgery alone and others promoting chemotherapy and radiation. Surgery is necessary in some cases to confirm the diagnosis. Surgical resection is curative in many patients with localized disease and can prevent bleeding or perforation in patients receiving radiotherapy or chemotherapy. Moreover, more accurate staging is obtained at surgery. An attempt should always be made to resect the entire lymphoma while leaving uninvolved stomach intact. Negative margins, however, are not necessary for cure. Several studies have shown adjuvant radiotherapy to be of no benefit.

Many patients with GI lymphoma receive chemotherapy in addition to resection. In fact, cure rates of 70% have been seen in patients with stage IE and IIE gastric lymphoma treated by chemotherapy alone. Other studies have found no survival benefit with adjuvant chemotherapy. Still other authors believe that patients will benefit from a combination of radiotherapy and chemotherapy without any need for surgery. Talamonti et al. reported a 5-year survival rate of 82% with surgery alone for stage I and II patients, whereas radiotherapy only produced a 50% 5-year survival rate in similar patients.

At M. D. Anderson, patients with gastric lymphoma are initially treated with a chemotherapeutic regimen based on doxorubicin and cyclophosphamide (Cytoxan). A complete response has been documented in more than 90% of patients treated by this aggressive protocol. Radiotherapy and surgery are reserved for those patients who do not achieve a complete response to chemotherapy or who have recurrent disease.

Selected References

Abe M, Takahashi M. Intraoperative radiotherapy: The Japanese experience. *Int J Radiat Oncol Biol Phys* 7:863, 1981.

Ajani JA, Ota DM, Jessup M, et al. Resectable gastric carcinoma. *Cancer* 68:1501, 1991.

Alexander HR, Grem JL, Pass HI, et al. Neoadjuvant chemotherapy for locally advanced gastric adenocarcinoma. *Oncology* 7:37, 1993.

Bonenkamp JJ, Songun I, Hermans J, et al. Randomised comparison of morbidity after D1 and D2 dissection for gastric cancer in 996 Dutch patients. *Lancet* 345:745, 1995.

Bozzetti F, Bonfanti G, Bufalino R, et al. Adequacy of margins of resection in gastrectomy for cancer. *Ann Surg* 196:685, 1982.

Brady MS, Rogatko A, Dent LL, et al. Effects of splenectomy on morbidity and survival following curative gastrectomy for carcinoma. *Arch Surg* 126:359, 1991.

Cady B, Rossi RL, Silverman ML, et al. Gastric adenocarcinoma. *Arch Surg* 124:303, 1989.

Cook AO, Levine BA, Sirinek KR. Evaluation of gastric adenocarcinoma: abdominal computed tomography does not replace celiotomy. *Arch Surg* 121:603, 1986.

Correa P, Shiao YH. Phenotypic and genotypic events in gastric carcinogenesis. *Cancer Res* 54(Suppl):1941s, 1994.

Estape J, Grau J, Alcobendas F, et al. Mitomycin C as an adjuvant treatment to resected gastric cancer. A 10-year follow-up. *Ann Surg* 213:219, 1991.

Fujimoto S, Shrestha RD, Kokubun M, et al. Positive results of combined therapy of surgery and intraperitoneal hyperthermic perfusion for far-advanced gastric cancer. *Ann Surg* 212:592, 1990.

Gunderson LL, Sosin H. Adenocarcinoma of the stomach: Areas of failure in a re-operation series clinicopathologic correlation and implications for adjuvant therapy. *Int J Radiat Oncol Biol Phys* 8:1, 1982.

Hamazoe R, Maeta M, Kaibara N. Intraperitoneal thermochemotherapy for prevention of peritoneal recurrence of gastric cancer. Final results of a randomized controlled study. *Cancer* 73:2048, 1994.

Hermans J, Bonenkamp JJ, Boon MC, et al. Adjuvant therapy after curative resection for gastric cancer: Meta-analysis of randomized trials. *J Clin Oncol* 11:1441, 1993.

Jatzko GR, Lisborg PH, Denk H, et al. A 10-year experience with Japanese-type radical lymph node dissection for gastric cancer outside of Japan. *Cancer* 76:1302, 1995.

Kelson D. Adjuvant therapy of upper gastrointestinal tract cancers. *Semin Oncol* 18:543, 1991.

Kodama Y, Sugimuchi K, Soejima K, et al. Evaluation of extensive lymph node dissection for carcinoma of the stomach. *World J Surg* 5:241, 1981.

Koga S, Hamazoe R, Maeta M, et al. Prophylactic therapy for peritoneal recurrence of gastric cancer by continuous hyperthermic peritoneal perfusion with mitomycin C. *Cancer* 61:232, 1988.

Komaki S, Toyoshima S. CT's capability in advanced gastric cancer. *Gastrointest Radiol* 8:307, 1983.

Landry J, Tepper JE, Wood WC, et al. Patterns of failure following curative resection of gastric carcinoma. *Int J Radiat Oncol Biol Phys* 19:1357, 1990.

Lawrence M, Shiu MH. Early gastric cancer. *Ann Surg* 213:327, 1991.

Lightdale CJ. Endoscopic ultrasonography in the diagnosis, staging, and follow-up of esophageal and gastric cancer. *Endoscopy* 24 (Suppl 1):297, 1992.

Lowy AM, Mansfield PF, Leach SD, Ajani J. Laparoscopic staging for gastric cancer. *Surgery* 119:611, 1996.

MacDonald JS. Gastric cancer: Chemotherapy of advanced disease. *Hematol Oncol* 10:37, 1992.

MacDonald JS, Steele G, Gunderson LL. Cancer of the stomach. In VT DeVita, S Hellman, SA Rosenberg (eds.), *Cancer: Principles and Practice of Oncology* (3rd ed). Philadelphia: Lippincott, 1989.

Maehara Y, Okuyama T, Kakeji Y, et al. Postoperative immunochemotherapy including streptococcal lysate OK-432 is effective for patients with gastric cancer and serosal invasion. *Am J Surg* 168:36, 1994.

Moertel C, Childs D, O'Fallon J. Combined 5-FU and radiation therapy as a surgical adjuvant for poor prognosis gastric carcinoma. *J Clin Oncol* 2:1249, 1984.

Normura, A, Stermmermann, GN, Chyou, PH, et al. *Helicobacter pylori* infection and gastric carcinoma in a population of Japanese-Americans in Hawaii. *N Engl J Med* 325:1132, 1991.

Oiwa H, Maehara Y, Ohno S, et al. Growth pattern and p53 overexpression in patients with early gastric cancer. *Cancer* 75(Suppl): 1454, 1995.

Ota DM, Mansfield PF, Ajani JA. Operative and adjuvant treatment strategies for gastric carcinoma. *Cancer Bull* 44:286, 1992.

Parker SL, Tong T, Bolden S, Wingo PA. Cancer Statistics, 1997. *CA Cancer J Clin* 47:5, 1997.

Rugge M, Cassaro M, Leandro G, et al. *Helicobacter pylori* in promotion of gastric carcinogenesis. *Dig Dis Sci* 41:950, 1996.

Sawyers JL, Gastric carcinoma. *Curr Probl Surg* 32:101, 1995.

Shiu MH, Moore E, Sanders M, et al. Influence of the extent of resection in survival after curative treatment of gastric carcinoma: A retrospective multivariate analysis. *Arch Surg* 122:1347, 1987.

Shiu MH, Perrotti M, Brennen MF. Adenocarcinoma of the stomach: A multivariate analysis of clinical, pathologic, and treatment factors. *Hepatogastroenterology* 36:7, 1989.

Smith JW, Brennen MF. Surgical treatment of gastric cancer. *Surg Clin North Am* 72:381, 1992.

Smith JW, Shiu MH, Kelsey L, et al. Morbidity of radical lymphadenectomy in the curative resection of gastric carcinoma. *Arch Surg* 126:1469, 1991.

Tahara, E. Genetic alterations in human gastrointestinal cancers. The application to molecular diagnosis. *Cancer* 75(Suppl 6):1410, 1995.

Talamonti MS, Dawes LG, Joehl RJ, et al. Gastrointestinal lymphoma. A case for primary surgical resection. *Arch Surg* 125:972, 1990.

Wanebo HJ, Kennedy BJ, Chmiel J, et al. Cancer of the stomach. A patient care study by the American College of Surgeons. *Ann Surg* 218:583, 1993.

Wanebo HJ, Kennedy BJ, Winchester DP, et al. Gastric carcinoma: Does lymph node dissection alter survival? *J Am Coll Surg* 183:616, 1996.

Yonemura Y, Fujimura T, Nishimura G, et al. Effects of intraoperative chemohyperthermia in patients with gastric cancer with peritoneal dissemination. *Surgery* 119:437, 1996.

Small-Bowel Malignancies and Carcinoid Tumors

Emily K. Robinson, James C. Cusack, Jr., and Douglas S. Tyler

Epidemiology

Malignancies of the small intestine are rare, with only 4,600 new cases estimated in the United States in 1995. The small intestine represents 75% of the length and 90% of the surface area of the alimentary tract, accounting for only 1% of gastrointestinal (GI) neoplasms. The incidence of this rare malignancy is 0.7–1.6 per 100,000 population, with a slight male predominance. Mean age at presentation is 57 years. Associated conditions include familial polyposis, Gardner's syndrome, Peutz-Jeghers syndrome, adult (nontropical) celiac sprue, von Recklinghausen's neurofibromatosis, and Crohn's disease. In addition, immunosuppressed patients (e.g., immunoglobulin [Ig] A deficiency) are thought to be at increased risk of developing small-bowel malignancies. As many as 25% of affected patients have synchronous malignancies, including neoplasms of the colon, endometrium, breast, and prostate.

The peak incidence of carcinoid tumors is in the sixth and seventh decades of life, although these tumors have been reported in patients as young as 10 years. The sites of origin of carcinoid tumors are shown in Table 10-1. Approximately 85% of carcinoid tumors are found in the GI tract, with the appendix being the most common site. Nonintestinal sites include the lungs, pancreas, biliary tract, thymus, and ovary. Ileal carcinoids are the most likely to metastasize, even when small, in contrast to appendiceal carcinoids, which rarely metastasize.

Risk Factors

Several distinctive characteristics of the small intestine may explain its relative sparing from malignancy. Benzopyrene hydroxylase, an enzyme that converts benzopyrene to a less carcinogenic compound, is found in large amounts in the mucosa of the small intestine. In contrast, anaerobic bacteria, which convert bile salts into potential carcinogens, are generally lacking in the small intestine. Unlike the stomach or colon, the small intestine is protected from the tumorigenic effects of an acidic environment and from the irritating effects of solid GI contents. In addition, the rapid transit of liquid succus entericus through the small bowel is thought to reduce its tumorigenicity by minimizing the contact time between potential enteric carcinogens and the mucosa. Secretory IgA, also found in large quantities in the small intestine, safeguards against oncogenic viruses.

Table 10-1.   Site of origin of carcinoid tumors

Tumor site	Percentage of cases
Stomach	2.8
Duodenum	2.9
Jejunoileum	25.5
Appendix	36.2
Colon	6.0
Rectum	16.4
Bronchus	9.9
Ovary	0.5
Miscellaneous	0.2
Unknown primary	3.3

GI dysfunction may predispose the small intestine mucosa to tumorigenesis. Stasis secondary to partial obstruction or blind loop syndrome leads to bacterial overgrowth and has been implicated in the development of small-intestine malignancies.

Clinical Presentation

SMALL-BOWEL MALIGNANCY

Seventy-five percent of patients with malignant lesions of the small bowel will develop GI symptoms, compared with only 50% of patients with benign tumors. Sixty-five percent will present with intermittent abdominal pain that is dull and crampy and radiates to the back, 50% with anorexia and weight loss, and 25% with signs and symptoms of bowel obstruction. Only 10% of patients with small-bowel malignancies will develop bowel perforation, most commonly among patients with lymphomas or sarcomas. A palpable abdominal mass is present in 25% of patients.

The nonspecificity of symptoms, when present, frequently results in a 6- to 8-month delay in diagnosis. The correct diagnosis is established preoperatively in only 50% of cases. Late detection and inaccurate diagnosis contribute not only to the advanced stage of disease at the time of surgery but also to a 50% rate of metastasis at presentation and thus to the overall poor prognosis for patients with malignant tumors of the small intestine.

CARCINOID TUMORS

The presentation of carcinoids varies, depending not only on their physical characteristics and site of origin but also on whether they are producing substances that are hormonally active. In general, most carcinoids are small, indolent tumors that remain asymptomatic and undetected while the patient is alive. Carcinoid tumors are categorized either pathologically by microscopic features or according to their embryologic site of origin.

The embryologic classification of carcinoids is more commonly used and is outlined in Table 10-2. This classification system subdivides carcinoids into those of the foregut (stomach, pancreas, and lungs), midgut (small bowel and appendix), or hindgut (colon and rectum). Foregut carcinoids are more commonly associated with an atypical presentation due to secretion of peptide hormone products other than serotonin, such as gastrin, adrenocorticotropic hormone, or growth hormone. Gastric carcinoids, when symptomatic, cause abdominal pain or bleeding. Patients with bronchial carcinoids may present with hemoptysis, wheezing, or postobstructive pneumonitis. Midgut carcinoids produce symptoms of hormone excess only when bulky or metastatic. The vast majority of appendiceal carcinoids are found incidentally, but carcinoids rarely may be the cause of appendicitis. Patients with small-bowel carcinoids usually present with symptoms similar to those described for other small-bowel tumors. Not uncommonly, as a small-bowel carcinoid progresses, it induces fibrosis of the mesentery, which may by itself cause intestinal obstruction as well as lead to varying degrees of mesenteric ischemia. Hindgut carcinoids tend to be clinically silent tumors that rarely produce serotonin even in the presence of metastatic disease. Patients with hindgut tumors most commonly present with bleeding but occasionally also have abdominal pain.

The hormonal manifestations of carcinoid tumors ("carcinoid syndrome") are seen in only 10% of patients and occur when the secretory products of these tumors gain direct access to the systemic circulation and avoid metabolism in the liver. This clinical syndrome occurs in the following situations: (1) when hepatic metastases are present; (2) when there is extensive retroperitoneal disease with venous drainage directly into the paravertebral veins; and (3) when the primary carcinoid tumor is outside the GI tract, as with bronchial, ovarian, or testicular tumors. Ninety percent of the cases of carcinoid syndrome are seen in patients with midgut tumors.

Table 10-2. Characteristics of carcinoid tumors based on their embryologic site of origin

Characteristics	Foregut	Midgut	Hindgut
Location	Bronchus Stomach Pancreas	Jejunum Ileum Appendix	Colon Rectum
Histology	Trabecular	Nodular, solid Nests of cells	Trabecular
Secretion:			
Tumor 5-HT	Low	High	None
Urinary 5-HIAA	High	High	Normal
Carcinoid syndrome	Yes	Yes	No
Other endocrine secretions	Frequent	Frequent	No

5-HT = 5-hydroxytryptamine; 5-HIAA = 5-hydroxyindoleacetic acid.

Table 10-3.   Clinical symptoms of carcinoid syndrome and tumor products suspected of causing them

Symptom	Tumor product
Flushing	Bradykinin
	Hydroxytryptophan
	Prostaglandins
Telangiectasia	VIP
	Serotonin
	Prostaglandins
	Bradykinin
Bronchospasm	Bradykinin
	Histamine
	Prostaglandins
Endocardial fibrosis	Serotonin
Glucose intolerance	Serotonin
Arthropathy	Serotonin
Hypotension	Serotonin

VIP = vasoactive intestinal polypeptide.

The main symptoms of carcinoid syndrome are watery diarrhea, flushing, sweating, wheezing, dyspnea, abdominal pain, hypotension, and/or right heart failure due to tricuspid regurgitation or pulmonic stenosis caused by endocardial fibrosis. The flush is often dramatic and is an intense purplish color on the upper body and arms. Facial edema is often present. Repeated attacks can lead to the development of telangiectasias and permanent skin discoloration. The flush can be precipitated by consuming alcohol, blue cheese, chocolate, red wine, and exercise. The mediators of these symptoms are shown in Table 10-3.

A life-threatening form of carcinoid syndrome called *carcinoid crisis* is usually precipitated by a specific event such as anesthesia, surgery, or chemotherapy. The manifestations include an intense flush, diarrhea, tachycardia, hypertension or hypotension, bronchospasm, and alteration of mental status. The symptoms are usually refractory to fluid resuscitation and administration of vasopressors.

Diagnostic Work-up

SMALL-BOWEL MALIGNANCIES

A high index of suspicion is essential to the early diagnosis and treatment of small-intestine malignancies. The patient presenting with nonspecific abdominal symptoms should undergo a complete history, physical examination, and screening for occult fecal blood. Laboratory work-up should include a complete blood count, measurement of serum electrolytes, and liver function tests. Further laboratory testing, including measurement of urinary 5-hydroxyindoleacetic acid (5-HIAA), should be directed by clinical suspicion.

Retrospective reviews report that 50–60% of small-intestine neoplasms are detected using conventional radiographic techniques, including upper GI series with small-bowel follow-through (UGI/SBFT) and enteroclysis. Hypotonic duodenography, using anticholinergic agents or glucagon to reduce duodenal peristalsis, may enhance diagnostic yield to as high as 86% for more proximally located duodenal malignancies. Upper GI endoscopy, when performed to the ligament of Treitz, was diagnostic in eight of nine patients with duodenal malignancies reviewed by Ouriel and Adams. Traditionally, computerized tomography (CT) was not felt to be helpful in diagnosing small-bowel neoplasms. However, several recent reviews have shown that CT was able to detect abnormalities in 97% of patients with small-bowel tumors. Angiography demonstrates a tumor blush in specific subtypes of small-bowel malignancies, most notably carcinoid and leiomyosarcoma, but is rarely indicated in the initial diagnostic work-up.

Enteroscopy should be considered when all previous diagnostic studies are negative. Lewis et al. reviewed the experience at Mt. Sinai Medical Center in New York with two endoscopic techniques—push enteroscopy and small-bowel enteroscopy—in 258 patients with obscure GI bleeding. Push enteroscopy uses a pediatric colonoscope that is passed orally and then pushed distally through the small intestine, facilitating intubation of the jejunum 60 cm distal to the ligament of Treitz. This technique established a diagnosis in 50% of patients examined. Small-bowel enteroscopy using a 120-degree, forward-viewing, 2,560-mm, balloon-tipped endoscope that is carried distally by peristalsis permitted intubation of the terminal ileum in 77% of cases within 8 hours.

Most retrospective studies report only moderate success in diagnosing small-bowel neoplasms preoperatively, with large series reporting a correct preoperative diagnosis in only 50% of cases, with the remainder diagnosed at laparotomy. Exploratory laparotomy remains the most sensitive diagnostic modality in evaluating a patient suspected of having a small-bowel neoplasm and should be considered in the diagnostic evaluation of a patient with occult GI bleeding, unexplained weight loss, or vague abdominal pain. Because most tumors will present as large, bulky lesions with lymph node metastasis, laparoscopy is potentially useful for establishing the diagnosis of malignancy when the work-up is otherwise negative and for obtaining adequate tissue samples if a diagnosis of lymphoma is suspected. Early detection and treatment remain the most significant variables in improving outcome from small-bowel malignancy, necessitating the thoughtful and expedient diagnostic work-up of patients presenting with vague abdominal symptoms.

CARCINOIDS

The diagnosis of carcinoid tumor is made using a combination of biochemical tests and imaging studies. Overall, about 50% of patients with carcinoids will have elevated urinary levels of

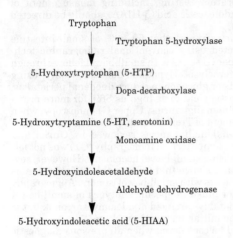

Tryptophan

Tryptophan 5-hydroxylase

5-Hydroxytryptophan (5-HTP)

Dopa-decarboxylase

5-Hydroxytryptamine (5-HT, serotonin)

Monoamine oxidase

5-Hydroxyindoleacetaldehyde

Aldehyde dehydrogenase

5-Hydroxyindoleacetic acid (5-HIAA)

Fig. 10-1. Biochemical steps in the production of 5-hydroxy-tryptamine (5-HT, serotonin) and 5-hydroxyindoleacetic acid (5-HIAA).

5-HIAA, irrespective of whether they have symptoms of carcinoid syndrome. When urinary 5-HIAA levels are nondiagnostic, a more extensive work-up should be undertaken, consisting of measurement of urinary 5-hydroxytryptamine (5-HT, serotonin) and 5-hydroxytryptophan (5-HPT), plasma 5-HPT, platelet 5-HT, and serum levels of other secretory products such as chromogranin A, neuron-specific enolase, substance P, and neuropeptide K. An overview of serotonin metabolism is shown in Fig. 10-1.

Localization of the tumor also may help confirm the diagnosis. Bronchial carcinoids are best visualized with a chest radiograph or CT scan. Gastric, duodenal, colonic, and rectal carcinoids are usually seen on endoscopy and barium studies. Small-intestine carcinoids are initially evaluated as described for other small-bowel malignancies. Abdominal CT scan is most useful for assessing mesenteric fibrosis, involvement of the retroperitoneum, and presence of liver metastasis.

Nuclear medicine scans have also been used in localization. Scans using metaiodobenzylguanidine (MIBG) radiolabeled with ^{131}I or [121]I can identify primary or metastatic carcinoid tumors approximately 50% of the time, when MIBG is taken up by the tumor and stored in its neurosecretory granules. Tyr-3-octreotide, a somatostatin analog, radiolabeled with ^{123}I, has also been used in an attempt to take advantage of the finding that most carcinoids display receptors for somatostatin. Scans with this analog appear useful in localizing 70–80% of carcinoids but are not widely available.

On occasion, a patient may benefit from angiography or selective venous sampling if other diagnostic maneuvers prove unsuccessful.

Table 10-4. AJCC staging of small-intestine malignancies

Primary tumor (T)

T1	Tumor invades lamina propria or submucosa
T2	Tumor invades muscularis propria
T3	Tumor invades through the muscularis propria into the subserosa or into the nonperitonealized perimuscular tissue (mesentery or retroperitoneum) with extension ≤2 cm
T4	Tumor perforates the visceral peritoneum or directly invades other organs or structures (includes other loops of the small intestine, mesentery, or retroperitoneum >2 cm, and the abdominal wall by way of the serosa; for the duodenum only, includes invasion of the pancreas)

Regional lymph nodes (N)

N0	No regional lymph node metastasis
N1	Regional lymph node metastasis

Distant metastasis (M)

M0	No distant metastasis
M1	Distant metastasis

Staging

Stage I	T1–T2	N0	M0
Stage II	T3–T4	N0	M0
Stage III	Any T	N1	M0
Stage IV	Any T	Any N	M1

Source: Adapted from OH Beahrs, DE Henson, RVP Hutter, et al. (eds). *AJCC Manual for Staging of Cancer* (4th ed). Philadelphia: Lippincott, 1992.

Staging

Only recently has the American Joint Committee on Cancer (AJCC) published a staging system for small-bowel malignancies (Table 10-4).

Malignant Neoplasms

The distribution of small-bowel malignancies (reported by Weiss and Yang in a review of nine population-based cancer registries participating in the National Cancer Institute's Surveillance, Epidemiology, and End Results [SEER] Program) is shown in Table 10-5. Information on tumor biology, modes of lymphatic spread, and patterns of recurrence for small-bowel malignancies is limited.

The most common histologic types of malignant tumors of the small intestine are adenocarcinoma (45.3%), carcinoid (29.3%),

Table 10-5.   Distribution of primary malignant neoplasms in the small intestine by subsite of cancer and histologic type as a percentage of total ($N = 1,413$)

Subsite specified	Adenocarcinoma	Carcinoid	Lymphoma	Sarcoma
Duodenum	21.9	1.3	0.8	1.8
Jejunum	14.7	2.5	5.1	5.0
Ileum	8.7	25.5	8.9	3.6
Total	45.3	29.3	14.8	10.4

Source: Adapted from NCI SEER Registries 1973–82. In NS Weiss, C Yang. Incidence of histologic types of cancer of the small intestine. *J Natl Cancer Inst* 78:653, 1987.

lymphoma (14.8%), and sarcoma (10.4%). Adenocarcinoma is the most common malignancy in the proximal small intestine, whereas carcinoid is the most common malignancy in the ileum. Sarcoma and lymphoma may develop throughout the small intestine but are more prevalent in the distal small bowel.

ADENOCARCINOMA

Pathology

Adenocarcinoma of the small intestine occurs most commonly in the duodenum, with 65% of these neoplasms clustered in the periampullary region. These tumors infiltrate into the muscularis propria and may extend through the serosa and into adjacent tissues. Ulceration is common, causing occult GI bleeding and chronic anemia. Obstruction may develop from progressive growth of apple core lesions or large intraluminal polypoid masses. It manifests itself as gastric outlet obstruction in cases of duodenal lesions or severe cramping pain in cases of more distally located lesions. Adenocarcinoma of the small bowel follows a pattern of tumor progression similar to that of colon cancer, with similar survival rates when compared stage for stage. Seventy to eighty percent of small-bowel lesions are resectable at the time of diagnosis, with a 5-year survival rate of 20–30% reported for patients undergoing resection. Approximately 35% of patients will have metastasis to regional lymph nodes at the time of diagnosis, with an additional 20% having distant metastasis. Mural penetration, nodal involvement, distant metastasis, and perineural invasion correlate with a poor prognosis.

Treatment

Wide excision of the malignancy and surrounding zones of contiguous spread is performed to provide complete tumor clearance for lesions located in the jejunum and ileum. Treatment strategies ranging from pancreaticoduodenectomy to local excision have been proposed for the management of duodenal adenocarcinoma. Pancreaticoduodenectomy has been touted as a superior operation for duodenal adenocarcinoma because of its more radical clearance of the tumor bed and regional lymph nodes. In fact, some authors, including Lai et al., continue to recommend pancreaticoduodenectomy for all primary duodenal adenocarcinomas. However, segmental resection for adenocarcinoma of the duodenum satisfies the principles of en bloc resection, without the morbidity of a pancreaticoduodenectomy, and should be considered when technically feasible.

Unlike pancreatic cancer, which diffusely infiltrates into the surrounding soft tissues, adenocarcinoma of the duodenum extends into adjacent tissues as a more localized process. Therefore tumor-free resection margins, critical to a curative extirpation, may be accomplished without necessarily resecting a generous portion of the surrounding soft tissues and adjacent organs; however, the tumor-free status of resection margins must be confirmed on frozen-section evaluation of the resected specimen.

In a comparison of pancreaticoduodenectomy to segmental resection for management of duodenal adenocarcinoma at the University of Texas M. D. Anderson Cancer Center, Barnes et al. found no significant difference in survival rates but did find a difference in 5-year local control rates—76% versus 49% for pancreaticoduodenectomy and segmental resection, respectively. Several other reviews—including those of Lowell et al., Joestling et al., and vanOoijen and Kalsbeek, which compared survival following pancreaticoduodenectomy or segmental resection for lesions in the third and fourth portion of the duodenum—have demonstrated no significant difference in 5-year survival. In these studies, a more limited resection, with less associated morbidity and mortality, provided a survival benefit equal to that of a more extensive resection.

At M. D. Anderson, a Whipple pancreaticoduodenectomy is performed for lesions involving the proximal duodenum to the right of the superior mesenteric artery (SMA). A segmental resection is performed for duodenal lesions to the left of the SMA. Local excision is considered for small lesions on the antimesenteric wall of the second portion of the duodenum.

Experimental Therapy

Electron beam intraoperative radiotherapy (EB-IORT) and external beam radiotherapy have been administered at M. D. Anderson in a limited number of cases of microscopic involvement of resection margins or unresectable disease. However, adenocarcinoma of the small intestine is generally considered to be radioresistant. Chemotherapy, based on 5-fluorouracil (5-FU) and nitrosoureas, has been recommended in both the adjuvant setting and cases of unresectable disease, yet most retrospective studies have failed to demonstrate a significant response to chemotherapy. Because most centers have only limited experience treating adenocarcinoma of the small intestine, the efficacy of chemotherapy needs further study, and patients should continue to be enrolled in prospective randomized trials.

CARCINOID

Pathology

Carcinoids are known mainly for their ability to secrete serotonin and are the most common endocrine tumors of the GI system.

They arise from enterochromaffin cells, which are located predominantly in the GI tract and mainstem bronchi. In addition to serotonin, these tumors can secrete a number of biologically active substances (Table 10-6), including amines, tachykinins, peptides, and prostaglandins.

Carcinoid tumors occur most frequently in the appendix (40%), small intestine (27%), rectum (15%), and bronchus (11%). Small-bowel carcinoids occur most commonly in the terminal 60 cm of the ileum as tan, yellow, or gray-brown intramural or submucosal nodules. The presence of multiple synchronous nodules in 30% of patients mandates careful inspection of the entire small intestine in these patients.

Primary carcinoid tumors are indolent, slow-growing lesions that become symptomatic late in the course of the disease. Rarely ulcerative, these tumors infiltrate the muscularis propria and may extend through the serosa to involve the mesentery or retroperitoneum and to produce a characteristically intense desmoplastic reaction.

Metastatic disease, present in 90% of symptomatic patients, correlates not only with the depth of invasion but also with the size of the primary lesion. For carcinoids <1 cm, the risk of metastasis is 2% for appendiceal, 15–18% for small-bowel, and 20% for rectal primaries. If carcinoid tumors are >2 cm, 33% of appendiceal, 86–95% of small-bowel, and almost all rectal primaries have metastasized.

Distant sites of metastases include the liver and, to a lesser degree, the lungs and bone.

Table 10-6.   Biologically active substances that can be secreted by carcinoid tumors

Amines
5-HT
5-HIAA
5-HTP
Histamine
Dopamine

Tachykinins
Kallikrein
Substance P
Neuropeptide K

Others
Prostaglandins
Pancreatic polypeptide
Chromogranins
Neurotensin
HCGa
HCGb

5-HT = 5-hydroxytryptamine; 5-HIAA = 5-hydroxyindoleacetic acid;
5-HTP = 5-hydroxytryptophan; HCG = human chorionic gonadotropin.

Treatment of Localized Disease

Surgical extirpation is the definitive treatment for localized primary carcinoid tumors. The extent of resection is determined by the size of the primary lesion and is based on the likelihood of mesenteric lymph node involvement. The incidence of metastasis depends on the location of the tumor, its depth of invasion, and its size.

Appendiceal carcinoids smaller than 1 cm rarely metastasize and are adequately treated by appendectomy alone unless the base of the appendix is involved, in which case a partial cecectomy may be necessary. Because the incidence of metastasis increases with size, treatment of appendiceal carcinoids between 1 and 2 cm is more controversial. In general, most authors recommend appendectomy alone for lesions smaller than 1.5 cm and right hemicolectomy for lesions larger than 1.5 cm or for any lesion with invasion of the mesoappendix, blood vessels, or regional lymph nodes.

In contrast to appendiceal carcinoids, carcinoids of the small bowel are more likely to metastasize even when smaller than 1 cm. As a result, most surgeons recommend a wide en bloc resection that includes the adjacent mesentery and lymph nodes. Such a resection may be difficult at times if fibrosis and foreshortening of the mesentery are present. Although some surgeons advocate local excision for small midgut carcinoids, up to 70% of these tumors will metastasize to the lymph nodes. Therefore a wide resection not only may cure many of these patients but also should provide better local disease control. Because of the slow-growing nature of these tumors, wide excision is advocated even when distant metastases are present. In addition, approximately 40% of patients with midgut carcinoids have a second GI malignancy. Therefore the entire bowel and colon should be evaluated prior to any planned surgical intervention.

Rectal carcinoids <1 cm are adequately treated by wide local excision alone. Tumors between 1 and 2 cm should be locally resected by a wide, local, full-thickness excision with abdomino-perineal resection (APR) or low anterior resection recommended for tumors that invade the muscularis propria. The treatment of patients with rectal carcinoids >2 cm remains controversial. Even though major cancer operations were once recommended for rectal carcinoids >2 cm, it is now appreciated that the risk of distant metastasis is so high that radical surgery should not be entertained if the tumor can be removed by wide local excision. Every attempt should be made for sphincter preservation in patients with carcinoids of the rectum of >2 cm because of the high likelihood of distant relapse and the marginal benefit obtained from radical local therapy.

Treatment of Advanced Disease

The role of surgery for unresectable and metastatic disease is not clearly defined, but it appears that surgery may benefit patients. When metastatic disease is present, it is necessary to establish whether the patient has symptoms of carcinoid syndrome and whether curative resection is possible. If there are no contraindications to surgery, then an attempt at complete extirpation should be made because it may lead to prolonged disease-free survival as well as symptomatic relief. Patients with metastatic carcinoid should all begin receiving octreotide therapy preoperatively to pre-vent a carcinoid crisis (see later). The duration of effective relief from these palliative procedures is generally less than 12 months, and no survival benefit has been consistently demonstrated.

Patients with mildly symptomatic carcinoid syndrome can be treated medically. Diarrhea can usually be controlled with loper-amide, diphenoxylate, or the serotonin receptor antagonist cypro-heptadine. Flushing can frequently be controlled with either adre-nergic blocking agents (e.g., clonidine or phenoxybenzamine) or a combination of type 1 and 2 histamine receptor antagonists. Albu-terol (a beta-adrenergic blocking agent) and aminophylline are effective in relieving bronchospasm and wheezing.

For patients whose symptoms cannot be controlled with these conservative measures or who develop a carcinoid crisis, the somatostatin analog octreotide has shown tremendous promise. A trial from the Mayo Clinic found that flushing and diarrhea could be controlled in the vast majority of patients with as little as 150 mg of octreotide administered subcutaneously three times per day. The duration of the responses was on the average more than 1 year. Interestingly, a number of studies have now shown that octreotide is also able to slow tumor growth significantly in more than 50% of patients and to cause tumor regression for vari-able periods in another 10–20% of individuals.

Because such good results can be obtained with octreotide, interferon, and/or hepatic artery chemoembolization (see later), surgical debulking procedures, which used to be recommended for patients with symptomatic carcinoid syndrome and liver metas-tasis, are rarely required. Patients with unresectable disease, if asymptomatic, should just be monitored. Local complications related to the tumor can be addressed if and when they develop. Our current indications for surgical intervention in unresectable and widely metastatic disease include complications of bulky car-cinoid tumors such as obstruction and perforation. In addition, surgical debulking is considered for severe intractable symptoms unresponsive to medical treatment, if a dominant mass or liver metastasis can be identified.

Despite the advanced stage of disease at presentation and the limited effectiveness of currently available therapies, the natural history of carcinoids affords affected patients a better prognosis than other malignancies of the small bowel. The 5-year survival rate for localized disease approaches 100% after complete resec-tion. Resection of metastatic disease is associated with a 68% 5-year survival rate, whereas unresectable disease has a 38% 5-year survival rate.

Experimental Therapy

A number of chemotherapeutic agents have been tried in patients with carcinoid tumors. Results of chemotherapy trials with such agents as doxorubicin, dacarbazine, and streptozotocin, either alone or in combination, have been disappointing. Most chemotherapy trials show response rates of less than 30%, with the duration of these responses being only a few months. The role of chemotherapy is still investigational, but for patients with advanced disease that cannot be controlled with standard mea-sures, monitored clinical trials should be recommended.

One biologic agent, interferon, in both the alpha-2a and alpha-2b forms, has shown promising results in diminishing urinary levels of 5-HIAA as well as symptoms of carcinoid syndrome. Most patients in most studies had either a partial regression or stabilization of their disease for a prolonged period. Unfortunately, objective responses with reduction of tumor size occurred in only about 15% of patients.

In some centers, hepatic artery chemoembolization has been used with some success to diminish the size of liver metastases and decrease levels of biologically active mediators of carcinoid syndrome.

Although external beam radiation has not proven effective in treating carcinoid tumors, targeted radiation in the form of radioactive iodine coupled to either MIBG or octreotide are two therapeutic strategies that may hold some promise for the future.

SARCOMA

Pathology

Sarcomas of the small intestine are typically slow-growing lesions; they occur more frequently in the jejunum and ileum than in the duodenum. Sharing a similar growth pattern with other GI sarcomas, these malignancies invade adjacent tissues, with metastasis occurring predominantly via the hematogenous route to the liver, lungs, and bones. The most common clinical presentations are pain (65%), abdominal mass (50%), and bleeding. More than 75% of tumors exceed 5 cm in diameter at diagnosis, with extramural extension, rather than intramural or intraluminal extension, representing the typical growth pattern. For this reason, obstruction is rarely a manifestation of this disease process.

CT of these lesions typically demonstrates a heterogeneous mass with focal areas of necrosis where the tumor has outgrown its nutrient blood supply and formed localized abscesses.

Leiomyosarcoma accounts for 75% of small-intestine sarcomas; fibrosarcoma, liposarcoma, and angiosarcoma are seen less frequently. In summary, sarcoma represents only 10% of small-bowel malignancies, yet the various subtypes encompass a broad range of biologic behavior, the scope of which exceeds this review.

Treatment

Surgical resection is the primary treatment modality for sarcoma of the small bowel. Because sarcoma infrequently metastasizes to regional mesenteric lymph nodes, unlike adenocarcinoma and carcinoid, an extensive mesenteric lymphadenectomy is unnecessary and will not improve survival. En bloc resection of the lesion with tumor-free margins is recommended for a potentially curative resection; however, at the time of diagnosis, 50% of lesions are unresectable and most exceed 5 cm in diameter. Local resection should be considered in the presence of widely metastatic disease for control of bleeding and relief of obstruction.

Experimental Therapy

There is no clearly defined benefit from chemotherapy or radiotherapy when used in the adjuvant setting, for leiomyosarcomas of the small bowel. Combined chemotherapy and radiotherapy should only be offered to patients with leiomyosarcomas as part of an experimental protocol in an attempt to downstage the disease and/or possibly make an unresectable lesion resectable. Chemotherapy can be used in the treatment of recurrent or metastatic disease, but again, only as part of an experimental protocol. Currently at M. D. Anderson, chemoembolization with cisplatin is used in patients with metastatic disease to the liver. Sarcomas of other histologic subtypes should be treated as discussed in Chapter 5.

LYMPHOMA

Pathology

The distribution of lymphoma in the small intestine parallels the distribution of lymphoid follicles in the small intestine, with the lymphoid-rich ileum representing the most common location of small-bowel lymphoma. Lymphoma arises from the lymphoid aggregates in the submucosa; infiltration of the mucosa can result in ulceration and bleeding. The tumor may also extend to the serosa and adjacent tissues, producing a large obstructing mass associated with cramping abdominal pain. Perforation occurs in as many as 25% of patients. Lymphoma may arise as a primary neoplasm or as a component of systemic disease with GI involvement. As with sarcoma, bulky disease is a characteristic of lymphoma, with approximately 70% of tumors larger than 5 cm in diameter.

Primary tumors are staged according to the Kiel classification (see Chapter 16) as low-, intermediate-, or high-grade, with high-grade lesions being diagnosed most frequently. Prognostic factors include tumor grade, extent of tumor penetration, nodal involvement, peritoneal disease, and distant metastasis. The 5-year survival rate ranges from 20% to 33%.

Treatment

Extended surgical resection of the primary lesion and accompanying regional mesenteric lymph nodes is the mainstay of treatment for lymphoma of the small bowel. Because of the extensive submucosal infiltration of lymphoma, frozen section should be performed to microscopically confirm tumor-free margins. Lymph node metastases are frequent, necessitating an en bloc resection of the adjoining mesentery. Resection alone provides adequate therapy for low-grade lymphomas, whereas resection combined with adjuvant chemotherapy is indicated for intermediate- and high-grade lymphomas. The first-line chemotherapy regimen currently used at M. D. Anderson is cyclophosphamide, doxorubicin, vincristine, and prednisone (CHOP).

Experimental Therapy

Chemoradiation has been used at some institutions for nodal metastasis, positive resection margins, and unresectable disease. However, a survival benefit from such treatment regimens has not been demonstrated. The use of radiotherapy alone has been associated with significant tumor necrosis, bleeding, and bowel perforation but may be considered in elderly patients unable to tolerate the toxicity of chemotherapy.

METASTATIC MALIGNANCIES

Pathology

Metastases are the most common form of malignancy in the small intestine and develop as a result of hematogenous or lymphatic spread from a primary tumor to the mucosa or submucosal lymphatics of the small intestine. The primary tumors that most commonly metastasize to the small bowel include ovarian, colon, lung, and melanoma. Metastatic melanoma is unique in that once localized in the small bowel, the metastatic focus may further disseminate to the small-bowel mesentery and draining lymph nodes. In general, however, small-bowel metastases remain localized to the bowel wall, and they may produce small-bowel obstruction or perforation.

Although the typical presentation of metastatic lesions is obstruction or perforation, the more common cause of obstruction and perforation in patients who have previously undergone resection of a GI primary tumor is related to the initial procedure—that is, either recurrence of the primary tumor or adhesions resulting from the initial exploration.

Segmental bowel resection is the primary treatment for small-bowel metastases. Except for melanoma metastases, which may function as a source of further lymphatic dissemination, a regional lymphadenectomy is not performed for metastatic tumors of the small intestine.

PALLIATION

At the time of diagnosis, most small-bowel malignancies are locally advanced, with significant bulky disease and/or metastases. When the advanced stage of disease precludes surgical resection, enteric bypass should be performed to prevent obstruction. In the event of bleeding from an unresectable small-bowel malignancy, intra-arterial embolization of nutrient arteries may be considered, but the benefits must be weighed against the significant risks of this procedure. Our experience with this technique at M. D. Anderson Cancer Center has been discouraging because of the significant rate of bowel ischemia and perforation associated with embolization of the small-bowel mesentery.

Chemotherapy or combined chemoradiation may offer effective control of locally advanced unresectable disease, particularly in the case of lymphoma, and should be considered among palliative treatment options.

Surveillance

Routine follow-up for patients should include a complete history and physical examination, complete blood count, serum electrolyte determination, and liver function tests performed at regular intervals. A chest radiograph should be obtained every 6 months for the first 3 years after resection, followed by subsequent yearly exams. Assessment of locoregional recurrence in patients who have undergone a right hemicolectomy for ileal malignancy or segmental resection for duodenal malignancy should include endoscopy at 6-month intervals. Assessment for recurrence at other sites may include CT, UGI/SBFT, angiography, or enteroscopy and must be directed by clinical suspicion based on patient history and physical and laboratory findings.

Selected References

Ajani JA, Carrasco H, Samaan NA, et al. Therapeutic options in patients with advanced islet cell and carcinoid tumors. *Reg Cancer Treat* 3:235, 1990.

Ashley SW, Wells SA. Tumors of the small intestine. *Semin Oncol* 15:116, 1988.

Barnes G, Romero L, Hess KR, et al. Primary adenocarcinoma of the duodenum: Management and survival in 67 patients. *Ann Surg Oncol* 1:73, 1994.

Bomanji J, Mather S, Moyes J, et al. A scintigraphic comparison of iodine-123 metaiodobenzylguanidine and iodine-labeled somatostatin analog (tyr-3-octreotide) in metastatic carcinoid tumors. *J Nucl Med* 33:1121, 1992.

Carrasco CH, Charnsangavej C, Ajani J, et al. The carcinoid syndrome palliation by hepatic artery embolization. *Am J Roentgenol* 147:149, 1986.

Cattell RB, Braasch JW. A technique for the exposure of the third and fourth portions of the duodenum. *Surg Gynecol Obstet* 11:379, 1960.

Cheek RC, Wilson H. Carcinoid tumors. *Curr Probl Surg* Nov:4, 1970.

Crist DW, Sitzman JV, Cameron JL. Improved hospital morbidity, mortality, and survival after the Whipple procedure. *Ann Surg* 206:358, 1987.

Cubilla AL, Fortner J, Fitzgerald PJ. Lymph node involvement in carcinoma of the head of the pancreas area. *Cancer* 41:880, 1978.

Donohue JH. Malignant tumors of the small bowel. *Surg Oncol* 3:61, 1994.

Farouk M, Niotis M, Branum GD, et al. Indications for and the techniques of local resection of tumors of the papilla of Vater. *Arch Surg* 126:650, 1991.

Godwin JD II. Carcinoid tumors: An analysis of 2837 cases. *Cancer* 36:560, 1975.

Hanson MW, Feldman JE, Blinder RA, et al. Carcinoid tumors: Iodine-131 MIBG scintigraphy. *Radiology* 172:699, 1989.

Joestling DR, Beart RW, van Heerden JA, et al. Improving survival in adenocarcinoma of the duodenum. *Am J Surg* 141:228, 1981.

Johnson AM, Harman PK, Hanks JB. Primary small bowel malignancies. *Am Surg* 51:31, 1985.

Kvols LK, Moertel CG, O'Connell MJ, et al. Treatment of the malignant carcinoid syndrome: Evaluation of a long acting somatostatin analogue. *N Engl J Med* 315:663, 1986.

Lai EC, Doty JE, Irving C, et al. Primary adenocarcinoma of the duodenum: Analysis of survival. *World J Surg* 12:695, 1988.

Lamberts SW, Bakker WH, Reubi JC, et al. Somatostatin-receptor imaging in the localization of endocrine tumors. *N Engl J Med* 323:1246, 1990.

Lewis BS, Kornbluth A, Waye JD. Small bowel tumors: Yield of enteroscopy. *Gut* 32:763, 1991.

Lowell JA, Rossi RL, Munson L, et al. Primary adenocarcinoma of third and fourth portions of duodenum. *Arch Surg* 127:557, 1992.

Maglinte DT, O'Connor K, Bessette J, et al. The role of the physician in the late diagnosis of primary malignant tumors of the small intestine. *J Gastroenterol* 86:304, 1991.

Martin RG. Malignant tumors of the small intestine. *Surg Clin North Am* 66:779, 1986.

Moertel CG, Weiland LH, Nagorney DM, et al. Carcinoid tumor of the appendix: Treatment and prognosis. *N Engl J Med* 317:1699, 1987.

Motojima K, Tsukasa T, Kanematsu T, et al. Distinguishing pancreatic cancer from other periampullary carcinomas by analysis of mutations in the Kirsten-ras oncogene. *Ann Surg* 214:657, 1991.

Oberg K, Eriksson B. The role of interferons in the management of carcinoid tumors. *Br J Haematol* 79:74, 1991.

O'Rourke MG, Lancashire RP, Vattoune JR. Lymphoma of the small intestine. *Aust NZ J Surg* 56:351, 1986.

Ouriel K, Adams JT. Adenocarcinoma of the small intestine. *Am J Surg* 147:66, 1984.

Rothmund M, Kisker, O. Surgical treatment of carcinoid tumors of the small bowel, appendix, colon and rectum. *Digestion* 55(Suppl 3):86, 1994.

Strodel WE, Talpos G, Eckhauser F, et al. Surgical therapy for small-bowel carcinoid tumors. *Arch Surg* 118:391, 1983.

Thompson GB, van Heerden JA, Martin JK Jr, et al. Carcinoid tumors of the gastrointestinal tract: Presentation, management, and prognosis. *Surgery* 98:1054, 1985.

vanOoijen B, Kalsbeek HL. Carcinoma of the duodenum. *Surg Gynecol Obstet* 166:343, 1988.

Vinik AI, Thompson N, Eckhauser F, et al. Clinical features of carcinoid syndrome and the use of somatostatin analogue in its management. *Acta Oncol* 28:389, 1989.

Weiss NS, Yang C. Incidence of histologic types of cancer of the small intestine. *J Natl Can Inst* 78:653, 1987.

Welch JP, Malt RA. Management of carcinoid tumors of the gastrointestinal tract. *Surg Gynecol Obstet* 145:223, 1977.

Willett CG, Warshaw AL, Connery K, et al. Patterns of failure after pancreaticoduodenectomy for ampullary carcinoma. *Surg Gynecol Obstet* 176:33, 1993.

Cancer of the Colon, Rectum, and Anus

Gregory P. Midis and Barry W. Feig

Colorectal Cancer

EPIDEMIOLOGY

Colorectal cancer comprises 13% of all cancers and is responsible for 10% of all deaths from cancer. In 1997, 131,000 cases were diagnosed and 54,900 Americans died of this disease.

The age-specific incidence of colorectal cancer increases steadily from the second through the eighth decades of life, with a male predominance. At diagnosis, 10% of patients will have *in situ* disease, one-third will have local disease, and one-third will have regional disease; 20% of patients will have distant disease.

The overall 5-year survival rate for colorectal cancer is 50%. However, when stratified by local, regional, and distant disease, the survival rates are 90%, 58%, and 5%, respectively. The age-adjusted death rate increased steadily for males and females from 1930 to 1950. Since 1950, the death rate in females has declined slightly, whereas that of males has remained constant.

RISK FACTORS

Diet

Dietary factors may promote or inhibit carcinogenesis. Consumption of red meat and animal fat, as well as the presence of high fecal levels of cholesterol, correlate with and may be causally related to an increased risk of colorectal carcinoma. There is weak data to support the use of vitamin C and beta-carotene to reduce colorectal cancer. Vitamin E may help prevent colorectal cancer. There is good evidence from epidemiologic studies that fiber is associated with a reduction in risk for cancer of the colon and rectum. Increased intake of fiber, calcium, and selenium decreases the incidence of colorectal carcinoma.

Polyps

Colorectal polyps are classified histologically as either neoplastic (adenomatous) polyps (which may be benign or malignant) or non-neoplastic (including hyperplastic, mucosal, inflammatory, hamartomatous). The National Polyp Study showed that colonoscopic removal of adenomatous polyps significantly reduced the risk of developing colorectal cancer. Adenomatous colorectal polyps are common, occurring in approximately 30% of adults in Western countries. Most colon carcinomas arise from polyps. Most lesions are less than 1 cm in size, with 60% of people having a single adenoma and 40% having multiple lesions. Sixty percent of lesions will be located distal to the splenic flexure.

Polyps coexist with colorectal cancer in 60% of patients and are associated with an increased incidence of synchronous and metachronous colonic neoplasms. Patients with a primary cancer and a solitary associated polyp have a lower incidence of synchronous and metachronous lesions when compared with patients with multiple polyps (7.3% and 2.7% versus 14.6% and 12.4%, respectively). The natural history of polyps supports an aggressive approach to their treatment: 24% of patients with polyps left untreated will develop invasive cancer at the site of that polyp within 20 years.

There are three histologic variants of adenomatous polyps. *Tubular adenomas* represent 75–87% of polyps and are found with equal frequency throughout all segments of the bowel. Less than 5% of tubular adenomas are malignant. *Tubulovillous adenomas* constitute 8–15% of polyps. They are also equally distributed throughout the bowel, and 20–25% are malignant. The remaining 5–10% of polyps are *villous adenomas,* which are usually localized to the rectum; 35–40% of these polyps are malignant. Besides histology, the size of a polyp and the degree of dysplasia have been associated with malignant potential. Malignancy was found in 1.3% of adenomas <1 cm, 9.5% between 1 and 2 cm, and 46% >2 cm. Similarly, 5.7% of mild, 18% of moderate, and 34.5% of adenomatous polyps with severe dysplasia were found to have malignant cells upon complete excision of the polyp. Therefore although only 2–5% of adenomatous polyps harbor malignancy at the time of diagnosis, the histology, size, and degree of dysplasia can help predict which polyps will be malignant.

The terms *carcinoma in situ* (CIS) and *intramucosal carcinoma* are used to describe severely dysplastic adenomas that have not invaded the muscularis mucosae and therefore have no risk of lymph node metastases. Approximately 5–7% of adenomatous polyps contain CIS. If a polyp containing CIS is completely excised endoscopically, the patient should be considered cured.

Overall, 8.5–17% of polyps harboring invasive carcinoma will develop metastases to regional lymph nodes. Four unfavorable pathologic features of malignant colorectal polyps are known to increase the probability that regional lymph nodes will be involved with tumor: (1) poor differentiation, (2) vascular and/or lymphatic invasion, (3) invasion below the submucosa, and (4) positive resection margin. Poorly differentiated lesions (grade 3) are associated with a higher incidence of lymphovascular involvement and recurrent disease when compared with well- and moderately differentiated lesions (grades 1 and 2). Approximately 4–8% of malignant polyps will be poorly differentiated. Vascular invasion is uncommon; when it occurs, it is associated with recurrent disease or lymphatic invasion in about 40% of patients. Lymphatic invasion occurs in 12% of malignant polyps and carries a poor prognosis. Either type of invasion and/or poor differentiation is an indication for evaluation for surgical resection. Depth of invasion may be the single most important prognostic factor for mesenteric lymph node involvement with invasive cancer arising in a polyp. Haggitt et al. approached this depth issue by assigning level 0–4 values for invasion from the head of the polyp to the submucosa of the bowel wall (between the stalk and the muscularis propria). Because pathologic studies have shown that lymphatic channels do not penetrate above the muscularis mucosa, they determined that level 4 invasion was the only significant prognostic factor in a multivariate analysis of risk factors for invasive carcinoma in a polyp. Although these findings have been confirmed by other studies, there are frequently multiple adverse prognostic factors seen in patients with higher levels of invasion (i.e., levels 3–4), which makes it difficult to assign depth as the most important factor. A negative resection margin has consistently been shown to be associated with a decreased adverse outcome (recurrence, residual carcinoma, lymph node metastases, decreased survival). Twenty-seven percent of patients with positive or indeterminate margins will have adverse outcomes, compared with 18% with negative margins and poor prognostic features and 0.8% with negative margins and no other poor prognostic features. Therefore a negative margin is important but only a component of the risk factor assessment.

Although clinical factors such as age, location, number of polyps, and gender are collectively known to be prognostic factors, only age greater than 60 years has been identified as an independent risk factor for invasion.

Treatment

When adenomatous polyps are found by sigmoidoscopy, we recommend complete colonoscopy with colonoscopic removal of the polyp and colonoscopic surveillance every 3 years until the exam is normal. Colonoscopic polypectomy is a safe, effective treatment for nearly all pedunculated polyps. Those polyps not amenable to safe polypectomy are biopsied and referred for surgical resection (usually large sessile villous lesions). Fungation, ulceration, and distortion of the surrounding bowel wall are indicative of invasion of the bowel wall and are contraindications to polypectomy. The surgical oncologist will become involved in decisions regarding the necessity of surgical resection after polypectomy. Colectomy is indicated for patients with residual carcinoma and for those at high risk for lymph node metastases despite complete endoscopic polypectomy. The high-risk pathologic features previously described (positive margin or margin <2 mm, poor differentiation, increased depth of invasion (level 4), and vascular/lymphatic invasion) and the resultant increased risk of lymph node metastasis must be weighed against the risk of surgical resection. Therefore an elderly patient with a completely excised pedunculated polyp with negative margins who has medical factors that increase the risk for open surgery may be best served by endoscopic polypectomy alone. In a review of 17 studies to evaluate the frequency of lymph node metastases or residual carcinoma in low-risk patients with pedunculated polyps, only a 1% incidence was found. In sessile polyps with low-risk features, the incidence was increased to 4.1%. Because the incidence of nodal metastases is higher in sessile polyps with invasive cancer, those patients at low operative risk should be considered for resection even if no high-risk pathologic features are observed. Stalk invasion in pedunculated polyps is not considered an adverse histologic feature, and treatment of polyps with stalk invasion is the same as that of polyps without stalk invasion (based on risk stratification). Polypoid cancers (almost all the polyp is invaded with carcinoma) are treated no differently from other malignant polypoid lesions. The decision for colectomy must depend on the presence and number of high-risk pathologic factors present in the polyp weighed against the patient's operative risks. Large villous adenomas of the rectum may be amenable to transanal local excision. This provides a complete diagnostic evaluation for malignancy, and if excised with negative margins (with other favorable prognostic features) may be the only therapeutic procedure needed.

Hereditary Polyposis Syndromes

Hereditary polyposis represents a constellation of syndromes rather than a single disease entity. All are characterized by multiple intestinal polyps as well as associated extraintestinal manifestations.

Familial adenomatous polyposis (FAP) is the best characterized of the syndromes; 1–2% of patients diagnosed with colon carcinoma will have FAP. The genetic alteration associated with FAP has been determined to be a point mutation in the adenomatous polyposis coli (APC) gene located on the long arm of chromosome 5 in band q21. It is inherited in an autosomal dominant pattern, with 90% penetrance. Affected individuals develop polyps throughout the gastrointestinal (GI) tract but most commonly in the colon. Without prophylactic colectomy, nearly all affected individuals will develop colorectal cancer by the sixth decade of life. Commercial genetic testing can identify an APC gene mutation in approximately 80% of FAP families. Once the specific mutation is identified in a family, the test can differentiate affected from unaffected individuals with 100% accuracy, thereby aiding in surveillance and surgical planning.

Gardner's syndrome is also inherited in an autosomal dominant pattern and is thought to represent a variant of FAP (including mutation of the APC gene). It is characterized by colonic and small-bowel adenomas, lipomas, abdominal desmoids, sebaceous cysts, osteomas, and fibromas. *Oldfield's syndrome* is associated with multiple sebaceous cysts, polyps, and carcinomas. Patients with *Turcot syndrome* experience intestinal polyposis and associated central nervous system tumors. This syndrome occurs less frequently than the others and has an autosomal recessive pattern of inheritance.

Although the hereditary syndromes are rare, the identification of a genetic alteration in patients with familial polyposis has provided a unique opportunity to investigate the molecular events involved in the pathogenesis of colon cancer.

Hereditary Nonpolyposis Syndromes

Hereditary nonpolyposis colorectal cancer (HNPCC), also classically known as the Lynch I and II syndromes, is a nonpolyposis autosomal dominant disease that occurs five times more frequently than familial polyposis. HNPCC appears to account for between 1% and 5% of colon cancers. Isolated colonic involvement occurs in the Lynch I syndrome. Colonic, breast, pancreatic, and endometrial tumors characterize the Lynch II syndrome. There is an approximately 80% lifetime risk of colon cancer. Compared with patients with sporadic colon cancer, patients with HNPCC have cancers that are more right-sided (60–70% occur proximal to the splenic flexure), occur earlier (about 45 years of age), have a lower stage, have better survival, and have an increased rate of metachronous and synchronous tumors (20%).

The genetic mutations causing HNPCC are in DNA mismatch repair genes that prevent replication errors (RER), and hence genetic instability. Although many genes have been associated with HNPCC, most cases seem to be due to defects in two genes: MLH1 and MSH2. Mutations in tumor suppressor genes such as p53, DCC, and APC can be associated with HNPCC because RER are produced in these tumor suppressor genes. Genetic testing is carried out to (1) identify risk within a known family by identifying the specific genetic defect and screening subsequent members, and (2) investigate sporadic cancers suspicious for HNPCC by first identifying RER mutations in cancers, then screening for the specific genetic defect.

Inflammatory Bowel Disease

Ulcerative colitis carries a risk of colorectal carcinoma that is 30 times greater than that of the general population. The incidence rises steadily with increasing duration of disease. After 30 years, the risk of colorectal cancer rises to 35% in this population. Crohn's disease is also associated with an increased risk of cancer, although the risk is hard to quantify. The risk associated with IBD underscores the importance of surveillance in this patient population.

Previous Colon Carcinoma

Patients with a history of colon cancer are three times more likely than the general population to develop a second primary colon carcinoma; 5–8% of these patients develop metachronous lesions.

History of First-Degree Relatives with Bowel Cancer

People with a first-degree relative with colorectal cancer have a 1.8–8-fold higher risk of developing colorectal cancer than the general population. The risk is higher if more than one relative is affected, and higher if the relative developed cancer at a young age (<45).

SCREENING

Screening can be defined as stratification of risk among apparently asymptomatic, average-risk individuals. Those with a positive screen are subjected to surveillance, and those with a positive surveillance test or symptoms are subjected to a diagnostic evaluation. Recently, screening for colorectal cancer has become a subject of much debate.

As many as 19% of the general population are at risk of developing adenomatous polyps, and 5% of sporadic polyps may progress to colorectal carcinoma. These data make it likely that screening patients for polyps and early cancers and treatment of these lesions could decrease overall mortality from colorectal carcinoma. Recently, this reduction in mortality has been shown in prospective, randomized trials.

Fecal occult blood testing (FOBT) (using Hemoccult or Hemo-quant) and endoscopy are the most widely employed screening tools for colorectal cancer. However, few studies have been able to document a significant impact of these tests on overall survival. Several factors have contributed to this finding. Compliance rates with FOBT are reported to vary between 40% and 68%. There is also an inherent error from random sampling of stool and improper specimen handling. The sensitivity and specificity of FOBT for the detection of colorectal cancer varies from 30% to 90%, and from 90% to 99%, respectively, and depends on whether the specimens are rehydrated or not (increases sensitivity but decreases specificity, which increases the numbers of colono-scopies). Nevertheless, there is proof from three randomized tri-als that FOBT detects cancers at an earlier stage than those detected in populations without testing and that there is a reduc-tion in colorectal cancer mortality. Rehydration of specimens is not recommended at this time. Early cost/benefit analyses in the 1980s did not show that FOBT was cost-effective. However, although the data conflict, there is more evidence that screening with FOBT, and subsequent colonoscopy, can be cost-effective.

Although the introduction of flexible sigmoidoscopy has improved patient comfort and decreased risk compared with rigid sigmoid-oscopy, the incidence of cancers proximal to the splenic flexure has increased, especially in women, which decreases the sensitivity of the test. Despite this, flexible sigmoidoscopy and polyp clearance has resulted in a decreased incidence of colorectal cancer, and hence a decreased mortality from this disease.

The value of colonoscopy in screening can be appreciated if one considers that approximately 40% of colon cancers arise proximal to the splenic flexure and that 75% of proximal colon cancers do not have an index lesion within reach of the flexible sigmoidoscope. Most studies using screening colonoscopy in average-risk patients report an average of 30% of neoplastic lesions detected. Cost is an important issue, however, if colonoscopy is considered the ultimate screening tool. Currently, screening colonoscopy is cost-effective if a 10-year interval is used once the colon is cleared of polyps.

Double-contrast barium enema (DCBE) is used less frequently than colonoscopy for screening and can detect colorectal carcinoma and polyps >1 cm with an accuracy equal to that of colonoscopy. It is used in patients who refuse or cannot have full colonoscopy to the cecum, as an adjunct to flexible sigmoidoscopy to evaluate the remainder of the colon, and for difficult-to-visualize turns in the colon.

The study of Winawer et al. from Memorial Sloan-Kettering Cancer Center (MSKCC) showed a reduction in mortality (43%) in people who were screened with fecal occult blood testing and rigid sigmoidoscopy, but this was not statistically significant ($p = .053$). Other prospective randomized trials have shown that tumors identified in screened populations tend to be earlier-stage tumors at the time of diagnosis, as compared with tumors found in control groups of unscreened patients. However, a sig-nificant reduction in cancer-specific mortality has been demon-strated to date in only one study, the Minnesota Colon Cancer Control Study. Other studies, including three European random-ized trials that have shown a significant decrease in the stage of detected cancers compared with the control group, may show a reduction in mortality when the data are more mature. A recent meta-analysis of the randomized trials indicates that Hemoccult testing is associated with a 19% reduction in the mortality rate from colorectal carcinoma.

Carcinoembryonic antigen (CEA) has no role in screening for primary lesions. The sensitivity ranges from 30% to 80%, depending on the stage of disease. False-positive results occur in benign disease (lung, liver, and bowel) as well as malignancies of the pancreas, breast, ovary, prostate, head and neck, bladder, and kidney. The CEA level is also elevated in smokers. Overall, 60% of tumors will be missed by CEA screening alone.

Screening Recommendations

Recently, an expert panel, after reviewing all pertinent data to late 1996, made the following recommendations regarding screening (Winawer et al.):

Symptomatic patients:
  Diagnostic studies
Average risk, asymptomatic (age ≥ 50):
  FOBT each year (full colonoscopy or DCBE/flex sig if +)
  Flex sig every 5 years (full colonoscopy if +, except tubular adenomas < 1 cm)
  FOBT + flex sig (as described earlier)
  Alternative: DCBE every 5–10 years
  Alternative: colonoscopy every 10 years
Increased risk, asymptomatic (close relatives with colorectal cancer or polyps):
  Same recommendations for average-risk patients, begin at 40 years of age
Increased risk, family history of FAP:
  Genetic counseling and possible testing
  Gene carriers or indeterminate cases—flex sig every 12 months, begin at puberty
  Polyps present: consider timing of colectomy
Increased risk, family history of HNPCC:
  Full colonoscopy every 1–2 years starting between the ages of 20 and 30
  Full colonoscopy every year after age 40
Increased risk, history of adenomatous polyps:
  1-cm polyp or multiple polyps found, repeat initial exam in 3 years
  2nd exam = normal, or single, small, or tubular adenoma, repeat exam in 5 years
  2nd exam = multiple, or large polyps, etc.; repeat exam per clinician judgment
Increased risk, history of colorectal cancer:
  Complete resection, full colonoscopy within 1 year of surgery
  2nd exam = normal, repeat exam in 3 years
  3rd exam = normal, repeat exam in 5 years

Abbreviations: FOBT= fecal occult blood testing; Flex sig = flexible sigmoidoscopy; DCBE = double-contrast barium enema; FAP = familial adenomatous polyposis; HNPCC = hereditary nonpolyposis colorectal cancer.

PATHOLOGY

Histologically, more than 90% of colon cancers are adenocarcinomas. On gross appearance, there are four morphologic variants of adenocarcinoma. Ulcerative adenocarcinoma is the most common configuration seen and is most characteristic of tumors in the descending and sigmoid colon. Exophytic (also known as polypoid or fungating) tumors are most commonly found in the ascending colon, particularly in the cecum. These tumors tend to project into the bowel lumen, and patients often present with a right-sided abdominal mass and anemia. Annular (scirrhous) adenocarcinoma tends to grow circumferentially into the wall of the colon, resulting in the classic apple core lesion seen on barium enema x-ray study. Rarely, a submucosal infiltrative pattern can be observed that is similar to linitis plastica seen with gastric adenocarcinoma.

Other epithelial histologic variants of colon cancer that are occasionally seen include mucinous (colloid) carcinoma, signet-ring cell carcinoma, adenosquamous carcinoma, and undifferentiated carcinoma. Other rare tumors include carcinoids and leiomyosarcomas (to be discussed later in the chapter).

The most commonly used grading system is based on the degree of formation of glandular structures, nuclear pleomorphism, and number of mitoses. Grade 1 tumors have the most developed glandular structures with the fewest mitoses, grade 3 is the least differentiated with a high incidence of mitoses, and grade 2 is intermediate between grades 1 and 3.

STAGING

The Dukes and TNM staging systems for colorectal carcinoma are presented in Tables 11-1 and 11-2.

CLINICAL PRESENTATION

Patients with colorectal cancer present with bleeding, abdominal pain, change in bowel habits, anorexia, weight loss, nausea, vomiting, fatigue, and anemia. Pelvic pain and or tenesmus in rectal cancer may be associated with an advanced stage of disease

Table 11-1. Modified Astler-Coller classification of the Dukes staging system for colorectal cancer

Stage	Description
A	Lesion not penetrating submucosa
B1	Lesion up to, but not through, serosa
B2	Lesion through serosa, with involvement of adjacent organs
C1	Lesion up to, but not through, serosa; regional lymph node metastasis
C2	Lesion through serosa, with involvement of adjacent organs; regional lymph node metastasis
D	Distant metastatic disease

Table 11-2.   TNM staging classification of colorectal cancer

Primary tumor (T)	
T1	Invades submucosa
T2	Invades muscularis propria
T3–T4	
Serosa	
T3	Invades into subserosa, but not through serosa
T4	Invades through serosa into free peritoneal cavity or into contiguous organ
Serosa	
T3	Invades through muscularis propria
T4	Invades contiguous organs
Regional lymph nodes (N)	
N0	No lymph node metastases
N1	Lymph node metastases in 1–3 nodes
N2	Lymph node metastases in 4 or more nodes
N3	Lymph node metastases in central nodes
Distant metastases (M)	
M0	No distant metastases
M1	Distant metastases present

indicating involvement of pelvic nerves. The incidence of complete obstruction in newly diagnosed colorectal cancer is 2–11%. Fifty percent of splenic flexure and 15% of rectal lesions present with obstructions. Obstruction increases the risk of death from colorectal cancer 1.4-fold and is an independent covariate in multivariate analyses. Similarly, although a less common presentation, perforation increases the risk of death from cancer 3.4-fold. Two-thirds of patients will have Duke's stage B and C lesions; one-third will have Duke's stage D lesions.

DIAGNOSIS

Colon Cancer

Clinical evaluation of carcinoma of the colon should include colonoscopy and biopsy, air contrast barium enema (BE), chest radiograph, complete blood count, CEA determination, urinalysis, and liver function tests (LFTs). BE and colonoscopy are complementary tests. The colonoscope allows evaluation of the distal 2–3 cm of the anorectal canal that is obscured by the BE catheter balloon, and the BE facilitates the visualization of the splenic and hepatic flexures, which may be obscured during colonoscopy. In addition, polypectomy or biopsy can be performed during colonoscopy.

The use of abdominopelvic computed tomography (CT) in the preoperative evaluation of patients with colon cancer remains controversial. The extracolonic abdomen should be evaluated with CT in patients with large, bulky lesions to detect involvement of contiguous organs, para-aortic lymph nodes, and the liver. Some authors only recommend CT scan when preoperative LFTs are abnormal. Both lactate dehydrogenase (LDH) and alkaline phosphatase (AP) levels are useful for detecting hepatic involvement. However, abnormal LFTs are present in only approximately 15% of patients with liver metastases. In contrast, the false-positive rate for elevated LFTs is close to 40%. Therefore a significant number of unnecessary CT scans would be performed if all patients with abnormal LFTs underwent CT scan. The preoperative CEA level can also reflect disease extent and prognosis: CEA levels surpassing 10–20 ng/ml are associated with increased chances of disease failure for both node-negative and node-positive patients. Some surgeons believe that preoperative evaluation of the liver is important because 15–20% of liver metastases will be nonpalpable at the time of surgery. However, 10–15% of lesions will be missed by combined preoperative and operative evaluation. Intraoperative ultrasonography has been shown to be the most accurate method of detecting liver metastasis.

Most patients with colon cancer will require an operative procedure even in the presence of liver metastasis; surgery is the best method to prevent the complications of colon tumors, such as obstruction and bleeding. Therefore the only advantages of a preoperative CT scan are in helping to plan possible treatment options for metastatic disease to the liver and/or to plan operative procedures when contiguous organ involvement is present. At the University of Texas M. D. Anderson Cancer Center, we do not routinely obtain preoperative CT scans in patients with colon tumors. The decision to perform a preoperative CT scan is individualized based on the results of physical examination, LFTs, and CEA level.

The role of routine preoperative urinary tract evaluation is controversial. Patients who are symptomatic or have large, bulky lesions should have a preoperative intravenous pyelogram or CT scan to evaluate the urinary tract. Up to 40% of these patients will have urinary tract abnormalities.

Rectal Cancer

In addition to the history and physical examination, chest x-ray, complete blood count, LFTs, electrolytes and urinalysis, endorectal ultrasound (EU), proctoscopic examination, full colonoscopy, and abdominopelvic CT scan should be performed to accurately stage patients with rectal cancer. Symptomatic patients undergo evaluation of their urinary tract as described earlier for colon cancer.

Accurate preoperative staging tools are critical in rectal cancer because disease stage may influence treatment decisions such as transanal resection or preoperative multimodality therapy. EU is the most accurate tool in determining tumor (T) stage. All layers of the rectal wall can be identified with 69–93% accuracy. The EU characteristics of T1 and T3 tumors make them relatively easy to differentiate. Unfortunately, the distinction between T2 and T3 tumors is not as well defined, yet it is vital in determining treatment planning. Limitations of EU include operator experience, differentiating lymph nodes from blood vessels and other structures, differentiating T2/T3 tumors, differentiating peritumoral edema from tumor, evaluating a tumor after radiation therapy, and overstaging (10–15%) or understaging (1–2%) errors. EU evaluation of depth of bowel wall penetration is superior to that of either CT

(52–83% accuracy) scanning or magnetic resonance imaging (MRI) (59–93% accuracy). CT and MRI are most valuable for locally advanced tumors because they can delineate the relationship of the tumor to surrounding viscera and pelvic structures. Neither CT nor MRI is more useful for the evaluation of locoregional disease after neoadjuvant chemoradiation treatment because radiation changes cannot be accurately differentiated from tumor.

Lymph node staging in rectal cancer has proven more difficult than primary tumor staging, with EU accuracies of 32–95%, CT accuracies of 35–73%, and MRI accuracies of 39–84% reported. Despite descriptions of methods to radiologically predict metastases in lymph nodes, only nodal enlargement can be detected with most current technologies. Fifty to seventy-five percent of positive lymph nodes in rectal cancer may be normal in size, thereby limiting accurate evaluation. Similarly, lymph nodes may be enlarged from inflammation, giving false-positive results. Accuracy can be increased by combining size and ultrasonographic characteristics. Lymph nodes that are greater than 3 mm and hypoechoic are more likely to contain metastatic deposits. In addition, it is possible to perform fine-needle aspiration of suspicious lymph nodes under EU guidance. EU is invaluable when evaluating patients for preoperative adjuvant therapy, but it cannot accurately assess response to preoperative adjuvant therapy due to the obliteration of tissue planes by edema and fibrosis.

Abdominopelvic CT scanning is important in assessing the presence of distant spread of disease and involvement of adjacent organs. In the management of rectal cancer it is extremely important to accurately assess the local spread of disease, including the potential involvement of the levator muscles and other pelvic structures. Although EU is superior to CT in detecting depth of penetration, CT provides a better assessment of contiguous organ involvement. MRI may provide better delineation of contiguous organ involvement than CT scan (e.g., bladder, blood vessel involvement); however, this advantage has not been definitively established.

The staging of recurrent rectal cancer is complicated by radiation and postoperative changes that are often difficult to distinguish from tumor. At the present time, EU is not useful in distinguishing scar from recurrent tumor. Similarly, there is poor correlation of postradiotherapy EU in preoperative regimens to final pathology (postresection), indicating the limited value of EU in assessing tumor in an irradiated milieu. CT is useful to assess extent of disease and adjacent organ involvement if recurrent tumor is obvious. MRI is equally useful and can provide sagittal images that may provide additional information on resectability. In cases where recurrence is unknown but suspected, CT is more useful if a baseline study is available for comparison. PET scanning has recently been introduced with early reports of increased accuracy in distinguishing postoperative changes from recurrent tumor. Further studies are required before this test can be recommended for use on a routine basis. Currently at M. D. Anderson Cancer Center, we obtain both a CT and MRI of the pelvis in cases of isolated recurrent rectal carcinoma, because we believe these studies are complimentary in their provision of critical staging and resectability information.

MANAGEMENT OF COLON CANCER

The goal of primary surgical treatment of colon carcinoma is to eradicate disease in the colon, the draining nodal basins, and contiguous organs. Careful surgical planning is essential. Patient age, stage of disease, extent of tumor, and presence of synchronous colonic tumors are significant factors in determining the optimal surgical approach. Overall medical condition is also important because most perioperative deaths result from cardiovascular or pulmonary complications.

Anatomy

Thorough knowledge of the arterial, venous, and lymphatic anatomy of the colon and rectum is essential to appropriate surgical management (Fig. 11-1). The ascending and proximal transverse colon are embryologically derived from the midgut and receive their arterial blood supply from the superior mesenteric artery via the ileocolic, right, and middle colic arteries. The distal transverse, descending, and sigmoid colon are hindgut derivatives whose arterial blood supply arises from the inferior mesenteric artery (IMA) through the left colic and sigmoid arteries. The rectum, also a hindgut derivative, receives its blood supply to the upper third from the IMA via the superior hemorrhoidal artery. The middle and lower thirds of the rectum are supplied by the middle and inferior hemorrhoidal arteries, which are branches of the hypogastric artery. Collateral blood supply for the colon is provided through the marginal artery of Drummond. The venous drainage of the colon and rectum parallels the arterial supply, with the majority draining directly into the portal venous system. This provides a direct route for metastatic spread of tumor to the liver. The only minor anatomic variation in the venous drainage compared with the arterial supply is that the inferior mesenteric vein (IMV) joins the splenic vein prior to emptying into the portal system. The rectum has dual venous drainage; the upper rectum drains into the portal system, and the distal one-third of the rectum drains into the inferior vena cava via the middle and inferior hemorrhoidal veins, providing a direct route for hematogenous spread outside of the abdomen.

The lymphatic drainage of the bowel is more complex than the vascular supply. Lymphatics begin in the bowel wall as a plexus beneath the lamina propria and drain into the submucosal and intramuscular lymphatics. The epicolic lymph nodes drain the subserosa and are located in the colon wall. This nodal group runs along the inner bowel margin between the intestinal wall and the arterial arcades. These nodes in turn drain into the paracolic nodes, which follow the routes of the marginal arteries. The epicolic and paracolic nodes represent the majority of the colonic lymph nodes and are the most likely sites of regional metastatic disease. The paracolic nodes drain into the intermediate nodes, which follow the main colic vessels. Finally, the intermediate nodes drain into the principal nodes, which begin at the origins of the superior and inferior mesenteric arteries and are contiguous with the para-aortic chain.

The route of lymphatic flow parallels the arterial and venous distribution of the colon. The right colon will drain to the superior mesenteric nodes through the intermediate nodes or to the portal

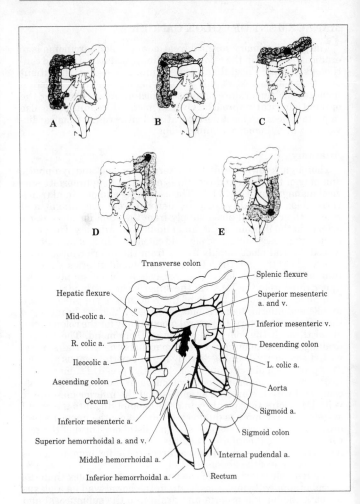

Transverse colon

Splenic flexure

Hepatic flexure

Superior mesenteric
a. and v.

Mid-colic a.

Inferior mesenteric v.

R. colic a.

Descending colon

Ileocolic a.

L. colic a.

Ascending colon

Aorta

Cecum

Sigmoid a.

Inferior mesenteric a.

Sigmoid colon

Superior hemorrhoidal a. and v.

Internal pudendal a.

Middle hemorrhoidal a.

Inferior hemorrhoidal a.

Rectum

Fig. 11-1. Anatomy of colonic blood supply along with a pictorial description of the various anatomic resections used for colon carcinoma. (A) Right hemicolectomy. (B) Extended right hemicolectomy. (C) Transverse colectomy. (D) Left hemicolectomy. (E) Low anterior resection. (From PH Sugarbaker, J MacDonald, L Gunderson. Colorectal cancer. In VT DeVita, S Hellman, SA Rosenberg [eds.], *Cancer: Principles and Practice of Oncology* [3rd ed.]. Philadelphia: Lippincott, 1984.)

system via the lymphatics of the superior mesenteric vein. The left colon's lymphatic drainage follows the marginal artery to the left colic intermediate nodes and finally to the inferior mesenteric nodes. The lymphatic drainage of the upper third of the rectum follows the IMV, whereas the lower two-thirds drain into the hypogastric nodes, which, in turn, drain into the para-aortic nodes. The lower third of the rectum can also drain along the pudendal vessels to the inguinal nodes.

Surgical Options

At laparotomy or laparoscopic resection, the primary tumor and its lymphatic, venous, and arterial supply are extirpated, as well as any contiguously involved organs. Our current use of intra-operative ultrasound is limited to the evaluation of palpable hepatic abnormalities or preoperatively identified lesions if a CT scan was obtained (to identify tumor extent, number of lesions, proximity to major vessels, etc.). We do not believe that the "no-touch" isolation technique is necessary; we do support high ligation of appropriate vessels (with involved lymphatics) in colon cancer resections.

The various surgical options, as well as their indications and major morbidities, are briefly discussed next.

A. *Right hemicolectomy*. Removal of the distal 5–8 cm of the ileum, right colon, hepatic flexure, and transverse colon just proximal to the middle colic artery. This procedure is indicated for cecal, ascending colonic, and hepatic flexure lesions. Major morbidities include ureteral injury, duodenal injury, and bile acid deficiency (rarely seen and only with extensive resection of the terminal ileum).

B. *Right radical hemicolectomy*. Removal of the transverse colon (including resection of the middle colic artery at its origin) in addition to the structures removed in the right hemicolectomy. Indications for the procedure are hepatic flexure or transverse colon lesions. Morbidities include anastomotic dehiscence and diarrhea in addition to the complications associated with right hemicolectomy.

C. *Transverse colectomy*. Segmental resection of the transverse colon. This procedure is indicated for middle transverse colon lesions. The major morbidity is anastomotic dehiscence. At M. D. Anderson this procedure is rarely performed because of the difficulty in achieving a tension-free anastomosis with adequate blood supply (as the marginal artery of Drummond is sacrificed). We prefer to perform an extended right radical hemicolectomy with an ileosigmoid anastomosis.

D. *Left hemicolectomy*. Removal of the transverse colon distal to the right branch of the middle colic artery and the descending colon up to but not including the rectum, plus IMA ligation and division. Indications for the procedure are left colon lesions. Morbidities include anastomotic dehiscence.

E. *Low anterior resection*. Removal of the descending colon distal to the splenic flexure, sigmoid colon, upper two-thirds of the rectum, and ligation of IMA (and IMV) at its origin. The procedure is indicated for sigmoid and proximal rectal lesions. Morbidities include anastomotic dehiscence and bowel ischemia (secondary to inadequate flow through the marginal artery of Drummond).

F. *Subtotal colectomy*. Removal of right, transverse, descending, and sigmoid colon with ileorectal anastomosis. This procedure is indicated for multiple synchronous colonic tumors and distal transverse colon lesions in patients with a clotted IMA. Morbidities include diarrhea, perineal excoriation, and anastomotic dehiscence.

The *surgical treatment of the familial polyposis syndromes* depends on the age of the patient and the polyp density in the rectum. Total abdominal colectomy and ileorectal anastomosis has a low complication rate, gives good functional results, and is a viable option for younger patients and those with few polyps in the rectum. These patients must be followed with 6-month-interval proctoscopic examinations to remove polyps and detect signs of cancer. If rectal polyps become too numerous, a trial of sulindac or conversion to an ileoanal pouch is warranted. The risk of cancer in the retained rectal stump increases to approximately 8% at 50 years of age and 29% at 60 years of age. It is clear that the age of the patient and not the follow-up time dictates the risk of rectal cancer. Older patients and those who were initially treated with an ileorectal anastomosis are best treated with an ileoanal pouch procedure (including mucosectomy). It should be remembered that proctocolectomy is only a small part of the gastrointestinal and abdominal management of these patients.

Laparoscopic Resection for Colorectal Carcinoma
Recent studies have confirmed that laparoscopy for colorectal carcinoma resection is technically feasible, is safe, and yields an equivalent number of resected lymph nodes. It may reduce hospital stay, be less morbid, and decrease convalescence, although this has yet to be proven in a randomized prospective trial. Despite reports of equivalent lymphadenectomies being performed laparoscopically, only prospective randomized studies with long-term follow-up will determine whether this translates into equivalent local and distant recurrence rates, and disease-specific survival. Laparoscopy clearly has a role in performing diverting ostomies in colorectal and anal carcinoma, in palliative resections in patients with metastatic disease, and in the resection of large polyps. Several single and multi-institutional prospective randomized trials are under way to answer the critical questions regarding laparoscopic versus open resection for colorectal carcinoma, including the issue of port-site recurrences, survival compared with equivalent open procedures, and economic issues. Until the results are disseminated, patients should only be offered laparoscopic resection with curative intent in the context of one of these trials.

Obstructing Colorectal Cancers
Historically, these patients were treated with a three-stage procedure. They are now more commonly treated in two stages: resection and Hartmann's procedure, followed by colostomy takedown and reanastomosis (colocolostomy). An alternative is a one-stage procedure with either subtotal colectomy and primary anastomosis or segmental resection and intraoperative colonic lavage for carefully selected patients. (Contraindications include multiple primary cancers, advanced peritonitis, hemodynamic instability, poor general health, steroid therapy or immunosuppressed state.) In the SCOTIA prospective randomized trial using these two

treatment modalities in 91 patients with malignant left-sided colonic obstruction, the morbidity and mortality rates were similar. There are reports of laser treatment and endoscopic stenting of obstructive lesions to allow for bowel preparation and subsequent single-step resection. Obstructing right-sided cancers can be effectively treated with resection and anastomosis in one stage.

Survival

Nodal involvement is the primary determinant of 5-year survival. In node-negative disease, the 5-year survival rate is 90% for patients with T1 and T2 lesions and 80% for those with T3 lesions. For node-positive cancers, the 5-year survival ranges from 69% (one positive node) to 27% with six or more positive nodes. Other factors that are proven prognostic indicators include grade, bowel perforation, and obstruction. Patients who present with unresectable metastatic disease have an overall 5% 5-year survival rate.

Adjuvant Therapy

Adjuvant therapy for colon cancer is an evolving and controversial subject. 5-fluorouracil (5-FU) is the most effective single agent for colon carcinoma, with response rates of 15–30% when it is used alone as treatment for patients with advanced disease.

History

Based on early studies that showed some anticancer activity for 5-FU, there have been numerous studies of 5-FU in combination therapies. Adjuvant trials using 5-FU and semustine (MeCCNU) (Gastrointestinal Tumor Study Group [GITSG]) or MeCCNU, vinblastine, and 5-FU (National Surgical Adjuvant Breast and Bowel Project, project C-01) have failed to demonstrate any survival benefit when compared with surgery alone.

5-FU / Levamisole

The failure of these chemotherapeutic combinations led to trials of 5-FU in combination with levamisole, an antihelminthic agent with immunostimulatory properties. The use of levamisole in the adjuvant setting was based on initial studies in patients with advanced stages of colon cancer that showed this agent had some activity when used as single-agent therapy. Later studies showed that 5-FU/levamisole was more effective than levamisole alone. Prospective randomized studies comparing 5-FU and levamisole with surgery alone were conducted by both the North Central Cancer Treatment Group (NCCTG) and the Intergroup trial (Moertel et al.) in patients with stage II and III disease. These studies demonstrated a 41% decrease in recurrence and a 33% decrease in mortality for patients with stage III disease compared with surgery alone. Additionally, the data suggested an improvement in disease-free and overall survival for patients with stage II colon carcinoma; however, statistical significance was not reached for this group of patients in either study. Based on these studies, the National Institutes of Health (NIH) Consensus Conference in 1991 recommended that all patients with stage III colon carcinoma receive adjuvant chemotherapy with 5-FU and levamisole. A final report by the Intergroup trial demonstrated a persistence in the one-third reduction in mortality at 6.5 years. Adjuvant chemotherapy for patients with stage II colon carcinoma remains controversial.

5-FU/Leucovorin

The addition of leucovorin to 5-FU has been shown to increase antitumor activity in both *in vitro* and *in vivo* models. Leucovorin works by stabilizing the 5-FU thymidylate synthase complex, thus prolonging the inhibition of thymidylate synthase and increasing tumor cytotoxicity. Early prospective randomized studies showed an increased survival rate in patients with advanced-stage colon cancer treated with combination 5-FU and leucovorin. This led to numerous prospective randomized trials comparing this combination of agents with various other single-agent and combination regimens in the adjuvant setting. Early results show increased disease-free and overall survival rates for all patients. Subset analysis for patients with stage II and III disease has not yet been done. Other studies are under way to confirm these results and to establish the optimal dosing and scheduling of these agents. 5-FU/leucovorin is a reasonable alternative to 5-FU/levamisole in patients with stage III colon cancer.

Completed/Ongoing Investigations

Recently completed trials (data not yet mature) will define the relative efficacy of 5-FU/levamisole versus 5-FU/leucovorin in both Duke's A and B carcinomas. Ongoing trials involve altering the dose of leucovorin in combination with 5-FU, using 5-FU/levamisole in the perioperative period (compared with 4 weeks following surgery) and combinations of 5-FU/leucovorin/levamisole (compared with standard therapy).

Treatment of Locally Advanced Colon Cancer

Colon cancers that are adherent to adjacent structures have a 36–53% chance of local failure after complete resection. Approximately 10% of carcinomas present in this fashion. Strategies designed to reduce local recurrence would benefit these patients.

Surgical Strategy

Resection of colorectal cancer that has invaded adjacent structures involves en bloc resection of all involved structures; failure to do so results in significantly increased local recurrence and decreased survival. Of importance, all adhesions between the carcinoma and adjacent structures should be assumed to be malignant and not taken down because 33–84% are malignant when examined histologically. The victim organ should have resection limited to the involved area with a rim of normal tissue. A patient who has a margin-negative multivisceral resection has the same survival as a patient with no adjacent organ involvement on a stage-matched basis.

Adjuvant Therapy

Retrospective series have shown subsets of patients who have benefited from postoperative radiotherapy with or without 5-FU-based chemotherapy. Unfortunately, there are no consistent criteria to use in assessing increased risk of local failure. The value of adjuvant radiotherapy after complete resection of high-risk colon cancer is currently being evaluated in a randomized prospective fashion by the North Central Cancer treatment Group (NCCTG 91-46-52). In this trial, patients with MAC B3 or C3 tumors are randomized to receive postoperative 5-FU/levamisole or 5-FU/ levamisole and radiotherapy. Patients with subtotally resected cancers fare worse than those with positive microscopic disease, as one would expect. It has been found that radiotherapy is more effective in microscopic than in macroscopic disease, and that it is more effective when combined with 5-FU. In a recent retrospective Mayo Clinic study of 103 mostly MAC B3 and C3 patients in which 49% had no residual disease, 17% had microscopic residual disease, and 34% had gross residual disease, the local failure rate was 10% for patients with no residual disease, 54% for those with microscopic residual disease, and 79% for those with gross residual disease. If there is any question regarding the ability to achieve a margin negative resection, surgical clips should be used to outline the area of the tumor bed. If the margin is positive on final pathology, radiation should be administered with concomitant 5-FU-based chemotherapy.

Management of Rectal Cancer

There are four goals in the successful management of rectal cancer: (1) cure; (2) local control (negative margin resection of tumor, and resection of all draining lymph nodes); (3) restoration of intestinal continuity; (4) preservation of the anorectal sphincter, sexual function, and urinary function. Because of the anatomic constraints of the bony pelvis, it may be difficult at times to achieve adequate sphincter, sexual, and urinary function without compromising cure and local control.

Local control is clearly related to the adequacy of the surgical procedure. Although local control is critical for increasing the chances of cure, many patient- and tumor-related factors are associated with overall outcome. Data suggest that there is a significant surgeon-related and center-related variability in patient outcome after treatment for rectal cancer. The Stockholm Rectal Cancer Study Group found that "specialists" and centers with higher volumes of rectal cancer cases had lower local failure rates and increased survival rates. It is not unusual to see local recurrence rates of 3.7–43% reported in various series for curative surgical resection, with or without adjuvant therapy. Obviously, other factors are involved, such as methods of adjuvant therapy, patient selection, and disease factors. These varying results have hindered an accurate assessment of the vital components of an adequate oncologic operation and prevented an accurate assessment of the value of adjuvant chemoradiation in rectal cancer. Consequently, there are some who believe that with an adequate oncologic procedure by an experienced surgeon, only large T3 and T4 (fixed) lesions need adjuvant chemoradiation treatment. Treating all other T3 patients and those with N1–N2 disease merely makes up for "bad surgery." Others contend that the significant decrease in local recurrence and possibly some improvement in survival associated with adjuvant radiation or chemoradiation justify its application in all patients with T3 or greater, or those with node-positive disease. Nevertheless, surgical technique is critical to the success of the treatment of rectal cancer.

When planning surgical treatment of a rectal cancer, the rectum can be divided into three regions in relation to the anal verge. The upper rectum is defined as 11–12 cm from the anal verge.

Tumors >12 cm behave like colonic cancers (low local recurrence rates) and are therefore generally considered to be distal sigmoid or "rectosigmoid" cancers. Tumors 6–10 cm from the anal verge are defined as middle rectal cancers, and tumors from 0–5 cm are defined as low rectal cancers. Note that low rectal cancers can be associated with the internal and external sphincters, anal canal, or levator muscles, or can be above the pelvic floor.

Surgical Aspects

In addition to understanding the anatomic site of the tumor, it is important to understand the principles influencing the extent of radical extirpative surgery regardless of the type of resection planned.

Resection Margin.   Optimal treatment of all malignancies requires an adequate margin of resection. Histologic examination of the bowel wall distal to the gross rectal tumor reveals that only 2.5% of patients will have submucosal spread of disease greater than 2.5 cm. In addition, patients with distal submucosal disease spread greater than 0.8 cm have a poor prognosis and will probably not benefit from more radical surgery. At M. D. Anderson we try to obtain distal resection margin of at least 2 cm. Although irrigation of the rectal stump is performed routinely at other institutions, we do not use this technique in rectal cancer surgery.

Lymphadenectomy.   An adequate lymphadenectomy should be performed for accurate staging and local control. Spread from the primary tumor occurs in a lateral and upward direction, with distal spread occurring in less than 5% of patients. Controversy surrounds the definition of an adequate lymphadenectomy. The technique involves sharp excision and extirpation of the mesorectum by dissecting outside of the investing fascia of the mesorectum (total mesorectal excision [TME]). It is important to note that TME optimizes the oncologic operation by not only removing draining lymph nodes, but also maximizing lateral resection margins around the tumor. Although no randomized prospective trial has compared TME with conventional mesorectal excision, some institutions have shown a significant decrease in the local recurrence rate compared with historical controls using conventional surgery (to the range of 6.3–7.3%). This dissection can be facilitated by ligation of the IMA (and IMV) at or near its origin ("high ligation"). The data on whether high ligation also results in a decreased local recurrence remain equivocal. Data do suggest that negative lateral (radial) margins are major determinants of survival that may be more important than longitudinal resection margins. Lateral margin clearance can be maximized by sharp dissection outside the mesorectum on the endopelvic fascia. The bony pelvis, which inherently limits the maximal extent of lateral dissection, may serve as the best explanation of why distal rectal cancers have a higher local recurrence rate than their more proximal counterparts when comparing patients with tumors of similar stage. It is controversial whether the entire mesorectum must be excised for all rectal cancers or whether the mesorectum can be sharply divided at the distal resection margin. At MDACC we excise the mesorectum to the distal resection margin, which would include nearly the entire mesorectum for lower and the lower half of middle rectal cancers, while preserving a portion of the mesorectum for the upper and upper half of middle rectal cancers. It is our belief that this does not compromise an adequate oncologic operation and may lessen the complication rate (anastomotic leak from devascularization of the rectal stump). It is important to remember that although a 2-cm distal mucosal margin is adequate, local control of rectal cancer requires maximal extirpation of the mesorectal and lateral pararectal tissues. A proven benefit of sharp mesorectal excision in a defined anatomic plane is the ability to perform an adequate cancer operation with preservation of the pelvic autonomic nerves. No benefit in survival or local disease control has been attainable with the use of more extended lymphadenectomy (iliac/periaortic nodes, pelvic sidewall, etc), and the complication rates are higher with these more extensive surgical procedures.

Surgical Approaches to Rectal Cancer

Surgical approaches to the rectum include transabdominal procedures (abdominoperineal resection [APR], low anterior resection [LAR], coloanal anastomosis [CAA]), transanal approaches, and transsacral approaches (York-Mason, Kraske). These latter two approaches will be discussed in detail in the section on local treatment of rectal cancer. APR was the only treatment in the past for all rectal cancers and is now reserved for cancers in the lower third of the rectum that do not have adequate tumor clearance for sphincter-preservation surgery (usually 0–3 cm). It is also indicated for patients with involvement of the levator muscles and those with poor preoperative sphincteric function.

Sphincter-Preservation Procedures

Besides local excision, sphincter-preservation procedures include LAR and proctectomy/CAA either alone or combined with neoadjuvant radiation and chemoradiation. Another option includes the addition of a colonic reservoir for improved function. These procedures can only be performed if the oncologic result is not compromised and the functional results are acceptable. It was demonstrated as early as 20 years ago that there is no difference in local recurrence rate or survival in patients with mid-rectal cancers who undergo LAR rather than APR. The technical feasibility of LAR in this setting was increased with the advent of circular stapling devices and the knowledge that distal margins of resection of 2 cm were adequate. Survival was found to depend on the distance of the tumor from the anal verge, the presence of positive lymph nodes, and the lateral extent of dissection. Therefore many studies comparing the two procedures included high-risk low rectal cancers treated by APR, and higher, lower-risk rectal cancers treated with LAR. More recently, a retrospective study (Rullier et al.) in 106 patients with low to middle rectal cancers treated by APR or LAR showed no difference in local recurrence or survival, confirming earlier results with middle and upper rectal cancers. An alternative to LAR is proctectomy with CAA. Originally, this was utilized for technically difficult LAR procedures in mid-rectal cancers. It is used now for low middle rectal cancers and very select low rectal cancers, with the stapled or hand-sewn anastomosis between the dentate line and the anorectal ring (within the surgical anal canal). Most surgeons use temporary fecal diversion when this procedure is performed. The use of proctectomy and CAA for low rectal cancers is usually in the context of preoperative radiation or chemoradiation protocols. Using either LAR or proctectomy with CAA (and adjuvant therapy), local recurrence rates of 3–6.5% have been reported by MDACC and Memorial Hospital. Functional results have been good with 60–86% patients attaining continence by 1 year, with 10–15% requiring laxative use, and some with mild soiling at night. Preoperative chemoradiation seems to not have a negative impact on these functional results. Obviously, the lower the anastomosis (i.e., coloanal), the greater the bowel dysfunction. More information is presented on neoadjuvant chemoradiation treatment in the adjuvant therapy of rectal cancer section.

Data, mostly retrospective, show that the oncologic results of proctectomy with coloanal anastomosis is similar to that of anterior proctectomy with TME with and without sphincter preservation: a local recurrence rate of 7–22% and a 5-year survival rate of 69–73%.

Colonic J Pouch

Although continence can be maintained in patients with a coloanal anastomosis, there is a degree of incontinence in some patients, and others require antidiarrheal agents. This is probably due to lack of compliance in the neorectum. This led to the introduction of the colonic J pouch for low rectal cancers that showed better results in terms of stool frequency, urgency, nocturnal movements and continence than straight coloanal anastomoses. There is some reduction in functional advantage of the pouch at 1 year, particularly regarding difficulty in pouch evacuation (20% of patients). Prospective randomized studies carried out to 3 years show superior functional advantage of the colonic J pouch to straight reconstructions. As in anterior resection, the functional outcome of patients with CAA (with or without a J pouch) may take 1–3 years to stabilize and is related to the level of the anastomosis (lower anastomoses tend to have poorer function). The pouch is usually constructed with a 6- to 8-cm efferent limb. Studies have shown that postoperative radiotherapy does not adversely affect pouch function.

Proximal diversion after sphincter preservation is indicated in the following circumstances: (1) anastomosis less than 5 cm above the anal verge; (2) patients have received preoperative radiotherapy; (3) patients are on corticosteroids; (4) when the integrity of the anastomosis is in question; (5) any case of intraoperative hemodynamic instability.

Local Approaches to Rectal Cancer

Local treatment alone as definitive therapy of rectal cancer was first applied to patients with severe coexisting medical conditions unable to tolerate radical surgery. Currently, conservative, sphincter-saving local approaches are being more widely considered. Early studies of local excision demonstrate up to a 97% local control rate and 80% disease-free survival for properly selected individuals. Local treatment is best applied to rectal cancers within 10 cm of the anal verge, tumors less than 3 cm in diameter involving less than one-fourth of the circumference of the rectal wall, exo-

Recommended surgical treatment strategy for rectal cancer

Location	T-stage	Resection	Mesorectal excision to
Upper Rectum	T1	TEM or Kraske	—
	T2 or >	LAR*	Distal resection margin
Middle Rectum	T1	TAE, Kraske, TEM	—
	T2	LAR	Distal resection margin or entire
	T3 or >	CXRT/LAR	Distal resection margin or entire
Low Rectum	T1	TAE	—
	T2	Proctectomy/ CAA,[†] (± J pouch), APR	Entire
	T3 or >	CXRT/Proctectomy/ CAA[†] (± J pouch), APR	Entire

* LAR distal resection margin ≥2 cm.
[†] CAA hand-sewn; protective ileostomy.
TEM = transanal endoscopic microsurgery; LAR = low anterior resection;
TAE = transanal excision; CXRT = preoperative chemoradiation;
APR = abdominoperineal resection; CAA = coloanal anastamosis.

phytic tumors, tumors staged less than T2 by EU, highly mobile tumors, and tumors of low histologic grade. The decision to use local excision alone or to employ adjuvant therapy after local excision is based on the pathologic characteristics of the primary cancer (with negative margins) and the potential micrometastases in draining lymph nodes. T1 lesions have positive lymph nodes in 5–10% of cases, whereas the rate for T2 and T3 lesions is 10–20% and 30–70%, respectively. T2 tumors treated with local resection alone can have local recurrence rates of 15–44%. Most authors recommend adjuvant chemoradiation after local excision of T2 or greater lesions, and select T1 lesions with poor prognostic features. A phase II intergroup study of 113 T1–T2 low to middle rectal cancers was performed where T1 cancers received no further therapy, whereas all T2 cancers received postoperative chemoradiation treatment. After a median follow-up of 24 months, only two patients had isolated local recurrences, furnishing evidence that these treatment recommendations provide adequate cancer control without loss of sphincter function.

Local therapy of distal rectal cancers can be accomplished by transanal excision, posterior proctectomy, fulguration, or endocavitary irradiation. *Transanal excision* is the most straightforward approach to removing distal rectal cancers. The deep plane of the dissection is the perirectal fat. Tumors should be excised with an adequate circumferential margin. *Posterior proctotomy* (Kraske procedure) can be used for tumors in the middle and upper rectum and is more suitable for larger, low rectal lesions. In this procedure a perineal incision is made just above the anus, the coccyx is removed, and the fascia is divided. The rectum can then be mobilized for a sleeve resection, or a proctotomy is performed for excision of the tumor. The disadvantages of this procedure are fistula formation and the potential to seed the posterior wound with malignant cells. *Fulguration* uses either standard electrocautery or laser to ablate the tumor. *Endocavitary radiation* is a high-dose, low-voltage irradiation technique that applies contact radiation to a small rectal cancer through a special proctoscope. Fulguration and endocavitary radiation have the disadvantage of not providing an intact specimen for histologic analysis. *Transanal endoscopic microsurgery* (TEM) provides accessibility to tumors of the middle and upper rectum that would otherwise require a laparotomy or transsacral approach, with improved visibility and instrumentation. Almost any adenoma 15–20 cm from the anal verge is amenable to this approach. The procedure requires special training and equipment, which is expensive and therefore has limited its acceptance in the United States. This procedure is not recommended for tumors within 5 cm of the anal verge. These tumors are optimally treated with a standard transanal approach. Patient selection is important and it is recommended that patients have preoperative EU to select superficial lesions. Patients with deeper lesions and metastatic disease or comorbid conditions that would preclude laparotomy are also candidates. TEM is now used at MDACC for carefully selected patients. Although local procedures have become more commonly used, few randomized prospective trials have evaluated oncologic and functional outcomes compared with anterior resection or APR. Winde et al. prospectively randomized 50 patients with T1 adenocarcinoma of the rectum to either anterior resection or TEM. Similar local recurrence and survival rates, as well as decreased morbidity rates, were found in the two study arms, confirming the advantages of local excision.

At MDACC, transanal excision is used for low rectal cancers, whereas a Kraske procedure or TEM is used for higher rectal lesions. Optimal local excision includes at least a 1-cm resection margin circumferentially, a full-thickness excision, and an excision that is not fragmented or piecemeal. An inadequate local excision mandates an alternate resection strategy, not merely the addition of adjuvant therapy. If preoperative T stage is increased after pathologic evaluation following local excision, the appropriate standard resection is recommended. T1 tumors are treated with local therapy alone unless any of the following poor prognostic features are identified: tumor >4 cm, poorly differentiated histology, lymphatic or vascular invasion, clinical or radiologic evidence of enlarged lymph nodes. Those T1 tumors with poor prognostic features and tumors T2 and greater are treated with adjuvant radiotherapy with or without concomitant chemotherapy. T3 cancers are treated with local excision alone only if the patient refuses standard resection. Adjuvant chemoradiation treatment is strongly recommended postoperatively.

Treatment for Locally Advanced Rectal Cancer

Occasionally, patients will present with involvement of adjacent structures (bladder, vagina, ureters, seminal vesicles, sacrum, etc.). These patients with stage T4, N1–N3, M0 disease clearly benefit from multimodality therapy, including pre- or postoperative chemoradiation treatment, IORT, and/or brachytherapy. The goal of surgical therapy is resection of the primary tumor, with en bloc resection of adjacent involved structures to obtain negative margins. The confines of the pelvis and the proximity to nerves and blood vessels that cannot be resected decrease the resectability rate of rectal tumors compared with locally advanced colon cancer. Increased resectability rates and margin-negative resections have been demonstrated for locally advanced rectal cancers after preoperative chemoradiation treatment. Furthermore, in patients requiring pelvic exenteration for locally advanced rectal cancer, the addition of preoperative radiotherapy decreases the locoregional recurrence rates. At the Mayo Clinic, the addition of IORT to standard external beam radiotherapy with 5-FU in patients with locally advanced rectal cancer has shown significantly improved local disease control and possibly some improvement in survival (Gunderson et al.). The best chance of cure in patients with locally advanced disease appears to involve preoperative chemoradiation treatment, maximal surgical resection, and IORT; randomized, controlled trials are needed to confirm these findings.

In the situation of unresectable locally advanced disease, significant rates of resectability have been reported after preoperative radiation therapy. Moreover, patients who are resected with negative margins have improved survival over those resected with close or positive margins.

At MDACC, preoperative chemoradiation is standard treatment for locally advanced rectal cancer. An evaluation of 40 patients (29 with locally advanced disease; 11 with recurrence) requiring pelvic exenteration for local disease control with negative margins demonstrated that chemoradiation may significantly improve survival and that chemoradiation response and S-phase fraction were important determinants of survival (Meterissian et al.). Patients with low-risk factors had a 65% 5-year survival, whereas high-risk patients had only a 20% survival.

Survival After Surgical Therapy

Seventy-five to ninety percent of node-negative rectal cancers are cured by radical surgical resection. Only one-third of patients with regional lymph node metastases will survive 5 years. As mentioned previously, 25% of patients who fail will fail in the pelvis alone. However, local failure will occur in up to 75% of patients succumbing to their disease.

The survival rate after local therapy varies from 70% to 86%, with recurrence rates of 10–50%. The overall local recurrence rate is 30%, and increasing recurrence rates are seen with increasing stage of disease and decreasing distance from the anal verge. Many of these patients can be salvaged with radical surgery after a local recurrence. When analyzing the results of local therapy, it must be remembered that this represents a carefully selected group of patients.

Complications of Surgical and Adjuvant Therapy for Rectal Cancer

Complications of surgical and adjuvant therapy for rectal cancer include all the complications associated with major abdominal surgery (bleeding, infection, adjacent organ injury, ureteral injury, and obstruction), with the addition of some complications that are unique to pelvic surgery. Specifically, anastomotic leak occurs in 5–10% cases overall, with increasing rates seen in lower anastomoses, those associated with immunocompromised states, and those associated with preoperative radiation therapy. The incidence of anastomotic leak is decreased with a defunctioning stoma. At MDACC, a defunctioning loop ileostomy is used in all anastomoses below the peritoneal reflection in patients who have received preoperative radiotherapy and in patients with CAA. Autonomic nerve preservation is part of all pelvic dissections unless tumor involvement necessitates the sacrifice of these structures. With careful dissection during TME, 75–85% of patients have a return to preoperative sexual and urinary function. Other complications include stoma dysfunction, perineal wound complications, hemorrhage from presacral vessels, and anastomotic stricture. The mortality rate from surgical resection varies from 2% to 6%.

The complications associated with chemoradiation treatment include radiation enteritis and dermatitis, hematologic toxicity, stomatitis (mostly with continuous 5-FU infusions), and venous access infections. The frequency and intensity of these complications depend on multiple factors, including radiotherapy total dosing, fractionation, field technique, and whether the radiotherapy is given preoperatively or postoperatively. There are no good predictors of which patients will have these complications and to what degree they will have them.

Adjuvant Therapy of Rectal Cancer

The two main components of adjuvant therapy for rectal cancer are radiotherapy to the pelvis and 5-FU-based chemotherapy. The goal of chemotherapy is to increase tumor radiosensitivity and to decrease the chance of distant failure. The goal of radiotherapy is to increase local control, and in the preoperative setting to increase margin-negative resection rates and sphincter preservation. It must be emphasized that successful multimodality treatment of rectal cancer requires close collaboration between radiotherapists, medical oncologists, and surgeons.

Postoperative Radiation

Three randomized trials have been performed comparing surgery alone with surgery plus postoperative radiotherapy for T3 and/or N1–N2 rectal cancer. The only trial to show a decrease in local recurrence rate was the NSABP R-01 trial. Local recurrence was decreased from 25% in the surgical arm to 16% in the postoperative radiotherapy arm ($p = .06$). Several nonrandomized trials have shown a decrease in local recurrence rates to the 6–8% level; the differences between these trials may reflect radiotherapy dosing and patient selection. These trials showed that postoperative radiotherapy could reduce local recurrence, but total radiotherapy dose and technique were important to achieve this effect. Higher radiation doses are proportional to higher local control rates. Despite the performance of several large prospective trials, survival, local pelvic control, and extrapelvic recurrence rates have not been improved consistently by radiation doses of 45–50 Gy. This prompted the addition of chemotherapy to radiation therapy in the postoperative period (see later).

Preoperative Radiotherapy (± Chemotherapy)

Several theoretical advantages to the use of preoperative radiotherapy have led to its extensive use in recent trials:

1. A reduction in the size of the tumor increases the potential for sphincter preservation.
2. There is a decreased risk of local failure and distant metastasis from cells shed at operation.
3. There is a decreased risk of late radiation enteritis because the small bowel can be excluded from the radiation field.
4. Some tumors considered unresectable may become resectable with therapy.
5. Tumor cells are well oxygenated when treated preoperatively because there has been no surgical manipulation of the blood supply to the tumor. Well-oxygenated cells are thought to have increased radiosensitivity, and therefore tumor cell killing may be increased.
6. There is no delay of therapy as in some cases of postoperative therapy due to operative morbidity.
7. Systemic therapy is initiated earlier than in postoperative therapy.
8. Preoperative radiotherapy may be more dose efficient than postoperative radiotherapy. Postoperatively, 15–20 Gy may be needed to equal the same effect given preoperatively.

Until now there have been 10 randomized trials evaluating the role of preoperative radiotherapy in resectable rectal cancer. Although five report significant decreases in local recurrence, only one study identifies a significant survival advantage for the total patient group (Swedish Rectal Cancer Trial, 1997). In this trial, 25 Gy was delivered in five fractions (1 week), followed by curative resection to one group, whereas the control group received curative surgery only. The local recurrence rate and 9-year disease-specific survival were 11% and 74%, respectively, versus 27% and 65% for the control group. In the United States, preoperative radiotherapy trials have usually included chemotherapy in a more protracted course. Although there has not been a significant increase in survival, there have been reports of increased sphincter preservation rates, decreased local recurrence, and acceptable toxicities. Many nonrandomized studies demonstrate local recurrence rates of 8–15% for T1–T3 disease in either long- or short-course 40–50 Gy total dose radiotherapy without chemotherapy. Three-fourths of patients initially declared to need APR have been found in some trials to be able to receive sphincter preservation, with 75–80% of these patients having good to excellent sphincter function postoperatively. Factors shown to be predictive of tumor downstaging have included higher total radiation dose, tumor differentiation, and a longer interval before surgery.

Given the increased success of combined chemotherapy and radiation therapy compared with radiation therapy alone in the postoperative setting as well as the increased morbidity from short-course preoperative radiotherapy, recent trials have included combined modality therapy over a protracted preoperative period. Several nonrandomized trials, including an MDACC trial (described later), have shown that preoperative 5-FU-based chemoradiation regimens for resectable T2–T3 rectal cancer results in a 4–5% local failure rate, and up to a 93% 5-year survival rate, with tolerable toxicities. An important advance in this area has been the appreciation that infusional 5-FU versus bolus treatment may enhance the radiotherapy effect while reducing combined treatment-induced toxicity. It has also been shown that the pathologic response rate can be correlated with the local control rate; this has not been definitely proven for disease-free and overall survival.

The addition of leucovorin to 5-FU in the preoperative period has recently been evaluated at MSKCC in 32 patients (Grann et al.). There was an 85% sphincter preservation rate in those patients initially thought to need an APR, with no local failure (median follow-up 22 months), a 60% 3-year disease-free survival rate, and a 9% complete pathologic response rate. Pending trials NSABP R-03 and INT 0147 compare preop to postop 5-FU with leucovorin chemoradiation therapy and should allow answers to which treatment modality is optimal. Functional data are also being collected to address this often overlooked aspect of adjuvant therapy in rectal cancer.

IORT

IORT is used for both recurrent and locally advanced rectal cancer. Its advantages include increased local control in high-risk cancers, accurate treatment of focal areas at risk, ability to adjust the depth of the radiation beam, and ability to shield sensitive structures. Even preoperative chemoradiation in high-risk tumors can result in high local recurrence rates. IORT allows treatment of areas with close or microscopically positive margins in this situation. At the Massachusetts General Hospital, IORT is used for focal areas of tumor adherence, close or positive margins, and areas of gross residual disease. IORT dosing depends on the clinical situation: 10–13 Gy is given for close margins (<5 mm), 15 Gy is given for microscopically positive margins, and 17–20 Gy is used for areas of gross residual disease. In a recent 2-year analysis of IORT in the RTOG study of locally advanced disease, the local control rate was 77%, with a 2-year survival of 88% and a complication rate of 16%. For facilities able to deliver this type of therapy, there is a clear advantage in local control in select patients with advanced and recurrent disease. At MDACC, IORT (10–20 Gy) is used selectively in patients with locally advanced or recurrent disease where there is a close or positive margin as demonstrated by frozen section. Another option is brachytherapy, particularly in areas where the IORT beam cannot be focused due to anatomic constraints of the pelvis.

Postoperative Radiotherapy and Chemotherapy

The addition of chemotherapy to radiation therapy has been utilized to enhance the radioresponsiveness of tumors and impact on distant disease. Several studies have shown not only a reduction in local recurrence, but increases in survival. Two large studies of postoperative chemotherapy and radiotherapy conducted by

GITSG and NCCTG have provided evidence that combination therapy may affect local control and distant failure. In the GITSG trial there was a decrease in pelvic failure for the group treated by surgery and postoperative chemoradiotherapy (11% versus 24% for surgery alone). In addition, a statistically significant survival advantage was found at 7 years using the combination of resection, radiation, and chemotherapy. The NCCTG trial did not have a surgery-alone control. However, there was a significant decrease in pelvic recurrence (14% versus 25%) and a significant decrease in cancer-related deaths for the group treated by resection, radiation, and chemotherapy compared with the group treated with resection and radiotherapy.

The findings from these studies prompted the publication of a clinical advisory by the NCI Consensus Conference in 1990 recommending adjuvant treatment for patients with Duke's B2 and C rectal carcinoma (T3–T4, N0; T3–T4, N1–N3) consisting of six cycles of fluorouracil-based chemotherapy and concurrent radiation therapy to the pelvis. This regimen has remained the standard by which all current adjuvant rectal cancer protocols are compared. In the United States, postoperative chemoradiation is by far the most common mode of delivering adjuvant therapy. This is usually given as a continuous infusion of 5-FU and approximately 55 Gy of irradiation delivered to the pelvis in 1.8–2.0 Gy fractions (6-week treatment). Although the trend in Europe is treatment with XRT and no chemotherapy, the addition of chemotherapy in the United States has been shown to decrease the rate of distant metastases, something not attainable with XRT alone. In addition, there has consistently been a 10–15% survival advantage when XRT is compared with XRT with chemo. The Intergroup 0114 trial has recently demonstrated that there is no statistically significant advantage to the addition of levamisole in the postoperative period to 5-FU and pelvic radiation; the results for modulation with leucovorin are unclear at this point.

M. D. Anderson Experience

Our preferred management of T3–T4, or any T, N1 or greater rectal cancer is to use preoperative radiotherapy with a protracted intravenous infusion of 5-FU. We deliver 45 Gy of preoperative radiotherapy with standard fractionation 1.8 Gray/Fraction (Gy/fxn). A continuous infusion of 5-FU at a dose of 300 mg m^{-2} day^{-1} is given 5 days per week. Surgery is performed 6–8 weeks after completion of therapy. In patients with T3 disease, 61% had either a complete response or microscopic residual disease. Sixty-six percent of patients could have sphincter-preserving procedures, with a local control rate of 96%, and a negative-margin resection rate of 99%. Grade 3–4 toxicity was seen in only 3–4% of patients, and the 3-year survival was 88%. In patients with fixed T3–T4 tumors, the same regimen was used with the addition of IORT boost for positive or close margins. The local control rate was 97% with an 82% 5-year survival. The use of this regimen for recurrences will be presented in that section.

Future Trends in Multimodality Treatment

Although some institutions will advocate TME alone for most rectal cancers, surgeons globally are now looking to identify those patients who will benefit most from adjuvant therapy, what therapy should be used (chemotherapy and radiation therapy dosing), and what setting (pre- or postoperative) is best. Ongoing studies are investigating whether there is an advantage to continuous or bolus 5-FU and whether 5-FU should be combined with leucovorin or levamisole. Lower radiation doses (e.g., 25 Gy) are being utilized in shorter preoperative courses to see if a lower preoperative dose confers the same advantage of decreased local recurrence. Some centers are exploring the use of IORT and brachytherapy as adjuncts to neoadjuvant chemoradiation treatments to increase the local disease control in select patients who are at high risk for local recurrence. Various molecular markers are being evaluated in fresh or archival specimens to aid in identifying patients who will benefit from treatment.

RECURRENT AND METASTATIC DISEASE

Two-thirds of patients who undergo curative surgery for colorectal cancer have tumor recurrences. Of the patients who have recurrences, 85% do so during the first 2.5 years after surgery. The remaining 15% recur during the subsequent 2.5 years. The risk of recurrence is higher with stage II or III disease, anaplasia, aneuploidy, or adjacent organ invasion. Recurrences may be local, regional, or distant. Distant disease recurrence, the most common presentation, occurs either alone or concomitantly with locoregional recurrence. Local recurrence develops in 20–30% of patients who undergo initial curative resections for rectal cancer, and in 50–80% of these patients the local recurrence is the only site of disease. Recurrence isolated to the anastomosis (intramural) is rare and usually indicates inadequate surgical resection. Liver involvement occurs in approximately 50% of patients with colon cancer, whereas lung, bone, and brain involvement occurs in 10%, 5%, and less than 5%, respectively. Symptomatic recurrences present with a constellation of symptoms ranging from the vague and nonspecific to the clinically overt.

CEA is invaluable for postoperative monitoring. It is most useful in patients whose levels are elevated preoperatively and return to normal following surgery. Levels should be determined preoperatively, 6 weeks postoperatively, and then according to the schedule described in the surveillance section. The absolute level and rate of rise and the patient's clinical status are important in determining prognosis and treatment. Postoperative levels that do not normalize within 6 weeks to 4 months suggest incomplete resection or recurrent disease, although false-positive results do occur. Levels that normalize postoperatively and then start to rise are indicative of recurrence. This may represent occult or clinically obvious disease. A rapidly rising CEA level suggests liver or lung involvement, whereas a slow, gradual rise is associated with locoregional disease. Despite the reliability of an elevated CEA level in predicting tumor recurrence, 20–30% of patients with locoregionally recurrent tumors have a normal CEA level. Poorly differentiated tumors may not make CEA, which is one explanation for such false-negative results. In contrast, CEA is elevated in 80–90% of patients with hepatic recurrences. A prospective randomized trial of the value of CEA in follow-up was undertaken in 311 patients (McCall et al.). The survival data have not matured, but some valuable information is available. The study followed asymptomatic patients with elevated CEAs until symptoms developed; then a full work-up was initiated. The purpose was to define the "natural history" of an elevated CEA. The sensitivity, specificity, and positive predictive values of an elevated CEA were 58%, 93%, and 79%. The median lead time of the elevated CEA to detection by other means was 6 months, a result found in other studies. The data on survival benefit from CEA detection are not mature. It should be noted that 7% of patients who had an elevated CEA failed to have recurrent disease on work-up. This and other newer studies call into question the cost-effectiveness and value of CEA monitoring. At MDACC, we routinely monitor CEA values because of the potential to detect liver metastases—a subgroup of patients who may benefit from early recurrence detection.

Management of the asymptomatic patient with an elevated CEA level can be challenging. An elevated level should be confirmed by a repeat CEA determination approximately 1 month later. A thorough clinical investigation that includes LFTs, CT scan of the abdomen, pelvis, and chest, colonoscopy, and, if clinically indicated, bone scan or CT of the brain should be performed. If the CEA is rising and the radiologic work-up is negative, attention should be directed to a radiolabeled monoclonal antibody study or a PET scan.

Radiolabeled monoclonal antibodies (MAbs) directed against tumor-specific antigens and CEA have been approved for imaging the extent and location of extrahepatic metastases. This modality is particularly useful in the evaluation of recurrent disease where postsurgical or postradiation changes are not easily differentiated from tumor on CT or MRI. One agent OncoScint CR/OV (Cytogen Corp., Princeton, NJ) is an Indium-111-labeled MoAb B72.3 that targets the tumor-associated glycoprotein TAG-72, which is reactive with approximately 83% of colorectal tumors. An anti-CEA preparation that is technetium labeled is also available (CEA-Scan). These agents were found to be superior to CT in evaluating extrahepatic and pelvic disease, whereas CT was better for detecting metastatic disease to the liver. Most studies of labeled MoAbs show a sensitivity range of 70–86%, with a higher specificity, and positive predictive values >90%. These studies are most useful for the detection of recurrent disease in a patient with a rising CEA and negative radiologic work-up, or to rule out metastatic disease in a patient with locoregional recurrence who may be suitable for surgical therapy (i.e., hepatic resection/cryotherapy, pelvic exenteration, etc.). Side effects occur in less than 4% of patients, and antimurine antibody formation is more problematic and may limit the ability to rescan patients (dose related). In the future the use of antibody fragments or peptides may resolve the problem of murine antibodies and shorten imaging times.

PET Imaging relies on the increased metabolic uptake of glucose (fluorine-labeled analog of 2-deoxyglucose or FDG) in tumors compared with normal tissues. Its value may lie in distinguishing postsurgical and postradiation changes from tumor, in measuring tumor response to chemo- or radiation therapy, or in evaluating the source of an elevated CEA in the patient with a negative radiologic work-up. Initial studies have been promising. Limitations of this technology include expense and limited access to PET scanners in the United States.

If the metastatic evaluation is negative in the face of an elevated CEA level, a second-look laparotomy should be performed. About 60–90% of patients with asymptomatically elevated CEA levels will have recurrent disease at laparotomy; 12–60% of these patients will have resectable disease at the time of laparotomy; and 30–40% will survive 5 years following resection of the recurrence. Early detection of asymptomatic disease results in a higher resectability rate than when resection is performed for symptomatic disease (60% versus 27%). The liver is the most common site of recurrence, followed by adjacent organs, the anastomotic site, and the mesentery. Resectability rates correspond to the level of CEA elevation, with CEA levels less than 11 ng/ml being associated with higher resectability rates.

In recent years, radioimmuno-guided surgery (RIGS) has been used to detect recurrences intraoperatively. This technique is useful in directing the surgeon to disease sites that would otherwise be left behind. In addition, it is especially useful in patients with resectable liver lesions who have extranodal disease that is otherwise not detectable. ^{125}I-labeled monoclonal antibodies directed against CEA are injected 6 weeks before the second-look surgery. The antibodies localize to the tumor sites and can be detected intraoperatively by a hand-held gamma probe. Tumor is accurately detected in 81% of patients. Sixteen percent of patients will have tumor that is detected by RIGS alone. Despite this novel modality for detecting and treating disease in the asymptomatic patient, no study has demonstrated a survival advantage with this technique.

Treatment

The appropriate treatment of resectable recurrent disease depends on the location of disease. If two disease sites are detected that are completely resectable, this is undertaken in select patients. Otherwise, individual treatment modalities are used as needed for palliation of pelvic symptoms. As in locally advanced disease, potentially resectable recurrent disease is treated in a multimodality fashion using preoperative chemotherapy (with our without radiation), surgery, IORT, if available, and brachytherapy. For recurrence involving the sacrum, en bloc sacral resection can sometimes result in 4-year survival rates of 30%. Contraindications to sacral resection include pelvic sidewall involvement, sciatic notch involvement, higher than S2 involvement, encasement of iliac vessels, and extrapelvic disease. A review of pelvic recurrence at MSKCC revealed that there were no predictors either in the initial tumor or in the recurrent tumor to indicate survival. Complete resection of the recurrence, however, improved survival. Symptoms of recurrent disease could be adequately palliated with surgery. At MDACC, potentially resectable pelvic recurrences are treated with preoperative chemoradiation, followed by surgery and the use of IORT and brachytherapy as needed for close or positive margins. Using this approach in 43 patients, the overall resection rate was 77%, with an 88% margin-negative resection rate, a 64% local control rate, and a 58% 5-year survival. Although the usual surgical procedure for resectable recurrent rectal cancer is APR, select cases can be treated with sphincter preservation.

Liver

Close to 70% of patients who die of colon cancer have hepatic involvement. The liver is the site of metastatic or recurrent disease in 50% of patients and is the primary determinant of patient survival. (See Chapter 12 for the management of colorectal hepatic metastasis.)

Lung

Pulmonary metastases occur in 10–20% of patients with colorectal cancer. They are most commonly seen in the setting of a large hepatic tumor burden or extensive metastatic disease. Isolated pulmonary metastases occur most commonly with distal rectal lesions, as the venous drainage of the distal rectum bypasses the portal system and allows metastasis to travel directly to the lungs.

The finding of a solitary lesion on a chest radiograph should prompt evaluation with thoracic CT scanning and, for a centrally located lesion, bronchoscopy with biopsy. Peripheral lesions may be amenable to CT-guided needle biopsy or video-assisted thoracoscopic surgery (VATS). Fifty percent of patients with solitary pulmonary nodules will have primary lung tumors rather than colorectal metastases.

Patients with locally controlled primary tumors, no evidence of metastases elsewhere, good pulmonary reserve, and good medical condition are candidates for resection. Patients with solitary metastases experience the best survival, but patients with as many as three lesions (unilateral or bilateral) can experience up to a 40% 5-year survival. The optimum surgical approach is a median sternotomy to allow for bilateral pulmonary exploration, because contrast-enhanced CT scan has up to a 25% false-negative and false-positive rate for the detection of metastases. As in liver resection for metastatic disease, the optimum surgery involves the minimal procedure to obtain negative margins (i.e., wedge resection versus pneumonectomy).

The overall 5-year survival rate following resection of pulmonary metastases ranges from 20% to 40%. In newer series involving only colorectal cancer metastases, the rate is closer to 40–43% 5-year survival. Age, sex, location of the primary disease, disease-free interval, or involvement of hilar or mediastinal lymph nodes does not seem to influence survival. The number of metastases in most series is inversely correlated with 5-year survival. Recurrence confined to the lung postresection is an indication by some for repeat resection.

Bone and Brain

Metastatic disease to the brain is uncommon and usually occurs after established lung involvement. Symptomatic solitary lesions can be treated by palliative craniotomy and resection. In a very small subpopulation of patients, cranial disease may be the only site of involvement, and excision in this setting may increase survival. Bone metastases are quite uncommon and are best managed with radiation therapy.

Ovary

Because 1–7% of women who undergo potentially curative resections subsequently develop ovarian metastases, it has been suggested that prophylactic oophorectomy may benefit these patients. Unfortunately, it has never been proven that removal of ovarian micrometastatic disease, or the potential for metastases at this site, improves survival. In most cases ovarian metastases develop in the presence of widespread disease, and it would not be expected that prophylactic oophorectomy would alter survival. In the postmenopausal patient with isolated unilateral or bilateral metastatic disease to the ovaries, a bilateral oophorectomy is performed. In the premenopausal patient with unilateral involvement, a unilateral oophorectomy is performed. Prophylactic oophorectomy is not performed routinely at the MDACC when resecting potentially curable colorectal carcinoma.

Pelvis

Local recurrence in the pelvis is a major problem after treatment for rectal cancer. These patients are infrequently saved by additional surgery. Radiation affords good palliation; however, if the patient has previously received adjuvant radiotherapy, external beam radiotherapy may no longer be an option. Radical surgical procedures, including pelvic exenteration and sacrectomy, may benefit a select group of patients whose disease can be completely extirpated by these procedures. IORT and brachytherapy may be useful adjuvants in the setting of radical surgery for recurrent disease.

SURVEILLANCE

Patients with a history of colon carcinoma require close surveillance. The data to support this, however, are lacking. In a recent Danish prospective randomized study in 597 colorectal cancer patients, patients had either close follow-up (every 6 months for first 3 years) or yearly for 3 years (including exam/stool heme test, colonoscopy, labs [except CEA], and CXR). The frequency of recurrent cancer was the same in both groups, but it was diagnosed earlier in the close follow-up group. The close follow-up group had more resections for curative intent (local and distant), but there was no cancer-specific survival difference. Other studies, mostly retrospective, show similar findings.

History and physical examination, Hemoccult stool testing, and laboratory tests (complete blood count, CEA determination, LFTs) are performed at M. D. Anderson every 3 months for the first 3 years after surgery, every 6 months during years 4 and 5, and yearly thereafter. Colonoscopy should be performed after 1 year, and then at 3 years if normal. A baseline CT scan of the abdomen and pelvis is obtained 3–4 months after resection of rectal carcinoma. Because of the 47% false-positive rate, the utility of routine CT scanning in surveillance is controversial. However, in the presence of symptoms or abnormal laboratory tests, CT should be performed. A chest radiograph is obtained every 6 months for the first

2 years and yearly thereafter. It has traditionally been proposed that patients should be monitored closely for local recurrence during the first 2 years postoperatively (time at which most local recurrences appear). Recent data show that the addition of adjuvant radiotherapy may extend this period of vulnerability such that 50% of local recurrences may occur greater than 2 years from surgery.

UNCOMMON COLORECTAL TUMORS

Lymphoma

Lymphoma is an uncommon tumor that occurs in 0.4% of patients with intestinal lymphoma between the second and eighth decades. Almost all are non-Hodgkin's lymphomas. Twenty-five percent of patients may present with fever, occult blood loss, anemia, a palpable mass, or an acute abdomen. The diagnosis is often made intraoperatively. A history of abdominal pain, fever, and weight loss in a patient who is younger than the expected age for a colorectal tumor should raise the suspicion of intestinal lymphoma.

Abdominal CT and endoscopy with biopsy are the most useful diagnostic tests because lesions are often missed on BE. A thickened bowel, adjacent organ extension, or nodal enlargement may be seen. If the lesion is intraluminal, biopsy will make the diagnosis. Most of these lesions are intermediate to high-grade B-cell lymphomas. If a diagnosis is made preoperatively in an otherwise asymptomatic patient, bone marrow biopsy should be performed. A primary lesion is defined as a lesion with no associated organ or lymphatic involvement, negative chest CT, and a negative peripheral blood smear and bone marrow.

Surgery is performed in the clinical setting of obstruction, bleeding, perforation, or an uncertain diagnosis. Surgery is also performed, although not consistently, for complete resection of a primary lesion. A thorough exploration is performed and all suspicious nodes or organs are biopsied to assess the stage of disease. The primary intestinal lesion should be resected with negative margins whenever possible. The bowel mesentery should be resected with the tumor so that regional nodes can be pathologically assessed. Intestinal continuity should be restored whenever possible. If a large tumor is found to be unresectable and is not obstructing the bowel, a bypass can be performed. Surgical clips should be placed to facilitate identification of the tumor by the radiation oncologist.

Intestinal lymphoma requires a combined-modality approach using surgery and chemotherapy with or without radiation. For rectal lymphoma, complete resection is followed by radiation treatments to the pelvis. Chemoradiation is used if the resection was incomplete. The overall survival for stage I and II disease is about 80%. This decreases to 35% with advanced disease.

Leiomyosarcoma

Leiomyosarcomas comprise less than 1% of colonic tumors. The peak incidence occurs in the sixth decade. Most of these tumors present as large intraluminal masses. They may invade the mesenteric and pericolic fat, prostate, vagina, and ischiorectal fossa.

Patients can present with pain, bleeding, obstruction, nausea, vomiting, anemia, tenesmus, or hematuria. A thorough clinical evaluation should be conducted to exclude metastatic disease. Excision with wide surgical margins is the treatment of choice. Colonic tumors are excised with adjacent mesentery. Wide nodal excision is not indicated in the absence of clinically evident disease. Small tumors of the rectum and anal canal can be removed transrectally or endoscopically.

As with other sarcomas, prognosis depends on tumor size, grade, and presence or absence of adjacent organ involvement. The 5-year survival rate with tumors less than 5 cm is 71%, compared with 25% in tumors greater than 5 cm. Survival decreases to 28% at 5 years with adjacent organ involvement. Grade is the most important prognostic factor. Survival with low-grade tumors is 62%, whereas that with high-grade tumors is only 12%. The liver and peritoneum are the most common sites of recurrence, followed by lymph nodes. Prognosis is poor in recurrent disease. Neither radiation nor chemotherapy is of proven benefit in the management of this disease.

Carcinoid

Carcinoids are neuroendocrine tumors derived from Kulchitsky's cells, which are uncommonly found in the colon and rectum. They constitute 11–50% of all alimentary tract carcinoids. They are usually discovered incidentally unless they are large. Size and depth of invasion are the best predictors of clinical behavior. Tumors in this location almost never produce the carcinoid syndrome. Although large tumors may present with bleeding, obstruction, or constipation, tumors <2 cm are frequently asymptomatic. Diagnosis is made by endoscopic biopsy. In general, tumors <1 cm rarely metastasize, whereas those >2 cm usually metastasize; in the 1- to 2-cm range, 10–20% will metastasize. This makes treatment decisions for tumors in the 1- to 2-cm range problematic. Small lesions (<1 cm) are commonly well differentiated and can be adequately treated with endoscopic excision. Tumors greater than 1 cm have associated lymphatic and distant metastases in 90% and 60% of cases, respectively. Lesions <2 cm can be treated with local excision. It is recommended that larger lesions, those that demonstrate invasion through the muscle wall, or inadequate resection margins be treated with standard resection techniques using either an anterior approach or APR. However, a recent retrospective review from this institution on 44 rectal carcinoids revealed that extensive surgery offered no survival advantage over local excision. At MDACC, we locally excise tumors <2 cm and resect those >2 cm if sphincter preservation is possible. The experience with radiation and chemotherapy in rectal carcinoids is not extensive enough to make recommendations regarding its use.

Squamous Carcinoma of the Anus
Epidemiology and Etiology

Anal cancers constitute 1–2% of all large-bowel malignancies and 2–4% of anorectal cancers. Anal cancer occurs most frequently during the sixth decade of life. Groups reported to be at increased risk of anal cancer include northern Brazilian females, homosexual males regardless of human immunodeficiency virus (HIV) status, women practicing receptive anal sex, and post-transplantation patients.

Anal cancers are divided into two groups that differ in epidemiology, histology, and prognosis. Anal canal cancers (tumors proximal to the anal verge) make up 67% of anal cancers. These cancers are three to four times more common in women than in men. Anal margin cancers (tumors distal to the anal verge) are more common in males. There are significantly more cases of anal margin cancers in homosexual males.

Anal cancer is associated with poor personal hygiene, chronic anal irritation, infection, and immune suppression. Other risk factors for the development of anal cancer include genital condyloma acuminatum, a history of gonorrhea in men, cigarette smoking, herpes simplex virus type I seropositivity, and a history of *Chlamydia trachomatis* infection. The presence of human papillomavirus (HPV) infection—especially serotypes 16, 18, and 31—has been strongly linked to anal squamous carcinoma. Up to 54% of HIV-positive patients have HPV DNA in their anal canal, which may account for the increased incidence of anal cancers seen in this group.

Pathology

More than 80% of malignant anal lesions are histologically squamous cell carcinomas. With the exception of melanoma (see later), small cell carcinoma, and anal adenocarcinoma, all other histologic subtypes behave similarly and are treated according to their anatomic location. Basaloid carcinoma (basal cell carcinoma with a massive squamous component), mucoepidermoid carcinoma (originating in anal crypt glands), and cloacogenic carcinoma are all variants of squamous carcinoma. Malignant anal tumors may be preceded by or coexist with premalignant dysplasia or anal intraepithelial neoplasia.

The prognosis of anal margin cancers is favorable. The rate of local recurrence is higher than the rate of distant metastases, which are rare. When they do occur, metastases most commonly are found in the superficial inguinal lymph nodes (approximately 15% of cases). It is unusual for anal margin cancers to metastasize to mesenteric or internal iliac nodes.

Anal canal cancers are associated with aggressive local growth and if untreated will extend to the rectal mucosa and submucosa, subcutaneous perianal tissue and perianal skin, ischiorectal fat, local skeletal muscle, perineum, genitalia, lower urinary system, and even the pelvic peritoneum and the broad ligament. Historically, mesenteric lymph node metastases have been detected in 30–50% of surgical specimens. More than 50% of patients present with locally advanced disease. The most common sites of distant metastases are the liver, lung, and abdominal cavity. However, most cancer-related deaths are due to uncontrolled pelvic or perineal disease.

Diagnosis

The initial symptoms of anal cancer include bleeding, pain, and local fullness. These symptoms are similar to those caused by the common benign anal diseases, which accompany anal cancer in more than 50% of cases. A detailed history, including previous anal pathology and sexual habits, should precede a meticulous physical examination. Physical examination should attempt to identify the lesion, its size and anatomic boundaries, and any associated scarring or condylomata. It is also important to determine the resting and voluntary anal sphincter tone. Occasionally, an examination under general anesthesia may be necessary to complete the local evaluation. Pelvic and abdominal CT scans and a chest radiograph are important in assessing extent of local disease and distant spread. Proctosigmoidoscopy is essential to assess the proximal extent of disease and to obtain tissue for biopsy. Palpable inguinal lymph nodes should be evaluated by fine-needle aspiration.

Staging

The current AJCC staging system for anal margin and anal canal cancers is depicted in Tables 11-3 and 11-4.

Treatment

Anal Margin Cancer.   SCCA of the anal margin is defined currently by the AJCC as a lesion originating in an area between the anal margin and 5 cm in any direction onto the perianal skin. Note that the data supporting the treatment of these uncommon, heterogeneous lesions derive from small, single-institution, mostly retrospective studies. Moreover, many of these studies include lesions of the lower anal canal (dentate to anal verge) that were included previously in older definitions of the anal margin. The rationale for any modality of therapy derives from the proportional increase in chance of metastases with increasing tumor size; in tumors <2 cm, LN metastases are rarely found. For lesions between 2 and 5 cm, and those >5 cm the rates are 24% and 25–67%, respectively.

Small (<5 cm), superficial (T1–T2) anal margin cancers that do not invade the sphincter complex can be treated by a negative-margin wide local excision alone, with a 5-year survival rate greater than 80%. Wide local excision may include parts of the superficial internal and external anal sphincters without compromising anal continence. Radiation as primary treatment for these smaller cancers can produce similar survival rates, but the complication rates are higher. The acceptance of high recurrence rates in this group of patients is supported by the excellent salvage results with further excision or APR.

Larger T2, T3–T4, or T1–T2, N-positive lesions are best treated with multimodality therapy, as in anal canal cancers, given the higher local recurrence rate. Prophylactic inguinal node radiation is given to patients with T3–T4 N0 lesions, and higher doses of radiation are given to patients with positive inguinal nodes. Lymph node dissection is reserved for those patients with residual or recurrent disease. It is not known if the treatment of inguinal disease translates into improved survival. T3–T4 patients with poor sphincter function are given APR. For all patients, the 5-year disease-specific survival is 71–88%, and the local control rate after initial therapy is 70–100%.

Anal Canal Cancer.   Until the 1980s, APR with permanent colostomy was the recommended treatment for all anal canal cancers. This treatment, however, was attended by low survival rates as a result of distant failure. Radiotherapy in the range of 50–60 Gy

Table 11-3.   AJCC staging of anal canal cancer

Primary tumor (T)

TX	Primary tumor cannot be assessed
T0	No evidence of primary tumor
Tis	Carcinoma *in situ*
T1	Tumor ≤2 cm in greatest dimension
T2	Tumor >2 cm but not >5 cm in greatest dimension
T3	Tumor >5 cm in greatest dimension
T4	Tumor of any size invades adjacent organ(s)

Lymph nodes (N)

NX	Regional lymph nodes cannot be assessed
N0	No regional lymph node metastasis
N1	Metastasis in perirectal lymph node(s)
N2	Metastasis in unilateral internal iliac and/or inguinal lymph node(s)
	Metastasis in perirectal and inguinal lymph nodes and/or bilateral internal iliac and/or inguinal lymph nodes

Distant metastasis (M)

MX	Presence of distant metastasis cannot be assessed
M0	No distant metastasis
M1	Distant metastasis

Stage grouping

0	Tis	N0	M0
I	T1	N0	M0
II	T2	N0	M0
	T3	N0	M0
IIIA	T1	N1	M0
	T2	N1	M0
	T3	N1	M0
	T4	N0	M0
IIIB	T4	N1	M0
	Any T	N2	M0
	Any T	N3	M0
IV	Any T	Any N	M1

Table 11-4. AJCC staging of anal margin cancer

Primary tumor (T)

TX	Primary tumor cannot be assessed
T0	No evidence of primary tumor
Tis	Carcinoma *in situ*
T1	Tumor ≤2 cm in greatest dimension
T2	Tumor >2 cm but not >5 cm in greatest dimension
T3	Tumor >5 cm in greatest dimension
T4	Tumor invades deep extradermal structures (i.e., cartilage, skeletal muscle or bone)

Lymph nodes (N)

NX	Regional lymph nodes cannot be assessed
N0	No regional lymph node metastasis
N1	Regional lymph node metastasis

Distant metastasis (M)

MX	Presence of distant metastasis cannot be assessed
M0	No distant metastasis
M1	Distant metastasis

Stage grouping

0	Tis	N0	M0
I	T1	N0	M0
II	T2	N0	M0
	T3	N0	M0
III	T4	N0	M0
	Any T	N1	M0
IV	Any T	Any N	M1

was also used as definitive treatment of these cancers, with recurrence and survival rates similar to those seen using APR. The pioneering chemoradiation protocol developed by Nigro et al., which has since been confirmed and modified by others, has radically changed the approach to this disease. Currently, surgery is reserved for (1) T1 and small T2 lesions, which may be locally excised; (2) salvage treatment for patients with persistent disease (within 6 months of chemoradiation) or recurrent disease (after 6 months); (3) severely symptomatic patients (perineal sepsis, intractable urinary or fecal fistulae, intolerable incontinence); (4) inguinal lymph node dissection for persistent inguinal disease, recurrent inguinal disease (treated first with radiotherapy unless associated with local recurrence), or primary disease in the inguinal basin where the disease is bulky or fungating; and (5) temporary fecal diversion in patients with nearly obstructing lesions.

Since the initial work of Nigro et al., studies have been performed to dissect out the vital components and doses of the chemoradiation treatments to optimize treatment. There is evidence that (1) higher doses of radiation produce better local control rates using a constant MMC dose (Rich); (2) 5-FU and MMC with XRT produces better local control rates than XRT alone; (3) 5-FU, MMC with XRT produces better local control rates than 5-FU with XRT; and (4) cisplatin with 5-FU and XRT produces local control and survival rates similar to 5-FU, MMC, and XRT, possibly with less toxicity.

The current regimen for primary treatment of anal canal cancer and large anal margin cancers is chemoradiation therapy (Table 11-5). This has recently been changed from a 5-FU, mitomycin, radiotherapy protocol (45–55 Gy, with boosts up to 60 Gy) because of improved response rates, decreased toxicity, and similar survival data. Complete responses with this treatment can be expected in up to 90% of patients, with 5-year survival rates approaching 85%.

Controversial issues involving the surgical oncologist include when to perform a biopsy after completion of the chemoradiation protocol and what therapy to initiate. It has been shown that a persistent mass after therapy will demonstrate cancer on biopsy in 18–34% cases. Moreover, the longer the time after completion of treatment, the higher the chances a mass will be a cancer on biopsy. There are reports of positive biopsies 6–8 weeks after therapy (persistent disease), which will revert to negative biopsy in patients who have refused surgery. This implies that there may be a delayed radiation effect for up to several months after treatment. At MDACC we do not routinely biopsy the treated tumor site; instead we wait for clinical evidence of locally recurrent disease in close follow-up.

Patients with local recurrence or persistent disease are almost all salvaged with APR. However, cisplatin-based chemotherapy with additional XRT has been used successfully to salvage up to one-third of patients with locally recurrent disease. These findings may allow a nonsurgical option, or a combined modality approach to recurrent or persistent disease.

SURVEILLANCE

Patients should be followed for detection of local and systemic failures as well as treatment complications. Local inspection, digital examination, anoscopy, and biopsy of any suspicious area are recommended every 3 months after chemoradiation treatment for 2 years, and twice a year thereafter. Early detection of local recurrence may enable less extensive salvage surgical procedures. Dis-

Table 11-5. Treatment protocol for anal canal cancer

Days 1–4	5-FU, 750–1,000 mg/m^2 over 24-hour continuous IV infusion
Day 1	Mitomycin C, 10–15 mg/m^2, IV bolus (alternatively, bleomycin, 15 units once a week, or cisplatin, 4 mg m^{-2} day^{-1} with 5-FU dose reduced to 250–300 mg/m^2)
Days 1–35	Radiation therapy 5 days/week for total dose of 45–55 Gy. Boosts of up to 60 Gy may be given to the anus and or inguinal basins
Days 29–32	5-FU, 750–1,000 mg/m^2 over 24-hour continuous IV infusion

tant failures of epidermoid cancer are responsive to radiotherapy, and up to 30% of patients respond to second-line chemotherapy. Therefore chest radiography, LFTs, and pelvic CT are recommended every 6–12 months for 2–3 years after initial therapy. Patients with anal margin cancers should have careful, close follow-up, given the indolent nature of these tumors and the benefits of further local therapy.

Paget's and Bowen's Disease

Although not cancers, the uncommon lesions of Paget's and Bowen's disease are precancerous. Paget's disease is an intraepithelial adenocarcinoma that occurs mostly in elderly women. The lesion—well-demarcated, eczematoid plaque—is usually characteristic; however, morphologic variations can occur, making the diagnosis difficult by inspection alone. The diagnosis is made histologically by the presence of large, vacuolated Paget's cells, which stain PAS positive (from high mucin content). There is some evidence for the association of perianal Paget's disease with other invasive carcinomas, but this relationship is not as strong as that seen with Paget's of the breast. Invasion can develop rarely in these lesions, and the prognosis is poor.

Bowen's disease is an intraepithelial squamous cell carcinoma that develops in mostly middle-aged women. The lesion is raised, irregular, scaly, plaquelike, with eczematoid features. Histologically, large atypical haloed cells (Bowenoid cells) are seen that stain PAS negative. As in Paget's disease, there is an association in some studies with invasive carcinomas, suggesting the need for colonoscopy or BE.

The treatment for these rare lesions is not completely uniform, given their rarity. However, most small series report excellent long-term results with complete excision (minimal clear margins). Local recurrence is common, but reexcision provides excellent local control. Because the lesion can microscopically extend beyond the visible boundary, perianal mapping is suggested to outline all involved areas and to help plan the local excision (four quadrant biopsies at anal margin, anal verge, and dentate line). Because of the increased incidence of these lesions in immunocompromised patients, particularly HIV patients, other treatments have been used successfully, including 5-FU topical cream. This treatment is also useful in patients with widespread perianal disease where excision would be too morbid.

Anorectal Mucosal Melanoma

EPIDEMIOLOGY

Primary melanoma of the anus or rectum is a rare tumor, accounting for 0.4–1.6% of all melanomas and less than 1.0% of all tumors of the anorectum. The overall prognosis for patients with anorectal melanoma is dismal. The reported 5-year survival rate is only 6–17%, and the median survival time is only 19–25 months.

PATHOLOGY

Melanomas arising from the true rectum are less common than those developing at the squamocolumnar junction in the anal canal. Nodal metastases in the pelvis are more commonly associated with rectal tumors, whereas inguinal node disease is more likely to result from anal lesions. Most patients present with a clinically localized but advanced polypoid or nodular primary tumor. Prognosis is related to tumor thickness, as with cutaneous melanomas.

DIAGNOSIS

Patients most commonly present with rectal bleeding. Some patients will complain of a painful rectal mass. Occasionally, melanoma will be an incidental pathologic finding after hemorrhoidectomy. Physical examination should include evaluation of the rectal mass as well as palpation of the inguinal nodes. A chest radiograph and LFTs should be performed to determine whether distant metastases are present. Abdominal and pelvic CT scans are helpful in determining the extent of local and regional disease.

TREATMENT

Although most patients will die of their disease regardless of therapy, there may be a group with disease confined to the primary site (smaller lesions) or mesenteric nodes that may benefit from more aggressive local therapy (APR). It has been found that, unlike epidermoid carcinoma of the anal canal, melanoma may preferentially spread to mesenteric rather than to inguinal lymph nodes. This argues in favor of APR rather than local excision because there is no better way to select patients for less aggressive, potentially curative surgery. On the other hand, sphincter-saving approaches have been advocated because, despite higher local recurrence rates, the overall outcome of these patients is the same. Certainly, APR is the treatment of choice for large, bulky tumors and recurrent disease. Therapeutic inguinal node dissection is indicated for palpable nodal disease. Because of the high incidence of local recurrence and inguinal nodal disease, regardless of treatment used, postoperative adjuvant irradiation of the tumor bed and nodal basins may be warranted.

Selected References

Arbman G, Nilsson E, Hallbrook O, et al. Local recurrence following total mesorectal excision for cancer. *Br J Surg* 83:375, 1996.

Blend MJ, Abdel-Nabi H. New methods for the staging of colorectal cancer using noninvasive techniques. *Semin Surg Oncol* 12:253, 1996.

Brady MS, Kavolius JP, Quan SHQ. Anorectal melanoma: A 64-year experience at Memorial Sloan-Kettering Cancer Center. *Dis Colon Rectum* 38:146, 1995.

Burt RW. Screening of patients with a positive family history of colorectal cancer. *Gastrointest Endosc Clin North Am* 7:65, 1997.

Cawthorn SJ, Parums DV, Gibbs NM, et al. Extent of mesorectal spread and involvement of lateral resection margin as prognostic factors after surgery for rectal cancer. *Lancet* 335:1055, 1990.

Cohen AM, Minsky BD, Friedman MA. Rectal cancer. In VT DeVita, S Hellman, SA Rosenberg (eds.), *Cancer: Principles and Practice of Oncology* (5th ed). Philadelphia: Lippincott, 1997.

Cohen AM, Minsky BD, Schilsky RL. Colon cancer. In VT DeVita, S Hellman, SA Rosenberg (eds.), *Cancer: Principles and Practice of Oncology* (5th ed). Philadelphia: Lippincott, 1997.

Cranley, JP. Proper management of the patient with a malignant colorectal polyp. *Gastrointest Endosc Clin North Am* 3:661, 1993.

Enker WE. Sphincter-preserving operations for rectal cancer. *Oncology* 10:1673, 1996.

Enker WE, Paty PB, Minsky BD, et al. Restorative or preservative operations in the treatment of rectal cancer. *Surg Oncol Clin North Am* 1:57, 1992.

Farouk R, Nelson H, Gunderson LL. Aggressive multimodality treatment for locally advanced irresectable rectal cancer. *Br J Surg* 84:741, 1997.

Fisher B, Wolmark N, Rockette H, et al. Postoperative adjuvant chemotherapy or radiation therapy for rectal cancer: Results from the NSABP Protocol R-01. *J Natl Cancer Inst* 90:21, 1988.

Fleshman JW, Myerson RJ. Adjuvant radiation therapy for adenocarcinoma of the rectum. *Surg Clin North Am* 77:15, 1997.

Franklin, ME, Rosenthal D, Medina DA, et al. Prospective comparison of open vs. laparoscopic colon surgery for carcinoma. *Dis Colon Rectum* 39:S35–46, 1996.

Fuchs CS, Mayer RJ. Adjuvant chemotherapy for colon and rectal cancer. *Semin Oncol* 22:472, 1995.

Gerard A, Buyse M, Nordlinger B. Preoperative radiotherapy as adjuvant treatment in rectal cancer: Final results of a randomized study of the European Organization for Research and Treatment of Cancer (EORTC). *Ann Surg* 208:606, 1988.

Gastrointestinal Tumor Study Group. Prolongation of the disease free interval in surgically treated rectal carcinoma. *N Engl J Med* 312:1465, 1985.

Grann A, Minsky BD, Cohen AM, et al. Preliminary results of preoperative 5-fluorouracil, low dose leucovorin, and concurrent radiation therapy for clinically resectable T3 rectal cancer. *Dis Colon Rectum* 40:515, 1997.

Gunderson LL, Nelson H, Martenson JA, et al. Locally advanced primary colorectal cancer: Intraoperative electron and external beam irradiation ± 5-FU. *Int J Radiol Oncol Biol Phys* 37:601, 1997.

Haggitt RC, Glotzbach RE, Soffer EE, et al. Prognostic factors in colorectal carcinomas arising in adenomas: Implications for lesions removed by endoscopic polypectomy. *Gastroenterology* 89:328, 1985.

Jessup JM, Bothe A, Stone MD, et al. Preservation of sphincter function in rectal carcinoma by a multimodality treatment approach. *Surg Oncol Clin North Am* 1:137, 1992.

Jones DJ, James RD. Anal cancer. *Br Med J* 305:169, 1992.

Kafka NJ, Coller, JA. Endoscopic management of malignant colorectal polyps. *Surg Oncol Clin North Am* 5:633, 1996.

Kjeldsen BJ, Kronberg O, Fenger C, Jorgensen OD. A prospective randomized study of follow-up after radical surgery for colorectal cancer. *Br J Surg* 84:666, 1997.

Koura A, Giacco G, Curley S, et al. Carcinoid tumors of the rectum. *Cancer* 79:1294, 1997.

Lowy AM, Rich TA, Skibber JM, et al. Preoperative infusional chemoradiation, selective intraoperative radiation, and resection for locally advanced pelvic recurrence of colorectal adenocarcinoma. *Ann Surg* 223:177, 1996.

Markowitz AJ, Winawer, SJ. Management of colorectal polyps. *CA Cancer J Clin* 47:93, 1997.

McCall JL, Black RB, Rich CA, et al. The value of serum carcinoembryonic antigen in predicting recurrent disease following curative resection of colorectal cancer. *Dis Colon Rectum* 37:875, 1994.

McCormack PM, Burt ME, Bains MS, et al. Lung resection for colorectal metastases: 10-year results. *Arch Surg* 127:1403, 1992.

Mendenhall WM, Zlotecki RA, Vauthey J-N, et al. Squamous cell carcinoma of the anal margin. *Oncology* 10:1843, 1996.

Meterissian SH, Skibber JM, Giacco GG, et al. Pelvic exenteration for locally advanced rectal carcinoma: factors predicting improved survival. *Surgery* 121:479, 1997.

Milsom JW. Pathogenesis of colorectal cancer. *Surg Clin North Am* 73:6, 1993.

Minsky BD. Multidisciplinary management of resectable rectal cancer. *Oncology* 10:1701, 1996.

Moertel CG, Fleming TR, MacDonald JS, et al. Levamisole and fluorouracil for adjuvant therapy of resected colon carcinoma. *N Engl J Med* 322:352, 1990.

Moertel CG, MacDonald JS. Fluorouracil plus levamisole as effective adjuvant therapy after resection of stage III colon carcinoma: a final report. *Ann Intern Med* 122:321, 1995.

Nelson, RL, ed. Anal and perianal cancer. *Semin Colon Rectal Surg* 6:131, 1995.

Nigro ND, Sydel HG, Considine B, et al. Combined preoperative radiation and chemotherapy for squamous cell carcinoma of the anal canal. *Cancer* 51:1286, 1983.

NIH Consensus Conference. Adjuvant therapy for patients with colon and rectal cancer. *JAMA* 264:1444, 1990.

Nivatvongs S, Rojanasakul A, Reiman HM, et al. The risk of lymph node metastases in colorectal polyps with invasive adenocarcinoma. *Dis Colon Rectum* 34:323, 1991.

Ota DM, Skibber R, Rich TA. MD Anderson Cancer Center experience with local excision and multimodality therapy for rectal cancer. *Surg Oncol Clin North Am* 1:147, 1992.

Papillon J, Gerard JP. Role of radiotherapy in anal preservation for cancer of the lower third of the rectum. *Int J Radiat Oncol Biol Phys* 19:1219, 1990.

Petros JG, Lopez MJ. Pelvic exenteration for carcinoma of the colon and rectum. *Surg Oncol Clin North Am* 3:257, 1994.

Philipshen SJ, Heilweil M, Quan SHQ, et al. Patterns of pelvic recurrence following definitive resections of rectal cancer. *Cancer* 53:1354, 1983.

Phillips RKS. Familial adenomatous polyposis: The surgical treatment of the colorectum. *Semin Colon Rectal Surg* 6:33, 1995.

Quirke P, Durdey P, Dixon MF, et al. Local recurrence of rectal adeno-carcinoma due to inadequate surgical resection. *Lancet* 11:996, 1986.

Ranshoff DF, Lang CA. Screening for colorectal cancer with the fecal occult blood test: A background paper. *Ann Intern Med* 126:811, 1997.

Rich TA. Infusional chemoradiation for operable rectal cancer: Post-, pre-, or nonoperative management? *Oncology* 11:295, 1997.

Rich TA, Skibber JM, Ajani JM, et al. Preoperative infusional chemoradiation therapy for stage T3 rectal cancer. *Int J Radiat Oncol Biol Phys* 32:1025, 1995.

Rowe VL, Frost DB, Huang S. Extended resection for locally advanced colorectal carcinoma. *Ann Surg Oncol* 4:131, 1997.

Rullier E, Laurent C, Charles J, et al. Local recurrence of low rectal cancer after abdominoperineal and anterior resection. *Br J Surg* 84:525, 1997.

Saclarides TJ, Bhattacharyya AK, Britton-Kuzel C, et al. Predicting lymph node metastases in rectal cancer. *Dis Colon Rectum* 37:52, 1994.

Schild, SE, Gunderson, LL, Haddock, MG, et al. The treatment of locally advanced colon cancer. *Int J Radiat Oncol Biol Phys* 37:51, 1997.

SCOTIA Study Group. Single-stage treatment for malignant left-sided colonic obstruction: A prospective randomized clinical trial comparing subtotal colectomy with segmental resection following intraoperative irrigation. *Br J Surg* 82:1622, 1995.

Scott N, Jackson P, Al-Jaberi T, et al. Total mesorectal excision and local recurrence: A study of tumor spread in the mesorectum distal to rectal cancer. *Br J Surg* 82:1031, 1995.

Smith LE, Ko ST, Saclarides T, et al. Transanal endoscopic micro-surgery—USA Registry results. *Dis Colon Rectum* 38:P33, 1995.

Soreide O, Norstein J. Local recurrence after operative treatment of rectal carcinoma: A strategy for change. *J Am Coll Surg* 184:84, 1997.

Steele GD, Herndon JE, Burgess AM, et al. Sphincter sparing treatment for distal rectal adenocarcinoma: A phase II intergroup study. *Proc ASCO* 16:256, 1997.

Stockholm Colorectal Cancer Study Group. Randomized study on pre-operative radiotherapy in rectal carcinoma. *Ann Surg Oncol* 3:423, 1996.

Swedish Rectal Cancer Trial. Improved survival with preoperative radiotherapy in resectable rectal cancer. *N Engl J Med* 336:980, 1997.

Tempero M, Brand R, Holdeman K, et al. New imaging techniques in colorectal cancer. *Semin Oncol* 22:448, 1995.

Tepper JE, O'Connell MJ, Petroni GR, et al. Adjuvant postoperative fluorouracil-modulated chemotherapy combined with pelvic radiation therapy for rectal cancer: Initial results of Intergroup 0114. *J Clin Oncol* 15:2030, 1997.

Wanebo HJ, Koness RJ, Vezeridis MP, et al. Pelvic resection of recurrent rectal cancer. *Ann Surg* 220:586, 1994.

Weinstein GD, Rich TA, Shumate CR, et al. Preoperative infusional chemoradiation and surgery with or without an electron beam intraoperative boost for advanced primary rectal cancer. *Int J Radiat Oncol Biol Phys* 32:197, 1995.

Winawer SJ, Fletcher RH, Miller L, et al. Colorectal cancer screening: Clinical guidelines and rationale. *Gastroenterology* 112:594, 1997.

Wolmark N, Rockette H, Fisher B, et al. The benefit of leucovorin modulated fluorouracil as postoperative adjuvant therapy for primary colon cancer: Results from National Surgical Adjuvant Breast and Bowel Project Protocol C-03. *J Clin Oncol* 11:1879, 1993.

Hepatobiliary Cancers

Francis R. Spitz, Michael Bouvet,
and Alan M. Yahanda

Surgical Anatomy of the Liver

A basic knowledge of the anatomy of the liver is essential to the management of hepatic or biliary tract neoplasms. On the most elementary level, the liver can be divided into right and left lobes (Fig. 12-1) by an imaginary line drawn between the gallbladder bed and the vena cava (Cantlie's line). The left lobe is further divided by the falciform ligament into the medial segment (that portion between the falciform ligament and Cantlie's line) and the lateral segment (that portion to the left of the falciform ligament). The right lobe is divided into anterior and posterior segments.

Most surgeons further conceptualize the segmental anatomy of the liver in the manner described by Couinaud. Each of the eight segments of the liver is defined by its distinct and separate arterial and portal vascular supplies and its hepatic venous and biliary drainage (Fig. 12-2). A thorough understanding of these vascular structures and their locations within the liver is mandatory to perform a safe hepatic resection.

Anatomic variations of the hepatic artery are frequent. At the University of Texas M. D. Anderson Cancer Center, hepatic arterial variants are divided into 10 types (Table 12-1). By far the most common types are I, II, and III, constituting approximately 76% of all cases.

Liver resections can be classified as a trisegmentectomy (removal of the right lobe and the medial segment of the left lobe, or removal of the left lobe and either the anterior or posterior segment of the right lobe), a lobectomy (removal of the entire left or right lobe), a segmentectomy (removal of an anatomic segment of the liver, based on Couinaud's segmental anatomy), and a subsegmental or nonanatomic resection (see Fig. 12-1). An additional type of resection is a total hepatectomy, which obviously can be done only in the setting of liver transplantation.

Primary Hepatocellular Carcinoma

EPIDEMIOLOGY

Primary hepatocellular carcinoma (HCC) is relatively rare in the United States, with an annual incidence of less than five cases per 100,000. It is ranked as the twenty-second most common type of cancer in the country. Globally, however, HCC stands as one of the most common and deadly of all tumors. This striking geographic variation in the incidence of HCC is thought to be related

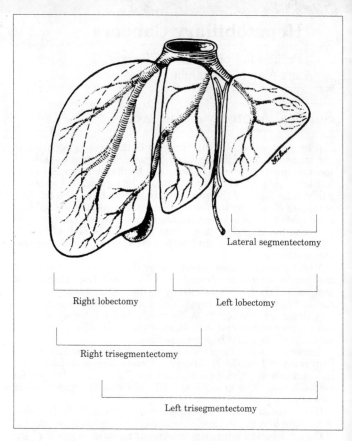

Right lobectomy

Left lobectomy

Lateral segmentectomy

Right trisegmentectomy

Left trisegmentectomy

Fig. 12-1. Liver anatomy with the description of common anatomic hepatic resections. (From S Iwatsuki, DG Sheahan, TE Starzl. The changing face of hepatic resection. *Curr Probl Surg* 26:291, 1989.)

to the varying prevalence of chronic hepatitis B virus (HBV) infections. Patients with HCC have a rate of chronic HBV infection that is much higher than that seen in the general population. It has been found that in countries where chronic HBV infection is not endemic, a number of patients with HCC will, in fact, be positive for antibodies to the hepatitis C virus (HCV).

In addition to hepatitis virus infection, a number of other risk factors have been implicated in HCC. Alcohol-related cirrhosis is probably the leading cause of HCC in the United States, Canada, and Western Europe. Dietary intake of aflatoxins is elevated in several countries where the incidence of HCC is high. HCC has also been reported in association with several metabolic disorders, such as hemochromatosis and tyrosinemia. The resultant cirrhosis or chronic hepatocellular injury may be the common etiologic factor.

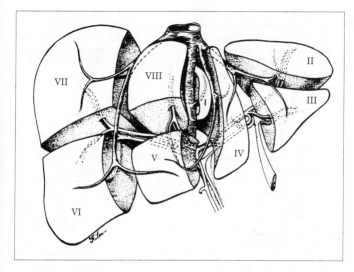

Fig. 12-2. Segmental liver anatomy as originally described by Couinaud. Each of the eight segments is based on its separate and distinct blood supply and biliary drainage. (From S Iwatsuki, DG Sheahan, TE Starzl. The changing face of hepatic resection. *Curr Probl Surg* **26:291, 1989.)**

Table 12-1. Hepatic arterial variations

Type I	RHA, MHA, and LHA arise from the CA (55%)
Type II	RHA and MHA arise from the CA, replaced LHA from the LGA (10%)
Type III	MHA and LHA arise from the CA, replaced RHA from the SMA (11%)
Type IV	MHA arises from the CA, replaced RHA from the SMA and replaced LHA from the LGA (1%)
Type V	RHA, MHA, LHA arise from the CA, accessory LHA from the LGA (1%)
Type VI	RHA, MHA, LHA arise from the CA, accessory RHA from the SMA (7%)
Type VII	RHA, MHA, LHA are from the CA, accessory LHA from the LGA, and accessory RHA from the SMA (1%)
Type VIII	Replaced RHA and an accessory LHA; or replaced LHA and an accessory RHA (2%)
Type IX	Absent celiac HA. Entire hepatic trunk arises from the SMA (4.5%)
Type X	Absent celiac HA. Entire hepatic trunk arises from the LGA (0.5%)
Type X (variant)	Double celiac HA (no common HA)

CA = celiac artery; LGA = left gastric artery; LHA = left hepatic artery; HA = hepatic artery; MHA = middle hepatic artery; RHA = right hepatic artery; SMA = superior mesenteric artery.

Men are affected by HCC more frequently than women. In high-incidence areas, the male-to-female ratio is approximately 4:1, and in low-incidence areas, the ratio is 2:1. Increasing age has also been associated with HCC. More important than the actual age of the patient, however, is the chronicity of the HBV infection or the cirrhosis.

PATHOLOGY

The majority of primary malignancies of the liver are HCC (85–90%), with cholangiocarcinoma, angiosarcoma, and hepatoblastoma being much less common.

The histologic variations of HCC are of little importance in determining the treatment and prognosis of a patient. There are, however, two exceptions. The first, fibrolamellar carcinoma (FLC), is found in younger patients and is thought to carry a better prognosis. The second exception is adenomatous hyperplasia. This premalignant lesion develops within a regenerating nodule in a cirrhotic liver. Therefore complete resection of adenomatous hyperplasia is curative.

HCC will frequently spread by local extension to the diaphragm and adjacent organs and into the portal and hepatic veins. Metastatic spread occurs most often to regional lymph nodes (periportal), lungs, bone, adrenals, and brain.

CLINICAL PRESENTATION

Most patients with HCC have a history of HBV infection, alcoholic liver disease, or cirrhosis. Common presenting symptoms include upper abdominal pain or discomfort, a palpable right upper quadrant mass, weight loss, ascites, or other sequelae of portal hypertension. Jaundice is relatively uncommon. On physical examination, one may find firm, nodular hepatomegaly, a hepatic rub, or an arterial bruit in the right upper quadrant. Numerous paraneoplastic complications have been described, including hypoglycemia, hypercalcemia, erythrocytosis, and hypertrophic pulmonary osteoarthropathy.

DIAGNOSIS

Certain laboratory and radiologic findings should raise one's suspicion for HCC. Alpha-fetoprotein (AFP) is elevated in 50–90% of all patients with HCC, with the highest levels usually found in those with large tumors or rapidly growing tumors. Consequently, a patient with a small HCC may have minimal or even no elevation of AFP. Transient increases in AFP may also be seen in benign chronic liver diseases such as cirrhosis. Serum AFP measurements are used to monitor patients for tumor recurrence, as levels should fall to normal after curative resection.

Radiologic confirmation of a mass in the liver can be made by either ultrasound (US) or computed tomography (CT). US, which is as sensitive and specific as CT for detecting small lesions (<3 cm in diameter), has the advantage of being relatively inexpensive. As a result, US has been used extensively as a screening tool in regions where the incidence of HCC is high.

Conventional CT can detect larger lesions in the liver and assess the presence of extrahepatic disease. Sensitivity can be improved by using CT angiography, in which a contrast agent is injected into the hepatic artery during the study. The blood supply to HCC is derived almost entirely from the hepatic artery; thus the tumor will appear as a hyperdense area on the scan. The accuracy of the study depends on the uniform distribution of contrast agent to both lobes of the liver. Unfortunately, this is not always possible in a diseased, cirrhotic liver or with variant hepatic arterial anatomy.

CT with arterial portography (CTAP) has proved to be the best method to study mass lesions in the liver. In CTAP, a contrast agent is injected into the superior mesenteric artery or the splenic artery prior to the scan, and delayed images are then taken when contrast has entered into the portal venous system. Because it is not well perfused by the portal system, HCC is seen as a low-density area against the surrounding liver parenchyma. The sensitivity of CTAP in identifying liver lesions is reported to be as high as 97%.

More recently, magnetic resonance imaging (MRI) with magnetic resonance angiography (MRA) has demonstrated sensitivity and provides good information concerning anatomic relations of the tumor and major vessels.

Lipiodol has been used in Asia and Europe to aid in evaluating small HCCs. Lipiodol, an oily derivative of the poppy seed combined with iodine contrast medium, is retained by HCC cells. It is injected into the hepatic artery, and a CT scan is performed 1–2 weeks later. Lesions as small as a few millimeters can be detected using this technique.

The histologic diagnosis of HCC can be obtained by percutaneous needle biopsy or fine-needle aspiration of the mass, usually under US guidance. The risk of hemorrhage following this procedure is not insignificant, as most HCCs are hypervascular, and patients may have ascites or some degree of coagulopathy. Tumor seeding of the biopsy track, a rare event, has been reported. Therefore a preoperative liver biopsy is unnecessary unless the work-up has demonstrated the lesion to be unresectable and tissue is needed to plan appropriate alternative therapy.

The evaluation of the patient is completed with a chest radiograph to exclude pulmonary metastases. Further studies, such as a CT scan of the brain or bone scan, are not indicated unless there is clinical suspicion of metastases to these areas.

STAGING

The current American Joint Committee on Cancer (AJCC) staging system for HCC is shown in Table 12-2.

EVALUATION OF OPERATIVE RISK

Before contemplating major surgery, let alone hepatic resection, in a patient with a diseased liver, one must determine whether the patient has adequate liver function to tolerate surgery and anesthesia. In addition, one must try to predict whether the remaining liver will have adequate hepatic function following resection of the tumor. This assessment has been plagued by the lack of specific

Table 12-2.   AJCC staging system for primary liver cancer

Primary tumor (T)

Tx	Primary tumor cannot be assessed
T0	No evidence of tumor
T1	Solitary tumor ≤2 cm without vascular invasion
T2	Solitary tumor ≤2 cm with vascular invasion; or multiple tumors ≤2 cm, limited to one lobe without vascular invasion; or solitary tumor >2 cm without vascular invasion
T3	Solitary tumor >2 cm with vascular invasion; or multiple tumors ≤2 cm, limited to one lobe with vascular invasion; or multiple tumors, any >2 cm, limited to one lobe, with or without vascular invasion
T4	Multiple tumors in more than one lobe; or tumor involving a major branch of the portal or hepatic vein(s)

Regional lymph nodes (N)

Nx	Regional lymph nodes cannot be assessed
N0	No regional lymph node metastasis
N1	Regional lymph node metastasis

Distant metastasis (M)

Mx	Presence of distant metastasis cannot be assessed
M0	No distant metastasis
M1	Distant metastasis

Stage grouping

Stage I	T1	N0	M0
Stage II	T2	N0	M0
Stage III	T3	N0	M0
	T1–3	N1	M0
Stage IVa	T4	Any N	M0
Stage IVb	Any T	Any N	M1

Source: OH Beahrs et al. *Manual for Staging Cancer* (4th ed). Philadelphia: Lippincott, 1997.

tests to determine hepatic function and hepatic reserve. Traditionally, the Child-Pugh classification or its modifications have been applied to liver resection in the same manner in which they were used originally in portosystemic shunt surgery. The parameters measured in this classification scheme give a rough estimation of the gross synthetic and detoxification capacity of the liver. Numerous studies have validated this system as a predictor of survival in cirrhotic patients. To better evaluate liver function, several other tests have been devised, including the urea-nitrogen synthesis rate, galactose elimination capacity, indocyanine green (ICG) clearance, and bromsulphalein and aminopyrine breath tests. A ratio of liver function to liver volume can be determined by radionuclide imaging using technetium-labeled N-pyridoxyl-5-methyltryptophan; the uptake of tracer by the anticipated liver remnant is compared with that of the whole liver. A more invasive, but more accurate, method is to determine the ICG clearance rate of the liver remnant by injecting the dye directly into the hepatic artery supplying that particular portion of the liver. Bruix et al. have demonstrated that portal hypertension (hepatic venous pressure >10 mmHg) is the best predictor of unresolved postoperative hepatic decompensation.

Despite modern surgical techniques and perioperative care, hepatic resection carries an operative mortality as high as 20%. Most perioperative deaths are due to liver failure, hemorrhage, and sepsis.

The preoperative evaluation of liver function at M. D. Anderson is based primarily on the Child-Pugh classification scheme. The age of the patient is taken into consideration. Coexisting medical problems such as ischemic heart disease and chronic obstructive pulmonary disease are investigated, as these are known to be poor prognostic factors. The CTAP and accompanying arteriogram (or MRI/MRA) are used to determine the presence and extent of cirrhosis and portal hypertension. We do not use any other tests, such as the aminopyrine breath test or ICG clearance, in the preoperative work-up of liver function.

SURGICAL THERAPY

The definitive treatment for resectable HCC remains surgery. Unfortunately, of the patients presenting with HCC, only 10–30% will be eligible for surgery, and of those patients who undergo exploration, only 50–70% will have a resection with curative intent. The criteria that render a tumor unresectable include (1) the presence of extrahepatic disease, (2) evidence of severe hepatic dysfunction, (3) extensive tumor that would leave too little liver remaining following extirpation, and (4) tumor involvement of the portal vein or vena cava. The latter criterion has become more of a relative contraindication, as many surgeons are now resecting portions of involved portal vein and hepatic artery.

The operative approach to the patient with a potentially resectable HCC should begin with a thorough surgical exploration of the abdomen, searching for any evidence of extrahepatic disease. In particular, care is taken to evaluate the periportal lymph nodes, as well as the nodes in the hepatoduodenal ligament. The liver is then completely mobilized to allow full examination of the organ. Intraoperative US should be used to define both the size of the tumor and its relationship to the major vascular and biliary structures.

Once the tumor has been determined to be resectable, the decision must be made as to how much liver to remove. This will depend, in part, on the size of the mass, the number of nodules, the tumor's proximity to vascular structures, and the severity of the liver disease. Most surgeons believe a 1-cm margin of uninvolved tissue around a tumor is adequate. Larger HCCs, especially those in cirrhotic livers, should have the widest margin possible that will leave a sufficient amount of remnant tissue. In such cases, it may be necessary to compromise on the 1-cm tumor-free margin. A segmentectomy is usually practical only for small tumors. Several series have demonstrated that for HCCs smaller than 3 cm, the best operation is a segmentectomy. More radical surgeries for these lesions are accompanied by higher operative morbidity and mortality without any reduction in the recurrence rate or improvement in survival. On the other hand, lesser operations, such as wedge resections, should be discouraged, as they are associated with high rates of recurrence. The extent of the resection is often limited by the concomitant presence of cirrhosis and impaired liver function. In these cases, nonanatomic or subsegmental resections are useful to preserve as much liver as possible.

Recurrence rates following hepatic resection range between 30% and 70% in the literature. The site of the recurrence is usually intrahepatic. Tumor size and number are by far the most significant factors predicting tumor recurrence. Other risk factors include capsular or vascular invasion by tumor cells, high histologic grade, absence of a pseudocapsule, presence of cirrhosis, and tumor located deep in the liver.

Survival data vary, depending on the patient population. In those series in which all stages are evaluated, the 5-year survival rate following hepatic resection is 15–30%. Better survival rates have also been reported in patients with small HCCs. Zhou et al. achieved a 100% 5-year survival rate in patients with stage I disease treated by radical resection.

The role of orthotopic liver transplantation (OLT) in the treatment of HCC is still not completely defined. In theory, total hepatectomy seems advantageous, as it would remove the entire diseased organ, thereby reducing recurrences and improving survival. In the larger series reported in the literature, the survival rates for patients undergoing OLT for HCC range from 15% to 35% at 5 years and are no better, or are even worse, than those reported for subtotal resection. Likewise, the tumor recurrence rates with OLT are similar to those for subtotal hepatic resection. There are, however, several subpopulations for which OLT may confer improved survival. The Pittsburgh group found that when HCC was associated with cirrhosis, OLT provided a significant survival advantage over subtotal resection at each tumor stage. This survival advantage was absent in the noncirrhotic patients. More recent studies have demonstrated that if OLT is restricted to patients with solitary HCC <5 cm or to patients with less than three tumor nodules each <3 cm, recurrence is low and 4-year survival rates are 75%. The Pittsburgh group has reported a small series in which patients with advanced HCC first underwent at least three cycles of intra-arterial chemotherapy before OLT. Although the follow-up was short, the 1-year survival rate was 91% in the treated patients. This result was in contrast to patients undergoing OLT without chemotherapy, who had a 1-year survival rate of 43%.

Cryosurgery has been advocated as an alternative to resection for HCC. With this technique, liquid nitrogen is circulated through a vacuum-insulated metal probe placed in the tumor. Placement of the probe and treatment are monitored by intraoperative ultrasound. Each freezing takes 15–20 minutes, and multiple areas may be treated, particularly for larger tumors. This technique has generally been reserved for patients with unresectable tumors, although it can be used in combination with a resection. Cryosurgery has the advantage of treating the tumor and a small area of surrounding liver parenchyma. Its disadvantage is that it necessitates both an anesthetic and a laparotomy. Zhou et al. (1992) have reported treatment of 87 patients with HCC with cryosurgical therapy. The 1-, 3-, and 5-year survival rates were 60%, 32%, and 20%, respectively.

The management of previously resected HCC that recurs in the liver is difficult. Most often, further liver resection is not possible without subjecting the patient to certain postoperative liver failure. Most patients should be treated with surgical therapies that do not require resection, such as cryosurgery, or nonoperative therapies, such as percutaneous ethanol injection or chemoembolization. As mentioned previously, OLT can be considered in highly selected cases.

Percutaneous ethanol injection (PEI) has been used with some success in cirrhotic patients who are ineligible for surgery. With this technique, US is used to direct the placement of a needle in the tumor. Through this needle, 8–10 ml of 95% ethanol is injected. These treatments are repeated once or twice a week on an outpatient basis. Several studies have documented survival rates following this treatment that are similar to, or even better than, those with hepatic resection. The largest series reported is by Livarghi et al., who treated 207 cirrhotic HCC patients using PEI. These patients were deemed to have unresectable tumors or to be at too high a surgical risk, or they refused surgery. Most of the patients were Child's class A (66%) and had lesions <5 cm in diameter. The 3-year survival rates for patients with single and multiple lesions were 63% and 31%, respectively. Currently, HCC <3 cm in size and fewer than three in number are candidates for PEI. In an effort to treat larger tumors, some authors have evaluated using larger volumes of ethanol for injection under general anesthesia or combining PEI with chemoembolization. However, survival benefits of these approaches are unknown.

CHEMOTHERAPY

Systemic chemotherapy has little activity against HCC. The results of single-agent clinical trials demonstrate response rates under 20%. The most active agent appears to be doxorubicin, with an overall response rate, pooled from several trials, of 19%. Multiagent chemotherapeutic regimens have been equally disappointing.

A variety of regional treatments have been studied in an effort to improve the poor results with systemic chemotherapy. Intra-arterial infusion of chemotherapeutic agents is advantageous for several reasons. As mentioned previously, the blood supply to HCC is derived from the hepatic arteries. Intra-arterial infusion allows the delivery of high concentrations of cytotoxic drugs directly to the tumor. In addition, because these agents are metabolized in the liver, their systemic levels can be minimized.

Numerous studies have been performed using intra-arterial infusion of single and multiple chemotherapeutic agents. Although there appears to be some survival benefit from intra-arterial therapy, there have been few prospective trials comparing it with standard IV systemic chemotherapy. Intra-arterial doxorubicin, alone or in combination with other agents, has produced the best response rates.

Hepatic artery ligation or occlusion has been used as a palliative treatment for unresectable HCC. It can offer significant symptomatic relief in some patients. This palliation, however, is usually transient, as collateral vessels quickly revascularize the liver.

Transcatheter arterial embolization (TAE) is basically a combination of both intra-arterial infusion chemotherapy and hepatic artery occlusion. Chemotherapeutic agents are either infused into the liver prior to embolization or impregnated in the gelatin sponges used for the embolization. Lipiodol has also been used in conjunction with TAE. When it is combined with cytotoxic drugs or radionuclides and injected into the hepatic artery, lipiodol will remain selectively in HCC tissue for an extended period, delivering locally concentrated therapy. The treatment protocols that have produced the highest survival rates are TAE with gelatin sponges containing the chemotherapeutic agent or TAE with gelatin sponges and lipiodol mixed with the chemotherapeutic agent. There was a slight survival difference in favor of those treated by the former regimen, with 2-year survival rates of 55% and 43%, respectively. However, prospective randomized trials have failed to demonstrate an advantage for chemoembolization over embolization.

RADIOTHERAPY

External beam radiotherapy has limited use in the treatment of HCC. The dose that can be safely delivered to the liver is about 30 Gy; higher doses cause radiation hepatitis. Radiotherapy can, however, provide palliative, symptomatic relief in cases of unresectable HCC. Alternatively, locally concentrated doses of radiation can be delivered with intra-arterial infusion of lipiodol or antiferritin antibodies that are coupled with radioactive iodine.

MULTIMODALITY THERAPY

Combinations of surgical and nonsurgical therapies are currently the state of the art in the treatment of HCC. Some tumors that were previously considered unresectable can now be rendered resectable with intra-arterial chemotherapy and radiotherapy. A variety of chemotherapeutic agents have been studied in the neoadjuvant setting, including doxorubicin, 5-fluorouracil (5-FU), mitomycin C, and cisplatin. Furthermore, tumor recurrence may be prevented by the administration of adjuvant intra-arterial chemotherapy following surgical resection, ethanol injection, or cryosurgery.

Metastasis to the Liver

Virtually every malignant tumor has been known to metastasize to and proliferate in the liver. Most of these metastases are from gastrointestinal primary tumors, especially from the colon and rectum. In collected series of resected noncolorectal metastases to the liver, there are few 5-year survivors. However, in series of highly selective groups of patients with noncolorectal metastases, 5-year survivals of 40% have been reported. These patient series represent a small percent of patients with non-colorectal metastasis, and presently there are no well-defined criteria for which patients should be considered candidates for surgical resection. The exceptions to this appear to be metastases from neuroendocrine tumors, Wilms' tumor, and, to a lesser extent, renal cell carcinoma. In the case of neuroendocrine tumors, even a subtotal resection of gross disease can lead to significant palliation by decreasing the volume of hormone-secreting tumor. Given that the vast majority of metastases to the liver considered for resection are from colorectal primary tumors, the remainder of this discussion is concerned with their management.

EPIDEMIOLOGY AND ETIOLOGY

Of the 150,000 patients newly diagnosed with colon cancer each year, approximately 50% will have recurrences within 5 years following surgical resection of the primary tumor. Of those who have recurrences, only 20% will have the liver as the sole or predominant site, and fewer still will have lesions amenable to surgical resection. It has been estimated that fewer than 5,000 patients a year are potential candidates for resection of their liver metastases.

The discovery of metastatic disease in the liver is made at the time of the initial presentation for the primary lesion (synchronous lesions) in approximately 25% of patients. The remainder will have their metastatic disease found some time following resection of the primary (metachronous) lesions. Metachronous lesions are associated with a Duke's C primary tumor in approximately 60% of cases, and the disease-free interval is usually less than 2 years.

CLINICAL PRESENTATION

Symptoms or clinical signs suggesting metastatic disease in the liver are usually late occurrences. Consequently, findings such as ascites, jaundice, right upper quadrant pain, and elevation of liver function values are associated with a poor prognosis.

DIAGNOSIS

In the vast majority of patients, metastases to the liver are found through routine postoperative carcinoembryonic antigen (CEA) screening or radiologic imaging following resection of their colorectal primary tumor. Any patient with a rising CEA level should undergo a thorough diagnostic evaluation, including a chest radiograph and a contrast-enhanced CT scan of the abdomen and pelvis. In addition, the colon should be examined by either a barium enema or, preferably, colonoscopy to exclude the presence of a metachronous colon or rectal primary tumor as the source of the rising CEA.

DETERMINING RESECTABILITY

In cases in which the initial evaluation suggests the metastatic disease is isolated to the liver, one must determine whether the patient is a candidate for surgical resection. Patients should be further studied using CTAP to better visualize small lesions that might have been missed by standard CT. The rationale for CTAP in this setting is the same as that for primary tumors of the liver: Metastatic lesions derive the majority of their blood supply from the hepatic artery, not the portal vein. At the time of CTAP, visceral angiography is performed to exclude tumor encasement of major blood vessels and the presence of any hepatic arterial anomalies.

Magnetic resonance imaging (MRI) has been gaining increasing usage. In the T_1-weighted images metastases are low intensity, and angiographic or three-dimensional reconstructive images can demonstrate the relationship of the tumor to major blood vessels.

Many investigators have attempted to identify the group of patients who will benefit from hepatic resection. Several factors that impact on resectability can be gleaned from these studies. An absolute contraindication to hepatic resection includes the presence of common bile duct or celiac lymph node involvement, which is associated with a poor prognosis (5-year survival <5%). Other relative contraindications to hepatic resection include size greater than 10 cm (5-year survival = 14%); presence of four or more metastatic lesions, even if all are located within the same lobe (5-year survival = 24%); preoperative CEA level over 200 ng/ml (5-year survival = 26%); and presence of coexisting serious medical problems. In a recent report by Fong et al. (1997) age greater than 70 was not associated with a worse prognosis (5-year survival = 36%). A positive surgical margin has been consistently associated with a poor prognosis (5-year survival = 17%). The presence of extrahepatic metastases has traditionally been considered another contraindication to hepatic resection. Hughes et al. (1988) found that patients with extrahepatic metastases resected simultaneously with the hepatic resection did not have statistically significant reduced overall survival. The disease-free survival, however, was significantly shorter. Therefore at M. D. Anderson, we believe that in the presence of extrahepatic metastases, hepatic resection should be considered only in good surgical candidates when all metastases (hepatic and extrahepatic) can be removed safely and completely with negative surgical margins.

In patients whose liver metastases are deemed resectable by preoperative evaluation, there is no need to seek histologic identification of the mass prior to exploration. Percutaneous biopsy of lesions under US or CT guidance may be necessary prior to initiation of alternative therapies in patients for whom surgical resection is not indicated.

EVALUATION OF OPERATIVE RISK

Patients undergoing surgery for metastases to the liver differ from those with HCC in that cirrhosis is not frequently present. This does not relieve the surgeon of the responsibility of determining the preoperative condition of the liver parenchyma and the expected adequacy of hepatic reserve following resection of the tumor. The preoperative evaluation of liver function is the same as outlined for patients with HCC.

SURGICAL THERAPY

Once the metastases have been determined to be potentially resectable, the patient should undergo a thorough exploratory laparotomy. Particular attention should be paid to the presence of any extrahepatic disease and enlarged portal and celiac lymph nodes. The colon should be examined for any local recurrences of the primary tumor. The liver is examined, first by visual inspection and palpation, then by intraoperative US. This study will help define the relationship of the tumor(s) to the portal veins, hepatic veins, and vena cava. In addition, it can identify small lesions that were not palpable or demonstrable on preoperative imaging studies. Suspicious areas can be sampled by fine-needle aspiration under US guidance. Complete exploration combined with intraoperative US will determine that nearly half of all patients have unresectable disease. In a prospective trial conducted by the Gastrointestinal Tumor Study Group (GITSG), 42% of patients who underwent surgical exploration were found to have unresectable tumors, and only 46% underwent curative resection. More than two-thirds of the patients had tumors deemed unresectable as a result of anatomic constraints, such as the proximity of the tumor to major blood vessels or the presence of bilobar disease.

The type of resection performed will depend on the size, number, and location of the lesions. In all cases, the resection must achieve at least a 1-cm tumor-free margin. Thinner margins are invariably associated with local recurrences and shorter survival. Solitary lesions smaller than 4 cm can usually be extirpated with either a nonanatomic resection or a segmentectomy. Larger lesions should be approached with an anatomic lobectomy, if at all possible. Lesser procedures for these lesions result in a poor prognosis, probably because of the inability to achieve an adequate tumor-free margin around the large tumor. Lesions that are situated in proximity to major intrahepatic vascular structures are best removed with a lobectomy, even though they may be small.

The presence of bilobar metastases is not necessarily a contraindication to resection. Patients with multiple unilobular metastases have no survival advantage or prolongation of disease-free survival compared with patients with a comparable number of bilobar metastases. What dictates resectability will be the amount of normal, functioning liver parenchyma that will remain following removal of the lesions. Small lesions are best treated with multiple segmentectomies; these can be safely performed in up to three isolated segments. Larger bilobar lesions or those involving more than three segments should be removed with a trisegmentectomy if their locations and the patient's hepatic reserve allow such a major procedure.

The operative mortality reported in most major series ranges from 5% to 10%. Postoperative complications occur in 12–43% of all patients. The most common sources of morbidity are hepatic failure, bile leak (biloma or biliary fistula), intra-abdominal hemorrhage, and subphrenic or intra-abdominal abscess. In most reported series of hepatic resection for colorectal metastases, the 5-year survival rate ranges from 25% to 40%.

Despite surgical removal of all gross tumor, most patients will have a tumor recurrence following hepatic resection. In the two large series compiled by Hughes (1986) and by Fong (1997), the recurrence rates were 70% and 51%, respectively. Results from the GITSG study were better, with a reported recurrence rate of 49%.

The patterns of recurrence have been described in detail by Hughes et al. (1986). Of 607 patients treated with hepatic resection, 316 had initial recurrences at one site. The liver (47%) and lung (23%) were the most common sites of initial recurrence. Analysis of late recurrences showed a similar distribution, with involvement of the liver in 43% of patients and the lungs in 31%. In only 16% of patients was the late recurrent disease in the liver alone. Fong et al. (1997) have reported the liver as the first site of recurrence in 41% of their patients. As a result, those patients who have recurrences following hepatic resection for liver metastases are seldom candidates for further resective surgery. Nevertheless, several authors have reported results of hepatic surgical resections for recurrent colorectal metastasis, with median survivals ranging from 23 to 39 months.

Synchronous liver metastases found at the time of surgery for a primary tumor should, in general, not be resected in the same operation. The exception would be a solitary, small, peripherally located lesion in a healthy, hemodynamically stable patient that could be adequately excised with a wedge resection. Lesions that are larger or that will require a major hepatic resection are best approached during a second operation after further evaluation and staging. A delay of weeks to months between surgeries has not been shown to have a negative impact on survival. Obviously, at the time of the initial operation, a thorough exploration should be conducted to rule out the presence of extrahepatic metastases. The liver should also be examined by intraoperative US, if available.

Cryosurgical ablation as described in the previous section has been applied to colorectal cancer liver metastases. Several studies have shown the efficacy and safety of hepatic cryosurgery. Ravikumar et al. reported 32 patients who underwent cryosurgery. The histology of these tumors was as follows: colorectal, 24 patients; hepatoma, three patients; neuroendocrine tumors, two patients; and others, three patients. The median follow-up was 24 months and the median hospital stay was 6 days. The 5-year actuarial disease-free survival and overall survival were 24% and 62%, respectively. There were no operative mortalities. Bleeding from the probe sites was controlled with packing of thrombogenic materials. Transient elevation of temperature, liver function enzymes, and white blood cell count were seen, but normalized in the postoperative period. Onik et al. recently reviewed 57 patients with colorectal metastatic disease to the liver. These patients were treated with cryosurgery with or without surgical resection. The overall and disease-free survival were 62% and 36%, respectively, at 23 months. Additional studies have demonstrated similar efficacy and morbidity, with operative mortality ranging from 0 to 3%. Significant complications that have been reported include myoglobinurea, renal failure, cracking of the liver surface, and hemorrhage. Thrombocytopenia and transient evidence of disseminated intravascular coagulation have also been reported. At M. D. Anderson we are continuing to investigate this form of therapy for patients who are not candidates for surgical resection. Our present eligibility criteria include:

1.   An age greater than 18 years;
2.   Biopsy-proven metastatic disease, or suspicious lesion on CT scan;

3. Intraoperative ultrasound that demonstrates lesions are unresectable;
4. No extrahepatic disease; and
5. Ability to ablate all disease with either cryosurgery or cryosurgery in combination with surgical resection.

Patients with PTs greater than 14 seconds, bilirubin greater than 2, white blood cell count below 2,000, or platelet count below 100,000 are excluded.

An analysis of our first 40 patients demonstrated a 25% complication rate, with a majority of these being pleural effusions; one patient developed ATN, two patients developed abscess, and one patient developed hepatic failure. With a median follow-up of 17 months, our disease-free survival was 65%. Recurrences have occurred in the liver and have been extrahepatic. Investigations of cryosurgery in combination with hepatic artery chemotherapy are ongoing for this high-risk population of patients without other viable treatment options.

CHEMOTHERAPY

Systemic chemotherapy has been studied extensively in the treatment of liver metastases from colorectal carcinoma. Clinical trials using single or multiple chemotherapeutic agents have been disappointing, with response rates ranging from 0 to 45%. In addition, the duration of the responses has been short. Almost all regimens are based on 5-FU, an agent that has been one of the most active against colorectal cancer. The most active regimen is 5-FU in combination with leukovorin, with median survivals of 10–14 months.

Patients with unresectable metastatic disease confined to the liver may be considered for regional chemotherapy, administered via a hepatic arterial infusion (HAI) pump. This option is attractive because it allows infusion of high concentrations of drug to the tumor while limiting systemic drug levels and therefore toxicity.

Prior to implantation of the HAI pump, it is imperative that the possibility of extrahepatic or nodal metastases be excluded. In addition, a good-quality arteriogram is necessary for the proper positioning of the catheter. Once the decision has been made to proceed with pump placement, a cholecystectomy should first be performed to prevent the development of chemical cholecystitis, a well-described complication of HAI. In the presence of normal hepatic arterial anatomy, the infusion catheter is placed into the gastroduodenal artery (GDA), in a retrograde direction, with its tip just at the take-off of this artery from the common hepatic artery. The right gastric artery and any accessory arteries distal to the GDA should be ligated to prevent inadvertent perfusion of extrahepatic tissues. The pump is usually positioned in a subcutaneous pocket in the right lower quadrant of the abdomen, with the catheter inserted through the anterior abdominal wall. Following placement of the catheter, a fluorescein dye study should be performed through the catheter. A Wood's lamp is used to confirm that no extrahepatic perfusion is present. Prior to the initiation of chemotherapy, a radionuclide pump study is performed during the postoperative period to reconfirm the proper functioning of the catheter.

Variant hepatic arterial anatomy must be recognized and defined clearly on the preoperative arteriogram. When present, accessory lobar vessels are ligated to prevent inhomogeneous perfusion of drug to that lobe. Replaced hepatic arteries are managed in several ways. Two catheters can be placed—one to infuse the main hepatic artery and the other to supply the replaced vessel. One or two infusion pumps may need to be used. The method used at M. D. Anderson is to ligate the replaced vessel and use a single catheter to infuse the main hepatic artery. The lobe with the ligated accessory artery will rapidly develop collateral flow from the other lobe, allowing it to be perfused with the drug.

Although 5-FU is the favored drug in systemic chemotherapy, its first-pass clearance by the liver is low. Consequently, the relative increase in hepatic exposure to the drug by HAI is estimated to be only five- to tenfold. A related pyrimidine antagonist, floxuridine (fluorodeoxyuridine [FUDR]), has a much higher extraction on the first pass through the liver. The estimated increase in exposure of the liver to this drug when delivered by HAI is 100- to 400-fold, making it an ideal drug for this use.

Interest in HAI increased after the development of the totally implantable Infusaid pump. This device allows both continuous and bolus injection of drug into the hepatic artery. Initial studies using this delivery system for the infusion of FUDR demonstrated remarkable response rates—as high as 83%. There have since been five major randomized trials comparing the efficacy of HAI to standard IV chemotherapy (Table 12-3). All studies showed significantly better response rates for patients receiving HAI chemotherapy. Because of differences in study design and length of follow-up, survival data are not as easily compared. All studies showed a tendency for longer survival in patients treated with HAI; however, only the NCI trial demonstrated a statistically significant improvement in

Table 12-3.   Major randomized trials comparing hepatic arterial infusion (HAI) and IV chemotherapy for liver metastases from colorectal cancer

Study	No. of patients	HAI Agent	HAI Response (%)	IV Agent	IV Response (%)
MSKCC	162	FUDR	50	FUDR	20
NCI	64	FUDR	62	FUDR	17
NCOG	115	FUDR	42	FUDR	10
Mayo	69	FUDR	48	5-FU	21
France	163	FUDR	43	5-FU	9

MSKCC = Memorial Sloan-Kettering Cancer Center (N Kemeny et al. *Ann Intern Med* 107:459, 1987); NCI = National Cancer Institute (AE Chang et al. *Ann Surg* 206:685, 1987); NCOG = Northern California Oncology Group (DC Hohn et al. *J Clin Oncol* 7:1646, 1989); Mayo = Mayo Clinic (JK Martin et al. *Arch Surg* 125:1022, 1990); France = multicenter French cooperative study (P Rougier et al. *J Clin Oncol* 10:1112, 1992.) 5-FU = 5-fluorouracil; FUDR = floxuridine.

survival rate. In this study, the 2-year survival rates for HAI and systemic regimens were 44% and 13%, respectively.

The efficacy of HAI therapy can be further evaluated by the patterns of responses and failures. In a Memorial Sloan-Kettering Cancer Center study, 82% of patients in the systemic group had disease progression in the liver, compared with 37% in the HAI group. On the other hand, 56% of patients who received HAI developed extrahepatic disease, compared with 37% of patients who received systemic chemotherapy. These data demonstrate, once again, that regional control of the disease alone may not be adequate, as most people treated with HAI ultimately die of extrahepatic disease.

This problem has been the impetus for several studies aimed at reducing the rate of extrahepatic failure in patients receiving HAI. One approach has been to infuse IV chemotherapy concomitantly with HAI infusion. Safi et al. compared patients treated with intrahepatic FUDR with those treated with both intrahepatic and IV FUDR. Both groups had comparable response rates and survival durations; however, the rates of extrahepatic failure differed between the two treatment groups. Extrahepatic metastases developed in 61% of patients in the HAI group and in 33% of patients in the HAI/IV group. Another approach that has been taken at M. D. Anderson is to alternate administration of FUDR and 5-FU via the HAI pump. The use of 5-FU not only reduces the toxicity to the liver but also, because of the lower first-pass clearance of that drug by the liver, allows significant systemic levels to be attained. This treatment has resulted in a 50% response rate and a prolongation of survival, compared with intrahepatic FUDR alone.

Presently, the most active regimen for HAI chemotherapy is a combination of FUDR, 5-FU, LV, and dexamethasone. Response rates of up to 80% have been reported with the use of this regimen.

There has been only one prospective, randomized study evaluating the use of HAI as an adjunct to surgical resection of hepatic metastases. Wagman et al. randomized patients with solitary, resectable lesions to receive surgery or surgery plus postoperative HAI with FUDR. A second group with multiple resectable lesions was randomized to surgery plus HAI or HAI alone. Patients from groups treated with surgery plus HAI had a longer disease-free interval; however, they did not have longer survivals.

Although HAI significantly decreases the systemic toxicity of chemotherapy, it is by no means a benign procedure. The locally concentrated dose of drug is associated with a number of complications, including chemical hepatitis, biliary sclerosis, gastritis, and gastric or duodenal ulcer disease. Permanent hepatic damage can be averted by careful monitoring of liver function during chemotherapy, and prompt reduction of the dose, should evidence of chemical hepatitis be noted.

Cancer of the Extrahepatic Bile Duct

EPIDEMIOLOGY AND ETIOLOGY

Cancer of the extrahepatic bile duct (cholangiocarcinoma) is extremely rare. In most reported series, the male-to-female incidence ratio is equal and patients are in their seventh decade. There is no significant geographic variation in the prevalence of the tumor.

The etiology of cholangiocarcinoma is unknown. Several diseases are associated with an increased incidence of such tumors: sclerosing cholangitis, ulcerative colitis, choledochal cysts, and infection with *Clonorchis sinensis*. The common cancer-causing factor in all these conditions is unclear, although chronic inflammation of the bile duct probably plays a role.

PATHOLOGY

Histologically, cholangiocarcinoma can be classified as papillary, nodular, or sclerosing adenocarcinomas. The papillary variety has a better prognosis than the other two types. Papillary tumors are usually well differentiated and can present with multiple lesions within the duct. The worst prognosis is associated with the sclerosing type, which is usually poorly differentiated.

Most cholangiocarcinomas are located in the proximal portion of the duct. A tumor arising at the confluence of the right and left hepatic ducts is termed a *Klatskin's tumor,* following the description of 13 such lesions by Klatskin in 1965.

Cholangiocarcinomas are slow growing and most often spread by local extension or metastasize to regional lymph nodes. Lesions of the proximal and middle thirds of the extrahepatic bile duct can compress, constrict, or invade the underlying portal vein or hepatic artery. In addition, proximal tumors can invade the liver parenchyma. It has been appreciated that hilar cholangiocarcinomas will involve the parenchyma of the caudate lobe in as many as 36% of patients. Distant metastases from cholangiocarcinomas are rare.

There are a number of pathologic findings important in predicting the outcome of patients with cholangiocarcinoma. These factors include infiltration to the serosa of the bile duct, lymph node metastases, vascular invasion, and perineural invasion.

CLINICAL PRESENTATION

The most common presenting symptom in patients with cholangiocarcinoma is obstructive jaundice. Rarely, a very proximal tumor may block a segmental or lobar bile duct without the occurrence of clinical jaundice. Other symptoms that may occur are pruritus, weight loss, fatigue, vague abdominal pain, and nausea. A patient may present with cholangitis and sepsis resulting from contamination of the obstructed bile. Except for the jaundice, the physical findings in a patient with bile duct cancer are nonspecific. In cases of middle or distal duct obstruction, a distended gallbladder may be palpable.

DIAGNOSIS

When extrahepatic bile duct obstruction is suspected, the first radiologic test that should be performed is US, as it can provide information about the level and nature of an obstructing lesion. CT is as sensitive as US in demonstrating bile duct dilation. Because of its higher cost, however, CT should not be used routinely as the initial diagnostic test. Should the US demonstrate extrahepatic bile duct dilation that is not a result of common bile duct stones, a CT should be obtained. CT has the advantage of being able to identify the actual tumor mass more often than US. In addition, CT is better able to define the relationship of the tumor to surrounding structures and to evaluate the remainder of the abdomen for metastatic spread.

The actual location of the tumor and, more important, its proximal extent must be defined before planning any surgical intervention. This goal can be accomplished in one of two ways: percutaneous transhepatic cholangiography (PTC) or endoscopic retrograde cholangiopancreatography (ERCP). If the point of obstruction is thought to be proximal, PTC is the preferred method for visualizing the biliary tract. For suspected distal bile duct lesions, ERCP is superior, as it will enable one to image both the bile duct and the pancreatic duct. Recently, MRI cholangiopancreatography has been demonstrated to be a noninvasive study able to diagnose pancreaticobiliary neoplasia and delineate the anatomy.

The work-up for a suspected cholangiocarcinoma is completed with visceral angiography and portography. As mentioned previously, these tumors have a tendency to involve the portal vein and the hepatic artery by local invasion. Evidence of encasement of these vascular structures would suggest that the lesion is unresectable. This criterion has become more a relative contraindication, as many surgeons are now resecting portions of involved portal vein and hepatic artery.

Obtaining tissue to confirm the diagnosis of bile duct cancer is difficult because of the location of such tumors and their small size. Fine-needle aspiration can be done under US or CT guidance. Cytologic evaluation of bile and of bile duct brushings is also possible, although the sensitivity of these tests is only about 30% and 40%, respectively. In most cases, the decision to operate is based on the preoperative radiologic examinations, not histologic confirmation.

The differential diagnosis for focal stenosis or obstruction of the bile duct is given in Table 12-4. Although the list is extensive, choledocholithiasis and cholangiocarcinoma are the most common causes.

STAGING

The current AJCC staging system for cholangiocarcinoma is shown in Table 12-5.

SURGICAL THERAPY

The definitive therapy for all extrahepatic bile duct carcinomas is surgical resection; however, only a fraction of these lesions will ultimately be resectable. Overall resectability rates range from 10% to 85%, depending on the series. Lesions of the lower third of the bile duct have the best rates of resectability, followed by those of the middle third. Proximal cholangiocarcinomas are technically difficult to approach, resulting in the lowest rate of resectability among bile duct tumors. Standard criteria that render a tumor

Table 12-4.   Differential diagnosis for focal bile duct obstruction

Malignant lesions
  Primary cholangiocarcinoma
  Mucoepidermoid carcinoma
  Direct invasion
    Hepatoma
    Gallbladder carcinoma
    Pancreatic carcinoma
    Retroperitoneal sarcoma
  Metastases to hilar or periportal lymph nodes
  Lymphoid tumors (Hodgkin's and non-Hodgkin's lymphoma)

Benign lesions
  Choledocholithiasis
  Sclerosing cholangitis
  Iatrogenic bile duct stricture
  Mirizzi's syndrome
  Idiopathic focal stenosis
  Tuberculosis
  Clonorchis or *Ascaris* infestation

unresectable are (1) lymph node involvement outside the hepatic pedicle, (2) distant metastases, (3) bilateral tumor extension into secondary hepatic ducts, or (4) bilateral extension of tumor into hepatic parenchyma. As stated earlier, many surgeons would resect involved portal vein, therefore making vascular involvement a relative contraindication.

The need for preoperative biliary drainage had been debated at length in the literature. Earlier reports noted that preoperative hyperbilirubinemia was a poor prognostic indicator and that normalization of the bilirubin level prior to surgery was associated with reduced morbidity and mortality. However, recent studies have found no benefit from, or have found deleterious effects of, preoperative biliary drainage. Nevertheless, Cameron advocates routine preoperative placement of biliary drainage catheters to facilitate identification and dissection of the bile duct during surgery and to aid the intraoperative placement of larger, softer Silastic transhepatic stents. We, along with the Memorial group, believe that these procedures can be performed safely and effectively without preoperative biliary drainage. Nevertheless, many patients have undergone preoperative ERCP and stenting prior to referral.

Resectable lesions of the lower third of the bile duct are best treated with a pancreaticoduodenectomy. The proximal bile duct should be resected to the point that the surgical margin is negative for tumor. Occasionally, this may require removal of most of the extrahepatic biliary tract with a high hepaticojejunostomy. The operative approach for a pancreaticoduodenectomy at M. D. Anderson is outlined in Chapter 13.

Lesions of the middle third of the bile duct are in proximity to the hepatic artery and the portal vein and have a tendency to invade these structures. If such a tumor has been deemed resectable, it is best treated by local excision and regional lymph node dissection.

Table 12-5. AJCC staging system for cancer of the extrahepatic bile duct

Primary tumor

Tx	Primary tumor cannot be assessed
T0	No evidence of primary tumor
Tis	Carcinoma *in situ*
T1	Tumor invades subepithelial connective tissue or fibromuscular layer
T1a	Tumor invades subepithelial connective tissue
T1b	Tumor invades fibromuscular layer
T2	Tumor invades perifibromuscular connective tissue
T3	Tumor invades adjacent structures: liver, pancreas, duodenum, gallbladder, colon, stomach

Regional lymph nodes

Nx	Regional lymph nodes cannot be assessed
N0	No regional lymph node metastasis
N1	Metastasis in cystic duct, pericholedochal and/or hilar lymph nodes (i.e., in the hepatoduodenal ligament)
N2	Metastasis in peripancreatic (head only), periduodenal, periportal, celiac, and/or superior mesenteric and/or posterior pancreaticoduodenal lymph nodes

Distant metastasis

Mx	Presence of distant metastasis cannot be assessed
M0	No distant metastasis
M1	Distant metastasis

Stage grouping

Stage 0	Tis	N0	M0
Stage I	T1	N0	M0
Stage II	T2	N0	M0
Stage III	T1–T2	N1–N2	M0
Stage IVA	T3	Any N	M0
Stage IVB	Any T	Any N	M1

Source: OH Beahrs et al. *Manual Staging Cancer* (5th ed). Philadelphia: Lippincott, 1997.

All efforts should be made to achieve a microscopically negative margin. Care must be taken not to disrupt the soft tissues containing the blood supply to the remaining proximal bile duct to which the hepaticoenteric anastomosis will be performed; otherwise one risks a postoperative bile duct stricture. Biliary drainage is reestablished using a Roux-en-Y hepaticojejunostomy.

The surgical management of proximal cholangiocarcinomas is challenging and remains controversial. Numerous reports have suggested that radical excision of the duct and any involved liver improves survival and quality of life. However, some surgeons think the morbidity and mortality associated with major hepatic resection

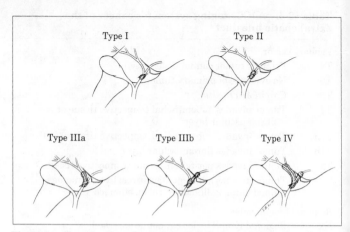

Fig. 12-3.   Classification of extrahepatic bile duct tumors according to the location of the obstructing lesion (Bismuth classification).

for this tumor are too high to justify its use. Part of the controversy involves the necessity of resecting the caudate lobe (segment I) en bloc with the bile duct. Proponents of this approach state that pathologic examination of resected specimens demonstrates direct invasion of tumor into the liver parenchyma or the bile ducts of the caudate lobe in as many as 35% of patients. In addition, the site of tumor recurrence following bile duct resection is often the caudate lobe. Therefore several surgeons have recommended routine caudate lobectomy with bile duct excision. Other surgeons believe the caudate lobe should be removed only if it is invaded by the tumor, citing equivalent survival data for those who had caudate lobectomy and those with similar lesions who did not. The difficulty and potential benefits of obtaining a negative margin have been demonstrated in a recent report by Burke et al. Twelve of 13 patients treated with potentially curative resection required concomitant hepatic resection; however, 83% of patients had microscopically negative margins. This translated into a 5-year survival rate of 40% in patients treated with potentially curative resection. This argues for an aggressive surgical approach in centers that can perform these procedures with acceptable morbidity and mortality.

A final area of controversy is the use of total hepatectomy and OLT for tumors with bilateral extension into secondary intra-hepatic biliary ducts. Thus far, there is no convincing evidence that liver transplantation is of benefit to these patients.

The surgical approach to proximal bile duct tumors at M. D. Anderson depends on their location relative to the confluence of the right and left bile ducts and on their proximal extension. Lesions in this region are classified according to the scheme described by Bismuth and Corlette (Fig. 12-3). Type I and II lesions are treated by local excision and local lymph node dissection. We do not perform routine caudate lobe resections for type II tumors unless invasion into the lobe can be demonstrated. Type IIIa and IIIb lesions undergo local excision and either right or left hepatic lobectomy, respectively. Type IV lesions are not considered resectable. We do not advocate the use of OLT in patients with such advanced disease.

Despite aggressive surgical management, most patients with bile duct carcinoma will succumb to their tumors. Survival rates are the best for lesions of the distal bile duct. Langer et al. reported mean survival times of 37, 32, and 28 months for patients with tumors in the distal, middle, and upper thirds of the bile duct, respectively. Reported 5-year survival rates range from 7% to 50%, depending on the tumor location, with distal lesions being associated with higher rates. Patients with negative lymph nodes and clear surgical margins have the best prognoses.

The optimal palliation for patients with unresectable tumors is unclear. If the tumor has been deemed unresectable prior to exploration, the bile duct can be intubated either percutaneously or endoscopically. The use of metallic in-dwelling stents, which are more durable than traditional stents, has made this option more appealing. If the tumor has been found to be unresectable at the time of exploration, the duct can be intubated using either transhepatic Silastic stents or a T tube following dilation of the lesion. When technically feasible, operative biliary bypass with or without concomitant tumor resection provides the best survival and quality of life for patients with unresectable tumors. Unresectable lesions at the bile duct confluence, especially Bismuth type III and IV lesions, can be particularly difficult to palliate. A left intrahepatic cholangioenteric anastomosis has been used with success in these situations. In this technique, the left hepatic duct branch is located between segments III and IV and is drained into a Roux-en-Y limb of jejunum.

CHEMOTHERAPY

There are no clearly effective chemotherapeutic agents for the treatment of cholangiocarcinoma. Single-agent trials using 5-FU have demonstrated response rates under 15%. Other agents, such as doxorubicin, mitomycin C, and cisplatin, used alone or in combination with 5-FU, have been no more successful.

RADIOTHERAPY

Radiotherapy has been demonstrated to be effective in the palliation of patients with unresectable bile duct cancers. Doses of 40–60 Gy have resulted in median survival rates of 12 months, as well as symptomatic improvement. At M. D. Anderson, postoperative chemoradiation is given to patients with resected bile duct cancers. Patients receive continuous-infusion 5-FU concomitantly with 54 Gy of radiation to the tumor bed. Although patient numbers are small and follow-up time is short, initial results suggest a prolongation of survival in treated patients when compared with untreated, historical controls. Intraoperative radiotherapy (IORT) has also been used at our institution in combination with external beam radiation. Again, because of the small numbers of patients treated at this and other institutions, no firm conclusion can be drawn regarding the benefit of IORT. There does appear to be a prolongation of survival in the limited number of patients who have received this therapy.

MULTIMODALITY THERAPY

At the M. D. Anderson Cancer Center we are currently investigating the role of preoperative chemoradiation in patients with proximal cholangiocarcinomas in an effort to improve local control and potentially improve resectability rates. The results of this approach are not available presently.

Periampullary Carcinoma

James Cusack

PATHOLOGY

Adenocarcinoma accounts for 95% of malignancies of the periampullary area and may develop from four different tissues of origin at this site: head of pancreas, ampulla of Vater, distal bile duct, and periampullary duodenum. Although the modes of presentation and treatment are similar, the prognosis for each of these malignancies is different. The 5-year survival rate for adenocarcinoma of the head of the pancreas is reported to be 18%; of the ampulla, 36%; of the distal bile duct, 34%; and of the periampullary duodenum, 33%. Determination of the tissue of origin is therefore critical, because it affects management decisions regarding potential for cure and extent of resection necessary to obtain tumor-free resection margins. The current American Joint Committee on Cancer (AJCC) staging system for ampullary tumors is shown in Table 12-6.

Determination of the tissue of origin may be made from fine-needle aspiration biopsy or endoscopic biopsy and is based on mucin production and the degree of cellular differentiation. Anatomic information based on thin-section CT and endoscopic retrograde cholangiopancreatography may also contribute to the determination of the tissue of origin. Detection of a mutation in the Kirsten (Ki)-ras proto-oncogene, which occurs in 75–90% of pancreatic adenocarcinomas, may be helpful in differentiating these neoplasms from other periampullary tumors.

Locoregional spread of periampullary adenocarcinoma results from lymphatic invasion and direct tumor extension to adjacent soft tissues. In a prospective study of regional lymph node metastases in patients undergoing pancreaticoduodenectomy for periampullary adenocarcinoma, Cubilla et al. found significant variability in both the frequency of lymph node metastases and the pattern of lymph node involvement, depending on the tissue of origin. Ampullary lesions metastasized to regional lymph nodes in only 33% of cases, typically involving only a single lymph node in the posterior pancreaticoduodenal group. Duodenal adenocarcinomas had an intermediate risk of nodal metastasis, with metastases to several lymph nodes in different subgroups of the paraduodenal area. Pancreatic adenocarcinoma, with its propensity to invade the rich lymphatic network of the pancreas and its ability to directly invade adjacent tissues, had the highest frequency of lymph node involvement (88%); metastases typically involved multiple lymph nodes, multiple subgroups, and distant sites.

Table 12-6. AJCC staging system for cancer of the ampulla of Vater

Primary tumor

Tx	Primary tumor cannot be assessed
T0	No evidence of primary tumor
Tis	Carcinoma *in situ*
T1	Tumor limited to the ampulla of Vater or sphincter of Oddi
T2	Tumor invades duodenal wall
T3	Tumor invades 2 cm or less into the pancreas
T4	Tumor invades more than 2 cm into pancreas and/or into other adjacent organs

Regional lymph nodes

Nx	Regional lymph nodes cannot be assessed
N0	No regional lymph node metastasis
N1	Regional lymph node metastasis

Distant metastasis

Mx	Presence of distant metastasis cannot be assessed
M0	No distant metastasis
M1	Distant metastasis

Stage grouping

Stage 0	Tis	N0	M0
Stage I	T1	N0	M0
Stage II	T2–T3	N0	M0
Stage III	T1–T3	N1	M0
Stage IV	T4	Any N	M0
	Any T	Any N	M1

Source: OH Beahrs et al. *Manual Staging Cancer* (5th ed). Philadelphia: Lippincott, 1997.

TREATMENT

The standard Whipple pancreaticoduodenectomy is thought to provide adequate tumor clearance in the case of nonpancreatic periampullary carcinoma because disease spread is usually localized. Although biopsy-proved paraduodenal lymphadenopathy is thought by most surgeons to preclude curative resection in patients with pancreatic adenocarcinoma, one may appropriately consider en bloc resection in patients with duodenal, ampullary, or distal bile duct tumors in the presence of regional lymph node metastasis if the disease is confined to the field of resection. A detailed description of operative technique is provided in Chapter 13.

The effectiveness of locoregional control of periampullary adenocarcinoma by surgery alone and the potential benefits of adjuvant chemoradiation continue to be examined. In a retrospective review of 41 patients with periampullary carcinoma, Willett et al.

identified patients with low-risk pathologic features (tumor limited to ampulla or duodenum, well- or moderately well-differentiated histology, negative resection margins, and uninvolved lymph nodes) who had significantly better 5-year actuarial local control and survival rates—100% and 80%, respectively. In contrast, patients with high-risk pathologic features (tumor invasion of pancreas, poorly differentiated histology, positive resection margins, and involved lymph nodes) had 5-year actuarial local control and survival rates of 50% and 38%, respectively. Based on these findings, the authors have proposed a course of preoperative chemoradiation to improve local disease control and survival rates in patients with locally advanced, poorly differentiated tumors.

Gallbladder Cancer

EPIDEMIOLOGY AND ETIOLOGY

Although carcinoma of the gallbladder is a rare tumor, it is actually the most common malignancy of the biliary system and the fifth most common cancer of the gastrointestinal tract. The tumor has been reported in almost all age groups but is most often found in patients in their seventh and eighth decades. There is a striking difference in the incidence of the tumor between the sexes; females are affected three to four times as often as males.

The exact etiology of carcinoma of the gallbladder is not known; however, there are several entities with which it is frequently associated. Cholelithiasis is found in the vast majority of gallbladders resected for carcinoma. Furthermore, gallbladder carcinoma can be found in 1–2% of all cholecystectomy specimens, a rate that is several times higher than that reported in autopsy studies. Chronic cholecystitis, especially cases in which the gallbladder is calcified (porcelain gallbladder), has also been associated with an increased risk of cancer, with an incidence as high as 61%.

PATHOLOGY

Adenocarcinoma of the gallbladder is a slow-growing tumor that usually arises in the fundus. Grossly, the gallbladder is firm and the walls are thickened. The tumor has a tendency to invade surrounding structures, including the liver, bile duct, and duodenum. The papillary subtype of gallbladder carcinoma characteristically grows intraluminally and spreads intraductally. It is a less aggressive tumor that, consequently, carries a better prognosis.

Lymph node metastases are found in 50–75% of gallbladder carcinoma cases. The cystic duct node, at the confluence of the cystic and hepatic ducts, is the initial focus of regional lymphatic spread. Invasion of the liver, either by direct extension or via draining veins that empty into segments IV and V, is seen in more than 50% of patients. Distant hematogenous spread is rare and is usually seen only in the later stages of the disease.

CLINICAL PRESENTATION

In most series, the most common presenting complaint is abdominal pain. Nausea, vomiting, weight loss, and jaundice are other common symptoms. Most patients have had symptoms for 3 months or less prior to presentation. On physical examination, patients may have right upper quadrant pain with hepatomegaly or a palpable, distended gallbladder. In advanced cases, patients may have jaundice, cachexia, and ascites.

DIAGNOSIS

Unfortunately, no laboratory or radiologic tests are routinely accurate in making the diagnosis of gallbladder carcinoma. That inconsistency, along with the paucity of clinical signs and symptoms, has made the tumor's preoperative diagnosis difficult. In fact, a correct preoperative diagnosis of gallbladder cancer is made in fewer than 10% of cases in most series. In the Roswell Park experience, none of the 71 patients reported were correctly diagnosed preoperatively. The most common preoperative diagnoses are acute and chronic cholecystitis and malignancies of the bile duct or pancreas.

In the rare event a diagnosis of gallbladder carcinoma is suspected preoperatively, US or CT may demonstrate a mass with local hepatic extension or suspicious portal adenopathy. Angiography may demonstrate encasement of the cystic or hepatic arteries or the portal vein. There may also be increased vascularity around the gallbladder. Cholangiography is of value in jaundiced patients because it allows the determination of the location and extent of biliary obstruction.

The most common staging system used for carcinoma of the gallbladder, as described by Nevin, is based on the depth of invasion and the spread of tumor (Table 12-7). The standard AJCC staging scheme is shown for comparison in Table 12-8. The bulk of the literature on gallbladder cancer uses the Nevin staging system.

SURGICAL THERAPY

The surgical treatment for gallbladder carcinoma is dictated by the stage of the tumor. In fact, in developing his staging system, Nevin found that survival was inversely correlated with the depth of invasion and the extent of spread. Patients with tumor confined to the mucosa and muscularis (stages I and II) all survived 5 or more years, whereas those who had transmural involvement or

TABLE 12-7.   Nevin's staging system for gallbladder carcinoma

Stage I	Intramucosal involvement only
Stage II	Involvement of the mucosa and muscularis
Stage III	Transmural involvement of gallbladder wall
Stage IV	Metastases to the cystic duct lymph nodes
Stage V	Involvement of the liver by direct extension or metastasis, or metastases to any other organ

Table 12-8.   AJCC staging system for cancer of the gallbladder

Primary tumor

Tx	Primary tumor cannot be assessed
T0	No evidence of primary tumor
Tis	Carcinoma *in situ*
T1	Tumor invades lamina propria or muscle layer
T1a	Tumor invades lamina propria
T1b	Tumor invades muscle layer
T2	Tumor invades perimuscular connective tissue; no extension beyond serosa or into liver
T3	Tumor perforates serosa (visceral peritoneum) or directly invades one adjacent organ, or both (extension 2 cm or less into liver)
T4	Tumor extends more than 2 cm into liver and/or into two or more adjacent organs (stomach, duodenum, colon, pancreas, omentum, extrahepatic bile ducts, any involvement of liver)

Regional lymph nodes

Nx	Regional lymph nodes cannot be assessed
N0	No regional lymph node metastasis
N1	Metastasis in cystic duct, pericholedochal and/or hilar lymph nodes (i.e., in the hepatoduodenal ligament)
N2	Metastasis in peripancreatic (head only), periduodenal, periportal, celiac, and/or superior mesenteric lymph nodes

Distant metastasis

Mx	Presence of distant metastasis cannot be assessed
M0	No distant metastasis
M1	Distant metastasis

Stage grouping

Stage 0	Tis	N0	M0
Stage I	T1	N0	M0
Stage II	T2	N0	M0
Stage III	T1–T2	N1	M0
	T3	N0–N1	M0
Stage IVA	T4	N0–N1	M0
Stage IVB	Any T	N2	M0
	Any T	Any N	M1

Source: OH Beahrs et al. *Manual Staging Cancer* (4th ed). Philadelphia: Lippincott, 1997.

spread to lymph nodes (stages III and IV) had a 5-year survival rate of only 10%. None of the stage V patients survived beyond 1 year.

Most patients with gallbladder carcinoma present with advanced disease (stage V). Standard criteria that make a tumor unresectable include (1) distant hematogenous or lymphatic metastases, (2) peritoneal implants, or (3) invasion of tumor into major vascular structures such as the celiac or superior mesenteric arteries, vena cava, or aorta. Tumors involving the hepatic artery or portal vein have been extirpated with an en bloc vascular resection and reconstruction, but such an extensive procedure would not be considered standard therapy. The dismal prognosis for patients with stage V cancers has made many surgeons advocate palliative procedures rather than resection.

The optimal treatment for patients with stage III and IVA tumors is an extended cholecystectomy. The components of this procedure are a cholecystectomy, regional lymph node dissection in the hepatoduodenal ligament, and a wedge resection of the gallbladder bed (including at least a 3-cm margin of normal parenchyma). Using this operative approach, Morrow reported mean survival times for patients with stage III and IV tumors of 48 and 5 months, respectively. Similarly, the Roswell Park group noted a median survival time of 13 months for patients with stage III cancers and 5.3 months for those with stage IV lesions. There are advocates of more extensive hepatic resection for stage IV disease, but the poor prognosis of these patients does not justify the more morbid operation.

Stage I carcinoma of the gallbladder can be adequately treated with cholecystectomy alone, with 5-year survival rates as high as 100% in several series. Hepatic resection and lymphadenectomy are not justified for patients with stage I disease.

The management of stage II tumors is not so clearly defined. Several studies suggest that cholecystectomy alone is sufficient treatment. On the other hand, a number of groups report higher rates of recurrence and lower survival rates for stage II patients treated with cholecystectomy alone. The treatment philosophy at M. D. Anderson involves extended cholecystectomy for most patients diagnosed with stage II disease. Patients with stage II disease not offered extended cholecystectomy include patients with tumors based on the anterior, or serosal, surface of the gallbladder (away from the liver) and patients in whom the medical risk of the procedure outweighs the potential benefit.

NONOPERATIVE THERAPY

The use of single and multiple chemotherapeutic agents either as primary therapy or as adjuvant therapy has been disappointing. Radiotherapy has shown some promise when used in the postoperative adjuvant setting, although most series are small. IORT has also been used with some success.

At M. D. Anderson, patients with gallbladder cancer are treated postoperatively with a combination of continuous-infusion chemotherapy and external beam radiation in a manner similar to treatment for patients with cholangiocarcinoma. It is too early to draw any conclusions regarding the impact of this regimen on survival.

Selected References

Bartlett DL, Fong Y, Fortner JG, et al. Long-term results after resection for gallbladder cancer. Implications for staging and management. *Ann Surg* 224(5):639, 1996.

Bismuth H, Corlette MB. Intrahepatic cholangioenteric anastomosis in carcinoma of the hilus of the liver. *Surg Gynecol Obstet* 140:170, 1975.

Bismuth H, Nakache R, Diamond T. Management strategies in resection for hilar cholangiocarcinoma. *Ann Surg* 215:31, 1992.

Blumgart LH, Kelley CJ. Hepaticojejunostomy in benign and malignant high bile duct stricture: Approaches to the left hepatic ducts. *Br J Surg* 71:257, 1984.

Bruix J, Castells A, Bosch J, et al. Surgical resection of hepatocellular carcinoma in cirrhotic patients: Prognostic value of preoperative portal pressure. *Gastroenterology* 111(4):1018, 1996.

Burke EC, Jarnagin WR, Hochwald SN, et al. Hilar cholangiocarcinoma: Patterns of spread, the importance of hepatic resection for curative operation, and a preoperative clinical staging system. *Am Surg* 1998, in press.

Cady B, Stone MD, McDermott WV, et al. Technical and biological factors in disease-free survival after hepatic resection for colorectal cancer metastases. *Arch Surg* 127:561, 1992.

Cameron JL, Broe P, Zuidema GD. Proximal bile duct tumors: Surgical management with Silastic transhepatic biliary stents. *Ann Surg* 196:412, 1982.

Cameron JL, Pitt HA, Zinner MJ, et al. Management of proximal cholangiocarcinomas by surgical resection and radiotherapy. *Am J Surg* 159:91, 1990.

Cubilla AL, Fortner J, Fitzgerald PJ. Lymph node involvement in carcinoma of the head of the pancreas area. *Cancer* 41:880, 1978.

Di Bisceglie AM, Rustgi VK, Hoofnagle JH, et al. Hepatocellular carcinoma. *Ann Intern Med* 108:390, 1988.

Feldman D, Kulling D, Kay C, et al. Magnetic resonance cholangiopancreatography (MRCP): A novel approach to the evaluation of pancreaticobiliary neoplasms. Abst. 55, 50th Annual Cancer Symposium of the Society of Surgical Oncology, 1997.

Fong Y, Cohen AM, Fortner JG, et al. Liver resection for colorectal metastases. *J Clin Oncol* 15(3):938, 1997.

Fong Y, Kemeny N, Paty P, et al. Treatment of colorectal cancer: Hepatic metastasis. *Semin Surg Oncol* 12(4):219, 1996.

Gagner M, Rossi RL. Radical operations for carcinoma of the gallbladder: Recent status in North America. *World J Surg* 15:344, 1991.

Groupe d'Etude et de Traitement du Carcinome Hepatocellulaire. A comparison of lipiodol chemoembolization and conservative treatment for unresectable hepatocellular carcinoma. *N Engl J Med* 332(19):1256, 1995.

Hohn DC, Stagg RJ, Friedman MA, et al. A randomized trial of continuous intravenous versus hepatic intraarterial floxuridine in patients with colorectal cancer metastatic to the liver: The Northern California Oncology Group Trial. *J Clin Oncol* 7:1646, 1989.

Hughes KS, et al. Resection of the liver for colorectal carcinoma metastases: A multi-institutional study of indications for resection. *Surgery* 103:278, 1988.

Hughes KS, Simon R, Songhorabodi S, et al. Resection of the liver for colorectal carcinoma metastases: A multi-institutional study of patterns of recurrence. *Surgery* 100:278, 1986.

Iwatsuki S, Sheahan DG, Starzl TE. The changing face of hepatic resection. *Curr Probl Surg* 26:283, 1989.

Iwatsuki S, Starzl TE, Sheahan DG, et al. Hepatic resection versus transplantation for hepatocellular carcinoma. *Ann Surg* 214:221, 1991.

Kanematsu T, Matsumata T, Shirabe K, et al. A comparative study of hepatic resection and transcatheter arterial embolization for the treatment of primary hepatocellular carcinoma. *Cancer* 71:2181, 1993.

Karl RC, Morse SS, Halpert RD, et al. Preoperative evaluation of patients for liver resection: Appropriate CT imaging. *Ann Surg* 217:226, 1993.

Kawai S, Okamura J, Ogawa M, et al. Prospective and randomized clinical trial for the treatment of hepatocellular carcinoma: A comparison of lipiodol-transcatheter arterial embolization with and without adriamycin (first cooperative study). The Cooperative Study Group for Liver Cancer Treatment of Japan. *Cancer Chemother Pharmacol* 31(Suppl):S1, 1992.

Kemeny N, Daly J, Reichman B, et al. Intrahepatic or systemic infusion of fluorodeoxyuridine in patients with liver metastases from colorectal carcinoma: A randomized trial. *Ann Intern Med* 107:459, 1987.

Klatskin G. Adenocarcinoma of the hepatic duct at its bifurcation within the portahepatis: An unusual tumor with distinctive clinical and pathological features. *Am J Med* 38:241, 1965.

Klempnauer J, Ridder GJ, Von Wasielewski R, et al. Resectional surgery of hilar cholangiocarcinoma: A multivariate analysis of prognostic factors. *J Clin Oncol* 15:947, 1997.

Langer JC, Langer B, Taylor BR, et al. Carcinoma of the extrahepatic bile ducts: Results of an aggressive surgical approach. *Surgery* 98:752, 1985.

Livarghi T, Bolondi L, Lazzaroni S, et al. Percutaneous ethanol injection in the treatment of hepatocellular carcinoma in cirrhosis: A study of 207 patients. *Cancer* 69:925, 1992.

Llovet JM, Bruix J, Fuster J, et al. Liver transplantation for hepatocellular carcinoma. Results of a restrictive policy. *Hepatology* 24:350A, 1996.

MacIntosh EL, Minuk GY. Hepatic resection in patients with cirrhosis and hepatocellular carcinoma. *Surg Gynecol Obstet* 174:245, 1992.

Mazzaferro V, Regalia E, Doci R, et al. Liver transplantation for the treatment of small hepatocellular carcinomas in patients with cirrhosis. *N Engl J Med* 334(11):693, 1996.

McPherson DAD, Benjamin IS, Hodgson HJF, et al. Preoperative percutaneous transhepatic biliary drainage: The results of a controlled trial. *Br J Surg* 71:371, 1984.

Morrow CE, et al. Primary gallbladder carcinoma: Significance of serosal lesions and results of aggressive surgical treatment and adjuvant chemotherapy. *Surgery* 94:709, 1983.

Nagorney DM, van Heerden JA, Ilstrup DM, et al. Primary hepatic malignancy: Surgical management and determinants of survival. *Surgery* 106:740, 1989.

Nevin JE, Moran TJ, Kay S, et al. Carcinoma of the gallbladder: Staging, treatment and prognosis. *Cancer* 37:141, 1976.

Ogura Y, Mizumoto R, Tabaya M, et al. Surgical treatment of carcinoma of the hepatic duct confluence: Analysis of 55 resected carcinomas. *World J Surg* 17:85, 1993.

Onik GM, Atkinson D, Zemel R, et al. Cryosurgery of liver cancer. *Semin Surg Oncol* 9:309, 1993.

Order SE, Stillwagon GB, Klein JL, et al. Iodine-131 antiferritin, a new treatment modality in hepatoma: A radiation therapy oncology group study. *J Clin Oncol* 3:1573, 1985.

Pitt HA, Somes AS, Lois JF, et al. Does preoperative percutaneous biliary drainage reduce operative risk or increase hospital cost? *Ann Surg* 201:545, 1985.

Ravikumar TS, Kane R, Cady B, et al. A 5-year study of cryosurgery in the treatment of liver tumors. *Arch Surg* 126:1520, 1991.

Rich TA. Adjuvant therapy for primary biliary and pancreatic cancer. In JE Niederhuber (ed.), *Current Therapy in Oncology*. St. Louis: Mosby-Year Book, 1993.

Rivera JA, Rattner DW, Fernandez-del Castillo C, et al. Surgical approaches to benign and malignant tumors of the ampulla of Vater. *Surg Oncol Clin North Am* 5(3):689, 1996.

Rougier P, Laplanche A, Huguier R, et al. Hepatic arterial infusion of floxuridine in patients with liver metastases from colorectal carcinoma: Long-term results of a prospective randomized trial. *J Clin Oncol* 10:1112, 1992.

Safi F, Bittner R, Rosher R, et al. Regional chemotherapy for hepatic metastases of colorectal carcinoma (continuous intraarterial versus continuous intraarterial/intravenous therapy): Results of a controlled clinical trial. *Cancer* 64:379, 1989.

Scheele J, Stangl R, Altendorf-Hofmann A. Hepatic metastases from colorectal carcinoma: Impact of surgical resection on the natural history. *Br J Surg* 77:1241, 1990.

Shirai Y, Yoshida K, Tsukada K, et al. Inapparent carcinoma of the gallbladder: An appraisal of a radical second operation after simple cholecystectomy. *Ann Surg* 215:326, 1992.

Silk YN, Douglass HO, Nava HR, et al. Carcinoma of the gallbladder: The Roswell Park experience. *Ann Surg* 210:751, 1989.

Sitzmann JV, Abrams R. Improved survival for hepatocellular cancer with combination surgery and multimodality treatment. *Ann Surg* 217:149, 1993.

Sitzmann JV, Coleman JA, Pitt HA, et al. Preoperative assessment of malignant hepatic tumors. *Am J Surg* 159:137, 1990.

Stagg RJ, Venook AP, Chase JL, et al. Alternating hepatic intraarterial floxuridine and fluorouracil: A less toxic regimen for treatment of liver metastases from colorectal cancer. *J Natl Cancer Inst* 83:423, 1991.

Stain SC, Baer HU, Denison AR, et al. Current management of hilar cholangiocarcinoma. *Surg Gynecol Obstet* 175:579, 1992.

Steele G Jr, Bleday R, Mayer RJ, et al. A prospective evaluation of hepatic resection for colorectal carcinoma metastases to the liver: Gastrointestinal Tumor Study Group protocol 6584. *J Clin Oncol* 9:1105, 1991.

Steele G Jr, Ravikumar TS. Resection of hepatic metastases from colorectal cancer: Biologic perspectives. *Ann Surg* 210:127, 1989.

Suenaga M, Nakao A, Harada A, et al. Hepatic resection for hepatocellular carcinoma. *World J Surg* 16:97, 1992.

Tuttle TM, Curley SA, Roh MS. Repeat hepatic resection as effective treatment of recurrent colorectal liver metastases. *Ann Surg Oncol* 4(2):125, 1997.

Wagman LD, Kemeny MM, Leong L, et al. A prospective, randomized evaluation of the treatment of colorectal cancer metastatic to the liver. *J Clin Oncol* 8:1885, 1990.

Wanebo HJ, Castle WN, Fechner RE. Is carcinoma of the gallbladder a curable lesion? *Ann Surg* 195:624, 1982.

Willett CG, Warshaw AL, Convery K, Compton CC. Patterns of failure after pancreaticoduodenectomy for ampullary carcinoma. *Surg Gynecol Obstet* 176:33, 1993.

Yu YQ, Xu DB, Zhou XD, et al. Experience with liver resection after hepatic arterial chemoembolization for hepatocellular carcinoma. *Cancer* 71:62, 1993.

Zhou X, Yu Y, Tang Z, et al. An 18-year study of cryosurgery in the treatment of primary liver cancer. *Asian J Surg* 15:43, 1992.

Zhou XD, Tang ZY, Yu YQ, et al. Solitary minute hepatocellular carcinoma: A study of 14 patients. *Cancer* 67:2855, 1991.

Pancreatic Adenocarcinoma

Francis R. Spitz, Michael Bouvet,
George M. Fuhrman, and David H. Berger

Epidemiology

Pancreatic cancer is the eighth most common malignancy and the fifth leading cause of adult cancer death in the United States. In 1996, 26,300 new cases of adenocarcinoma of the pancreas were diagnosed in the United States and 27,800 patients died of this aggressive malignancy. Only 1–4% of all patients diagnosed with pancreatic cancer can expect to survive 5 years. Thus incidence rates are virtually identical to mortality rates. Over the past decade the incidence of pancreatic cancer has increased slightly.

The etiology of pancreatic adenocarcinoma and the reason for the slight decrease in incidence are uncertain. Epidemiologic studies report cigarette smoking increases the risk of developing pancreatic cancer threefold. Coffee, alcohol, organic solvents, and petroleum products have been linked epidemiologically to pancreatic cancer. However, none of these agents is conclusively causal. Diabetes mellitus and chronic pancreatitis are complications of the neoplasm and may be etiologic factors. Because high-risk groups of patients have not been well defined, there is presently only a very limited role for screening programs.

Staging

The current American Joint Committee on Cancer Staging (AJCC) staging for pancreatic cancer is listed in Table 13-1.

Clinical Presentation

The presenting signs and symptoms of patients with pancreatic cancer are shown in Table 13-2. The most common presenting symptoms are weight loss, pain, and jaundice.

Pain is initially of low intensity, visceral in origin, and poorly localized to the upper abdomen. This pain may mimic peptic ulcer disease. Severe pain localized to the lower thoracic or upper lumbar area is more characteristic of advanced disease due to invasion of the celiac and superior mesenteric plexus.

Anorexia and weight loss are common in pancreatic cancer patients. Weight loss results from malabsorption and decreased caloric intake. The sudden onset of diabetes mellitus in nonobese

Table 13-1. AJCC staging of pancreatic cancer

Tis	Carcinoma *in situ*		
T1	Tumor limited to the pancreas 2 cm or less in greatest dimension		
T2	Tumor limited to the pancreas more than 2 cm in greatest dimension		
T3	Tumor extends directly into any of the following: duodenum, bile duct, peripancreatic tissues		
T4	Tumor extends directly into any one of the following: stomach, spleen, colon, adjacent large vessels		
N0	No regional lymph node metastasis		
N1	Regional lymph node metastasis		
M0	No distant metastasis		
M1	Distant metastasis		
Stage I	T1–T2	N0	M0
Stage II	T3	N0	M0
Stage III	T1–T3	N1	M0
Stage IVA	T4	Any N	M0
Stage IVB	Any T	Any N	M1

adults older than 40 years warrants evaluation for pancreatic cancer.

Painless jaundice as the sole presenting symptom is more frequently seen with ampullary or distal bile duct tumors but can be present with adenocarcinoma of the head or uncinate process of the pancreas. Courvoisier's sign, a palpable gallbladder at presentation, is seen in less than one-third of patients.

Table 13-2. Presenting signs and symptoms of patients with carcinoma of the head of the pancreas

Sign or symptom	Percentage of patients
Weight loss	90
Pain	75
Malnutrition	75
Jaundice	70
Anorexia	60
Pruritis	40
Courvoisier's sign	33
Diabetes mellitus	15
Ascites	5
Gastric outlet obstruction	5

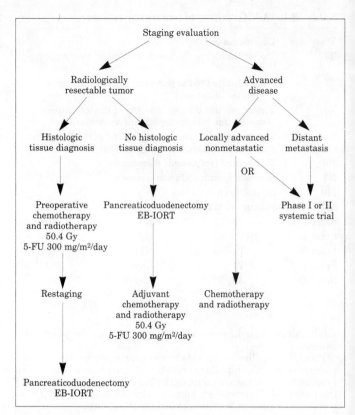

Fig. 13-1.   Algorithm for the management of pancreatic carcinoma. (EB-IORT = electron-beam intraoperative radiotherapy; 5-FU = 5-fluorouracil.)

Management

An algorithm for the current management of pancreatic adenocarcinoma at the MD Anderson Cancer Center is presented in Fig. 13-1.

PREOPERATIVE EVALUATION

Once the suspicion of pancreatic cancer is raised, radiologic confirmation should be attempted. Several large reviews of pancreatic cancer note delays in diagnosis of more than 2 months from the onset of symptoms in the majority of patients. Ultrasound should be the initial diagnostic test in the jaundiced patient to confirm extrahepatic biliary ductal dilatation and to assess the pancreatic head and liver.

Thin-section computed tomography (CT) scanning through the pancreas with an intravenous (IV) bolus injection of contrast remains the test of choice to evaluate the extent of disease and to assess tumor resectability. Local tumor resectability is most accurately assessed preoperatively. Laparotomy should be therapeutic, not diagnostic. We utilize objective, reproducible radiologic criteria to include only patients with potentially resectable disease, defined as (1) the absence of extrapancreatic disease, (2) the absence of direct tumor extension to the superior mesenteric artery (SMA) and celiac axis as defined by the presence of a fat plane between the low-density tumor and these arterial structures, and (3) a patent superior mesenteric-portal vein confluence. The accuracy of this form of radiographic staging is supported by our previous work and validated by the high resectability rate (94/118, 80%) and low rate of microscopic retroperitoneal margin positivity (17%) observed in the recent report by Spitz et al. The accuracy of CT in predicting unresectability and the inaccuracy of intraoperative assessment of resectability are both well established.

Endoscopic ultrasound with biopsy is emerging as a helpful diagnostic and staging tool. Although not frequently utilized at our institution, this technique may provide valuable information about the resectability of the tumor and its relation to the superior mesenteric vessels.

Endoscopic retrograde cholangiopancreatography (ERCP) is used to differentiate choledocholithiasis from malignant obstruction of the distal common bile duct when a mass is not seen on CT.

Angiography has been used to demonstrate encasement of the celiac or mesenteric vessels; however, this information is more accurately obtained by thin-section contrast-enhanced CT scan. Currently, the only indication for routine angiography in the work-up of these patients is to exclude the possibility of aberrant arterial anatomy. This information prevents iatrogenic arterial injury of a replaced right hepatic artery. Because a replaced right hepatic artery can be identified at laparotomy, we utilize angiography in the evaluation of patients who were operated on prior to referral in whom dissection is often more difficult.

Percutaneous CT-guided needle biopsy of pancreatic neoplasms is an effective method of obtaining cytologic confirmation of the diagnosis. Laparotomy can be avoided in patients with locally advanced unresectable disease who often require histologic diagnosis for the initiation of treatment. The possibility of shedding cancer cells into the peritoneal cavity during this procedure is theoretic. A study by Leach et al. at the M. D. Anderson Cancer Center examining peritoneal cytology demonstrated the risk of positive peritoneal cytology after percutaneous fine-needle aspiration biopsy (6%) was no greater than that when patients do not undergo percutaneous fine-needle aspiration biopsy (9%). In patients with potentially resectable disease, percutaneous needle biopsy should be considered in cases where pretreatment cytologic confirmation of the diagnosis is important, such as in patients being considered for preoperative multimodality therapy as part of a clinical trial.

Historically, preoperative biliary tract drainage was done in an attempt to lower the serum bilirubin level. It was believed that this approach would provide benefit by improving immunologic, hepatic, and renal function. However, randomized prospective trials in this country have failed to demonstrate a reduction in operative morbidity or mortality following routine preoperative biliary drainage. Currently, decompression can be recommended only as part of a clinical trial for patients with a total bilirubin level above 20 mg/dl or for patients with symptomatic jaundice who are to be treated with preoperative radiation or chemotherapy.

PATHOLOGY

Approximately 90% of pancreatic exocrine tumors arise from the pancreatic ductules, and 80% of these tumors are adenocarcinoma. Pancreatic adenocarcinomas arise in the head of the gland in 60–70% of cases. The remainder of the tumors are located in the body or tail, or diffusely throughout the pancreas.

Pancreatic adenocarcinoma grossly, on cut section, is firm and white with poorly defined margins. An associated surrounding area of pancreatitis is often present and can make pathologic diagnosis difficult. An intense desmoplastic reaction is identifiable on both gross and microscopic examination. Histologically, identification of mucin production is helpful in diagnosing an adenocarcinoma. Perineural invasion can be identified in most specimens. The degree of differentiation reported on microscopic examination is based on the degree of formation of tubular glandular structures.

SURGICAL TREATMENT

Surgical resection of carcinoma of the pancreatic head remains the only potentially curative treatment modality. Five surgical techniques are used to resect pancreatic cancer: (1) the standard pancreaticoduodenectomy, modified from Whipple's initial description in 1935; (2) pylorus-preserving pancreaticoduodenectomy; (3) total pancreatectomy; (4) regional pancreatectomy; and (5) the M. D. Anderson extended resection. The current standard of therapy for carcinoma of the head of the pancreas is either the Whipple procedure or the pylorus-preserving pancreaticoduodenectomy. Thorough abdominal exploration should precede resection. There is no role for resection of adenocarcinoma in the presence of metastatic disease. Exploration includes intraoperative inspection and palpation of the liver, peritoneal surfaces, para-aortic lymphatics, and root of the mesentery for spread of tumor.

The surgical resection is divided into the following six clearly defined steps (Fig. 13-2).

1. A Cattell-Braasch maneuver is performed by mobilizing the right colon and incising the visceral peritoneum to the ligament of Treitz. When complete, this maneuver allows cephalad retraction of the right colon and small bowel, exposing the third and fourth portions of the duodenum. Mobilization of the retroperitoneal attachments of the mesentery is of particular importance in patients who require venous resection and reconstruction. The omental bursa is entered by taking the greater omentum from the transverse colon. The middle colic vein is identified, ligated, and divided before its junction with the SMV. Routine division of the middle colic vein allows

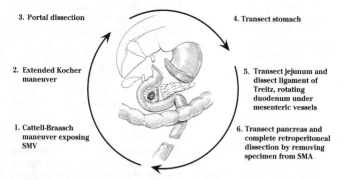

3. Portal dissection

4. Transect stomach

2. Extended Kocher maneuver

5. Transect jejunum and dissect ligament of Treitz, rotating duodenum under mesenteric vessels

1. Cattell-Braasch maneuver exposing SMV

6. Transect pancreas and complete retroperitoneal dissection by removing specimen from SMA

Fig. 13-2. Six surgical steps of pancreaticoduodenectomy (clockwise resection). (Tyler DS, Evans DB. Reoperative pancreaticoduodenectomy. *Ann Surg* 219:214, 1994.)

greater exposure of the infrapancreatic SMV and prevents iatrogenic traction injury during dissection of the middle colic vein–SMV junction.

2. The Kocher maneuver is begun at the junction of the ureter and right gonadal vein. The right gonadal vein is ligated and divided, and all fibrofatty and lymphatic tissue overlying the medial aspect of the right kidney and inferior vena cava is removed with the tumor specimen. The gonadal vein is again ligated at its entrance into the inferior vena cava. The Kocher maneuver is continued to the left lateral edge of the aorta, with careful identification of the left renal vein.

3. The portal dissection is initiated exposing the common hepatic artery proximal and distal to the gastroduodenal artery. The gastroduodenal artery is then ligated and divided. Two large lymph nodes are commonly encountered during portal dissection: one along the inferior border of the common hepatic artery, and one behind the portal vein seen after transection of the common bile duct. Removal of these lymph nodes (en bloc with the specimen) is necessary to mobilize the hepatic artery and portal vein. However, they rarely contain metastatic disease. Lymph node metastases from pancreatic cancer are commonly small and are almost always found by the pathologist rather than the surgeon. The gallbladder is dissected out of the liver bed and the common hepatic duct transected just cephalad to its junction with the cystic duct. The anterior wall of the portal vein is easily exposed following division of the common hepatic duct and medial retraction of the common hepatic artery. This connective tissue anterior to the portal vein is divided in a caudal direction to the junction of the portal vein and the neck of the pancreas. A constant venous tributary, the posterior pancreatic duodenal vein, can be located at the supralateral aspect of the portal vein. Bleeding caused by traction injury to the venous tributary may be difficult to control at the time of the operation. The portal

dissection is made more difficult in the presence of anomalous hepatic artery circulation. Rarely, the hepatic artery (distal to the origin of the gastroduodenal artery) courses posterior to the portal vein. More commonly, an accessory or replaced right hepatic artery arises from the proximal SMA and lies posterior and lateral to the portal vein. The common hepatic artery may arise from the SMA (type IX hepatic arterial anatomy). Fatal hepatic necrosis can result if this is unrecognized and the vessel is sacrificed. Identification of aberrant arterial anatomy is generally not difficult except in the reoperative portal dissections

4. The stomach is transected at the level of the third or fourth transverse vein on the lesser curvature and of the confluence of the gastroepiploic veins on the greater curvature. The omentum is divided at the level of the greater curvature transection.

5. The jejunum is transected approximately 10 cm distal to the ligament of Treitz, and its mesentery is sequentially ligated and divided. The duodenal mesentery is similarly divided to the level of the aorta; the duodenum and jejunum are then reflected beneath the mesenteric vessels.

6. After traction sutures are placed on the superior and inferior borders of the pancreas, the pancreas is transected with an electrocautery at the level of the portal vein. If there is evidence of tumor adherence to the portal vein or SMV, the pancreas can be divided at a more distal location in preparation for segmental venous resection. The specimen is separated from the SMV by ligating and dividing the small venous tributaries to the uncinate process and the pancreatic head. Complete removal of the uncinate process combined with medial retraction of the superior mesenteric–portal vein confluence facilitates exposure of the SMA, which is then dissected to its origin at the aorta. Total exposure of the SMA avoids iatrogenic injury and ensures direct ligation of the inferior pancreaticoduodenal artery.

Reconstruction proceeds in the counterclockwise direction, and again in a stepwise and orderly fashion (Fig. 13-3).

1. The pancreatic remnant is mobilized from the retroperitoneum and splenic vein for a distance of 2–3 cm. Failure to adequately mobilize the pancreatic remnant results in poor suture placement at the pancreaticojejunal anastomosis. The transected jejunum is brought through a small incision in the transverse mesocolon to the right or left of the middle colic vessels. A two-layer, end-to-side, duct-to-mucosa pancreaticojejunostomy is performed over a small Silastic stent. Following completion of the posterior row of 3-0 seromuscular sutures, a small, full-thickness opening in the bowel is made. The anastomosis between the pancreatic duct and small-bowel mucosa is completed with 4-0 or 5-0 monofilament sutures. Each stitch incorporates a generous bite of pancreatic duct and a full-thickness bite of jejunum. The posterior knots are tied on the inside, and the lateral and anterior knots are tied on the outside. Prior to the anterior sutures being tied, the stent is placed across the anastomosis so that it extends into the pancreatic duct and into the small bowel

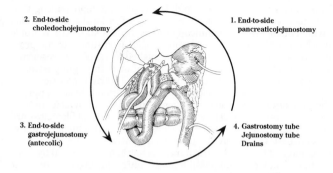

2. End-to-side
choledochojejunostomy

1. End-to-side
pancreaticojejunostomy

3. End-to-side
gastrojejunostomy
(antecolic)

4. Gastrostomy tube
Jejunostomy tube
Drains

Fig. 13-3.   Four surgical steps of counterclockwise reconstruction following standard pancreaticoduodenectomy. (Tyler DS, Evans DB. Reoperative pancreaticoduodenectomy. *Ann Surg* **219:214, 1994.)**

for a distance of approximately 2–3 cm. The anastomosis is completed with a placement of an anterior row of 3-0 seromuscular sutures. When the pancreatic duct is not dilated and/or the pancreatic substance is soft (not fibrotic), we prefer to perform a two-layer anastomosis that invaginates the cut end of the pancreas into the jejunum. The outer posterior row of 3-0 sutures is placed as outlined earlier. The bowel is then opened for its full length to the transverse diameter of the pancreatic remnant. Using a running, double-armed, 4-0 nonabsorbable monofilament suture, the pancreatic remnant is sewn to the jejunum. The anastomosis is completed with placement of an anterior row of 3-0 seromuscular sutures.

2. A single-layer biliary anastomosis is performed using interrupted, 4-0 absorbable monofilament sutures. It is important to align the jejunum with the bile duct to avoid tension on the pancreatic and biliary anastomosis. A stent is rarely used in the construction of the hepaticojejunostomy.

3. An anticolic, end-to-side gastrojejunostomy is constructed in two layers. Starting from the greater curvature, 6–8 cm of gastric staple line is removed. A posterior row of silk sutures is followed by a running, monofilament, full-thickness inner layer; the anterior row of silk sutures completes the anastomosis. The distance between the biliary and gastric anastomosis should allow the jejunum to assume its anticolic position (for the gastrojejunostomy) without tension. There is no harm in making a long (25–35 cm) afferent limb. The jejunum should be aligned so that the afferent limb is adjacent to the greater curvature of the stomach.

4. Gastrojejunostomy and feeding jejunostomy tubes are placed using the Witzel technique and then closed suction drains are placed.

The concept of pylorus-preserving pancreaticoduodenectomy was introduced by Traverso and Longmire in 1978 in an attempt to eliminate the postgastrectomy syndromes seen after antrectomy.

There are sufficient follow-up data available demonstrating that pylorus preservation does not adversely affect local control or survival. This operation technically differs from a standard Whipple procedure only in the preservation of the blood supply to the proximal duodenum. This can be accomplished by carefully preserving the right gastroepiploic arcade after ligation of the right gastroepiploic artery and vein close to their origin. The right gastric artery can be spared in some cases to provide additional blood supply to the duodenum. The most significant morbidity of pylorus preservation is transient gastric stasis. Operative time and blood loss are slightly reduced compared with classic pancreaticoduodenectomy.

Routine total pancreatectomy as definitive therapy for adenocarcinoma of the head of the pancreas has been advocated by some authors. They cite the possible multicentric nature of pancreatic cancer and the avoidance of a pancreatic anastomosis as justification for this approach. However, the incidence of pathologic documentation of multicentricity of pancreatic adenocarcinoma is less than 10% and does not justify the additional operative morbidity and life-long insulin dependence that results from total pancreatectomy. The significant operative morbidity and mortality from pancreaticoduodenectomy is historically attributed to pancreaticojejunal anastomotic leak. However, anastomotic complications are rare in centers experienced with this operation. Also, more effective management of pancreatic anastomotic leakage with hyperalimentation, percutaneous drainage, and somatostatin analog has reduced the magnitude of this problem. Total pancreatectomy is only indicated, in our opinion, if there is tumor at the pancreatic margin on serial frozen sections or if the pancreas is not suitable for an anastomosis.

Regional pancreatectomy includes an extensive retroperitoneal and hepatoduodenal lymph node dissection and sleeve resection of the SMV-portal venous confluence. Superior mesenteric and hepatic arterial resections have also been included by proponents of this more radical approach. The potential oncologic gain of regional pancreatectomy has been limited by increased morbidity and mortality.

We believe venous resection should be considered when the lesion has been deemed resectable, the pancreatic neck is divided, and, while dissecting the uncinate process from the SMV, the tumor is found to be adherent to the posterior-lateral portion of the vein. We believe vein resection is preferable to shaving the tumor from the portal-superior mesenteric venous confluence. In addition, we perform venous resection for any tumor involving the SMV–portal venous confluence as long as the vein has been demonstrated to be patent by preoperative CT. An interposition internal jugular vein graft is our preferred method of reconstruction. Unlike other recent reports, data from our institution suggest that resection of the superior mesenteric vein at the time of pancreaticoduodenectomy can be done safely, is not associated with retroperitoneal margin positivity (when high-quality preoperative imaging is performed), and does not negatively influence patient survival.

Intraoperative decision making in the surgical treatment of pancreatic cancer can challenge the most experienced surgeon. The morbidity and mortality associated with pancreaticoduodenectomy are greater than those seen after many other procedures and should be performed only by experienced surgeons. In support of this, Lieberman et al. reported the experience with pancreatico-duodenectomy in New York State from 1984 to 1991. More than 75% of patients who underwent pancreaticoduodenectomy had their operation performed at hospitals that reported less than seven of these operations per year. For patients who received their surgical care at these hospitals mean perioperative hospital stay was greater than 1 month, and the risk-adjusted perioperative mortality was 12–19%. Patients and their families must be informed preoperatively of the required complex postoperative care and potential complications of pancreaticoduodenectomy. This is most critical when there is no preoperative histologic confirmation of the diagnosis. Neoplasms of the pancreatic head can obstruct the pancreatic duct, resulting in pancreatitis, which makes definitive histologic diagnosis difficult. An intraoperative transduodenal biopsy that reveals inflammation does not exclude the possibility of malignancy. Because of this, many experienced pancreatic surgeons do not routinely perform intraoperative biopsies if malignancy is suspected. In our institution we do not routinely perform intraoperative biopsies in patients with radiographic (CT, ERCP) studies consistent with malignancy. Occasionally, a surgeon suspects that a malignancy exists but cannot establish radiologic or histologic confirmation. Every large series of pancreatic resections includes a few patients resected for benign disease. The potential morbidity of an unnecessary pancreatic resection is preferred to leaving a potentially curable lesion *in situ*. Repeated biopsy to obtain histologic confirmation of malignancy is inadvisable because of the risk of pancreatic fistula, pancreatitis, and hemorrhage. Patients should be aware of the potential need to perform a resection without histologic confirmation of malignancy.

SURGICAL RESULTS

Aggressive surgical resection of pancreatic head tumors has come under intense scrutiny, although presently, pancreatico-duodenectomy remains the only procedure capable of curing adenocarcinoma of the pancreatic head. Postoperative morbidity rates that were greater than 50% in reports from the late 1960s are now less than 25% in the most recently reported series. The most common complications are listed in Table 13-3. Postoperative mortality rates have also decreased, from a high of more than 20% in the early series to as low as 3% in the most recent reviews. Despite the improvement in morbidity and mortality, there has been little change in long-term patient survival. The 5-year survival rate following curative pancreaticoduodenectomy for carcinoma of the pancreatic head remains less than 25%, with a median survival of 20 months (Table 13-4).

Body and tail tumors are often considered to have a poorer prognosis than lesions of the pancreatic head, as these tumors frequently go undetected until they are locally advanced or metastatic. In our institution these lesions account for only 2% of the pancreatectomies performed. However, a Mayo Clinic report suggests that the rare patient with body or tail lesions amenable to resection for cure has similar long-term survival rates to patients

Table 13-3. Postoperative complications associated with pancreaticoduodenectomy

Sepsis	13%
Pancreatic fistula	10%
Biliary fistula	5%
Renal failure	13%
Gastrointestinal hemorrhage	10%
Pancreatitis	2%
Cardiac	5%
Myocardial infarction	
Congestive heart failure	
Arrhythmia	
Pulmonary	7%
Infection	
Embolus	

Table 13-4. Five-year survival, morbidity, and mortality after curative pancreaticoduodenectomy for adenocarcinoma of the pancreatic head

Author	Morbidity (%)	Mortality (%)	Survival (%)
Trede (Mannheim, Germany)	18	0	24
Cameron (Johns Hopkins)	36	2	19
Grace (UCLA)	26	2	13
Geer (Memorial Sloan-Kettering)	27	3	24

who have undergone complete resection of the more common carcinoma of the pancreatic head.

ADJUVANT THERAPY

Because the 5-year survival rate of patients with resected pancreatic cancer is poor, it is imperative to examine the potential benefit of adjuvant therapy in this disease. Autopsy series indicate that 85% of patients will experience recurrences in the field of resection. Furthermore, approximately 70% of patients will have metastasis to the liver. Therefore adjuvant therapy must address the possibility of distant disease (chemotherapy) as well as the possibility of local-regional recurrence (radiotherapy). The initial studies examining adjuvant therapy of pancreatic cancer were based on results from studies on patients with advanced disease.

Most widely used chemotherapeutic agents have limited activity against pancreatic cancer. 5-Fluorouracil (5-FU) is the only active agent, and its effect is marginal. Most studies report an overall response of 15–28% in patients with advanced disease. Studies of 5-FU have demonstrated the ability of this agent to act as a radiosensitizer—that is, to improve tumor responses to radiotherapy. Gemcitabine has demonstrated activity against pancreatic cancer. In a randomized trial of patients with advanced disease, patients treated with gemcitabine experienced a modest but statistically improved response rate and median survival and an improved quality of life compared with patients treated with 5-FU.

Combined 5-FU and radiation therapy have been reported to significantly increase survival in patients with locally advanced disease. In a study by the Gastrointestinal Tumor Study Group (GITSG) patients with unresectable pancreatic cancer were randomized to receive high-dose, postoperative radiotherapy (60 Gy) alone; high-dose, postoperative radiotherapy (60 Gy) plus concomitant 5-FU; or standard-dose, postoperative radiotherapy (40 Gy) and 5-FU. Patients receiving 5-FU and radiotherapy experienced a significant survival advantage compared with patients who received radiotherapy alone. Patients who received the higher dose of radiotherapy did not derive an additional survival advantage.

The combination of postoperative external beam radiotherapy and concomitant 5-FU as adjuvant therapy after resection was investigated by the Gastrointestinal Tumor Study Group (GITSG). Patients were randomized to receive surgery alone or surgery followed by radiotherapy (40 Gy delivered in two 20-Gy courses) and 5-FU (500 mg/m² by IV bolus delivered daily for the initial 3 days of each radiotherapy course and continued weekly for 2 years). Median survival was 20 months in the group that received adjuvant therapy; this was significantly longer than the 11-month median survival seen in patients treated with surgery alone.

In contrast to surgery in patients with adenocarcinoma of the esophagus, stomach, or colorectum, pancreaticoduodenectomy requires complete reconstruction of the upper gastrointestinal tract to include reanastomosis of the pancreas, bile duct, and stomach. The magnitude of the operation and its associated morbidity may result in a lengthy recovery period, preventing the timely delivery of postoperative therapy. In most large series approximately 25% of patients who undergo pancreaticoduodenectomy do not receive postoperative chemoradiation because of prolonged recovery.

The risk of delaying adjuvant therapy, combined with small preliminary experiences of successful pancreatic resection following external-beam radiation therapy, prompted many institutions to initiate studies in which chemoradiation was given before pancreaticoduodenectomy for patients with potentially resectable or locally advanced adenocarcinoma of the pancreas. The preoperative use of chemoradiation is supported by the following considerations:

1. Radiation therapy is more effective on well-oxygenated cells that have not been devascularized by surgery.
2. Peritoneal tumor cell implantation due to the manipulation of surgery may be prevented by preoperative chemoradiation.

3. The high frequency of positive-margin resections recently reported supports the concern that the retroperitoneal margin of excision, even when negative, may be only a few millimeters. Surgery alone may therefore be inadequate for local tumor control.

4. Patients with disseminated disease evident on restaging studies after chemoradiation will not be subjected to laparotomy and thereby spared the associated morbidity and risk of treatment-related mortality.

5. Because radiation therapy and chemotherapy are given first, delayed postoperative recovery will have no effect on the delivery of all components of the multimodality treatment, a frequent problem in postoperative adjuvant therapy studies.

Our standard-fractionation preoperative chemoradiation regimen is delivered over 5.5 weeks to a total dose of 50.4 Gy (1.8 Gy/fraction) concurrently with continuous infusion 5-FU at a dosage of 300 mg m^{-2} day^{-1}, 5 days per week, through a central venous catheter. To avoid the gastrointestinal toxicity seen with this standard 5.5-week program a rapid-fractionation program of chemoradiation was designed. Rapid-fractionation chemoradiation is delivered over 2 weeks to a total dose of 30 Gy (3 Gy/fraction) for 5 days per week. 5-FU is given concurrently by continuous infusion at a dosage of 300 mg m^{-2} day^{-1}, 5 days per week. This program is based on the principle that the total radiation dose required to obtain a given biologic effect decreases as the dose per fraction increases. Restaging with chest radiography and abdominal CT was performed 4 weeks following completion of chemoradiation. A recent review of our experience with preoperative and postoperative chemoradiation in patients who underwent potentially curative pancreaticoduodenectomy for adenocarcinoma of the pancreatic head revealed delivery of preoperative and postoperative chemoradiation resulted in similar treatment toxicity, patterns of tumor recurrence, and survival. Rapid-fractionation preoperative chemoradiation ensured the delivery of all components of therapy to all eligible patients with a significantly shorter duration of treatment than with standard-fractionation chemoradiation given either before or after pancreaticoduodenectomy. Prolonged recovery following pancreaticoduodenectomy prevents the delivery of postoperative adjuvant chemoradiation in up to one-fourth of eligible patients. Presently we are investigating the effectiveness of radiosensitizers other than 5-FU in this regimen.

Electron-beam intraoperative radiotherapy (EB-IORT) can be used to boost the radiation dose to the pancreatic bed and surrounding high-risk lymph node basins. EB-IORT for locally advanced unresectable tumors has been reported to reduce symptoms from advanced disease and to prolong survival. A National Cancer Institute–controlled prospective trial of adjuvant radiotherapy for pancreatic cancer examined the benefit of IORT (20 Gy) in addition to external beam radiotherapy (50 Gy) following resection. Although IORT did not have an impact on overall survival in this small study, patients who received IORT experienced prolonged disease-free survival and improved local control. At M. D. Anderson, complications are not increased in patients undergoing resection and EB-IORT.

The current M. D. Anderson approach to patients with resectable pancreatic cancer is preoperative chemoradiation, followed by en bloc resection of the tumor and draining lymph nodes and EB-IORT (10 Gy) to the pancreatic bed. Patients with a microscopic positive margin at the SMA origin on frozen section receive 15 Gy of EB-IORT following resection (see Fig. 13-4).

SURVEILLANCE

Patients should be seen at 3-month intervals following curative resection of pancreatic adenocarcinoma. Follow-up visits should include a thorough history and physical examination, a complete blood count, serum electrolyte determination, and liver function tests. A chest x-ray and abdominal CT should be obtained at 6- to 12-month intervals, or earlier if symptoms develop.

There have been numerous attempts to identify a tumor marker for pancreatic cancer. The most frequently measured antigens are CEA, CA 19-9, and pancreatic-oncofetal antigen (POA). Some encouraging results have been reported for using CA 19-9 to predict recurrence following resection of pancreatic adenocarcinoma.

Postoperatively, all patients receive some form of enteral nutritional supplementation via a jejunostomy tube for at least 6 weeks. Nutritional status should be carefully assessed at each clinic visit, including a serum albumin level, dietary history, and evaluation of general body habitus. Patients must also be evaluated for signs of malabsorption resulting from pancreatic enzyme insufficiency. This is readily treatable with pancreatic enzyme replacement.

PALLIATION

Patients with unresectable or recurrent pancreatic cancer frequently require palliative treatment for biliary obstruction, gastric outlet obstruction, and pain. Historically, palliation for these patients was undertaken at laparotomy after determining that a tumor was unresectable. Operative biliary bypass, gastric bypass, and splanchnicectomy are proven, effective methods of achieving palliation. However, with the advent of improved diagnostic techniques, unresectability can often be determined prior to laparotomy. Biliary diversion can then be achieved either endoscopically or percutaneously. Gastric outlet obstruction occurs in only 10–15% of patients and is often a preterminal event that does not mandate operative correction. CT-guided alcohol splanchnicectomy is an effective option in the palliation of pain for the occasional patient unresponsive to narcotics. Therefore the surgeon can avoid laparotomy in most patients with limited life expectancy.

Biliary Obstruction

Jaundice is a common presenting symptom in patients who have carcinoma of the head of the pancreas. Prolonged biliary obstruction leads to coagulopathy, hepatic dysfunction, malabsorption, and altered bile salt metabolism. Patients often complain of severe, disabling pruritis. Relief of biliary obstruction results in significant palliation of these problems and improve-

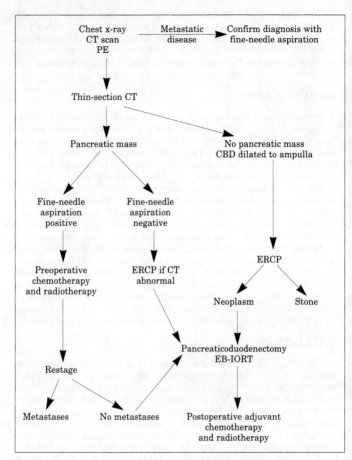

Fig. 13-4. Management of the patient with jaundice and extrahepatic ductal dilatation at M. D. Anderson. (PE = physical examination; CBD = common bile duct; ERCP = endoscopic retrograde cholangiopancreatography; EB-IORT = electron-beam intraoperative radiotherapy.)

ment in overall patient well-being. It is helpful to group pancreatic cancer patients into four separate categories when considering operative versus nonoperative biliary decompression:

1. Patients in poor health who would not tolerate laparotomy and are clearly best served by nonoperative palliative measures.
2. Patients with concomitant gastric outlet obstruction who require laparotomy for palliation of that symptom and for whom the benefit of avoiding the complications of a stent or transhepatic drain warrants the limited additional morbidity of adding an operative biliary bypass.

3. Patients undergoing operation for resection but who are found to have unsuspected unresectable disease; these patients are also best served by an operative biliary bypass.

4. Patients who have unresectable pancreatic cancer on diagnostic evaluation and are an acceptable medical risk for laparotomy; these patients are candidates for operative or nonoperative management, depending on the judgment of the surgeon and the expertise of the available endoscopist or invasive radiologist. (At M. D. Anderson these patients are successfully managed with nonoperative palliative measures.)

Surgical biliary diversion can be accomplished by either choledochoenteric or cholecystoenteric bypass. A Roux limb requires an additional anastomosis and longer operative time than a simple loop of small bowel for biliary bypass. Roux reconstruction is required when an unresectable tumor prevents a loop from reaching the right upper quadrant without tension. Most authorities advocate either loop choledochojejunostomy or cholecystojejunostomy for surgical palliation of malignant biliary obstruction. Cholecystojejunostomy has the advantage of being simple to perform; however, the possibility of recurrent biliary obstruction after this procedure also exists. The advantage of choledochojejunostomy is that it provides a more proximal biliary anastomosis and therefore obstruction by progressive extension of tumor is less likely. The high operative mortality and short median survival associated with each procedure are due to the aggressive nature of the malignancy rather than to the technique used. The choice of surgical option ultimately depends on local tumor considerations and the surgeon's experience.

Nonoperative palliative biliary decompression can be accomplished endoscopically or percutaneously. Experienced endoscopists report a success rate of more than 90%. In randomized studies comparing endoscopic biliary decompression with conventional surgical bypass, the procedures have resulted in identical survival and relief of jaundice. Total hospital stay is also similar for the two procedures because of the need for occasional readmissions to change stents after endoscopic decompression. Percutaneous transhepatic biliary drainage has provided successful palliation in 80–90% of patients. External catheters are being replaced by newer indwelling endoprostheses, which are associated with a lower rate of infectious complications. Hemobilia has been seen in up to 12% of percutaneously treated patients. Although endoscopic biliary decompression is the preferred method of nonoperative palliation, the choice of technique depends on the expertise available.

Gastric Outlet Obstruction

Patients with pancreatic cancer rarely present with duodenal obstruction. Furthermore, less than 15% of patients will require operative correction of gastric outlet obstruction prior to death. Clearly, patients with unresectable disease and gastric outlet obstruction require a gastrojejunostomy for palliation. Controversy exists as to whether all patients undergoing palliative laparotomy should undergo prophylactic gastroenterostomy. Complications resulting from the additional operative time and additional anastomosis are minimal. However, the incidence of subsequent duodenal obstruction in asymptomatic patients who undergo only biliary bypass is low. In addition, the development of gastric outlet obstruction is often a preterminal event not requiring treatment. At M. D. Anderson patients with symptoms of duodenal obstruction or operative or radiographic evidence of impending gastric outlet obstruction undergo palliative gastrojejunostomy at the time of biliary bypass.

Pancreatic Pain

Pain is the most disabling symptom of advanced pancreatic carcinoma. It occurs in most patients during the course of their disease. Sophisticated surgical neurotomies have been described but require prolonged operative time and are rarely used today.

Chemical splanchnicectomy is a much simpler approach and has been reported to provide pain relief in up to 80% of patients. This procedure can be performed surgically or percutaneously with CT guidance by injection of phenol and alcohol around the celiac axis. Limited morbidity is associated with this procedure. A randomized prospective trial of intraoperative celiac plexus alcohol injection versus placebo injection in patients with unresectable tumors is under way at The Johns Hopkins Hospital. This study should better define the role of chemical splanchnicectomy in the management of patients with pain from advanced pancreatic cancer.

Cystic Neoplasms

Cystic neoplasms of the pancreas account for approximately 1% of all pancreatic cancers and 10% of all pancreatic cystic lesions. Classically, these tumors are large, are located in the distal pancreas, and affect women three times more frequently than men. The diagnosis of a cystic neoplasm must be considered in patients with radiographic evidence of a pancreatic cyst and no prior symptoms or history of pancreatitis.

Cystic neoplasms with a cuboidal epithelial lining (serous cystadenoma) have no malignant potential. When a columnar epithelial lining is present in the cyst wall, the lesion is frankly malignant (mucinous cystadenocarcinoma) or premalignant (mucinous cystic neoplasm).

It is often impossible to distinguish malignant from benign cystic neoplasms preoperatively or intraoperatively, as the epithelial lining is often incomplete. Therefore all cystic neoplasms should be resected for potential cure. Patients with malignant cystic neoplasms who undergo complete resection have a 40–60% 5-year survival rate.

Selected References

Crist DW, Sitzman JV, Cameron JL. Improved hospital morbidity, mortality, and survival after the Whipple procedure. *Ann Surg* 206: 358, 1987.

Dalton RR, Sarr MG, van Heerden JA. Carcinoma of the body and tail of the pancreas: Is curative resection justified? *Surgery* 111:489, 1992.

Evans DB, Abbruzzese JL, Cleary KR, et al. Rapid-fractionation preoperative chemoradiation for malignant periampullary neoplasms. *J R Coll Surg Edinb* 40:319, 1995.

Evans DB, Abbruzzese JL, Rich TA. Cancer of the pancreas. In VT DeVita Jr, S Hellman, SA Rosenberg (eds.), *Cancer: Principles and Practice of Oncology* (5th ed.). Philadelphia: Lippincott, 1997.

Fortner JG. Regional pancreatectomy for cancer of the pancreas, ampulla, and other related sites. *Ann Surg* 199:418, 1984.

Foo ML, Gunderson LL, Nagorney DM, et al. Patterns of failure in grossly resected pancreatic ductal adenocarcinoma treated with adjuvant irradiation + 5 fluorouracil. *Int J Radiat Oncol Biol Phys* 26:483, 1993.

Fuhrman GM, Charnsangavej C, Abbruzzese JL, et al. Thin-section contrast-enhanced computed tomography accurately predicts the resectability of malignant pancreatic neoplasms. *Am J Surg* 167:104, 1994.

Fuhrman GM, Leach SD, Staley CA, et al. Rationale for en-bloc vein resection in the treatment of pancreatic adenocarcinoma adherent to the superior mesenteric-portal venous confluence. *Ann Surg* 223:154, 1996.

Gastrointestinal Tumor Study Group. Further evidence of effective adjuvant combined radiation and chemotherapy following curative resection of pancreatic cancer. *Cancer* 59:2006, 1987.

Geer RJ, Brennan MF. Prognostic indicators for survival after resection of pancreatic adenocarcinoma. *Am J Surg* 165:68, 1993.

Hatfield ARW, Tobias R, Terblanche J, et al. Preoperative external biliary drainage in obstructive jaundice: A prospective controlled trial. *Lancet* 2:896, 1982.

Itani KM, Coleman RE, Akwari OE, et al. Pylorus-preserving pancreaticoduodenectomy: A clinical and physiologic appraisal. *Ann Surg* 204:655, 1986.

Leach SD, Rose JA, Lowy AM, et al. Significance of peritoneal cytology in patients with potentially resectable adenocarcinoma of the pancreatic head. *Surgery* 118:472, 1995.

Lieberman MD, Kilburn H, Lindsey M, et al. Relation of perioperative deaths to hospital volume among patients undergoing pancreatic resection for malignancy. *Ann Surg* 222:638, 1995.

Lillemoe KD, Sauter PK, Pitt HA, et al. Current status of surgical palliation of periampullary carcinoma. *Surg Gynecol Obstet* 176:1, 1993.

Moertel CG, Frytak S, Hahn RG, et al. Therapy of locally unresectable pancreatic carcinoma: A randomized comparison of high dose (6000 rads) radiation alone, moderate dose radiation and 5-fluorouracil. *Cancer* 48:1705, 1981.

Moossa AR, Scott MH, Lavelle-Jones M. The place of total and extended total pancreatectomy in pancreatic cancer. *World J Surg* 8:895, 1984.

Moore M, Anderson J, Burris HA III, et al. A randomized trial of gemcitabine versus 5-FU as first-line therapy in advanced pancreatic cancer. *Proc Am Soc Clin Oncol* 14:198, 1995.

Shepherd HA, Royle G, Ross APR. Endoscopic biliary endoprosthesis in the palliation of malignant obstruction of the distal common bile duct: A randomized trial. *Br J Surg* 75:1166, 1988.

Sindelar WF, Kinsella TJ. Randomized trial of intraoperative radiotherapy in resected carcinoma of the pancreas. *Radiat Oncol Biol Physiol* 12:148, 1986.

Spitz FR. Abbruzzese JL, Lee JE, et al. Preoperative and postoperative chemoradiation strategies in patients treated with pancreaticoduodenectomy for adenocarcinoma of the pancreas. *J Clin Oncol* 15:928, 1997.

Warshaw AL, Compton CC, Lewandrowski K, et al. Cystic tumors of the pancreas. *Ann Surg* 212:432, 1990.

Warshaw AL, Swanson RS. Pancreatic cancer in 1988. *Ann Surg* 208:541, 1988.

Yeo CJ, Cameron JL, Lillemoe KD, et al. Pancreaticoduodenectomy for cancer of the head of the pancreas: 201 patients. *Ann Surg* 221:721, 1995.

Pancreatic Endocrine Tumors and Multiple Endocrine Neoplasia

Richard J. Bold, Jeffrey J. Sussman, and Douglas S. Tyler

Overview

Pancreatic endocrine tumors are relatively rare, with an incidence of approximately 1 per 100,000 patients, although some autopsy series have demonstrated a higher incidence. Most of these tumors are functional, and patients present with symptoms attributable to excesses of pancreatic endocrine hormones. The tumors tend to arise in the islet cells of the pancreas but can also be located in the small bowel, especially the duodenum, and the adrenal glands. Although the islet cells are thought to be of neural crest origin, more recent studies suggest they may be of endodermal origin.

Islet cell tumors are usually divided into tumors that are functioning and those that are nonfunctioning. More than 75% of the islet cell tumors diagnosed clinically are functioning and frequently secrete more than one hormone. The tumors are categorized by the major hormone producing the clinical syndrome. The hormones may include gastrin, insulin, glucagon, somatostatin, neurotensin, pancreatic polypeptide (PP), vasoactive intestinal peptide (VIP), and growth hormone–releasing factor (GRF). The tumors are considered entopic if they produce hormones or peptides usually found within the pancreas (e.g., insulinomas, glucagonomas, somatostatinomas, and PPomas) or ectopic if the hormones or peptides are not native to the normal pancreas (e.g., gastrinomas, VIPomas, GRFomas, and neurotensinomas). An overview of the characteristics of pancreatic endocrine tumors is shown in Table 14-1.

The diagnosis of pancreatic endocrine tumors is usually made by the recognition of the clinical syndrome caused by excess hormone production. However, PPomas and nonfunctioning islet cell tumors do not secrete clinically apparent hormones and hence are diagnosed as a result of mass-effect symptoms or on routine computed tomography (CT) scans of the abdomen. Histologic diagnosis of the islet cell tumor can be obtained with CT-guided fine-needle aspiration, although this is often not required, given the syndrome of pancreatic hormonal excess and a localizing study, such as a CT scan. (See Table 14-2 for the distribution of these tumors within the pancreas.) In general, pancreatic endocrine tumors are more indolent than ductal adenocarcinoma and carry a better prognosis; even patients with hepatic metastasis may have a mean survival of approximately 5 years.

Table 14-1. Characteristics of pancreatic endocrine neoplasms

Tumor name	Hormone secreted	Pancreatic cell type	Clinical syndrome	Malignant (%)	Association with MEN-I
Gastrinoma	Gastrin	D	Peptic ulcers Diarrhea	60–90	25%
Insulinoma	Insulin	B	Hypoglycemia	10–15	10%
VIPoma	Vasoactive intestinal peptide	H	Watery diarrhea Hypokalemia	60–80	Rare
Glucagonoma	Glucagon	A	Hyperglycemia Dermatitis	60–70	Rare
PPoma	Pancreatic polypeptide	PP	None	>60	Occasional
Somatostatinoma	Somatostatin	D	Hyperglycemia Steatorrhea Gallstones	90	Never
Nonfunctioning	None		None	>60	

MEN-I = multiple endocrineoplasia syndrome type.

Table 14-2. Anatomic distribution of pancreatic endocrine tumors within the pancreas (head, body, and tail) as well as the extrapancreatic tissue, including the duodenum

	Head (%)	Body (%)	Tail (%)	Extrapancreatic/ duodenal (%)
Gastrinoma	30	12	14	44
Insulinoma	25	41	33	1
Glucagonoma	23	37	40	0
PP-secreting tumor	52	14	14	20
Somatostatinoma	62	4	12	22

Adapted from Howard et al., 1990. (See references.)

Gastrinoma: Zollinger-Ellison Syndrome

In 1955, Zollinger and Ellison described a syndrome characterized by the triad of severe, atypical peptic ulceration; gastric hypersecretion and hyperacidity; and a non–insulin-producing islet cell tumor of the pancreas. They theorized that a humoral factor arising from the tumor was responsible for the syndrome. Several years later, the hormone gastrin was discovered and found to be the underlying cause of the peptic hyperacidity and the term *Zollinger-Ellison syndrome* was applied to these pancreatic tumors.

EPIDEMIOLOGY

Less than 0.1% of patients with duodenal ulcer disease and about 2% of patients with recurrent ulcers after appropriate medical therapy are found to have a gastrinoma. Approximately 75% of gastrinomas occur sporadically; the remaining 25% are associated with the multiple endocrine neoplasia type I syndrome (MEN-I). The mean age at onset of symptoms is 60 years, and about 60% of those diagnosed with Zollinger-Ellison syndrome are male. Gastrinomas that occur as part of MEN-I are more often benign, multicentric, and extrapancreatic, and occur at an earlier age than sporadic gastrinomas. Of patients with MEN-I syndrome, more than half of the pancreatic tumors are gastrinomas.

CLINICAL PRESENTATION

High levels of gastrin stimulate the parietal cells within the stomach to secrete excess acid in an unregulated state. This leads to the severe ulcer disease as well as to injury to the small-bowel mucosa well past the ligament of Treitz, resulting in various degrees of malabsorption. Profuse watery diarrhea occurs in up to 50% of patients because of the combination of acid hypersecretion and small-bowel mucosal injury. In addition to secreting gastrin, the majority of gastrinomas secrete at least one other peptide hormone, such as insulin, PP, or glucagon.

The clinical manifestations of gastrinomas are related predominantly to the elevated levels of gastrin. Ninety percent of patients have endoscopically documented ulcerations of the upper gastrointestinal (GI) tract. Most of these ulcers are accompanied by abdominal pain, with bleeding occurring in 30–50% and perforation occurring in 5–10%. As many as 50% will have secretory diarrhea, with 20% having it as their only manifestation of the syndrome. Patients with Zollinger-Ellison syndrome are often initially misdiagnosed, as shown by the fact that the mean duration of symptoms before diagnosis is more than 6 years. Clinical situations in which Zollinger-Ellison syndrome should be suspected are listed in Table 14-3.

BIOCHEMICAL DIAGNOSIS

The diagnosis of gastrinoma requires confirmation with laboratory studies. A fasting serum gastrin measurement is the first test obtained. A level of more than 1,000 pg/ml is usually diagnostic of a gastrinoma and is seen in about 30% of patients. Most patients with gastrinomas have fasting gastrin levels in the 200–1,000 pg/ml range (normal is 100–200 pg/ml). Typically, patients with gastrinomas have a basal acid output of more than 15 mEq/hour or greater than 5 mEq/hour if they have had a previous ulcer operation aimed at reducing gastric acid secretion. A basal acid output/maximal acid output ratio greater than 0.6 also helps support the diagnosis of gastrinoma.

Table 14-3. Clinical situations in which the patient should be suspected of having a gastrinoma and further screening evaluation may be warranted

Recurrent peptic ulcers

Failure of peptic ulcer to heal on medical therapy

Postoperative peptic ulcer (not gastritis)

Postbulbar or jejunal peptic ulcer

Multiple upper gastrointestinal ulcers

Family history of peptic ulcer disease

Peptic ulcer occurring with diarrhea

Diarrhea that persists without a clear etiology

Family history of known MEN-I, pancreatic islet cell tumor, pituitary adenoma, or hypercalcemia

Presence of peptic ulcers and history of parathyroid disease or pituitary tumor

Prominent gastric rugal folds (hyperplasia of fundus mucosa) associated with peptic ulcer disease

Recurrent peptic ulcers following an adequate acid-reducing operation

Provocative testing using the secretin stimulation test helps confirm the diagnosis in patients with borderline gastrin elevation and gastric acid secretion. After an overnight fast, the patient is given 2 units of secretin per kilogram of body weight IV. Serum gastrin levels are measured at 0, 2, 5, 10, and 20 minutes following injection. An increase in the serum level of gastrin by more than 200 pg/ml over baseline levels is diagnostic of gastrinoma. Patients with either antral G-cell hyperplasia or hypertrophy do not respond to secretin.

TUMOR LOCALIZATION

Tumor localization has become increasingly important in recent years with the demonstration that resection of gastrinomas is associated with an excellent prognosis and is frequently curative. A number of tests have been used for the localization of gastrinomas preoperatively, including CT scans, magnetic resonance imaging (MRI), octreotide scintigraphy, transabdominal ultrasound, selective visceral angiography, selective venous sampling of portal venous tributaries, intra-arterial secretin with hepatic venous sampling for gastrin, endoscopy, endoscopic ultrasound, and intraoperative ultrasound. CT scanning with thin sections and IV bolus contrast is usually the initial imaging study of choice, as it has the highest overall sensitivity (50%) and specificity (95%) in localizing primary gastrinomas and is approximately equal to MRI scanning in identifying metastatic gastrinoma. If the location of the tumor is still in question after CT, visceral angiography should be performed. Studies suggest that the sensitivity and specificity of visceral angiography are close to if not better than those with CT scanning. Both of these studies are good at excluding metastatic disease. Endoscopy rarely identifies gastrinomas, although endoscopic ultrasound holds some promise.

Because most gastrinomas are found in the gastrinoma triangle (an anatomic area bound by the neck of the pancreas medially, the junction of the second and third portion of the duodenum inferiorly, and the junction of the cystic duct and common bile duct superiorly), many surgeons think additional invasive testing does not add significantly to the findings of a high-quality CT scan and upper endoscopy with endoscopic ultrasound. Selective angiography or venous sampling provides little additional information, although in the hands of an experienced radiologist these tests can localize gastrinomas about 90% of the time. Another localizing study is the intra-arterial secretin test with hepatic venous sampling for gastrin. This test can be easily performed during the patient's localizing arteriogram. Finally, there is some evidence that octreotide scintigraphy may be useful in localization as well as staging, given that most pancreatic endocrine tumors possess high-affinity receptors for somatostatin.

Up to 50% of patients will undergo operative exploration without successful preoperative localization. However, the combined use of an extensive Kocher maneuver for bimanual palpation of the pancreatic head, intraoperative endoscopy with duodenal transillumination, intraoperative ultrasonography, and duodenotomy has allowed for identification of nearly all gastrinomas (including fairly small tumors) and essentially the elimination of the nonproductive laparotomy.

TREATMENT

Once the diagnosis of gastrinoma is made, the first step is to control the gastric acid hypersecretion. Total gastrectomy warrants only a historical note, as effective medical treatment is now readily available, whereas in the past, total gastrectomy served as the only modality to eliminate the sequelae of gastric hypersecretion. H_2-blockers initially control acid secretion in most patients with gastrinomas, but over time most of these individuals require increasing dosages. In addition, up to 65% of patients, depending on the series, will fail to respond to this form of medical therapy. On the other hand, omeprazole, a gastric proton pump inhibitor, is associated with a lower failure rate (0–7.5%) and a more convenient dosing schedule. As more experience is gained with omeprazole, it is becoming increasingly the drug of first choice. Octreotide acetate, the somatostatin analog, may also be useful in decreasing the release of gastrin and other peptide hormones from gastrinomas.

In a patient with a sporadic gastrinoma, surgical exploration with attempted curative resection should follow localization studies regardless of whether the tumor is identified preoperatively. Because as many as 10–40% of tumors may not be localized prior to surgery, a standardized approach to exploration needs to be undertaken. The exploration should be done through a bilateral subcostal incision and the abdomen completely explored for evidence of metastasis, especially the regional lymph nodes and the liver, as up to 50% of gastrinomas are malignant. A complete mobilization of the pancreas is essential to allow inspection and palpation of the gland. Any lymph node or suspicious mass should be evaluated by frozen-section examination, as it is unclear whether surgical resection in the presence of metastasis prolongs survival or alleviates medical management of gastric hypersecretion. Some groups do recommend aggressive debulking of all tumor deposits if they are unresectable, as survival may be improved and medical management of the acid disease may be better controlled. Intraoperative ultrasound may be helpful in identifying intrapancreatic lesions. Intraoperative endoscopy with transillumination of the duodenal wall may be done to identify duodenal gastrinomas. If no tumor is identified, a longitudinal duodenotomy should be made in the second portion of the duodenum. Careful bimanual examination of the bowel wall, along with its eversion, helps identify duodenal gastrinomas, which are frequently located submucosally. When the tumor is small (<2 cm), duodenal gastrinomas can be resected with a small margin of normal tissue, whereas pancreatic gastrinomas are usually enucleated. Larger tumors usually require some form of pancreatic resection such as a pancreaticoduodenectomy or distal pancreatectomy.

Despite extensive preoperative localizing studies and careful surgical exploration, the tumor of some patients cannot be identified at laparotomy. "Blind" pancreatic head resection is controversial. Patients with Zollinger-Ellison syndrome in whom no tumor is found have an excellent prognosis, with 5- and 10-year survival rates of more than 94% and 87%, respectively. If gastric hypersecretion is a problem despite maximal medical management, consideration may be given to performing a highly selective vagotomy. Total gastrectomy should be considered in patients who have had previous life-threatening complications from their ulcer disease despite appropriate medical management.

The role of surgery in patients with Zollinger-Ellison syndrome and MEN-I is more controversial. Resection of gastrinomas in patients with MEN-I rarely results in normal serum gastrin levels, suggesting that the probability of curing these patients with surgery is extremely low. As a result, many authorities have recommended that patients with MEN-I and gastrinomas do not undergo exploration. Other groups feel that resection of localized tumors may help reduce the risk of distant metastatic disease; therefore they recommend that patients with MEN-I undergo exploration.

METASTATIC DISEASE

Now that medical treatment of gastric acid hypersecretion in Zollinger-Ellison syndrome is so effective, patients rarely die from complications related to peptic ulcer disease. As a result, they live longer, only to die from metastatic disease. The larger series of gastrinoma patients report a 50–90% incidence of metastatic disease. Chemotherapy rarely results in cure, though some regimens have reasonable rates of response. The most promising regimen appears to be a combination of streptozocin and 5-fluorouracil, with or without doxorubicin; this combination gives response rates of 50–70%. The somatostatin analogs appear effective in controlling symptoms of gastrinomas but show a disappointing objective tumor response rate of 10–20%. Interferon has also been used and has shown some early promising results in patients refractory to chemotherapy.

Patients with isolated liver metastases have been treated with hepatic artery embolization, which may help decrease the size of these usually well-vascularized tumors. The role of local treatments for metastatic disease has been questioned in view of the finding that 12% of patients with liver metastases also have bone metastases. Tumor-debulking surgery has been advocated by some as a method of prolonging life expectancy; however, those in whom gross tumor is left behind do not benefit from debulking.

Insulinoma

EPIDEMIOLOGY

In most series, insulinomas are the most common islet cell tumors of the pancreas, with a reported incidence of 0.8–0.9 cases per 1 million people per year. These tumors occur slightly more often in women than in men. The average age at presentation is between 40 and 50 years. These tumors are almost always benign and overwhelmingly small, solitary lesions within the pancreas unless associated with MEN-I, when they tend to occur in a multicentric fashion.

CLINICAL PRESENTATION

The original diagnostic criteria for an insulinoma are known as Whipple's triad and were proposed by Whipple, who initially described the syndrome. This triad consists of (1) symptoms of hypoglycemia at fasting, (2) documentation of blood glucose levels less than 50 mg/dl, and (3) relief of symptoms following administration of glucose. However, Whipple's triad has proven not to be very specific. The clinical symptoms of insulinomas are due to the hypoglycemia induced by excess insulin secretion. A list of the common symptoms and their frequency is shown in Table 14-4. GI symptoms, including hunger, nausea, weight gain, and vomiting, are also reported occasionally.

BIOCHEMICAL DIAGNOSIS

The most reliable method of diagnosing an insulinoma is the provocative test of fasting. Blood glucose and insulin levels are measured every 4–6 hours during the fast. Eighty percent of patients with insulinoma become symptomatic within 24 hours of starting the fast, and almost all are symptomatic if the fast is continued for 72 hours. The presence of an elevated insulin level higher than 6 mU/ml along with concurrent hypoglycemia and an insulin–glucose ratio of more than 0.3 confirm the diagnosis. Measurement of the beta-cell products C-peptide and proinsulin is important because they both are usually elevated in patients with insulinoma. Patients who are surreptitiously administering insulin to themselves usually have low levels of C-peptide and proinsulin. Patients taking oral hypoglycemics have normal or elevated levels of C-peptide and proinsulin, so differentiation from an insulinoma is made by measurement of plasma levels of sulfonylureas.

TUMOR LOCALIZATION

Most insulinomas are small (<2 cm in diameter), and only about 10% of insulinomas are multicentric. There are no histo-

Table 14-4. **Symptoms associated with an insulinoma and their respective frequency**

Symptoms	Frequency (%)
Neuroglycopenic symptoms	
Visual disturbances	59
Confusion	51
Altered consciousness	38
Weakness	32
Seizures	23
Symptoms related to hypoglycemic catecholamine release	
Sweating	43
Tremulousness	23
Tachycardia	23

logic criteria of malignancy for insulinomas; therefore the diagnosis of a malignant tumor is based on the demonstration of metastatic disease, which is noted in 10% of cases. Much of the discussion of tumor localization for gastrinoma holds true for insulinoma and other pancreatic endocrine neoplasms; therefore the subsequent discussions will be limited, with only specific reference to yield of particular studies or additional modalities of localization. Dynamic CT scanning is usually the first localizing study done, because it can detect about two-thirds of the primary tumors and most metastatic lesions. When no tumor is seen with the CT scan, visceral angiography with digital subtraction techniques is successful in visualizing lesions about 60–90% of the time. Selective portal venous sampling is reserved mainly for patients whose tumors cannot be visualized with CT or angiography. Portal venous sampling is able to define the general area of the tumor in 90% of patients overall and about 75% of patients in whom other localizing tests are negative.

TREATMENT

At exploration, the pancreas must be completely mobilized as described previously for intrapancreatic gastrinomas. Small insulinomas located away from the main pancreatic duct can be enucleated. Small lesions in close proximity to the main pancreatic duct can be enucleated, but this requires intraoperative ultrasound to avoid injury to the duct. Distal pancreatectomy is recommended for small lesions near the pancreatic duct to minimize the risk of a pancreatic fistula. Large lesions in the head of the pancreas may require pancreaticoduodenectomy, whereas those in the body and tail can be treated with a distal pancreatectomy. Intraoperative ultrasound is useful to identify those tumors that could not be localized preoperatively using standard imaging techniques. Insulinomas are identified about 95% of the time at initial exploration. As with gastrinomas, blind resection of the pancreas is not recommended when no tumor is identified. If no tumor is identified, then pancreatic biopsy is recommended to rule out beta-cell hyperplasia, a condition that can be treated by subtotal pancreatectomy.

METASTATIC DISEASE

Patients with malignant metastatic disease should be considered for resection of the primary tumor and accessible metastatic lesions. Approximately 65% of patients with malignant tumors will have recurrences at a mean of about 2.8 years. Median disease-free survival is approximately 5 years in patients with malignant insulinoma who undergo curative resection. Although the chances for cure after resection are low in patients with malignant insulinoma, tumor debulking may improve control of hypoglycemic symptoms.

Palliation can be achieved with medical therapy as well as surgery. Diazoxide can control the endocrine symptoms of insulinomas in 50–70% of patients by inhibiting the release of insulin. Octreotide controls symptoms in 40–60% of patients. Of the chemotherapeutic agents used for patients with metastatic disease, streptozocin, dacarbazine, and doxorubicin have the best response rates.

VIPoma

EPIDEMIOLOGY

Although not a normal product of pancreatic islet cells, vasoactive intestinal peptide (VIP) can be secreted by islet cell tumors. The syndrome of excessive VIP secretion is associated with watery diarrhea, hypokalemia, and either hypochlorhydria or achlorhydria. First described in association with islet cell tumors in 1958, the syndrome has many names, including Verner-Morrison syndrome, pancreatic cholera, and WDHA (watery diarrhea, hypokalemia, and achlorhydria). Subsequently, it has been realized that only 80% of so-called VIPomas are located in the pancreas. Ten percent of the tumors are located elsewhere (retroperitoneum, lung, or esophagus), and 10% of the cases are due to islet cell hyperplasia. To date, only about 200 well-documented cases of VIPoma have been described, and in most cases the tumor is malignant.

CLINICAL PRESENTATION/TUMOR LOCALIZATION

Patients usually present with excessive secretory diarrhea that is aggravated by oral food intake and averages 3 liters per day. The patients become hypokalemic secondary to fecal potassium loss. The presence of a VIPoma is confirmed by demonstrating an elevated serum VIP level (>200 pg/ml) in the setting of secretory diarrhea. Pancreatic VIPomas are usually solitary, are greater than 3 cm in diameter, and most often are located in the tail of the pancreas. Diarrhea is such a nonspecific symptom that the evaluation should focus on eliminating more common causes (i.e., infectious, inflammatory, mechanical, etc.) first before proceeding to serum VIP levels or localization studies. Preoperative localization should include chest and abdominal CT scans followed by mesenteric arteriography if the tumor location is still in question.

TREATMENT

Surgical excision remains the only effective method of cure. Preoperative preparation should include adequate rehydration and correction of electrolyte imbalances. Control of the diarrhea preoperatively may be accomplished by the administration of steroids, indomethacin, or more effectively, octreotide. At exploration, most tumors are located in the distal pancreas and are amenable to a complete resection by a distal pancreatectomy. A careful evaluation of both adrenals is mandatory if no tumor is found in the pancreas. About 50% of the time, metastatic disease is found outside the pancreas at exploration. If curative resection is not possible, then surgical debulking is often indicated to help ease the clinical symptoms.

Streptozocin and interferon are currently the most active chemotherapeutic agents for advanced disease. Octreotide is useful for symptomatic relief from diarrhea in patients with metastatic disease.

Glucagonoma

Glucagonomas arise from the A cells in the pancreatic islets of Langerhans. The syndrome caused by this tumor is due to excess secretion of glucagon. In contrast to other pancreatic endocrine tumors, glucagonomas are frequently fairly large at diagnosis (>5 cm) and are rarely found outside the pancreas. Approximately 70% of these tumors are malignant.

CLINICAL PRESENTATION/DIAGNOSIS

Patients with glucagonoma usually present with mild diabetes that rarely requires insulin administration and a severe dermatitis called *necrolytic migratory erythema*. The skin rash is most often located on the lower abdomen, perineum, perioral area, and/or feet. Other symptoms often seen with this syndrome include malnutrition, anemia, weight loss, glossitis, and venous thrombosis.

The diagnosis is confirmed by documenting the presence of an elevated fasting serum glucagon level, almost always greater than 500 pg/ml (normal is 0–150 pg/ml). In addition, the diagnosis can be confirmed by the characteristic findings on biopsy of the skin rash.

TUMOR LOCALIZATION

CT scanning is the first localization study. Most tumors are large at the time of diagnosis, ranging from 5 to 10 cm, and occur most often in the body and tail of the pancreas. Given the large size of these lesions, additional localization studies are rarely needed, although angiography and portal venous sampling may be required for glucagonomas that are difficult to identify.

TREATMENT

Surgical exploration should be undertaken in any patient whose tumor is thought to be resectable. Sixty-eight percent of patients will have metastatic disease diagnosed by preoperative studies or at the time of exploration. Patients who are symptomatic due to metastatic disease frequently benefit from surgical resection. Patients with widely metastatic disease in whom surgical debulking is impossible can often benefit from medical therapy. Octreotide has been successful in controlling the diabetes and dermatitis in 60–90% of patients. Dacarbazine and streptozocin have had some success in treating unresectable or recurrent glucagonomas.

Somatostatinoma

Somatostatinomas arise from the D cells of the islets of Langerhans and are among the rarest endocrine neoplasms, with an estimated yearly incidence of one in 40 million. The syndrome associated with these tumors is marked by hyperglycemia, cholelithiasis, steatorrhea, and diarrhea. Early diagnosis is difficult because symptoms are frequently nonspecific. Most of these lesions are located in the head of the pancreas. More than 90% of the lesions are malignant, and metastatic disease is found in most cases. Patients taken to surgery for attempted curative resection should also have a cholecystectomy performed because of the high incidence of cholelithiasis.

Miscellaneous Functioning Tumors

Many islet cell tumors previously thought to be nonfunctioning have been found to secrete PP. Because this substance can now be measured, these tumors are referred to as *PPomas*. (Interestingly, 25–75% of all functioning pancreatic endocrine tumors secrete PP.) When an elevated level of PP is detected in conjunction with a pancreatic mass, the diagnosis of PPoma is made by excluding the possibility of other functioning islet cell tumors. The excess secretion of PP is not associated with any clearly defined clinical syndrome; thus these tumors are usually large at the time of diagnosis, presenting with symptoms related to local growth. Surgical excision is the treatment of choice for resectable tumors. PPomas are usually located in the head of the pancreas and are almost always malignant. Sixty percent are metastatic at the time of diagnosis. The 5-year overall survival rate is 44%.

Growth hormone-releasing factor (GRF) is another hormone that has recently been identified as a tumor product. Referred to as *GRFomas*, tumors that secrete GRF are located in the pancreas 30% of the time, lung 55% of the time, and intestine 15% of the time. About 30% of the lesions are malignant. Patients usually present with acromegaly, but these tumors also may secrete other products. Forty percent of patients have Zollinger-Ellison syndrome, and 40% have Cushing's syndrome. Although octreotide can significantly suppress the levels of circulating growth hormone in this syndrome, surgical excision, if possible, is the treatment of choice.

Other uncommon islet cell tumors include those that secrete neurotensin, adrenocorticotropic hormone (ACTH), or a parathyroid hormone (PTH)-like peptide.

Carcinoid

The classic carcinoid tumor of the pancreas is extremely rare, although anecdotal cases have been reported. Pancreatic carcinoids are grouped with foregut carcinoids and, as such, usually have normal serum levels of serotonin but commonly elevated urinary levels of 5-HIAA. Furthermore, the typical carcinoid syndrome is uncommon, even in the face of distant metastases. Therefore these tumors present due to mass-effect symptoms such as epigastric pain, weight loss, or jaundice from common bile duct compression. Localization has traditionally been by CT scan, as most of these tumors are several centimeters at the time of diagnosis, although octreotide scanning has shown promise as a method to diagnose and follow these patients after resection. Generally, carcinoid tumors grow slowly and invade adjacent organs late in the course of the disease, making resection possible in most patients. Unfortunately, almost 70% of patients have distant metastases at the time of diagnosis, preventing long-term survival. However, in the absence of distant metastases, complete resection of the primary offers excellent results for long-term survival.

Nonfunctioning Tumors

Approximately one-quarter of pancreatic islet tumors are found to be nonfunctioning in that they do not secrete any detectable levels of hormones. Instead of a well-defined clinical syndrome, the presentation of these tumors is similar to that of pancreatic ductal adenocarcinoma. Common symptoms include abdominal pain, weight loss, and jaundice. Most of these tumors are found in the head of the pancreas, and most are malignant. Diagnosis can be made by CT-guided fine-needle aspiration as well as by the characteristic hypervascular appearance on arteriography. Following localization studies, operative exploration for attempted curative resection is indicated. The prognosis for patients with nonfunctioning islet cell tumors is significantly better than that for those with pancreatic ductal adenocarcinoma, with the overall 5-year survival rate in the former group approaching 50%. Chemotherapy with streptozocin and 5-fluorouracil has shown some favorable responses.

Multiple Endocrine Neoplasia

OVERVIEW

There are currently three well-defined MEN syndromes (MEN-I, MEN-IIa, and MEN-IIb), characterized by a familial predisposition to develop tumors in various endocrine glands either metachronously or synchronously. An overview of the three syndromes is given in Table 14-5. Recently, specific genetic mutations have been identified as the likely causal event associated with the development of these syndromes. MEN-I has been mapped by linkage to chromosome 11q13, although the exact gene has yet to be determined. The gene involved in the development of MEN-II has been shown to be the receptor tyrosine kinase RET oncogene.

MEN-I

MEN-I, also known as Wermer's syndrome, is characterized by the development of parathyroid hyperplasia, pituitary tumors, and pancreatic islet cell tumors. Adenomas of the adrenal gland and thyroid can also occur. MEN-I is inherited in an autosomal dominant pattern, with nearly 100% penetrance, but there is

Table 14-5.   Features of multiple endocrine neoplasia sydromes (MEN) and the associated tumors (approximate incidence of tumor with each syndrome)

	MEN-I	MEN-IIa	MEN-IIb
Acronym	Wermer's syndrome	Sipple's syndrome	None
Genetic mutation	Chromosome 11q13	RET oncogene	RET oncogene
Tumors	Parathyroid (90%)	MTC (100%)	MTC (100%)
	Pancreas (80%)	Pheo (20–40%)	Pheo (20–40%)
	Pituitary adenoma (55%)	Parathyroid (20–60%)	Neuromas
	Adrenal adenomas (30%)		Skeletal deformities
	Thyroid nodules (10%)		

MTC = medullary thyroid carcinoma. Pheo = pheochromocytoma.

significant variability in the degree of gene expression. The clinical manifestations of the syndrome usually develop in the third or fourth decade and can vary significantly, depending on the endocrine tissue involved and the hormones produced. Thirty percent of patients with MEN-I develop adrenal tumors. Therefore prior to surgical resection of endocrine tumors, all MEN-I patients need to be screened by measuring urinary excretion of glucocorticoids, mineralocorticoids, catecholamines, vanillylmandelic acid, metanephrines, and sex hormones.

Hyperparathyroidism

Hyperparathyroidism is the most common endocrine abnormality seen in MEN-I and is usually the first to develop. Almost all patients develop hyperparathyroidism secondary to four-gland hyperplasia. The clinical presentation is similar to that seen in sporadic hyperparathyroidism, with most patients being asymptomatic. The diagnosis is made by measuring the serum calcium, phosphate, and PTH levels. Because there is a 15% incidence of thyroid neoplasms in patients with MEN-I, the thyroid needs to be examined carefully at the time of neck exploration as well as followed closely postoperatively.

There is some controversy over the appropriate surgical procedure in these patients. Many surgeons perform a three-and-one-half gland parathyroidectomy. With this technique, there is a 40–50% incidence of persistent or recurrent hyperparathyroidism, as well as a 25% incidence of hypoparathyroidism. Our preferred technique is to perform a four-gland excision and autotransplant pieces of the least hyperplastic gland into the brachioradialis muscle in the forearm. With this technique, the incidence of hypoparathyroidism is only about 5%. Although roughly 50% of patients develop graft-dependent hyperparathyroidism, it can be effectively managed by removing several pieces of parathyroid tissue from the forearm under local anesthesia, thus saving the patients a neck reexploration. In general, hyperparathyroidism associated with MEN-IIa is much easier to control and is associated with a less frequent recurrence rate after surgery when compared with MEN-I.

Pancreatic Tumors

The second most common neoplasms associated with MEN-I are the pancreatic islet cell tumors, which occur in approximately 60% of MEN-I patients. The clinical syndrome associated with these tumors results from the hormone secreted by them. The most common islet cell tumors are gastrinomas, followed by insulinomas. Rarely, glucagonomas, VIPomas, and somatostatinomas are found. MEN-I-associated pancreatic endocrine tumors are multifocal and may be located outside the pancreas, as is often the case with gastrinomas. The treatment of these tumors has been discussed in previous sections. Surgical correction of primary hyperparathyroidism should be performed first, because this may help decrease calcium-induced hormone release from pancreatic endocrine tumors.

Pituitary Neoplasms

Pituitary neoplasms occur in 30–50% of MEN-I patients, with benign prolactin-producing adenomas being the most common. Symptoms may be related directly to the tumor, such as headache and diplopia, or be related to the specific hormone overproduced. Excess prolactin causes galactorrhea and amenorrhea in women and impotence in men. Tumors may also produce growth hormone (30%) or ACTH (<10%), leading to acromegaly or Cushing's disease, respectively. Bromocriptine, a dopamine agonist, can be used to treat prolactinomas medically. Transsphenoidal hypophysectomy is reserved for patients who fail to respond to bromocriptine and who have non-prolactin-secreting tumors. All patients with MEN-I should be followed periodically with measurement of serum prolactin and growth hormone levels.

MEN-II

MEN-II consists of two syndromes, each inherited in an autosomal dominant pattern with 100% penetrance but variable expression. Both syndromes are marked by the presence of medullary thyroid carcinoma (MTC) and pheochromocytoma. In MEN-IIa, patients frequently also develop hyperparathyroidism secondary to four-gland hyperplasia. Patients with MEN-IIb tend to have a characteristic facies and marfanoid habitus. MEN-IIb is also marked by the development of multiple neuromas on the lips, tongue, and oral mucosa. In addition, IIb patients have a high incidence of skeletal abnormalities as well as diffuse ganglioneuromatosis of the GI tract, which can lead to a number of GI motility problems.

Medullary Thyroid Carcinoma

MTC makes up about 5–10% of all thyroid malignancies. The vast majority—approximately 80%—of these tumors occur sporadically; the remaining 20% are familial. MTC can occur in the familial setting without any other associated syndromes. Some features of sporadic and familial MTC are shown in Table 14-6. In the setting of MEN-II, MTC is usually the first endocrine abnormality to occur. MTC arises from the parafollicular or C cells of the thyroid and as a result has the capability to secrete not only calcitonin but also a variety of other hormonally active substances, such as serotonin, ACTH, prostaglandins, and melanin.

Clinical Presentation

MTC is often detected when it is clinically occult in patients screened for MEN-II. About 30% of the patients with MTC present with watery diarrhea, usually secondary to the stimulatory effect of high plasma calcitonin levels on intestinal fluid and electrolyte secretion. Symptoms such as hoarseness, dysphagia, and respiratory difficulty may be related to locally advanced disease. Presenting symptoms may also be secondary to metastatic disease, which is most commonly seen in the lungs, liver, and bones.

Diagnosis

The diagnosis of MTC can be made either pathologically or biochemically. When there is a palpable lesion, fine-needle aspiration can be performed. Histologically, MTC frequently shows sheets of uniformly round or polygonal cells separated by fibrovascular stroma. Immunohistochemical staining for calcitonin in the tumor cells is the most reliable way to confirm the diagnosis. Laboratory measurements for serum calcitonin are also important and usually demonstrate marked elevation, especially in patients with palpable tumors. Patients with clinically occult tumors, however, may have normal or minimally elevated serum calcitonin levels.

Provocative tests can be used to identify those patients who have MTC. In general, provocative testing is more reliable for MEN-IIa patients than for MEN-IIb patients. For this reason, MEN-IIb patients usually present with MTC as a palpable nodule and with more advanced disease. The original provocative test for diagnosing MTC was the calcium infusion test. With this test patients with MTC show a marked rise in calcitonin as compared with healthy persons, who have no rise at all. A more rapid method for making the diagnosis is the pentagastrin stimulation test. Pentagastrin is given by IV bolus, and serum calcitonin levels are measured within

Table 14-6.   Comparison of features of sporadic versus familial medullary thyroid carcinoma

Feature	Sporadic	Familial
Proportion of cases	80%	20%
Age at onset	40–60 years	10–30 years
Location	Unilateral	Bilateral

the next 5 minutes. Patients with MTC show a marked rise in serum calcitonin levels, often higher than those in the calcium infusion test. More recently, it has been shown that the highest stimulated serum calcitonin levels can be obtained with the sequential administration of calcium followed by an IV bolus of pentagastrin. Stimulated values of calcitonin above 300 pg/ml suggest MTC. Plasma values above 1,000 pg/ml are diagnostic.

Most authorities recommend that members of families at risk for MTC undergo provocative screening beginning at age 5 years and continuing through age 45. Increasingly, kindred of known MEN-II patients are undergoing genetic analysis for diagnosis and counseling. The role of prophylactic surgery, especially total thyroidectomy, in the setting of a known RET mutation and normal gastrin-stimulated calcitonin levels is evolving.

Treatment

Once the diagnosis of MTC is made, patients should be screened for pheochromocytoma and hyperparathyroidism. If a pheochromocytoma is found, it should be treated first (see Chapter 15). Surgery for the MTC is then done 2 weeks later. If hyperparathyroidism is diagnosed, it can be treated at the time of neck exploration for the MTC.

The appropriate treatment for MTC is total thyroidectomy and central neck dissection. In the MEN-II syndromes, MTC is frequently multicentric and bilateral, and metastasizes early to the cervical lymph nodes. The central neck dissection, which removes the lymphatic tissue between the jugular veins, the hyoid bone, and the sternal notch, helps eradicate microscopic metastatic disease. Patients with palpable lymphadenopathy should also undergo a functional neck dissection on the side of the enlarged pathologic nodes. Patients can be followed postoperatively with provocative testing to identify residual or recurrent MTC. Overall, the prognosis of MTC is good, with 60–80% 10-year survival rates being reported for MEN-IIa patients; MEN-IIb patients will usually present with more advanced disease (i.e., extrathyroidal extension or macroscopic nodal metastasis), and long-term survival is less common. In general, the course of the MTC determines the prognosis for patients with MEN-II. The average life expectancy for this group of patients is more than 50 years.

Metastatic Disease

Controversy exists over the appropriate management of patients with stimulated elevations of plasma calcitonin levels in the postoperative period. Such a finding implies the presence of residual disease in the neck or mediastinum or of undetected metastatic disease. Some clinicians think that these patients should be followed with observation only because MTC is slow-growing and the chance for cure with repeat neck exploration is low. Others recommend repeat neck exploration after selective catheterization of the neck veins and determination of stimulated plasma calcitonin levels. In experienced hands, a 30–40% normalization of plasma calcitonin levels by provocative testing can be achieved after repeat exploration. There are currently few options for patients with advanced disease; radioactive iodine ablation, thyroid suppression, radiotherapy, and chemotherapy have not been shown to be very effective for MTC. Because of the indolent nature of the tumor, many physicians do not treat metastatic disease aggressively.

Pheochromocytoma

Usually, pheochromocytoma associated with MEN-II appears between the ages of 10 and 30 years and is diagnosed concurrently or shortly after MTC. The pheochromocytomas associated with MEN-II are usually bilateral (60–80% of the time), limited to the adrenal medulla, and almost always benign. The adrenal gland appears to become hyperplastic before the pheochromocytoma develops. Further discussion of pheochromocytoma can be found in the chapter on adrenal tumors (Chapter 15).

The work-up and management of pheochromocytoma are discussed in more detail in Chapter 15. Patients with MEN-II should have a [I-131]Metaiodobenzylguanidine (MIBG) scan preoperatively in addition to other localizing studies. In this population of patients, the MIBG not only is the most sensitive (94%) and specific test (almost 100%), but also can help determine whether bilateral pheochromocytomas are present.

Because many years can separate the development of pheochromocytomas in opposite adrenal glands in MEN-II, some controversy exists about the optimal surgical procedure for patients who are initially found to have a unilateral pheochromocytoma. Although some surgeons recommend bilateral adrenalectomy in patients with MEN-II because up to 80% of these patients will develop bilateral tumors, a more conservative approach is followed by most to avoid as long as possible the need for lifetime glucocorticoid and mineralocorticoid replacement. This approach involves unilateral adrenalectomy and examination of the contralateral adrenal at the time of exploration. If no abnormality is found, the unaffected adrenal is left intact and the patient is followed closely for evidence of a contralateral tumor, which develops in approximately 50% of patients after 10 years of follow-up. In the event of bilateral pheochromocytoma, cortical-sparing adrenalectomy can be performed, thus avoiding chronic steroid replacement and the risk of Addisonian crisis. Long-term follow-up is indicated in all patients with MEN syndromes for the recurrence of any endocrine lesion.

Although laparoscopic adrenalectomy has become increasingly popular for benign adrenal lesions, the role of laparoscopy in the surgical treatment of pheochromocytoma has yet to be fully defined. Several groups have demonstrated the safety of laparoscopic adrenalectomy, although patients with pheochromocytoma may experience significant hypertensive crises during laparoscopy, even in the face of adequate preoperative medical treatment. This issue is further discussed in the chapter on adrenal tumors (Chapter 15).

Hyperparathyroidism

Hyperparathyroidism is the third and most variable component of the MEN-IIa syndrome. Most often the patients are asymptomatic and the diagnosis is made on routine follow-up laboratory tests. Occasionally, patients present with kidney stones. In patients with MEN-II, a work-up for hyperparathyroidism should be undertaken before neck exploration for MTC. In the vast majority of cases, the hyperparathyroidism is secondary to hyperplasia or multiple gland disease. If, at the time of exploration, the calcium levels are normal and the parathyroid glands appear normal, no parathyroidectomy is performed. If calcium and serum PTH levels are elevated or if the glands appear grossly abnormal and are hyperplastic on biopsy specimens at the time of neck exploration for MTC, a total parathyroidectomy should be performed. Transplantation of approximately one-half of the most normal-appearing parathyroid gland into the forearm should be carried out. If normal parathyroid tissue should become devascularized in the course of performing a total thyroidectomy for MTC in a patient with MEN-II, parathyroid autotransplantation should also be performed. Patients with MEN-IIa should have the autotransplant performed into the brachioradialis muscle of the forearm because the gland could become hyperplastic in the future and this placement facilitates later removal. In patients with MEN-IIb, because hyperparathyroidism rarely develops, the devascularized parathyroid glands can be transplanted into the sternocleidomastoid muscle in the neck.

Selected References

PANCREATIC ENDOCRINE TUMORS

Bieligk S, Jaffe BM. Islet cell tumors of the pancreas. *Surg Clin North Am* 75:1025, 1995.

Evans DB, Skibber JM, Lee JF, et al. Nonfunctioning islet cell carcinoma of the pancreas. *Surgery* 114:1175, 1993.

Fraker DL, Alexander HR. The surgical approach to endocrine tumors of the pancreas. *Semin Gastrointest Dis* 6:102, 1995.

Gibril F, Doppman JL, Jensen RT. Recent advances in the treatment of metastatic pancreatic endocrine tumors. *Semin Gastrointest Dis* 6:114, 1995.

Gower WR, Fabri PJ. Endocrine neoplasms (non-gastrin) of the pancreas. *Semin Surg Oncol* 6:98, 1990.

Harmon JW, Norton JA, Collen MJ. Removal of gastrinomas for the control of Zollinger-Ellison syndrome. *Ann Surg* 200:396, 1984.

Howard TJ, Stabile BE, Zinner MJ, et al. Anatomic distribution of pancreatic endocrine tumors. *Am J Surg* 159:258, 1990.

Krejs GJ. Gastrointestinal endocrine tumors. *Scand J Gastroenterol* 220(Suppl):121, 1996.

Lam KY, Lo CY. Pancreatic endocrine tumour: A 22-year clinico-pathological experience with morphological, immunohistochemical observation and a review of the literature. *Eur J Surg Oncol* 23:36, 1997.

Lee JE, Evans DB. Advances in the diagnosis and treatment of gastrointestinal neuroendocrine tumors. *Cancer Treat Res* 90:227, 1997.

Legaspi A, Brennan MF. Management of islet cell carcinoma. *Surgery* 104:1018, 1988.

Maton PN. The use of long-acting somatostatin analogue, octreotide acetate, in patients with islet cell tumors. *Gastroenterol Clin North Am* 18:897, 1989.

Maurer CA, Baer HU, Dyong TH, et al. Carcinoid of the pancreas: Clinical characteristics and morphologic features. *Eur J Cancer* 32A(7):1109, 1996.

Meko JB, Norton JA. Endocrine tumors of the pancreas. *Curr Opin Gen Surg* :186, 1994.

Norton JA. Neuroendocrine tumors of the pancreas and duodenum. *Curr Probl Surg* 31:77, 1994.

Norton JA, Doppman JL, Collen MJ, et al. Prospective study of gastrinoma localization and resection in patients with Zollinger-Ellison syndrome. *Ann Surg* 204:468, 1986.

Norton JA, Doppman JL, Jensen RT. Curative resection in Zollinger-Ellison syndrome: Results of a 10 year prospective study. *Ann Surg* 215:8, 1992.

Oberg K. Neuroendocrine gastrointestinal tumors. *Ann Oncol* 7:453, 1996.

Orbuch M, Doppman JL, Jensen RT. Localization of pancreatic endocrine tumors. *Semin Gastrointest Dis* 6:90, 1995.

Perry RR, Vinik AI. Diagnosis and management of functioning islet cell tumors. *J Clin Endocrinol Metab* 80:2273, 1995.

Sloan DA, Schwartz RW, Kenady DE. Surgical therapy for endocrine tumors of abdominal origin. *Curr Opin Oncol* 5:100, 1993.

Thompson GB, van Heerden JA, Grant CS, et al. Islet cell carcinomas of the pancreas: A twenty-year experience. *Surgery* 104:1011, 1988.

Venkatesh S, Ordonez NG, Ajani J, et al. Islet cell carcinoma of the pancreas. *Cancer* 65:354, 1990.

Zollinger RM, Ellison EC, O'Dorisio T, Sparks J. Thirty years' experience with gastrinoma. *World J Surg* 8:427, 1984.

MULTIPLE ENDOCRINE NEOPLASIA

Cance WG, Wells SA. Multiple endocrine neoplasia type IIa. *Curr Probl Surg* 22:1, 1985.

Carlson KM, Dou S, Chi D, et al. Single missense mutation in the tyrosine kinase catalytic domain of the RET protooncogene is associated with multiple endocrine neoplasia type 2B. *Proc Natl Acad Sci USA* 91:1579, 1994.

Clark OH. What's new in endocrine surgery. *J Am Coll Surg* 184:126, 1997.

Gagner M, Breton G, Pharand D, Pomp A. Is laparoscopic adrenalectomy indicated for pheochromocytomas? *Surgery* 120:1076, 1996.

Herfarth KK, Bartsch D, Doherty GM, Wells SA, Jr., Lairmore TC. Surgical management of hyperparathyroidism in patients with multiple endocrine neoplasia type 2A. *Surgery* 120:966, 1996.

Lairmore TC, Ball DW, Baylin SB, Wells SA. Management of pheochromocytomas in patients with multiple endocrine neoplasia type 2 syndromes. *Ann Surg* 217:595, 1993.

Lee JE, Curley SA, Gagel RF, Evans DB, Hickey RC. Cortical-sparing adrenalectomy for patients with bilateral pheochromocytoma. *Surgery* 120:1064, 1996.

Pipeleers-Mirichal M, Somers G, Willems G, et al. Gastrinomas in the duodenums of patients with multiple endocrine neoplasia type I and the Zollinger-Ellison syndrome. *N Engl J Med* 322:723, 1990.

Thompson JC, Lewis BG, Wiener I, Townsend CM, Jr. The role of surgery in Zollinger-Ellison syndrome. *Ann Surg* 197:594, 1983.

Wolfe MM, Jensen RT. Zollinger-Ellison syndrome: Current concepts in the diagnosis and management. *N Engl J Med* 317:1200, 1987.

Adrenal Tumors

Michael Bouvet, Douglas S. Tyler,
and Jeffrey E. Lee

The diagnosis and treatment of adrenal tumors require a sound fundamental knowledge of adrenal endocrine physiology. The clinical manifestations of hyperaldosteronism, hypercortisolism, and pheochromocytoma result from hypersecretion of adrenal endocrine products. Biochemical diagnosis and radiographic localization are required prior to surgical intervention. Adrenocortical carcinoma, a rare tumor that is potentially curable by surgery, must be differentiated from the more common metastatic tumors and computed tomography (CT)–detected "incidentalomas" of the adrenal glands, which rarely require surgical intervention.

Primary Hyperaldosteronism

Primary hyperaldosteronism (Conn's syndrome) is the clinical syndrome that results from hypersecretion of aldosterone. This condition is due to adrenal hyperplasia in about 40% of cases and to adrenal adenoma about 60% of the time. Other rare causes of primary aldosteronism include glucocorticoid-suppressible hyperaldosteronism, adrenocortical carcinoma, and aldosterone-secreting ovarian tumors. Primary hyperaldosteronism is responsible for approximately 0.5–1.0% of all cases of hypertension and roughly 5–10% of surgically correctable cases of hypertension.

CLINICAL MANIFESTATIONS

The main problem in diagnosing primary hyperaldosteronism is that the symptoms are usually mild and nonspecific. The most common symptoms are headache, fatigue, polydypsia, polyuria, and nocturia. Hypertension is almost always present but is frequently mild, with diastolic blood pressures below 120 mmHg in more than 70% of cases.

DIAGNOSIS

Patients suspected of having primary hyperaldosteronism should undergo a thorough evaluation. Initial laboratory findings that support the diagnosis, especially in patients not currently receiving diuretic therapy, include an elevated urine chloride level and hypokalemia accompanied by metabolic alkalosis. Initially, all nonessential medications should be stopped for at least 2 weeks. Estrogens and spironolactone should be discontinued for at least 6 weeks. Patients should then be placed on a salt-loading diet (10–12 g NaCl/day). During salt loading, urine should be collected over 24 hours and measurements made of aldosterone, sodium, potassium, and creatinine. Serum levels of aldosterone and electrolytes, and plasma renin activity should be measured. Patients with primary hyperaldosteronism do not have suppressed aldosterone production during the salt loading, but continue to have urinary aldosterone levels that are usually higher than 14 mg/day, a urinary potassium level higher than 10 µg/24 hours, and low plasma renin activity. Potassium supplementation should also be given during the period of salt loading because severe hypokalemia (K <3 mEq) can inhibit aldosterone production in some patients. A plasma aldosterone/plasma renin ratio of >30 (ng/dl : ng/ml/h) has been shown to be sensitive and specific in the screening and diagnosis of primary hyperaldosteronism. Other tests occasionally useful in the diagnosis of hyperaldosteronism include the Lasix stimulation test, the IV saline loading test, and the captopril suppression test.

Once the diagnosis of hyperaldosteronism is established, it is critical to differentiate unilateral adrenal adenoma from bilateral hyperplasia of the zona glomerulosa (idiopathic hyperaldosteronism). In patients with an aldosterone-producing adenoma, unilateral adrenalectomy corrects the hypokalemia and lowers the blood pressure in 70% of surgically treated patients. However, surgery is of little value in patients with idiopathic hyperaldosteronism. Patients with a unilateral adenoma usually have more severe hypertension, higher plasma aldosterone levels, and therefore more profound hypokalemia; however, these findings cannot accurately differentiate patients with unilateral adenoma from those with idiopathic hyperaldosteronism. Computed tomography (CT), magnetic resonance imaging (MRI), and selective venous sampling for aldosterone measurement can confirm the presence of a unilateral adenoma. However, the high frequency of nonfunctioning adenomas in the normal population (2–8%) means that the finding of a small adrenal mass on CT or MRI is not necessarily diagnostic of a unilateral aldosterone-producing adenoma. Because selective venous sampling is invasive and cannulation of the right adrenal vein is often difficult, the cause of the elevated aldosterone level may remain unclear even after the preceding studies. Therefore adrenal imaging is often combined with postural studies.

Postural studies are based on the principle that aldosterone-producing adenomas are not affected by changes in angiotensin II levels that occur with standing (unlike idiopathic hyperaldosteronism). The absence of the normal postural increase in aldosterone concentration supports the diagnosis of an aldosterone-producing adenoma. In fact, serum aldosterone levels in patients with aldosterone-producing adenomas (suppressed renin levels) usually fall in response to assuming an upright posture in the morning caused by the diurnal decline in corticotropin levels. However, to complicate matters further, rare patients with apparent unilateral aldosterone-producing adenomas may have results of postural studies more consistent with idiopathic hyperaldosteronism. Such patients have aldosterone-producing, renin-responsive adenomas and are often cured with unilateral adrenalectomy. Selective venous sampling can differentiate this rare disease from idiopathic (bilateral) hyperaldosteronism. Our approach to patients suspected of having primary hyperaldosteronism is shown in Fig. 15-1.

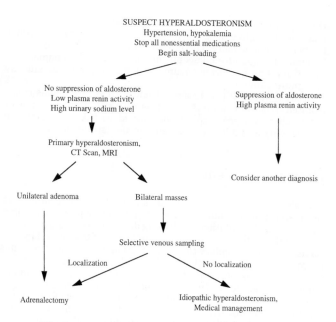

Fig. 15-1. Algorithm for the evaluation of the patient with suspected primary hyperaldosteronism.

TREATMENT

The treatment of primary hyperaldosteronism depends on the cause. Adrenal hyperplasia is best managed medically using the aldosterone antagonist spironolactone. Most patients can achieve adequate control of their blood pressure with this medicine alone or in conjunction with other antihypertensives. When a benign adenoma is diagnosed, the appropriate therapy consists of surgical resection. Preoperatively, patients should be placed on spironolactone and given potassium supplements to help normalize their fluid and electrolyte levels over a 3- to 4-week period.

A posterior flank incision has been the standard approach when excising an aldosterone-secreting adenoma. Adrenalectomy performed in this way is associated with minimal morbidity and mortality. The early results from surgical resection of an adenoma are good, with 95% of patients becoming normotensive and eukalemic. However, within 3 years 20–30% of the patients develop recurrent hypertension. The etiology of the hypertension is not clear, but it is usually not associated with hypokalemia. The long term cure rate is therefore approximately 70%.

Recently, laparoscopic adrenalectomy through either an anterior or a lateral approach has been described. The procedure may have several advantages over open adrenalectomy, including less postoperative pain, a shorter hospital stay, and a more rapid return to full activity. However, the mean operative time is longer than open adrenalectomy and uncontrollable hemorrhage, especially on the right side, is the most common reason for conversion to open adrenalectomy. The laparoscopic approach is best suited for small, benign adrenal neoplasms such as aldosteronomas, and its utility has not been documented for larger or potentially malignant tumors.

Approximately 2% or less of adrenocortical carcinomas cause isolated hyperaldosteronism. In this rare situation, an anterior approach to surgical exploration should be taken to facilitate resectability and allow assessment for metastatic disease.

Hypercortisolism

Cushing's syndrome refers to the state of hypercortisolism that can result from a number of different pathologic processes (Table 15-1). Cortisol regulation involves feedback loops on the pituitary gland and hypothalamus. Approximately 70% of the cases of hypercortisolism are secondary to hypersecretion of adrenocorticotropic hormone (ACTH) from the pituitary gland, a condition called *Cushing's disease*. Most of the time a small pituitary adenoma is found to be the cause. Hypersecretion of cortisol from the adrenal glands accounts for approximately 10–20% of cases of Cushing's syndrome. The underlying cause is an adrenal adenoma 50–60% of the time and an adrenocortical carcinoma 20–25% of the time. Bilateral adrenal hyperplasia accounts for the remaining 20–30% of cases. Although the etiology of autonomously functioning bilateral adrenal hyperplasia is unclear, several reports suggest that some cases may be due to an aberrant sensitivity of the adrenal glands to gastric inhibitory polypeptide, which is released in response to eating.

Ectopic secretion of ACTH, referred to as *ectopic ACTH syndrome*, causes about 15% of cases of Cushing's syndrome. Ectopic ACTH syndrome is usually caused by malignant tumors, with carcinoma of the lung, carcinoma of the pancreas, carcinoid tumors, and malignant thymoma accounting for 80% of such cases. Ectopic

Table 15-1.   Causes of Cushing's syndrome

Cushing's disease (due to pituitary adenoma)
    Associated with diffuse adrenal hyperplasia
    Associated with micronodular hyperplasia
    Associated with macronodular hyperplasia

Ectopic adrenocorticotropin syndrome

Ectopic corticotropin-releasing factor syndrome

Adrenal tumors
    Single adenoma
    Multiple adenomas
    Carcinoma

Primary adrenocortical hyperplasia

Exogenous steroids

secretion of corticotropin-releasing factor is exceedingly rare but has been reported in a few cases.

CLINICAL MANIFESTATIONS

Weight gain is the most common feature of hypercortisolism and occurs predominantly in the truncal area. Centripetal obesity combined with muscle wasting in the extremities, fat deposition in the head and neck region, and a dorsal kyphosis secondary to osteoporosis gives the patient a very characteristic habitus. Hypertension, striae, and virilization in females are three other common findings.

DIAGNOSIS

The work-up for Cushing's syndrome should be aimed first at establishing the diagnosis and then at determining the etiology. To establish the diagnosis, a state of hypercortisolism must be documented. The adult adrenal glands secrete on average 10–30 mg of cortisol each day. The secretion follows a diurnal variation: Cortisol levels tend to be high early in the morning and low in the evening. The variability of plasma cortisol levels requires that morning (8 A.M.) plasma cortisol levels be used as part of an overnight low-dose dexamethasone suppression test as screening for Cushing's syndrome. An alternative first-line screening test is measurement of 24-hour urinary-free cortisol; the normal level is generally below 80 µg/day.

To determine the etiology of the elevated cortisol level, plasma ACTH levels must be checked. ACTH secretion also follows a diurnal variation preceding that of cortisol by 1–2 hours. Suppressed levels of ACTH are seen in patients with adrenal adenomas, adrenocortical carcinomas, or autonomously functioning adrenal hyperplasia. In such cases, autonomous secretion of cortisol by the pathologic process in the adrenal gland inhibits ACTH release by the pituitary. Patients with Cushing's disease (i.e., a pituitary adenoma secreting ACTH) usually have plasma ACTH levels that are elevated or within the upper limits of normal. When there is an ectopic source of ACTH secretion, the plasma ACTH level is usually markedly elevated.

The most sensitive method for detecting hypercortisolism is the overnight dexamethasone suppression test. One milligram of dexamethasone is taken orally at 11:00 P.M.; normal individuals have a cortisol level of less than 5 mg/dl at 8:00 A.M. the following morning. Failure to suppress the 8:00 A.M. cortisol to <5 mg/dl is consistent with hypercortisolism; however, although this test has a false-negative rate of only 3%, the false-positive rate is 30%. Therefore although a normal overnight dexamethasone suppression test excludes clinically significant hypercortisolism, an abnormal test requires further investigation. Twenty-four-hour urine collection for urinary (unmetabolized) free cortisol is somewhat less sensitive than overnight dexamethasone suppression but more specific; urinary collection for 17-hydroxysteroids can also be used.

To confirm the presence of Cushing's syndrome, the low-dose and high-dose dexamethasone suppression test can be performed.

For this test, urine is collected over 24 hours for 6 consecutive days for measurement of free cortisol and 17-hydroxycortico-steroid (17-OHCS). During the first 2 days no dexamethasone is taken and urinary cortisol is measured to establish baseline values. During the third and fourth days, the patient takes 0.5 mg of dexamethasone every 6 hours. Hypercortisolism is confirmed if urinary cortisol levels do not decline below 20 mg/g creatinine/day and/or if urinary 17-OHCS levels stay above 2 mg/g creatinine/day. On the fifth and sixth days, the patient takes 2 mg of dexamethasone every 6 hours. Individuals who have Cushing's disease usually show a reduction in their urinary cortisol levels to 50% of the baseline obtained on days 1 and 2. The cortisol levels of patients with an ectopic ACTH syndrome or autonomously functioning adrenal pathology (neoplasm or hyperplasia) do not fall below 50% of the baseline.

The metyrapone test is also occasionally used to differentiate between the various etiologies of Cushing's syndrome. Metyrapone inhibits the enzyme 11b-hydroxylase, which converts 11-deoxy-cortisol to cortisol as well as converting 11-deoxycorticosterone to corticosterone and aldosterone. The inhibition of cortisol production in the normal adrenal gland by metyrapone is sensed in the pituitary gland and results in increased production of ACTH. The ACTH stimulates the adrenal cortex to produce cortisol precursors that can then be detected in either the blood or the urine. A decline in urinary and serum cortisol levels also occurs. On the day before the test begins, patients collect a baseline 24-hour urine sample and have blood drawn for baseline plasma cortisol and 11-deoxycortisol measurements. The patient then takes 30 mg/kg of metyrapone at midnight. Eight hours later the patient has plasma cortisol and 11-deoxycortisol levels rechecked. In addition, the patient collects another 24-hour urine sample. The pituitary gland of patients with Cushing's disease senses the decreased levels of cortisol; ACTH release is increased, which results in elevated serum deoxycortisol and urinary 17-OHCS levels accompanied by decreased serum cortisol levels. The pituitary gland of patients with ectopic ACTH syndrome or autonomously functioning adrenal tissue is chronically suppressed and does not respond to changes in cortisol levels. Therefore serum deoxycortisol and urinary 17-OHCS levels remain unchanged from the baseline values.

An overview of our approach to patients suspected of having Cushing's syndrome is shown in Fig. 15-2. Initial screening involves the 1-mg overnight dexamethasone suppression test. Patients with suppressed cortisol levels do not have Cushing's syndrome. Patients without suppressed cortisol levels receive a low-dose, high-dose dexamethasone test and/or a metyrapone test. Twenty-four-hour urine collections for measurement of free cortisol levels and measurement of morning and evening plasma cortisol levels are performed to determine whether the hormone has a diurnal variation. Patients whose cortisol levels are suppressed after the low-dose, high-dose dexamethasone test or who are metyrapone responsive have Cushing's disease and should have a CT scan of the head, with special focus on the pituitary region. In patients whose cortisol levels are not suppressed after the low-dose, high-dose dexamethasone test or

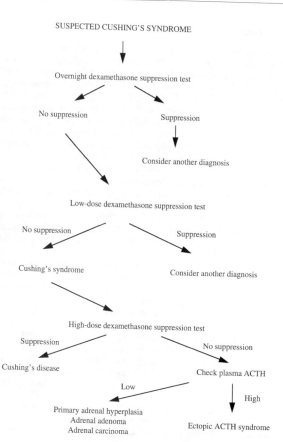

SUSPECTED CUSHING'S SYNDROME

Overnight dexamethasone suppression test

No suppression   Suppression

Consider another diagnosis

Low-dose dexamethasone suppression test

No suppression   Suppression

Cushing's syndrome   Consider another diagnosis

High-dose dexamethasone suppression test

Suppression   No suppression

Cushing's disease   Check plasma ACTH

Low   High

Primary adrenal hyperplasia
Adrenal adenoma
Adrenal carcinoma   Ectopic ACTH syndrome

Fig. 15-2. Algorithm for the evaluation and treatment of the patient with suspected Cushing's syndrome. (ACTH=adrenocorticotropin releasing hormone).

who are metyrapone unresponsive, we check the plasma ACTH level. High ACTH levels indicate ectopic ACTH syndrome. These patients should have a CT scan of the chest and abdomen in an attempt to identify the underlying malignancy. Patients with low plasma ACTH levels have adrenal pathology as the etiology of their Cushing's syndrome. An abdominal CT scan will help separate an adrenal neoplasm from primary adrenal hyperplasia. In selected cases, radioisotope imaging of the adrenals with labeled iodocholesterol can help distinguish primary adrenal hyperplasia, which should demonstrate bilateral uptake, from a cortisol-secreting adenoma, which leads to suppression of the contralateral gland and thus to uptake only by the adenoma. Adrenocortical carcinomas usually do not take up radiolabeled iodocholesterol.

TREATMENT

The appropriate management of Cushing's syndrome depends on the underlying etiology. Patients with Cushing's disease should undergo transsphenoidal resection of their pituitary adenoma when it is believed to be resectable. Remission of symptoms is seen in more than 80% of patients with a single adenoma but is less likely in the presence of extrasellar extension, macronodular disease of the pituitary, or pituitary corticotropic hyperplasia. Bilateral adrenalectomy is rarely indicated and should be reserved for patients who fail to respond to hypophysectomy. If bilateral adrenalectomy is performed, patients require not only perioperative steroid coverage (Tables 15-2 and 15-3) but also lifelong replacement of both glucocorticoids and mineralocorticoids. Some groups have advocated heterotopic autotransplantation of adrenal tissue after bilateral adrenalectomy as a way to minimize steroid utilization and prevent Nelson's syndrome. When this procedure is performed, approximately 4 g of each gland is sliced into 1- to 2-mm sections and placed into a muscle pocket in the paraspinous or rectus abdominis muscle.

Patients with a neoplasm of the adrenal gland, whether adenoma or carcinoma, should undergo resection of the involved side. Although almost all adenomas can be resected, adrenocortical carcinomas that secrete cortisol are resectable in only 25–35% of patients. Chemotherapy has been disappointing in patients with unresectable adrenocortical carcinoma. Symptomatic relief of the hypercortisol state can be achieved with various agents, including mitotane, aminoglutethimide, metyrapone, or ketoconazole.

Patients with autonomously functioning bilateral adrenal hyperplasia require bilateral adrenalectomy with or without heterotopic autotransplantation. To date, medical therapy has not been effective for this condition.

Finally, patients with ectopic ACTH syndrome should have the underlying malignant lesion resected if possible. Bilateral adrenalectomy should be reserved for the small group of patients

Table 15-2.   Recommendations for perioperative glucocorticoid coverage

Surgical stress	Examples	Hydrocortisone equivalent (mg)	Duration (days)
"Minor"	Inguinal herniorraphy	25	1
"Moderate"	Open cholecystectomy Lower-extremity revascularization Segmental colon resection Total joint replacement Abdominal hysterectomy	50–75	1–2
"Major"	Pancreaticoduodenectomy Esophagogastrectomy Total proctocolectomy Cardiac surgery with cardiopulmonary bypass	100–150	2–3

Table 15-3. Comparison of steroid preparations

Steroid	Half-life (hours)	Glucocorticoid activity (relative to cortisol)	Mineralocorticoid activity (relative to cortisol)
Cortisol	8–12	1	1
Cortisone	8–12	0.8	0.8
Prednisone	12–36	4	0.25
Prednisolone	12–36	4	0.25
Methylprednisolone	12–36	5	0
Triamcinolone	12–36	5	0
Betamethasone	36–72	25	0
Dexamethasone	36–72	30–40	0

whose primary tumor is unresectable and whose symptoms of cortisol excess cannot be controlled medically.

Pheochromocytoma

In large series of hypertensive patients, approximately 0.1–0.2% of patients are found to have pheochromocytomas. These neuroectodermal tumors arise from chromaffin cells in the adrenal medulla. About 10% of the time, pheochromocytomas can be found in both adrenal glands, with multiple tumors being present in some cases. Ten percent of pheochromocytomas can be found in extra-adrenal sites, where they are more appropriately called *paragangliomas* because of their close association with ganglia of the sympathetic nervous system. The most common extra-adrenal sites include the organ of Zuckerkandl (located between the inferior mesenteric artery and the aortic bifurcation), the urinary bladder, the thorax, and the renal hilum.

Histologic evidence of malignancy in pheochromocytomas can be demonstrated approximately 10% of the time; malignancy is more commonly seen with extra-adrenal lesions than with those arising in the adrenal glands. Documenting malignancy can be difficult because invasion of adjacent organs or metastatic disease must be present. Furthermore, both benign and malignant lesions may show tumor penetration of the gland's capsule, invasion of veins draining the gland, cellular pleomorphism, mitoses, and atypical nuclei. Familial pheochromocytomas account for about 10% of cases and are usually benign. The familial syndromes associated with pheochromocytomas include multiple endocrine neoplasia types IIa and IIb, in which bilateral tumors are common, as well as the neuroectodermal dysplasias consisting of neurofibromatosis, tuberous sclerosis, Sturge-Weber syndrome, and von Hippel-Lindau disease. Patients with these syndromes require close follow-up and periodic screening for pheochromocytoma, especially before any planned surgical procedure.

CLINICAL MANIFESTATIONS

The clinical manifestations of pheochromocytoma can be varied and at times quite dramatic. Hypertension, sustained or paroxysmal, is the most common clinical finding. Paroxysmal elevations in blood pressure can vary markedly in frequency and duration. A number of things can stimulate increases in blood pressure, ranging from heavy physical exertion to eating foods high in tyramine. Other common symptoms include excessive sweating, palpitations, tremulousness, anxiety, and chest pain. More than half of the patients have impaired glucose tolerance and may have symptoms of diabetes mellitus such as polydypsia and polyuria, but these are generally mild. Most symptoms appear secondary to the excess catecholamine secretion by the tumors. Patients with functioning tumors are rarely asymptomatic, and nonfunctioning tumors are extremely rare.

DIAGNOSIS

The diagnosis of pheochromocytoma is made by documenting the excess secretion of catecholamines. Twenty-four-hour urine collections should be tested for free catecholamines (dopamine, epinephrine, and norepinephrine) and their metabolites (normetanephrine, metanephrine, vanillylmandelic acid). Elevated levels of catecholamines or their metabolites are seen in more than 90% of patients with pheochromocytoma. Plasma levels of free catecholamines are also usually elevated. However, because plasma values frequently overlap those seen in essential hypertension, the urinary measurements are accepted as being more sensitive. The adrenal glands and the organ of Zuckerkandl produce the enzyme phenylethanolamine-N-methyl-transferase, which converts norepinephrine to epinephrine. Pheochromocytomas that arise elsewhere do not contain this enzyme and thus do not produce much, if any, epinephrine. As a result, extra-adrenal pheochromocytomas secrete predominantly dopamine and norepinephrine.

When the urinary values of catecholamines show only borderline elevation, the clonidine suppression test can help differentiate pheochromocytoma from other causes of hypertension. Clonidine should suppress the centrally mediated release of catecholamines in all patients except those with pheochromocytomas, in whom the tumors usually function autonomously. Plasma catecholamine levels are measured 3 hours after giving a PO dose of clonidine (0.3 mg). A pheochromocytoma can be ruled out in patients in whom the plasma catecholamine level is lower than 500 pg/ml at 3 hours.

Once the diagnosis of pheochromocytoma is made, localization studies can be carried out. CT can detect 95% of adrenal masses larger than 6–8 mm and is usually performed first because it can also identify extra-adrenal intra-abdominal pheochromocytomas. An MRI may also be useful because T2-weighted images can clearly identify chromaffin tissue and because MRI gives an adrenal-mass-to-liver ratio of more than 3. This ratio is much higher than would be seen for adenomas or adenocarcinomas of the adrenal. ^{131}I-Metaiodobenzylguanidine (MIBG) scanning is another imaging procedure that is helpful in localizing extra-adrenal, metastatic, and/or bilateral pheochromocytomas. The radiolabeled amine is selectively picked up by chromaffin tissue and can identify the majority of pheochromocytomas, regardless of their location. Using these techniques, it is rare to have a patient whose pheochromocytoma cannot be localized preoperatively.

TREATMENT

After diagnosis and localization of the pheochromocytoma, careful preoperative preparation is required to prevent a cardiovascular crisis during surgery caused by excess catecholamine secretion. The main focus of the preoperative preparation is adequate alpha-adrenergic blockade and complete restoration of fluid and electrolyte balances. Phenoxybenzamine is the alpha-adrenergic blocking agent of choice and is usually begun at a dose of 10 mg twice a day. The dosage is gradually increased over a 1- to 3-week period until adequate blockade is reached. The total dosage used should not exceed $1 \text{ mg kg}^{-1} \text{ day}^{-1}$. Alpha-methyltyrosine, a competitive blocker of tyrosine conversion to dihydroxyphenylalanine, is another drug that can be used alone or together with phenoxybenzamine to inhibit catecholamine synthesis by 50–80%. Use of a beta-adrenergic blocking agent is somewhat controversial. Proponents of beta blockade feel that it helps prevent tachycardia and other arrhythmias. When used, a dose of 10 mg of propranolol given PO three times a day is recommended for 3 days preoperatively. Dosages as high as 50 mg four times a day may be necessary if there is persistent tachycardia (heart rate >140 beats per minute). The beta blocker should not be given unless alpha blockade has been established; otherwise, the beta blocker would inhibit epinephrine-induced vasodilation, leading to more significant hypertension and left heart strain. In addition to requiring pharmacologic preparation, patients with pheochromocytoma may require correction of fluid volume depletion as well as any concurrent electrolyte imbalances.

The perioperative management of patients with pheochromocytoma can be difficult. Rarely is the alpha-adrenergic blockade complete. The anesthesiologist should be prepared to treat a hypertensive crisis with sodium nitroprusside and tachyarrhythmias with either a beta blocker or lidocaine. Central venous access and right heart catheterization should be established preoperatively. Surgical exploration has traditionally been performed via an anterior approach (bilateral subcostal incision) so that both glands can be evaluated and the abdomen examined for metastatic disease. However, if the contralateral adrenal gland is radiographically normal, we generally do not manually explore the opposite side. The surgeon should manipulate the tumor as little as possible, and ligate the tumor's venous outflow via the adrenal vein as early in the procedure as possible. The preoperative diagnosis and localization of pheochromocytomas has reached a level sufficient to permit either a posterior or a laparoscopic approach, but only if these approaches have been technically mastered and the patients have been carefully selected. Laparoscopic adrenalectomy for pheochromocytoma has been reported to be more difficult than for adrenal adenomas and is not recommended for tumors larger than 6 cm or when malignancy is suspected. A laparoscopic approach would be particularly appropriate for the multiple endocrine neoplasia type II syndrome (MEN-II) or von Hippel-Lindau (VHL) patient with a small, unilateral pheochromocytoma; a posterior approach, for the MEN-II or VHL patient with bilateral disease. Cortical-sparing adrenalectomy has been performed successfully in MEN-II or VHL patients with bilateral pheochromocytomas, avoiding chronic steroid hormone replacement and the risk of Addisonian crisis in most patients.

Postoperatively, patients should be monitored in an intensive care unit for 24 hours so they can be observed for arrhythmias, as well as hypotension secondary to compensatory vasodilation that can occur once the excess catecholamine secretion has been stopped. Sometimes hypertension can remain a problem postoperatively, especially in those patients who had sustained hypertension preoperatively.

The best currently available palliation for unresectable or metastatic disease is alpha blockade with phenoxybenzamine. Alpha-methyltyrosine can also be used, with good palliation. The most commonly used chemotherapy regimens for pheochromocytoma are high-dose streptozocin and a combination of cyclophosphamide, vincristine, and dacarbazine. The overall response rates with these regimens is approximately 50%. Radiation has been effective only for bony metastases. More recently, there has been some interest in treating metastatic lesions with therapeutic doses of ^{131}I-MIBG. Unfortunately, a high percentage of metastatic pheochromocytomas do not take up ^{131}I-MIBG; therefore the response rate, as manifested by a reduction in urinary catecholamines, is only about 50%. Objective responses as determined by imaging studies are seen even less frequently.

The 5-year survival rate for patients with malignant pheochromocytoma is approximately 43%, as compared with a 97% 5-year survival rate for benign lesions.

Adrenocortical Carcinoma

Adrenocortical carcinoma is a rare malignancy with approximately 150–200 new cases reported each year in the United States. There is a bimodal age distribution, with incidence peaking in young children and then again between 40 and 50 years of age.

CLINICAL MANIFESTATIONS

Patients with adrenocortical carcinoma usually present with vague abdominal symptoms secondary to an enlarging retroperitoneal mass or with clinical manifestations of overproduction of one or more steroid hormones. Most of these tumors are functional as measured by biochemical parameters. Fifty percent secrete cortisol, producing Cushing's syndrome. The work-up and management of patients with Cushing's syndrome are described in that section in this chapter. Another 10–20% of adrenocortical carcinomas produce various steroid hormones, causing varying degrees of virilization in females, feminization in males, and/or hypertension.

DIAGNOSIS

The work-up of these patients involves a careful biochemical screening, including a 24-hour urine collection to measure levels of cortisol, aldosterone, catecholamines, metanephrine, vanillyl-mandelic acid, 17-OHCS, and 17-keto-steroids. The results serve mainly to guide perioperative replacement therapy as well as to rule out pheochromocytoma.

High-resolution abdominal CT and MRI are the best ways to obtain images of the adrenal glands. CT can usually identify lesions as small as 7 mm. MRI may be especially helpful not only in identifying tumor extension up the inferior vena cava but also in differentiating between various lesions based on the adrenal-to-liver ratio on T2-weighted images. Adenomas usually have ratios of 0.7–1.4; malignant lesions, whether primary or metastatic to the adrenal gland, have ratios of 1.4–3.0; and pheochromocytomas usually have ratios greater than 3.0. Chest radiography is helpful in ruling out pulmonary metastasis. Adrenal arteriography and venography are usually reserved for selected patients who have large lesions that may distort the usual anatomy in the region of the tumor. The various staging systems for adrenocortical carcinomas are shown in Table 15-4.

TREATMENT

Surgery is the treatment of choice for adrenocortical carcinomas. Approximately 50% of the tumors are localized to the adrenal gland at the time of initial exploration. Radical en bloc resection that includes adjacent organs, if necessary, provides the only chance for long-term cure. Patients who undergo a complete resection of their tumor have a 5-year survival of approximately 40%; those who undergo incomplete resection have a median survival of less than 12 months.

Common sites of recurrence include lungs, lymph nodes, liver, peritoneum, and bone. Complete resection of recurrent disease, including pulmonary metastases, is associated with prolonged survival in some patients and can control symptoms related to excess hormone production. After a potentially curative resection, patients should be monitored closely with monthly urinary steroid profiles as well as abdominal and chest imaging. Adjuvant therapy for adrenocortical carcinoma (mitotane) has had minimal impact, if any, on disease progression.

Radiation can provide palliation for bone metastases and recurrent, unresectable abdominal tumors; however, it has failed to prolong survival. No chemotherapeutic agent or combination of agents has been shown to be consistently effective against unresectable disease. Mitotane has been one of the most commonly used chemotherapy agents against this neoplasm because of its ability to palliate the endocrine effects of the tumor. This drug is an isomer of DDT and not only inhibits steroid production but also leads to atrophy of adrenocortical cells. Mitotane is associated with a number of side effects in the gastrointestinal and neuromuscular systems. In addition, the drug appears to have a narrow therapeutic range and requires close monitoring of serum levels.

Table 15-4. Staging systems for adrenal cortical carcinoma

Stage	Macfarlane (1958)	Sullivan (1978)	Icard (1992)	Lee (1995)
I	T1 (≤5 cm), N0, M0	T1 (≤5 cm), N0, M0	T1 (≤5 cm), N0, M0	T1 (≤5 cm), N0, M0
II	T2 (>5 cm), N0, M0	T2 (>5 cm), N0, M0	T2 (>5 cm), N0, M0	T2 (>5 cm), N0, M0
III	T3 (local invasion without involvement of adjacent organs) or mobile positive lymph nodes, M0	T3 (local invasion), N0 M0 or T1–2, N1 (positive lymph nodes), M0	T3 (local invasion) and/or N1 (positive regional lymph nodes), M0	T3/T4 (local invasion as demonstrated by histologic evidence of adjacent organ invasion, direct tumor extension to IVC, and/or tumor thrombus within IVC or renal vein) and/or N1 (positive regional lymph nodes) M0
IV	T4 (invasion of adjacent organs) or fixed positive lymph nodes or M1 (distant metastases)	T4 (local invasion), N0, M0; or T3, N1, M0; or T1–4, N0–1, M1 (distant metastases)	T1–4, N0–1, M1 (distant metastases)	T1–4, N0–1, M1 (distant metastases)

IVC = inferior vena cava.

Incidentalomas

With the widespread use of abdominal CT, asymptomatic adrenal lesions are being discovered with increasing frequency. These lesions, termed *incidentalomas*, are seen in 0.6–1.3% of routinely performed abdominal imaging studies and in up to 9% of autopsy series. Although most of these lesions are benign adenomas, some cause problems either by being hormonally active or by becoming an invasive malignancy.

All patients with incidentalomas should have measurement of serum electrolyte levels and a 24-hour urine collection to determine levels of vanillylmandelic acid, metanephrine, catecholamines, cortisol, aldosterone, 17-OHCS, and 17-ketosteroids. Any hormonally active lesion, regardless of size, should be resected.

If the incidentaloma is nonfunctioning, the risk of its being malignant is related to its size. Lesions larger than 100 g, which corresponds to a diameter of approximately 6 cm, should be resected because as many as 35% may be malignant. Although observation is generally recommended for nonfunctioning lesions smaller than 3 cm in diameter, the management of tumors between 3 and 6 cm is more controversial. Tumors between 3 and 6 cm in diameter are most appropriately managed on an individual basis. The following may be helpful in evaluating such patients with intermediate-size nonfunctioning adrenal masses: (1) MRI scanning, (2) a more thorough endocrine evaluation, and (3) consideration of age and comorbidity. Figure 15-3 provides an overview of our approach to patients with incidentalomas.

Metastatic Lesions

The metastasis of tumors to the adrenal glands is relatively common. Based on autopsy studies, 42% of lung tumors, 16% of stomach tumors, 58% of breast tumors, 50% of malignant melanomas, and a high percentage of renal and prostate tumors have metastasized to the adrenals at the time of death. Only rarely are problems related to the metastases, such as adrenal insufficiency, encountered. It is generally held that more than 90% of the gland must be replaced before clinically detectable adrenal cortical hypofunction is appreciated. When adrenal insufficiency does occur, it is usually in the setting of grossly enlarged adrenal glands as detected by CT.

Surgery for metastases to the adrenal gland may be considered in good-risk individuals in whom there is an absence of extra-adrenal disease and in whom there is a history of favorable tumor biology. Evaluation of patients with favorable tumor biology includes consideration of those who have had a significant progression-free interval, those who have responded to systemic therapy, and those who have a history of isolated metachronous metastases. Selected pathologies that may be considered for resection include patients with metastatic melanoma, renal cell carcinoma, and colorectal cancer. Preoperative evaluation of the patient with an adrenal mass and a history of malignancy should include an evaluation for hormone production prior to fine-needle

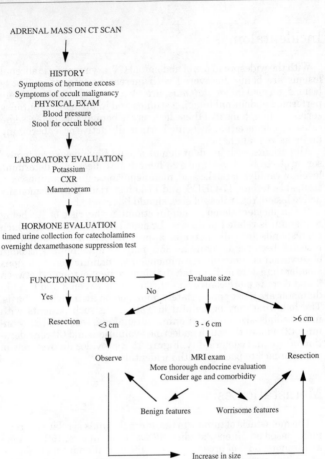

ADRENAL MASS ON CT SCAN

HISTORY
Symptoms of hormone excess
Symptoms of occult malignancy
PHYSICAL EXAM
Blood pressure
Stool for occult blood

LABORATORY EVALUATION
Potassium
CXR
Mammogram

HORMONE EVALUATION
timed urine collection for catecholamines
overnight dexamethasone suppression test

FUNCTIONING TUMOR   Evaluate size

Yes   No

Resection   <3 cm   3 - 6 cm   >6 cm

Observe   MRI exam   Resection
More thorough endocrine evaluation
Consider age and comorbidity

Benign features   Worrisome features

Increase in size

**Fig. 15-3. Algorithm for the evaluation and
treatment of the patient with an adrenal incidentaloma.**

aspiration biopsy, because some of these patients will have occult,
functioning adrenal tumors, including pheochromocytomas. In
addition, patients with known or suspected adrenal metastases
in whom surgical resection is contemplated should undergo
ACTH stimulation testing to document adequate adrenal cortical reserve prior to adrenalectomy. Fine-needle aspiration biopsy
may be helpful in selected cases to confirm the diagnosis of
metastasis preoperatively. Alternatively, surgical therapy can be
planned based solely on noninvasive imaging studies, such as the
T1-weighted chemical-shift MRI, in patients with a history of a
malignancy that commonly metastasizes to the adrenal glands,
favorable tumor biology, negative biochemical screening for hormone production, and a mass either fulfills size criteria for surgical excision or is radiographically suspicious for metastasis.

Selected References

PRIMARY HYPERALDOSTERONISM

Blumenfeld JC, Sealey JE, Schlussel Y, et al. Diagnosis and therapy of primary hyperaldosteronism. *Ann Intern Med* 121:877, 1994.

Lo CY, Tam PC, Kung AWC, Lam, KS, Wong J. Primary aldosteronism: Results of surgical treatment. *Ann Surg* 224:125, 1996.

Vallotton MB. Primary aldosteronism. Parts I and II. *Clin Endocrin* 45:47, 1996.

Weigel RJ, Wells SA, Gunnells JC, Leight GS. Surgical treatment of primary hyperaldosteronism. *Ann Surg* 219:347, 1994.

Weinberger MH, Fineberg NS. The diagnosis of primary aldosteronism and separation of two major subtypes. *Arch Intern Med* 153:2125, 1993.

HYPERCORTISOLISM

Lacroix A, Bolte E, Tremblay J, et al. Gastric inhibitory polypeptide-dependent cortisol hypersecretion: A new cause of Cushing's syndrome. *N Engl J Med* 327:974, 1992.

Orth DN. Cushing's syndrome. *N Engl J Med* 332:791, 1995.

van Heerden JA, Young, WF Jr, Grant CS, et al. Adrenal surgery for hypercortisolism: Surgical aspects. *Surgery* 117:466, 1995.

Zieger MA, Pass HI, Doppman JD, et al. Surgical strategy in the management of non–small cell ectopic adrenocorticotropic hormone syndrome. *Surgery* 112:994, 1992.

PHEOCHROMOCYTOMA

Gagner M, Breton JG, Pharand D, et al. Is laparoscopic adrenalectomy indicated for pheochromocytomas? *Surgery* 120:1076, 1996.

Lee JE, Curley SA, Gagel RF, et al. Cortical-sparing adrenalectomy for patients with bilateral pheochromocytoma. *Surgery* 120:1064, 1995.

Orchard T, Grant CS, van Heerden JA, et al. Pheochromocytoma: Continuing evolution of surgical therapy. *Surgery* 114:1153, 1993.

Peplinski GR, Norton JA. The predictive value of diagnostic tests for pheochromocytoma. *Surgery* 116:1101, 1994.

Werbel SS, Ober KP. Pheochromocytoma: Update on diagnosis, localization, and management. *Med Clin North Am* 79:131, 1995.

ADRENOCORTICAL MASSES AND CARCINOMA

Demeter JG, De Jong SA, Brooks MH, et al. Long-term results of adrenal autotransplantation in Cushing's disease. *Surgery* 108:1117, 1990.

Doppman JL, Reinig JW, Dwyer AJ, et al. Differentiation of adrenal masses by magnetic resonance imaging. *Surgery* 102:1018, 1987.

Herrera MF, Grant CS, van Heerden JA, et al. Incidentally discovered adrenal tumors: An institutional perspective. *Surgery* 110:1014, 1991.

Icard P, Chapuis Y, Andreassian BA, et al. Adrenocortical carcinoma in surgically treated patients: A retrospective study on 156 cases by the French Association of Endocrine Surgery. *Surgery* 112:972, 1992.

Lee JE, Berger DH, El-Naggar AK, et al. Surgical management, DNA content, and patient survival in adrenal cortical carcinoma. *Surgery* 118:1090, 1995.

Luton JP, Cerdas S, Billaud L, et al. Clinical features of adrenocortical carcinoma, prognostic factors, and the effect of mitotane therapy. *N Engl J Med* 322:1195, 1990.

McFarlane DA. Cancer of the adrenal cortex: The natural history, prognosis and treatment in a study of fifty-five cases. *Ann R Coll Surg Engl* 23:155, 1958.

Pommier RF, Brennan MF. An eleven-year experience with adrenocortical carcinoma. *Surgery* 112:963, 1992.

Ross NS, Aron DC. Hormonal evaluation of the patient with an incidentally discovered adrenal mass. *N Engl J Med* 323:1401, 1990.

Salem M, Tainsh RE, Bromberg J, et al. Perioperative glucocorticoid coverage: A reassessment 42 years after emergence of a problem. *Ann Surg* 4:416, 1994.

Sullivan M, Boileau M, Hodges CV. Adrenal cortical carcinoma. *J Urol* 120:660, 1978.

Vassilopoulou-Sellin R, Guinee VF, Klein MJ, et al. Impact of adjuvant mitotane on the clinical course of patients with adrenocortical cancer. *Cancer* 71:3119, 1993.

Carcinoma of the Thyroid and Parathyroid Glands

Paula M. Termuhlen

Thyroid Cancer

EPIDEMIOLOGY

Thyroid cancer constitutes approximately 1% of all human malignancies, with an estimated incidence in the United States of 16,100 in 1997. The majority of these cases—approximately 70%—occur in women. Carcinoma of the thyroid is considered an indolent disease, with many deaths occurring from other causes. An estimated 1,200 patients die annually of this disease. Overall, thyroid cancer is the most common endocrine malignancy.

The prevalence of thyroid nodules increases linearly with age, with spontaneous nodules occurring at a rate of 0.08% per year beginning early in life and extending into the eighth decade. Clinically apparent nodules are present in 4–7% of the adult population and occur more commonly in women.

Few environmental risk factors have been confirmed for thyroid carcinoma, with the exception of radiation exposure. A history of ionizing radiation in childhood is a major risk factor for thyroid malignancy, usually the papillary type. Approximately 9% of thyroid cancers are associated with prior radiation exposure. The risk of cancer from radiation increases linearly with doses up to 20 Gy, with thyroid ablation occurring at higher levels. The risk of developing thyroid cancer decreases rapidly with increasing age at exposure. Those 15 years of age and older do not have a demonstrable radiation-dose-dependent risk for thyroid cancer. In general, radiation-induced thyroid cancer is biologically similar to sporadic thyroid cancer and should be treated in the same manner. However, recent information regarding the high incidence of biologically aggressive thyroid cancer found in children exposed to radiation after the Chernobyl nuclear disaster suggests that radiation dose and tumor behavior may be linked.

Recently, associations have been described between thyroid cancer and several other inherited syndromes, such as familial polyposis, Gardner's syndrome and Cowden disease (familial goiter and skin hamartoma). In addition, papillary thyroid cancer may occur with increased frequency in some families with breast, ovarian, renal, or central nervous system malignancies. Medullary thyroid cancer occurs with a higher frequency in patients who have Hashimoto's thyroiditis. The mechanism of these associations is not well understood.

Within the last 5 years, rapid progress has been made in the identification of genes that are linked to thyroid cancer. Medullary thyroid cancer occurs as part of the multiple endocrine neoplasia type II (MEN-II) syndromes or as part of familial medullary thyroid carcinoma approximately 25–35% of the time. More than 90% of patients with MEN-IIa and MEN-IIb will develop medullary thyroid cancer. The identification of the RET proto-oncogene has made screening available for patients who have a genetic basis for their disease. By means of a point mutation, the normally expressed RET oncogene is activated to cause malignant transformation of the parafollicular C cells into medullary thyroid cancer. A rearrangement of the same RET proto-oncogene appears to make follicular cells express the papillary thyroid cancer oncogene (PTC1, PTC2, or PTC3), causing papillary thyroid cancer. The discovery of the RET oncogene has had significant clinical impact, affecting the screening and prophylactic treatment of patients who are members of the multiple endocrine neoplasia kindreds. Other oncogenes involved in the pathogenesis of thyroid neoplasias include Trk-T1, met, H-ras, K-ras, N-ras, myc, fos, and p53. The clinical significance of these oncogenes remains to be defined.

PATHOLOGY

Most malignant tumors of the thyroid gland are of glandular epithelial origin, with the remaining types arising from parafollicular C cells or from nonepithelial stromal elements. Primary carcinomas of the thyroid gland are often classified as differentiated thyroid cancer (papillary and follicular carcinomas), medullary thyroid carcinomas, and undifferentiated (anaplastic) thyroid carcinomas. Other, less common carcinomas include Hürthle cell (a follicular carcinoma variant), lymphomas, squamous cell carcinomas, sarcomas, and carcinomas metastatic from other sites.

Papillary carcinoma is the most well-differentiated form of thyroid carcinoma, representing 60% of all cases. Multifocality is a prominent feature of this pathologic type and has been documented in up to 80% of patients with papillary cancer. Papillary carcinoma occurs as an irregular solid or cystic mass that arises from follicular epithelium. It is nonencapsulated but sharply circumscribed. Microscopically, the hallmark is papillary fronds of epithelium. Rounded calcific deposits (psammoma bodies) can be found in 50% of lesions. Because papillary carcinomas are not encapsulated and invade regional lymphatics, cervical lymph node metastases are common. Papillary carcinoma is the predominant type found in patients with a history of prior radiation exposure.

Follicular carcinoma is the second most common malignancy of the thyroid and is considered a well-differentiated tumor, comprising 15–20% of thyroid cancers. It is often difficult to histologically confirm the diagnosis of follicular carcinoma because of its similarity to benign follicular adenomas. Follicular carcinoma is usually encapsulated and consists of highly cellular follicles; most are single, solid, and noncystic without central necrosis. This pathologic type is the most common found in association with endemic goiter. Hematogenous metastases rather than lymphatic metastases are more common with follicular carcinoma.

Hürthle cell neoplasms are thought to be variants of follicular carcinoma within the thyroid yet are distinct pathologic entities.

They represent 5% of thyroid carcinomas. The histopathologic diagnosis of malignancy, as in follicular carcinoma, is difficult to make without the presence of vascular or capsular invasion. The incidence of lymph node metastases is slightly higher in Hürthle cell carcinomas than in follicular carcinomas.

Medullary carcinomas arise from calcitonin-secreting parafollicular C cells of the thyroid gland. These lesions represent 5% of all thyroid cancers, with 20% of patients exhibiting an autosomal dominant inheritance pattern. The sporadic form usually occurs unilaterally, whereas familial forms are bilateral or are associated with C-cell hyperplasia in the contralateral lobe. In inherited forms, the bilateral or multicentric C-cell hyperplasia precedes and later undergoes transformation to medullary thyroid carcinoma. Histologically, medullary carcinoma is an ill-defined, nonencapsulated, invasive mass. It is composed of columns of epithelial cells and dense stroma that stains for amyloid and collagen. Calcitonin may be identified by immunohistochemical stains. These lesions are slow growing but metastasize by both lymphatic and hematogenous routes. Regional metastases occur early in the course of the disease, usually before the primary reaches 2 cm, and are present in 50% of patients at the time of diagnosis. Cervical and upper mediastinal lymph nodes are the usual sites involved. Overall 10-year survival rates are 90% with disease confined to the thyroid, 70% with cervical metastases, and 20% with distant metastases. Prognosis for medullary thyroid carcinoma falls between that of anaplastic tumors and well-differentiated tumors. Poor prognostic factors include age greater than 50 years, metastases at the time of diagnosis, and MEN-IIb. Seventy percent of the patients with MEN-IIb have metastasis at the time of diagnosis; less than 5% survive 5 years.

Anaplastic carcinoma is undifferentiated and represented by small cells of variable characteristics. These are rapidly growing tumors, usually greater than 6 cm and often inoperable. Anaplastic thyroid carcinoma is aggressive. These tumors invade local structures and metastasize locally and distantly. At the time of diagnosis, 25% are invading the trachea, 90% have regional metastases, and 50% have distant metastases to the lung. Although rare, it is considered one of the deadliest malignancies. The development of anaplastic thyroid carcinoma has been associated with previous well-differentiated thyroid cancer that has become undifferentiated with time or during a recurrence. Treatment seldom results in cure, with a mean survival of 6 months and a 5-year survival rate of 7%.

Lymphomas are also small cell tumors that enlarge rapidly. Lymphomas may be primary or secondary. In patients with disseminated lymphoma, 20% involve the thyroid at autopsy. Histologically, non-Hodgkin's, histiocytic lymphoma is the most common form of primary thyroid lymphoma. Thyroid lymphoma is rare, occurring with a peak onset in the seventh decade and a 6:1 female preponderance. Prognosis is related to the extent of disease at the time of diagnosis. When lymphoma is confined to the thyroid gland, the 5-year survival rate is 75–85% with radiation therapy. Survival at 5 years decreases to 35% with regional metastases and 5% with disseminated disease.

DIAGNOSIS

Most patients with thyroid cancer will have no specific symptoms. The most common presentation is the identification of a mass or nodule. A change in the size of a thyroid nodule or pain from hemorrhage into a nodule may occasionally bring the patient to the physician. Hoarseness, dysphagia, dyspnea, or hemoptysis are symptoms resulting from invasion of surrounding anatomic structures and are rare in well-differentiated thyroid carcinomas. Occasionally, the initial presentation may be that of a palpable lymph node in the neck.

A thorough physical examination is the most important diagnostic step. The presence of a single or dominant nodule, usually over 1 cm in diameter with a hard consistency and fixation, is characteristic of cancer. The presence of discrete 1- to 2-cm lymph nodes in conjunction with a thyroid nodule suggests malignancy. Palpable adenopathy is most often found along the middle and lower portions of the jugular vein but may be located lateral to the sternocleidomastoid muscle in the lower portion of the posterior cervical triangle. Physical findings of concern are vocal cord paralysis, fixation of the thyroid nodule, and tracheal deviation or invasion. Cervical spine flexibility should be assessed to ensure that the necessary hyperextension of the neck can be achieved for adequate operative exposure. Laryngeal function should be evaluated with either indirect mirror or flexible fiberoptic examination.

Various diagnostic tests are available to help distinguish benign from malignant disease. The ultimate goal is to avoid operating on benign lesions whenever possible. Initial evaluation of a patient with a single thyroid nodule consists of thyroid function studies, including thyroid-stimulating hormone, serum calcium measurement, thyroid antibodies, and a fine-needle aspiration (FNA). The FNA with an interpretation of cytology by an experienced pathologist is probably the single most useful procedure. This test is safe and cost-effective. When performed by an experienced cytopathologist, accuracy in the diagnosis of thyroid cancer is greater than 90%. The accuracy is greatest for lesions between 1 and 4 cm, because smaller lesions are difficult to sample and larger lesions have an increased sampling error as a result of the large area of the lesion. Lesions are generally classified as negative, positive, or suspicious for malignancy. Distinguishing a follicular adenoma from a follicular carcinoma is not possible with an FNA biopsy because pathologic examination demonstrating capsular or vascular invasion is required. Thus patients with the diagnosis of follicular neoplasm require surgical intervention for complete diagnosis. Individuals with a finding of benign colloid nodule or thyroiditis are observed with or without thyroid suppression. Growth of a nodule while on thyroid suppression is an indication for surgical removal. Specific indications for surgical intervention in thyroid abnormalities are listed in Table 16-1.

If a patient is diagnosed with thyroid cancer, a chest radiograph should be obtained to assess for pulmonary metastases and tracheal deviation. Patients diagnosed with medullary thyroid cancer will require additional testing to assess for the presence of other components of the multiple endocrine neoplasias.

Table 16-1.   Indications for surgical intervention for thyroid abnormalities

1. FNA of thyroid nodule suspicious for carcinoma or follicular adenoma

2. Thyroid nodule in a patient younger than 20 years, older than 60 years with FNA findings of atypia or in a patient with a history of irradiation

3. Thyroid mass associated with vocal cord paralysis, regional tissue invasion, cervical lymph node metastases or fixation to surrounding tissues

4. Hyperfunctioning thyroid nodule in a young patient

5. Solitary cold nodules or dominant nodules in a multinodular goiter that fail to respond to suppressive therapy

Ultrasonography of the thyroid is an accurate method for establishing the consistency of the nodule (solid or cystic), multicentricity, and presence of lymph node enlargement. Ultrasound can detect lesions as small as 1 mm; however, the percentage of these small lesions that are malignant is unknown. Unfortunately, interpretation depends on the experience of the imaging expert, and currently no specific sonographic criteria can distinguish benign from malignant nodules. Solid lesions have a 15–20% risk of malignancy. The risk in cystic lesions greater than 4 cm is 15% and is considered minimal in smaller lesions. In addition, ultrasound-assisted FNA is useful when the tumor is difficult to palpate or in a deep location. Ultrasonography is particularly useful in long-term management of patients with thyroid nodules.

Radionucleotide scintigraphy (^{99}Tc-pertechnetate, iodine ^{125}I or ^{131}I) was previously used as the first diagnostic step in evaluating palpable thyroid masses. Because most thyroid carcinomas and many benign thyroid nodules appear cold on scan, the main limitation of this imaging modality is its inability to distinguish between benign and malignant lesions. Approximately 16% of cold nodules, 9% of warm, and 4% of hot lesions harbor a malignancy. Although a cold lesion has the greatest probability of being malignant, the presence of a hot lesion on thyroid scan does not exclude malignancy. In general, the use of nuclear thyroid scans has been replaced by FNA for diagnosis.

Other diagnostic imaging studies are seldom needed for evaluation of a patient with a thyroid nodule. Computerized tomography (CT) and magnetic resonance imaging (MRI) are useful in large or recurrent cancers suspected of invasion into the surrounding soft tissue. When indicated by the history and physical findings, CT or MRI of the neck and upper mediastinum may be used to delineate extrathyroidal extension or to determine the presence of significant cervical and/or mediastinal metastases.

Preoperative laboratory assessment is similar to the testing obtained for the diagnosis of a nodule. It should include thyroid function testing and a serum calcium measurement. Thyroid function studies do not help in making the diagnosis of cancer, but the presence of hypothyroidism or hyperthyroidism in a patient with a thyroid nodule is important, particularly when considering general anesthesia. Parathyroid function should be assessed by measuring calcium level, as the incidence of parathyroid adenomas and other hyperfunctioning anomalies of the parathyroid gland are more frequent in the presence of thyroid nodules or carcinoma. Thyroid antibody tests are important when thyroiditis is a consideration. Serum calcitonin measurements are only indicated when a family history of medullary carcinoma is present or an MEN syndrome is likely. Serum thyroglobulin levels are useful mainly for follow-up studies following treatment of differentiated thyroid carcinoma and are not a part of the diagnostic evaluation.

TREATMENT

Controversy continues over what to do in the presence of a thyroid nodule, the extent of resection necessary in cases of papillary and follicular cancer, the role of postresection thyroid hormone suppression, and the appropriate use of postoperative therapeutic radioactive ^{131}I. Because of the length of time to recurrence and the overall good prognosis of most patients with thyroid cancer, prospective studies are in progress but have yet to be completed at the time of this writing. What follows are the general guidelines used at the University of Texas M. D. Anderson Cancer Center.

Staging and Prognosis

With respect to differentiated thyroid carcinoma, several classification and staging schemes have been introduced. However, no consensus has emerged favoring any one of these methods. The most commonly used are the AMES (Age, Metastasis, Extent, Size) system, which divides patients into low- and high-risk groups; the TNM (Tumor, Nodes, Metastasis), as used by the American Joint Commission on Cancer; the AGES (Age, Grade, Extent, Size) and MACIS (Metastasis, Age, Completeness of Resection, Invasion, Size), as proposed by the Mayo Clinic; and the University of Chicago system, which classifies patients from I to IV, depending on disease limited to the gland (I), lymph node involvement (II), extrathyroidal invasion (III), and distant metastases (IV). Given its relative ease of use, widespread availability, and superior predictive value, the TNM staging system is recommended as the standard staging scheme for clinical use (Table 16-2). Prognosis of patients with well-differentiated thyroid carcinoma who are stage I is excellent, with 20-year survival rates of nearly 100%. Patients with stage IV disease have a 5-year survival of only 25%. Within the group of well-differentiated thyroid cancer patients are a small number who have more aggressive disease and for whom none of the current staging systems apply. As molecular markers of disease are developed, these patients may be able to be identified at early stages and offered additional treatment.

In general, the prognosis for papillary thyroid carcinoma is influenced by age, gender, extent of disease, and volume of the primary tumor. More than 50% of patients have metastases to the regional lymphatics, and 10% develop hematogenous metastases. The prognostic significance of lymph node metastases continues to be debated; in patients with papillary cancer who are less than 40 years of age, the significance is considered negligible. The min-

Table 16-2.   TNM classification system for differentiated thyroid carcinoma

Definition

T1	Tumor diameter < 1 cm
T2	Primary tumor diameter 1–4 cm
T3	Primary tumor diameter >4 cm
T4	Primary tumor invasion beyond the thyroid gland capsule
TX	Primary tumor size unknown, but without extrathyroidal invasion
N0	No metastatic nodes
N1	Ipsilateral cervical node metastases
N2	Bilateral, midline, contralateral, or mediastinal node metastases
NX	Nodes not assessed at surgery
M0	No distant metastates
M1	Distant metastases
MX	Distant metastases not assessed

Stages

	Patient age < 45 years	Patients age 45 years or older
Stage I	Any T, any N, M0	T1, N0, M0
Stage II	Any T, any N, M1	T2, N0, M0
		T3, N0, M0
Stage III		T4, N0, M0
		Any T, N1, M0
Stage IV		Any T, any N, M1

imal effect of lymph node metastases on prognosis is reflected in the American Joint Committee on Cancer (AJCC) staging system (see Table 16-2). It is only for patients over 45 years of age that lymph node metastases are factored into the staging prognosis. The diminished importance of lymph node metastases is based on data suggesting that microscopic metastases are present in up to 80% of lymph nodes examined, yet only 10% of patients develop clinically significant disease. In addition, if long-term survival is examined in patients under 40 years of age, the presence of positive nodes is not a significant negative prognostic factor in papillary carcinoma. Survival for thyroid carcinoma according to stage is shown in Table 16-3.

The prognosis of follicular carcinoma is thought to be poorer than that of papillary carcinoma, perhaps because of the higher incidence of hematogenous metastases. However, treatment decisions and prognosis are based on well-differentiated thyroid malignancies as a group.

Surgical Resection

Surgical resection is the principal treatment used in thyroid cancer. Accepted surgical management varies from a thyroid

Table 16-3.   Ten-year survival rates for thyroid carcinoma by stage

Stage	10-year survival (%)
I	95
II	50–95
III	15–50
IV	<15

lobectomy and isthmusectomy to a total thyroidectomy and modified neck dissection.

The management of well-differentiated thyroid cancer is controversial. Proponents of total thyroidectomy argue that (1) this operation can be performed safely with a 2% incidence of permanent recurrent nerve injury or permanent hypoparathyroidism; (2) foci of papillary carcinoma are found in both thyroid lobes in up to 85% of patients, and 5–10% of recurrences occur in the contralateral lobe; (3) residual thyroid tissue left after less than total thyroidectomy hampers radioiodide ablation of thyroid bed remnants, treatment of metastatic disease, and use of thyroglobulin measurements as a tumor marker of recurrence; and (4) one-half of patients who die from recurrent thyroid carcinoma die from complications of central neck recurrence. Advocates of more conservative procedures such as thyroid lobectomy and isthmusectomy or near total thyroidectomy argue that (1) there is a decreased risk of recurrent laryngeal nerve and parathyroid gland injury with conservative surgery; (2) it is rare for a total thyroidectomy to remove all the thyroid gland; (3) occult foci of papillary carcinoma left behind with conservative surgery are rarely of clinical significance; (4) clinically significant recurrences after conservative surgery can be safely managed by reoperation. Retrospective studies suggest that the risk of recurrence of thyroid carcinoma within the thyroid bed is reduced by total thyroidectomy as compared with lesser procedures.

Lobectomy with isthmusectomy is an appropriate treatment for a small papillary cancer <1.0 cm in diameter and in patients at low risk of death from thyroid cancer (i.e., age less than 45 years and no metastasis). An incidental microscopic carcinoma found at the time of thyroidectomy for other reasons does not require further treatment.

At M. D. Anderson we perform a total thyroidectomy for all well-differentiated carcinomas >1.0 cm, extrathyroidal tumor extension, patients 45 years of age and more, or patients with metastases. Although total thyroidectomy is our treatment of choice for follicular carcinoma and Hürthle cell carcinoma, the diagnosis may not be ascertained by frozen-section examination at the time of surgery. Patients with a minimally invasive, small (<1 cm) follicular tumor or a single, well-encapsulated, benign Hürthle cell neoplasm may be treated by thyroid lobectomy and isthmusectomy. All other patients should undergo a total thyroidectomy. When the diagnosis of follicular carcinoma is confirmed postoperatively, a completion thyroidectomy should be performed in high-risk patients (i.e., age >45 years, lesions >1 cm, patients with distant metastasis). In well-differentiated carcinomas, total thyroidectomy is combined with a modified neck dissection when clinical evidence of lymph node metastases is present. Important structures such as the recurrent and superior laryngeal nerves, spinal accessory nerve, sternocleidomastoid muscle, parathyroid glands, esophagus, and trachea should be preserved unless invasion by tumor is present.

In medullary carcinoma, all patients should undergo a total thyroidectomy combined with a central paratracheal neck dissection to remove all disease. This procedure is important because medullary tumors do not concentrate radioiodine, the disease is multifocal, metastases occur early, and nonsurgical treatments are ineffective. Identifying C-cell hyperplasia in the contralateral lobe indicates a familial case and the need for family screening.

Anaplastic carcinoma is an aggressive lesion that is rarely resectable at presentation. The diagnosis is usually made by core-needle biopsy. Treatment consists of combination radiotherapy and chemotherapy. Resectable lesions are treated by total thyroidectomy and wide local excision of adjacent soft tissues. Resected patients are treated with postoperative adjuvant chemotherapy and radiotherapy.

Surgical Technique

Surgical resection of a possible thyroid cancer requires meticulous dissection of the ipsilateral thyroid compartment, identification and preservation of the recurrent laryngeal nerve, and complete resection of the affected lobe and thyroid isthmus. Identification of the ipsilateral parathyroid glands should be attempted, but preservation may be impossible if there is extensive invasion by cancer or clinical metastases in the paratracheal area. If the diagnosis of cancer is confirmed by frozen-section histologic examination of the specimen, total thyroidectomy is completed by resecting the opposite lobe, taking special care to identify and spare parathyroid glands and their blood supply. Once the thyroid gland is removed, the posterior surface is carefully inspected for any possible parathyroid tissue. If the parathyroid is identified, a portion is sent for frozen-section examination, with the remnant kept in physiologic solution. If parathyroid tissue is confirmed, the preserved portion is minced and implanted in a small pocket created in the sternocleidomastoid muscle.

The surgical procedure should be carried out under general anesthesia. The approach to the thyroid gland itself is through a transverse incision, approximately one or two finger breadths above the clavicles. Flaps are elevated superiorly to the level of the thyroid notch and inferiorly to the suprasternal notch in the subplatysmal plane. Separation of the fascia between the strap muscles and the sternocleidomastoid muscles is done to facilitate exposure of the gland and allow inspection of the lower jugular lymph nodes. The strap muscles are separated in the midline and can be divided on the side of the primary tumor if necessary. Portions of the strap muscles adherent to the gland are resected with the specimen. The thyroid compartment may be approached laterally along the anterior border of the sternocleidomastoid muscle or medially through the midline raphe of the strap muscles.

Palpable adenopathy or clinical suspicion of lymphatic metastasis in the high-risk patient requires that a neck dissection be performed. In these cases, all areolar and lymphatic tissue along the internal jugular vein and carotid vessels from the subdigastric area down to the supraclavicular fossa is resected. The middle thyroid veins are divided during this portion of the procedure. The dissection is continued medially, allowing for identification and dissection of the recurrent laryngeal nerve. All lymphoareolar tissue in the thyroid compartment and upper mediastinum to the level of the innominate vein is accessible through a collar incision. This tissue contains the lymph nodes of the central compartment and is dissected medially and superiorly in continuity with the specimen. A nonrecurrent laryngeal nerve on the right side may be recognized as it originates high from the vagus nerve. Nonrecurrent laryngeal nerves may be found in proximity to the superior thyroid vessels or the inferior thyroid artery.

The thyroid vessels are identified and ligated close to the gland. The superior pole vessels are individually transected with a small curved or right angle hemostat. The superior laryngeal nerve should be identified between the thyroid vessels as it crosses the constrictor muscle and enters the cricothyroid muscle. Caution is warranted, as the position of the superior nerve in relation to the vascular pedicle may vary.

Dissection of the gland is continued inferiorly on the posterior aspect of the gland, incising the fascia that secures the gland (visceral and suspensory ligament). The recurrent laryngeal nerve, if not previously located, is identified in the paratracheal groove inferior to the gland and is dissected superiorly. The inferior artery is identified and its branches are individually ligated as they enter the thyroid gland, taking care not to injure the recurrent nerve. The anatomic relationship of the nerve and the inferior artery is extremely variable. Also, the nerve may divide into several branches at the level of the inferior thyroid artery. All nerve branches should be preserved in the course of the dissection. Careful dissection is continued up to where the nerve enters the larynx. Eighty percent of superior parathyroid glands are located within 1 cm of the intersection of the recurrent laryngeal nerve and the inferior thyroid artery, usually within the thyroid fascia. About 15% are located within the thyroid capsule, and the remainder are in the retropharyngeal or retroesophageal spaces. The location of the inferior parathyroids is far more variable. They are usually anterior and lateral to the recurrent laryngeal nerves. Compromise of the blood supply to the parathyroid glands is the most common cause of hypoparathyroidism in the postoperative period. Careful attention to dissection of the inferior thyroid vessels and their branches is warranted. Often a small portion of thyroid tissue may have to be spared (subtotal resection) to preserve the vascular pedicle to the parathyroid tissue. Meticulous dissection of the parathyroid glands and their vascular supply, and autotransplantation of devascularized parathyroid tissue are important techniques that have contributed to a lower incidence of permanent hypoparathyroidism. All parathyroid-like tissue should be inspected and left attached to individual vascular pedicles. In addition, distinguishing between lymph nodes and parathyroid glands may be difficult. If confusion arises, biopsies should be taken and sent for frozen-section diagnosis. Dissection of the opposite lobe, when indicated, proceeds similarly to the dissection of the involved lobe.

Any extrathyroidal extension of carcinoma into surrounding tissues needs to be clearly delineated. Judicious resection of the invaded structure should be accomplished—including resection of laryngeal nerves, tracheal rings, or portions of the larynx—to ensure complete surgical extirpation. Local invasion of tissues surrounding the thyroid, though rare, is a source of significant morbidity and mortality. Uncontrolled local recurrence is a major cause of mortality from thyroid cancer, making local control a key issue in these patients. Fortunately, locally invasive thyroid carcinoma can often be resected with a much narrower margin than other carcinomas that arise in tissues surrounding the thyroid.

Neck Dissection

The necessity and extent of neck dissection for follicular and papillary carcinomas is another subject of controversy. Follicular carcinoma rarely metastasizes to the regional lymph nodes, whereas papillary carcinoma frequently spreads to regional nodes. Neck dissection is obviously indicated for palpable adenopathy. Elective neck dissections have not conclusively been proven to be more effective than observation and therapeutic dissection. Careful intraoperative assessment of the regional nodes and sampling or dissection of the central compartment lymph nodes is advisable, however, during surgical resection of papillary carcinomas to avoid the necessity of later repeat dissection for recurrent disease.

When neck dissection for differentiated thyroid carcinoma is indicated, all the nodal groups at highest risk for metastasis should be included. The central or interjugular tracheal compartment contains the first echelon of lymph nodes for the thyroid gland. The nodes along the jugular vein from the subdigastric area to the root of the neck are important metastatic sites. Another route of lymphatic spread for thyroid cancer is along the inferior thyroid artery as it courses behind the common carotid artery and to the lower portion of the posterior triangle of the neck. The classic radical neck dissection, with removal of internal jugular vein, sternocleidomastoid muscle, and accessory nerve, is seldom necessary. Most often, a comprehensive modified neck dissection sparing the above structures is the appropriate cancer operation for metastatic thyroid cancer. A central, bilateral neck dissection, clearing all lymphatic tissue from hyoid bone to the brachiocephalic vein and between the carotid arteries, is considered standard therapy in medullary carcinoma. A formal modified neck dissection is reserved for patients with positive nodes or on the ipsilateral side of patients with a thyroid mass and sporadic medullary thyroid cancer.

Adjuvant Therapy

As in the other aspects of diagnosis and treatment of well-differentiated thyroid carcinomas, controversy exists about the use of adjuvant treatment in the management of this disease. The goal of treatment is maximum disease-free survival. Retrospective studies of patient cohorts who have been followed postoperatively for many years (often more than 10–20 years) suggest that multimodality adjuvant therapy decreases local recurrence and may improve survival. The mainstay of adjuvant treatment in well-differentiated thyroid carcinoma is radioactive ^{131}I treatment and thyroid stimulating hormone suppression. The use of therapeutic radioactive ablation of remnant thyroid tissue after thyroidectomy is well established, though criteria for the use of postoperative radioactive iodine vary from institution to institution. Our practice after total thyroidectomy for follicular or papillary carcinoma of the thyroid is to delay thyroid hormone replacement for 4–6 weeks to maximize iodine uptake during scanning. For up to 2 weeks postoperatively, patients can receive short-acting thyroid hormone replacement (liothyronine) and then complete cessation of thyroid hormone replacement until after scanning and radioactive thyroid ablation. Most patients will develop some symptoms of hypothyroidism. A tracer dose of radioactive iodine is then administered and a whole-body scan is performed. This allows scintigraphic staging of disease and may show the presence and extent of metastases that are minimally recognizable by conventional techniques.

Most patients will have uptake of radioactivity in the thyroid bed. Thyroid remnant ablation is recommended for all patients with differentiated thyroid carcinoma who are 45 years of age or older, those whose primary tumor was >1 cm in diameter or was multifocal, and those with extrathyroidal disease due to tissue invasion or metastases. The standard ablative dose of ^{131}I for patients with papillary thyroid carcinoma whose tumor was less than 3 cm in diameter without extrathyroid invasion and few or no lymph nodes involved is 29 mCi, which can be administered as an outpatient. Remnant ablation in all other patients with well-differentiated thyroid carcinoma is 100 mCi, which requires overnight hospitalization.

Patients who have evidence of residual disease or metastases on their initial postoperative thyroid scan receive higher doses of ^{131}I in the range of 150–200 mCi. These doses or higher may be administered for recurrent or persistent disease if subsequent thyroid scans demonstrate the presence of cancer.

After surgery and subsequent ^{131}I ablation therapy, all patients receive hormonal replacement treatment (levothyroxin sodium) at a dose of 100–200 mg/day. The dose varies among patients and needs to be adjusted to suppress the thyrotropin (TSH) to low or undetectable levels. The dose typically requires modification 3–4 months after completion of treatment.

Adjuvant therapy for other types of thyroid cancers such as Hürthle cell, medullary, and anaplastic carcinoma is less effective. The problem with Hürthle cell and medullary carcinomas is their lack of consistent uptake of radioactive iodine. In addition, they arise from a tissue that does not contain TSH receptors, and thus they are not sensitive to suppression.

Overall cytotoxic chemotherapy has not been very effective in the treatment of thyroid carcinomas. However, radiation therapy combined with doxorubicin has been used in patients with anaplastic carcinomas with some response.

SURVEILLANCE

Most recurrences of well-differentiated thyroid carcinoma occur within the first 5 years after initial treatment, but recurrences can occur even decades later. More than 50% of patients with papillary carcinomas of the thyroid who die of their disease die with central neck disease, whereas most of the recurrences of follicular carcinomas occur distantly. Patients with papillary carcinoma of the thyroid have a high (40%) incidence of lymph node metastases. The most common sites of distant metastases for thyroid cancers are lungs, bone, soft tissues, brain, liver, and adrenal glands. Lung metastases more commonly occur in young patients, whereas bone metastases occur more commonly in older patients. A coordinated plan of follow-up for thyroid carcinomas must consider the varied presentations possible for recurrent disease. Most patients are seen every 6 months for 1–2 years postoperatively and then yearly. Follow-up visits typically include measuring the serum thyroglobulin level and a chest x-ray. Thyroglobulin values normally drop after thyroidectomy or ablation and serve as a sensitive indicator of recurrent or persistent disease. This protocol may vary, depending on the risk group of the patient and special circumstances. When indicated, a repeat ^{131}I scan is done after temporary (4–6 weeks) deletion of hormonal replacement. Subsequent therapeutic doses of radioactive iodine may be administered.

Follow-up for medullary carcinoma differs in that no scanning or thyroglobulin measurements are used. Instead, calcitonin or pentagastrin-stimulated calcitonin is used to follow these patients. Similarly, Hürthle cell, anaplastic carcinoma, and lymphoma cannot be followed by thyroid scanning and require regular physical exam and radiographic or ultrasound studies for follow-up.

Parathyroid Carcinoma

EPIDEMIOLOGY

Carcinoma of the parathyroid gland is a rare lesion. Its incidence as a cause of hyperparathyroidism varies from 0.5% to 4.0%. The incidence is equally divided between men and women and usually is diagnosed in the fifth decade. The rarity of this tumor has limited the accumulation of natural history data and etiologic factors that might cause it. Associations with familial hyperparathyroidism MEN-I syndrome, and chronic renal dialysis have been described. External irradiation has also been reported in association with parathyroid carcinoma.

The natural history of parathyroid carcinoma is one of a slow-growing, persistent, locally recurrent tumor. The local recurrence rate has been estimated to range from 36% to 69%, and overall survival is less than 50%. The major cause of death is hypercalcemia. Distant metastases tend to occur late, with lung, liver, bone, and pancreas being frequent sites.

CLINICAL PRESENTATION

The clinical presentation of patients with parathyroid carcinoma is usually severe hypercalcemia. The serum calcium level in carcinoma patients averages more than 14 mg/dl, compared with lower levels of 10 or 11 mg/dl seen with benign causes of hyperparathyroidism. As a result, renal (60%) and skeletal (50%) involvement in parathyroid carcinoma is significantly increased compared with benign causes of primary hyperparathyroidism, where renal and skeletal disease occur in 48% and 20% of patients, respectively. The presence of a palpable neck mass in a patient with hyperparathyroidism should raise the suspicion of parathyroid carcinoma.

DIAGNOSIS

Preoperative localization studies are useful in parathyroid carcinoma. Real-time ultrasound of the neck is an effective localization study. Malignancy is suggested by signs of gross invasion and marked irregularity of the tumor margins.

Unless the tumor is clinically virulent, it is difficult to differentiate benign from malignant. The findings of invasion of surrounding structures, metastases, or recurrent tumor point to malignancy. The histologic criteria for a diagnosis of parathyroid malignancy are (1) fibrous capsule and/or fibrous trabeculae, (2) a trabecular or rosettelike cellular architecture, (3) presence of mitotic figures, and (4) capsular or vascular invasion.

TREATMENT

Surgery is the most effective therapy for carcinoma of the parathyroid glands. Parathyroid cancer has a propensity for local recurrence and rarely metastasizes to regional nodes. Therefore resection should be performed as an en bloc procedure. En bloc in this case usually requires a thyroid lobectomy and excision of paratracheal alveolar tissue, local lymph nodes, and the thymic tongue. A neck dissection is not necessary at the time of the initial procedure unless clinically positive lymph node metastases are demonstrated.

METASTATIC DISEASE

Localization of metastatic foci is important if treatment of recurrent parathyroid cancer is planned. Thallium chloride scintiscanning and 99mTc-SestaMIBI are useful for locating cervical or upper mediastinal recurrence. CT scan is effective for identification and localization of mediastinal or pulmonary metastases. Venous catheterization and selective venous sampling are helpful in situations where noninvasive studies fail to show recurrent tumors.

The principal cause of death and the most difficult problem in the long-term management of patients with carcinoma of the parathyroid gland is hypercalcemia. Surgical excision of recurrent carcinoma offers the best palliation. There are no effective chemotherapeutic agents that inhibit tumor growth or affect the secretion of parathyroid hormone in parathyroid carcinoma; as a result, medical management is used only to control hypercalcemia.

Selected References

Anderson BJ, Samaan NA, Vassilopoulou-Sellin R, et al. Parathyroid carcinoma: Features and difficulties in diagnosis and management. *Surgery* 94:906, 1983.

Austin JR, El-Naggar AK, Goepfert H. Thyroid cancers II: Medullary, anaplastic, lymphoma, sarcoma, squamous cell. *Otolaryngol Clin North Am* 29:611, 1996.

Devine RM, Edis AJ, Banks PM. Primary lymphoma of the thyroid: A review of the Mayo Clinic experience through 1978. *World J Surg* 5:33, 1981.

Duh QY, Sancho JJ, Greenspan FS, et al. Medullary thyroid carcinoma: The need for early diagnosis and total thyroidectomy. *Arch Surg* 124:1206, 1989.

Gagel RF, Goepfert H, Callender DL. Changing concepts in the pathogenesis and management of thyroid carcinoma. *CA* 46:261, 1996.

Goldman ND, Coniglio JU. Thyroid cancers I: Papillary, follicular, and Hurthle cell. *Otolaryngol Clin North Am* 29:593, 1996.

Hay ID, Grant CS, Taylor WF, et al. Ipsilateral lobectomy versus bilateral lobar resection in papillary thyroid carcinoma: A retrospective analysis of surgical outcome using a novel prognostic scoring system. *Surgery* 102:1089, 1987.

Kenady DE, McGrath PC, Schwartz RW. Treatment of thyroid malignancies. *Curr Opin Oncol* 3:128, 1991.

Krubsack AJ, Wilson SD, Lawson TL, et al. Prospective comparison of radionucleotide, computed tomographic, sonographic, and magnetic resonance localization of parathyroid tumors. *Surgery* 106:639, 1989.

Maffioli L, Steens J, Pauwels E, et al. Applications of 99mTc-sestamibi in oncology. *Tumori* 82:12, 1996

Mazzaferri EL, Jhiang SM. Long-term impact of initial surgical and medical therapy on papillary and follicular thyroid cancer. *Am J Med* 97:418, 1994.

Mazzaferri EL, Robyn J. Postsurgical management of differentiated thyroid carcinoma. *Otolaryngol Clin North Am* 29:637, 1996.

McLeod MK, Thompson NW. Hürthle cell neoplasm of the thyroid. *Otolaryngol Clin North Am* 23:441, 1990.

Merino MJ, Boice JD, Ron E, et al. Thyroid cancer: A lethal endocrine neoplasm. *Ann Intern Med* 115:133, 1991.

Nel CJC, van Heerden JA, Goellner JR, et al. Anaplastic carcinoma of the thyroid: A clinicopathologic study of 82 cases. *Mayo Clin Proc* 60:51, 1985.

Niederle B, Roka R, Schemper M, et al. Surgical treatment of distant metastases in differentiated thyroid cancer: Indication and results. *Surgery* 100:1088, 1986.

Norton JA. Reoperative parathyroid surgery: Indication, intraoperative decision-making and results. *Prog Surg* 18:133, 1986.

Obara T, Fujimoto Y. Diagnosis and treatment of patients with parathyroid carcinoma: An update and review. *World J Surg* 15:738, 1991.

Parker SL, Tong T, Bolden S. Cancer statistics, 1997. *CA* 5, 1997.

Ron E, Saftlas AF. Head and neck radiation carcinogenesis: Epidemiologic evidence. *Head Neck Surg* 115: 403, 1996.

Rosen IB, Sutcliffe SB, Gospodarowicz MK, et al. The role of surgery in the management of thyroid lymphoma. *Surgery* 104:1095, 1988.

Samaan NA, Schultz PN, Hickey RC, et al. The results of various modalities of treatment of well differentiated thyroid carcinoma: A retrospective review of 1599 patients. *J Clin Endocrinol Metab* 75:714, 1992.

Sandelin K, Thompson NW, Bondeson L. Metastatic parathyroid carcinoma: Dilemmas in management. *Surgery* 110: 978, 1991.

Sherman SI. Clinicopathologic staging of differentiated thyroid carcinoma. *UpToDate in Medicine* [CD-ROM] Editor-in-Chief, Rose B. 5 (1) onwards, UpToDate, Wellesley, MA 1997.

Sherman SI. Management of differentiated thyroid carcinoma: An overview. *UpToDate in Medicine* [CD-ROM] Editor-in-Chief, Rose B. 5(1) onwards, UpToDate, Wellesley, MA 1997.

Sherman SI. Radioiodide treatment of differentiated thyroid cancer. *UpToDate in Medicine* [CD-ROM] Editor-in-Chief Rose B, 5(1) onwards, UpToDate, Wellesley, MA 1997.

Sherman SI. Surgery for differentiated thyroid carcinoma. *UpToDate in Medicine* [CD-ROM] Editor-in-Chief Rose B. 4(3) onwards, UpToDate, Wellesley, MA 1996.

Shortell CK, Andrus CH, Phillips CE, et al. Carcinoma of the parathyroid gland: A 30-year experience. *Surgery* 110:704, 1991.

Thomas CG. Role of thyroid-stimulating hormone suppression in the management of thyroid cancer. *Semin Surg Oncol* 7:115, 1991.

Vassilopoulou-Sellin R. Management of papillary thyroid cancer. *Oncology* 145, 1995.

Wynne AG, van Heerden JA, Carney JA, et al. Parathyroid carcinoma: Clinical and pathological features in 43 patients. *Medicine* 71:197, 1992.

Hematologic Malignancies and Splenic Tumors

James A. Reilly, Jr., and Ana M. Grau

Leukemia and lymphoma account for 6–8% of adult cancers and about 8% of the deaths from malignancy in the United States. In children younger than 15 years, leukemias are the most common malignancies, with non-Hodgkin's lymphoma fourth in frequency.

Leukemia and lymphoma patients are usually referred to a surgeon with a specific request: diagnostic biopsy, vascular access, staging laparotomy, or therapeutic splenectomy. Surgeons must be familiar with this group of disorders, both to perform the operation appropriately and to know the procedure's probability of success and risks. At times a major procedure is unlikely to achieve the desired result, or the patient's limited life expectancy makes such an operation unwise.

The Leukemias

The chronic proliferative diseases appear to be a spectrum of clonal hematopoietic stem cell disorders ranging in increasing severity from polycythemia vera and essential thrombocythemia to myeloid metaplasia to chronic myelogenous leukemia (CML). A few patients with polycythemia vera and essential thrombocythemia and a larger percentage of patients with myeloid metaplasia ultimately develop leukemia.

POLYCYTHEMIA VERA AND ESSENTIAL THROMBOCYTHEMIA

Polycythemia vera is associated with an autonomous expansion of the red blood cell mass and volume with a variable effect on white blood cells (WBCs) and platelets. The most accepted etiologic mechanism involves the existence of a clone with an abnormally high sensitivity to erythropoietin. Essential thrombocythemia is characterized by an increase in the megakaryocyte lineage, with a greatly increased platelet count and a variable effect on erythrocytes and WBCs. In both diseases there is an increased risk of thrombosis and, paradoxically, of hemorrhage. Three-fourths of patients with polycythemia vera have palpable splenomegaly, and about half have hepatic enlargement. Phlebotomy, low-dose chemotherapy, or a combination of these modalities is the primary treatment for patients with polycythemia vera and essential thrombocythemia. The goal is to obtain a hematocrit of 45% or less. Because of the risk of hemorrhage, any operation should be avoided in these patients until the polycythemia is under control. Rapid phlebotomy to a normal hematocrit and fluid replacement should be performed before emergency surgery. Plateletpheresis has been used to control thrombocytosis.

Although splenectomy has little or no role in the management of most patients with polycythemia vera or essential thrombocythemia, a small number of patients develop a condition similar to myeloid metaplasia and require splenectomy. The operative risks are greater and the survival is poorer in this group than in patients with myeloid metaplasia. Patients with polycythemia vera and essential thrombocythemia should be treated with aggressive nonoperative therapy and offered splenectomy only when pain, anemia, and thrombocytopenia are refractory to other treatment. Splenectomy does not increase the survival rate, but it may improve the quality of life.

MYELOID METAPLASIA

Myeloid metaplasia is characterized by fibrosis of the bone marrow and extramedullary hematopoiesis, chiefly in the spleen, liver, and lymph nodes. Fibrosis is polyclonal in nature and is thought to be a reactive process to growth factor release from the clonal cells. As the spleen enlarges, the hematopoietic function it serves may be overwhelmed by destructive hypersplenism (excessive destruction of one or more of the blood components, usually by an autoimmune mechanism).

Although some patients are asymptomatic, most present with fatigue, anorexia and weight loss, or symptomatic splenomegaly. Leukocytosis and thrombocytosis may be present; other hematologic abnormalities such as diminished WBC and platelet counts may result from passive splenic sequestration or active destruction. Active splenic destruction may be humorally mediated (related to specific antibody recognition) or cell mediated (probably by activated macrophages). Peripheral blood smears often demonstrate large platelets, nucleated red cells, anisocytosis, and immature myeloid elements. The diagnosis is made by bone marrow biopsy. In about 5% of cases myeloid metaplasia will progress to CML or acute myeloblastic leukemia.

Initial management may include transfusions, steroids, androgens, cytotoxic chemotherapy, and splenic irradiation. If these measures are not effective in treating the complications of hypersplenism, a splenectomy may be indicated. At the University of Texas M. D. Anderson Cancer Center, patients who have myeloid metaplasia with myelofibrosis are advised to undergo splenectomy under the following conditions: (1) for severe anemia due to hypersplenism when medical management is unsuccessful; (2) for chronically symptomatic splenomegaly; or (3) for the development of worsening congestive heart failure caused by a shunt effect through the spleen. Splenectomy for portal hypertension secondary to increased portal flow associated with splenomegaly has also been reported. Because splenectomy may inadvertently preclude the possibility of performing a splenorenal shunt, it is critical to eliminate hepatic portal hypertension as the etiology of the splenomegaly.

Adequate bone marrow activity must be verified before splenectomy is contemplated. If the spleen is the major site of hematopoiesis, splenectomy may result in severe pancytopenia. A bone marrow biopsy and nuclear medicine bone marrow scan may define the hematopoietic productivity of the marrow cavity. Full coagulation studies should be performed and occult disseminated intravascular coagulation should be controlled before surgery.

Splenectomy does not prolong survival but may improve the quality of life. The response rate for anemia varies from 75% to 95% following splenectomy. The morbidity of splenectomy ranges from 35% to 75% and the mortality rate, from 5% to 18%. Low-dose radiation to the spleen may be used in poor candidates for surgery.

CHRONIC MYELOGENOUS LEUKEMIA

Chronic myelogenous leukemia (CML), also known as chronic granulocytic leukemia, involves a clonal proliferation of myeloid stem cells. About 90% of patients will have a translocation of chromosomes 9 and 22; this translocation is called the *Philadelphia chromosome*. The Philadelphia chromosome may be followed clinically to help assess response to therapy.

CML has both a chronic benign phase and a phase of acute blastic transformation. Most patients present with symptoms of the chronic phase, which include fatigue, weakness, night sweats, low-grade fever, and abdominal pain. Splenomegaly may be an isolated finding during physical examination. The WBC and platelet count may be elevated; however, the platelets may not function normally. Hypersplenism may result in anemia or thrombocytopenia. Patients with the chronic phase of CML should be evaluated every 3–6 months. The median duration of the chronic phase is about 45 months, but some patients may live up to 20 years with this condition. CML will progress from the chronic benign phase to the acute leukemic transformation phase in about 80% of patients.

The acute or accelerated stage of CML may be heralded by progressive fatigue, high fevers, increasingly symptomatic splenomegaly, anemia, thrombocytopenia, basophilia, and bone or joint pain. In addition to the Philadelphia chromosome, other deletions and translocations may be detected. The WBC count may markedly increase and may not be readily controlled by medical means. Increased splenic destruction of blood components may be manifested by more frequent infections or bleeding episodes. Average survival is approximately 6 months, and during this period the disease may become resistant to chemotherapy. Blast crisis is heralded by large numbers of these immature cells in the circulation, with a decrease in other cellular components; this is usually a preterminal event.

Traditional treatment of CML included conventional chemotherapy with hydroxyurea or busulfan. These agents can achieve hematologic remissions, but no significant reduction of Philadelphia chromosome cells has been observed. Interferon-alpha (IFN-α) has been able to achieve hematologic as well as cytogenetic remissions in a significant number of patients and to prolong survival in patients who have shown cytogenetic response. Allogenic bone marrow transplant may be curative, but only a limited number of patients qualify for it.

Splenectomy is generally used as palliation for either painful splenomegaly or refractory anemia. Symptoms due to splenomegaly will likely be improved by splenectomy, but the response is variable when splenectomy is performed to correct dyscrasias. Removal of an enlarged spleen prior to bone marrow transplantation has failed to improve survival or to decrease the relapse frequency. In these patients, though, splenectomy may eliminate a focus of disease or decrease transfusion requirements. Prospective randomized trials will help define the role of splenectomy in the enhancement of bone marrow engraftment. For CML patients whose disease becomes resistant to IFN-α, a splenectomy may improve response to this therapy. Splenectomy does not delay blast transformation, and its effect on survival is controversial. A recent analysis of the M. D. Anderson experience with splenectomy in patients in the accelerated or blastic phase of the disease has shown that although the survival period in these patients may be limited, splenectomy, if indicated, can be performed safely in this phase of the disease and thrombocytopenia can be reliably reversed, minimizing transfusion requirements.

CHRONIC LYMPHOCYTIC LEUKEMIA

Chronic lymphocytic leukemia (CLL) is the most common leukemia in the Western Hemisphere. It is typified by an accumulation of long-lived, mature-appearing but functionally inactive B cells. The median age of onset is in the seventh decade, and the incidence continues to increase beyond that age.

CLL patients may present with enlarged, painless lymph nodes; weakness, weight loss; and anorexia. As the disease progresses, they may develop more pronounced lymphadenopathy and splenomegaly. There may be a decrease in red blood cell count due to either bone marrow infiltration with leukemic cells or a Coombs-positive hemolytic anemia. About 20% of patients will develop a second malignancy, most commonly lung cancer, melanoma, or sarcoma. CLL may have either an indolent or an aggressive course, with patient survival ranging from 1 to 20 years. CLL patients have a progressive loss of immune function, and infection is the most common cause of death.

Previously, treatment was withheld in the early stages until signs of progression occurred. Currently, at M. D. Anderson, treatment is not generally started in the Rai stage 0 patients (lymphocytosis only), but chemotherapy is used to treat other early-stage patients (Rai stage I or II) with poor prognostic signs and all patients with Rai stage III or IV disease (Table 17-1). Fludarabine is used in conjunction with granulocyte-macrophage colony stimulating factor (GM-CSF). Splenectomy may be recommended for patients refractory to fludarabine or with symptomatic splenomegaly and for patients with hypersplenism. Experience at M. D. Anderson has shown that splenectomy can provide an excellent hematologic response in patients with either isolated anemia or thrombocytopenia, but this response is relatively poor in patients presenting with both disorders, suggesting that an adequate hematopoietic reserve is required for a significant response. In addition, splenectomy significantly improves survival in selected subgroups of patients with advanced-stage CLL when compared with conventional chemotherapy. These subgroups include CLL patients with hemoglobin less than or equal to 10 g/dl or a platelet count less than or equal to 50×10^9/L.

Table 17-1.   Rai staging of chronic lymphocytic leukemia

Stage	Criteria
0	Lymphocytosis (WBC s > 15,000/ml with >40% lympho-cytes in the bone marrow)
I	Lymphocytosis with lymphadenopathy
II	Lymphocytosis with enlarged liver or spleen (lymphadenopathy not necessarily present)
III	Lymphocytosis with anemia. Anemia may be due to hemolysis or to decreased production (lymphadenopathy or hepatosplenomegaly need not be present)
IV	Lymphocytosis with thrombocytopenia (platelet count < 100,000/µl) anemia, and lymphadenopathy

WBC = white blood cell.

HAIRY CELL LEUKEMIA

Hairy cell leukemia (HCL) is a monoclonal lymphoproliferative disorder of mature B cells. It comprises only 2–5% of all leukemias, and there is a 3:1 male predominance. The pathognomonic hairy cells are named for their cytoplasmic projections; they may be found in both the bone marrow and the peripheral circulation.

Patients with HCL may complain of weakness and fatigue. Splenomegaly is almost universally present. About 10% of patients with HCL will have such mild symptoms that they never require treatment. Most patients will require therapy for neutropenia, splenomegaly, hypersplenism, or bone marrow failure. Infection related to neutropenia is the most common cause of death.

Early efforts to use chemotherapy to treat HCL were unsuccessful because the degree of associated myelosuppression was not tolerable. Splenectomy became the treatment of choice and was associated with increased survival. Since that time, more effective chemotherapeutic agents have become available. At M. D. Anderson splenectomy is not used in the routine management of patients with HCL. Instead, they are treated with IFN-α, deoxycoformycin, or chlorodeoxyadenosine. The overall response rate to IFN-α is between 80% and 90%. If relapse occurs, chlorodeoxyadenosine is usually effective in regaining control of the disease. The few patients who relapse after chlorodeoxyadenosine treatment can obtain second remissions with retreatment. Splenectomy may be considered in the rare cases of pure splenic form of the disease.

ACUTE LYMPHOCYTIC AND MYELOGENOUS LEUKEMIA

Except in cases of splenic rupture, splenectomy has no role in the management of patients with acute lymphocytic or acute myelogenous leukemia during induction chemotherapy or during relapse. In rare cases, patients in complete remission require splenectomy because of persistent fungal granulomas of the spleen.

SPLENIC RUPTURE IN LEUKEMIA

Splenic rupture is a rare event in leukemic patients and is almost always associated with some form of trauma. There is no increased risk with any particular type of leukemia, but patients with splenomegaly may be more susceptible to splenic trauma. The reported incidence of rupture from four series was 0.72%. Leukemic patients make up only 3.5% of those with spontaneous splenic rupture.

Signs and symptoms include abdominal tenderness and rigidity, shifting dullness, and tachycardia. The chest radiograph may demonstrate an elevated hemidiaphragm or a pleural effusion. A high index of suspicion is necessary in evaluating patients with splenomegaly and abdominal pain because the precipitating event may have been so minor as to not be remembered.

Survival rates vary with the rapidity of diagnosis and of performance of splenectomy. Patients who survive splenectomy following rupture have a life expectancy similar to that of other patients with the same type of leukemia.

The Lymphomas

HODGKIN'S DISEASE

The prognosis of patients with Hodgkin's disease (HD) has improved dramatically over the past 20 years. This advancement is due to increased knowledge of the biology of the disease and more effective use of radiotherapy and multiagent chemotherapy. The role of staging laparotomy continues to evolve as nonoperative staging becomes increasingly accurate and as subsets of patients are identified who are unlikely to benefit from the information laparotomy provides.

HD is characterized by the presence of multinucleated Reed-Sternberg (RS) cells or one of their variants. As opposed to non-Hodgkin's lymphoma, in which a monoclonal population of malignant lymphocytes usually predominates, in HD the malignant cells are a minority population outnumbered by inflammatory cells.

HD patients typically present with nontender lymphadenopathy. The cervical nodes are most commonly involved; other regions—including axillary, inguinal, mediastinal, and retroperitoneal nodes—are less frequently affected at presentation. The presence or absence of B symptoms should be elucidated from the patient's history. B symptoms include any one of the following: unexplained fever with temperature over 38°C, night sweats significant enough to require changing bed clothes, or weight loss of more than 10% of body weight over 6 months. Although classic for HD, the Pel-Ebstein fever, with progressively shortening intervals between fevers, is a relatively rare phenomenon.

The physical examination should include an evaluation of all lymph node–bearing areas, including Waldeyer's tonsillar ring, and palpation for liver or splenic enlargement. Initial work-up should include a complete blood count with differential count, liver function tests, and a chest radiograph. A bone marrow biopsy is useful to determine the extent of the disease. Excisional biopsy of the largest node that is likely to provide the diagnosis should be performed. Careful selection of the biopsy site is important because some areas, particularly the inguinal region, frequently contain nondiagnostic inflammatory nodes.

Other clinical staging tools include computed tomography (CT), nuclear medicine scans, and bipedal lymphangiography. CT is used to detect mediastinal and abdominal lymphatic enlargement; however, nodes containing HD often are not enlarged. Gallium scans have been useful in detecting mediastinal and peripheral nodal disease. Bipedal lymphangiography may detect changes in femoral, inguinal, external iliac, and retroperitoneal nodes. Use of lymphangiography has improved the staging of HD because this procedure identifies lymphatic enlargement as well as changes in the architecture of normal-sized nodes caused by neoplastic involvement.

The prognosis of patients with HD depends on the histologic subtype and stage of disease at presentation. The Rye modification of the Lukes-Butler classification of HD identifies four histologic subtypes: lymphocyte predominant, nodular sclerosis, mixed cellularity, and lymphocyte depleted. These subtypes are determined by the specific variant of RS cell, the ratio of these cells to the normal population, and the degree of sclerosis. The nodular sclerosis subtype has the best prognosis, followed by lymphocyte predominant, mixed cellularity, and finally lymphocyte depleted.

The Ann Arbor staging system (Table 17-2) is used for staging HD based on the extent of disease. Clinical staging includes all data from the history and physical examination and nonoperative diagnostic studies. Pathologic staging includes additional information obtained from a staging laparotomy. The Ann Arbor stages are subclassified to reflect lymphatic disease and involvement of extranodal areas designated by E, for involvement of an extralymphatic site (i.e., stomach or small intestine), or S, for

Table 17-2. Ann Arbor staging system for Hodgkin's disease

Stage	Criteria
I	Involvement of a single lymph node region (I) or a single extralymphatic organ or site (IE)
II	Involvement of two or more lymph node regions on the same side of the diaphragm (II) or of an extralymphatic organ and its adjoining lymph node site (IIE)
III	Involvement of lymph node sites on both sides of the diaphragm (III) or localized involvement of an extra-lymphatic site (IIIE), spleen (IIIS), or both (IIISE)
IV	Diffuse or disseminated involvement of one or more extralymphatic organs with or without associated lymph node involvement
A	Asymptomatic
B	Fever, night sweats, or weight loss of more than 10%

splenic involvement. Disease is further subclassified according to the presence or absence of systemic symptoms of the disease.

Increasing knowledge of the effect of patient characteristics, histologic subtype, and stage of disease have allowed more individualized treatment of patients, with dramatic improvements in survival. Staging laparotomy was first introduced to define disease extent in all presentations of HD. Subsequently, investigators performed staging by laparotomy to determine which patients had early-stage disease that could be treated by local irradiation and which had extensive disease requiring systemic therapy. Previously, up to 40% of patients who underwent staging laparotomy had a change in their clinical stage. Both improvements in the accuracy of radiologic diagnostic procedures and more intensive use of chemotherapeutic and radiation treatments earlier in the course of the disease have decreased the number of patients who require staging laparotomy.

Currently at M. D. Anderson, nonoperative staging and prognostic factors are used to guide therapy in about 80% of patients. Certain subsets of patients have been identified who almost never require staging laparotomy. An example is females with lymphocyte-predominant histology and stage IA disease. This group can be effectively treated with mantle radiotherapy (axilla, neck, and mediastinum) because they almost never have disease below the diaphragm. Patients who require chemotherapy with or without radiation because of extensive disease or poor prognostic factors also do not benefit from the information gained by a staging laparotomy. Conversely, other patients may benefit from the procedure if a negative staging laparotomy allowed treatment with radiation therapy alone. This group includes those without B symptoms, who have no hilar disease and whose mediastinal involvement is less than one-third of the chest diameter. Of note, in this subgroup of patients with favorable prognosis, acceptable results in terms of freedom from progression and survival can be achieved using radiation therapy without performing laparotomy. The increased risk of relapses is balanced by a high success in salvage and the absence of complications related to the laparotomy.

Most centers have eliminated staging laparotomy in pediatric patients with HD. This approach is supported by failure of long-term follow-up to show a significant difference in survival between clinical and surgical staging.

Components of a Staging Laparotomy

For staging laparotomy of HD, the abdomen is entered through a midline incision from the xyphoid process to below the umbilicus. A thorough exploration is performed to identify palpable abnormalities. This includes bimanual palpation of the liver, examination of the bowel and mesentery, and exploration of the major nodal groups. Lymph nodes containing disease are often normal in size. The areas most likely to contain disease include the spleen and the splenic, celiac, and portal lymph nodes.

Splenectomy and liver biopsies are performed early in the procedure so that ample time is available to ensure hemostasis. The spleen should routinely be removed because it may contain nonpalpable disease. In children, some surgeons advocate performing a partial splenectomy to prevent a lifetime risk of asplenic sepsis. Splenic nodes, along with the distal 3 cm of the splenic artery and vein, should be removed in continuity with the spleen. The ends of the splenic vessels are marked with titanium clips to guide future radiotherapy should it be necessary.

A wedge biopsy is obtained from one or both lobes of the liver, and a deeper biopsy with a Tru-cut core needle is done on both lobes. Additional wedge biopsies should be done on any grossly abnormal areas of the liver.

As each nodal group is dissected, it is sent as a separate specimen in sterile saline to the pathologist, and the area is marked with titanium clips. The gastrohepatic ligament is incised, and lymph nodes along the hepatic artery leading to the celiac axis are removed. The sentinel node at the junction of the portal vein with the duodenum, along with any other nodes along the porta hepatis, are excised. The transverse colon is retracted superiorly, and the small bowel is reflected to the patient's right to visualize the aorta. The retroperitoneum is incised over the aorta from the left renal vein down to the iliac bifurcation. The nodes between the aorta and the inferior mesenteric vein are excised. Nodes along the iliac vessels and within the mesentery seldom contain disease, but they should be sampled and submitted for review. Any lymph nodes that appeared abnormal on the lymphangiogram should also be removed.

If a bone marrow biopsy has not been performed preoperatively, it should be obtained from the iliac crest while the patient is under general anesthesia. Oophoropexy was once routinely performed in females of reproductive age, but currently its use is limited to patients with suspected iliac nodal involvement. Some surgeons recommend performing appendectomy during the staging procedure.

The morbidity rate is generally less than 10%, and deaths related to staging laparotomy are rare. Complications include wound problems, atelectasis, pneumonia, pulmonary embolus, and infection. Any complications that delay the initiation of needed systemic therapy or radiotherapy are potentially serious. Long-term complications include small-bowel adhesions, asplenic sepsis, and development of secondary leukemia.

Laparoscopic staging of lymphoma is currently being explored as a modality in the management of these patients. Case reports and small series of lymphoma patients staged laparoscopically have been reported in the literature. The indications have been the same as those for open staging, and absolute contraindications are portal hypertension and uncorrectable coagulopathy. The components of laparoscopic staging include percutaneous and wedge liver biopsies, lymph node biopsies, and splenectomy. Because the spleen needs to be removed intact to allow complete pathologic evaluation, a 6- to 8-cm midline incision is made to allow removal of the spleen. This midline incision is then used to complete the lymph node dissection under direct vision. Conversion to open procedure has most frequently been secondary to hemorrhage during splenectomy and varies from 0 to 20%. Diagnostic accuracy has been reported to be close to 90%. This procedure should be used with caution because there is a risk of spreading tumor cells and seeding of the trocar insertion ports as described for a patient with Burkitt lymphoma. Laparoscopic staging of lymphoma may result in a shorter hospital stay and recovery time, but the accuracy and morbidity of this technique cannot be known until more experience is available.

NON-HODGKIN'S LYMPHOMA

Patients in the United States with non-Hodgkin's lymphoma (NHL) characteristically have a monoclonal proliferation of lymphocytes, with 80% of cases being of B-cell derivation and the remainder originating from T cells. The diagnosis of various subsets of B-cell NHL depends on the identification of histopathologic markers using monoclonal antibodies and of cellular morphology; criteria assessed are a diffuse versus follicular (nodular) pattern of lymph node involvement, small versus large cell type, and cleaved versus noncleaved nuclear morphology. With this information, the lymphoma can be categorized according to the Working Formulation, which is a modification of the Lukes and Collins schema. Although an in-depth discussion of this classification system is beyond the scope of this chapter, the Working Formulation has simplified our understanding of the behaviors of these subtypes by placing them into one of three categories, depending on whether patients have a low, intermediate, or high risk of death due to the disease. The T-cell NHLs are much more difficult to identify precisely and to place into prognostic groups. More recently, the proposed European-American classification of lymphoid neoplasms, uses morphology, phenotype, and cytogenetics to classify these disorders. The clinical relevance of this classification is under study, but it might offer additional information to the Working Formulation.

Most NHL patients present with superficial adenopathy, most commonly in the cervical lymph nodes. These nodes are generally enlarged and not tender. The Ann Arbor system (see Table 17-2) is used to stage these patients, but it is less helpful in NHL than in HD because more than half of NHL patients present with stage III or IV disease and about 20% present with B symptoms.

Because NHLs do not spread in the orderly manner that HD does, the surgeon is generally asked to see NHL patients to perform a diagnostic biopsy, to establish vascular access for chemotherapy, or to treat complications of therapy. Staging laparotomy is not indicated in these patients. Splenectomy is necessary, though rarely, for hypersplenism, massive splenomegaly, or a persistent splenic focus of disease, usually in those with low-grade lymphomas. Although primary splenic lymphoma is unusual, splenectomy may be beneficial for patients with isolated splenic disease. This diagnosis is often made only after splenectomy is performed for hypersplenism or splenomegaly. If the lymphoma is localized to the spleen, the prognosis is similar to that of other stage I patients.

Diagnostic Biopsy for Lymphoma

When lymphoma is suspected, proper planning and execution of the biopsy are crucial to enable the pathologist to make a diagnosis. Because preservation of the architecture aids in histologic diagnosis, efforts should be made to avoid traction or cautery. The largest node found on physical examination should be biopsied. If several nodal areas are enlarged, biopsy of the cervical area is preferred to biopsy of an axillary node, which in turn is superior to biopsy of nodes from the inguinal region. In suspected extranodal disease or in the case of matted nodes, it is important to excise as generous an amount of tissue as possible. Communication with the pathologist is important to guarantee that adequate tissue is sent and that it is delivered in an acceptable fashion. In general, the specimen is sent fresh, is sent in saline, or is wrapped in a saline-soaked sponge. It is important that the specimen be sent directly to the pathologist and that there is an indication that the diagnosis of lymphoma is suspected. Needle biopsies rarely provide an adequate amount of tissue, although they may be helpful in ruling out a carcinoma or sarcoma or in suspected relapse of lymphoma when a tissue diagnosis is needed before treatment.

Miscellaneous Splenic Tumors

SPLENIC CYSTS

A splenic cyst may be confused with a neoplastic process when detected as a palpable abnormality or an unexpected radiologic finding. Patients often present with vague symptoms, possibly due to cyst enlargement. Although parasitic cysts are extremely rare in the United States, they are more common outside this country. Parasitic cysts are most commonly due to an echinococcal infection. Nonparasitic cysts make up 75% of splenic cysts in the United States and are classified as primary if they have a true cellular lining or secondary if they lack this layer. Primary splenic cysts may be congenital, due to an embryologic remnant, or neoplastic. The neoplastic cysts include epidermoid cysts, dermoid cysts, lymphangiomas, and cavernous hemangiomas. Secondary cysts are the more common type of nonparasitic cyst and are thought to be the result of splenic injury and resultant hematoma.

Splenic cysts rarely require treatment unless they become infected, hemorrhage, or perforate. Treatment may consist of a partial or total splenectomy; marsupialization or drainage procedures should be avoided.

INFLAMMATORY PSEUDOTUMOR

Inflammatory pseudotumor, also known as plasma cell granuloma, has histologic features of inflammation and mesenchymal repair. Such masses can be found in various locations in the body, including the respiratory system, gastrointestinal tract, orbit, and lymph nodes. When a pseudotumor is detected in the spleen, it may be mistaken for lymphoma. Pseudotumors are thought to occur at sites of previous trauma or infection. Unfortunately, the definitive diagnosis can be made only after excision. Immunohistochemical stains and flow cytometry studies of the specimen may be useful to rule out a lymphoproliferative disorder.

NONLYMPHOID TUMORS

The spleen is involved with various benign and malignant non-lymphoid tumors. Benign vascular tumors include hemangioma, lymphangioma, and hemangioendothelioma. Lipoma and angiomyolipoma are also encountered. Angiosarcoma of the spleen confers a poor prognosis; this tumor has been associated with exposure to thorium dioxide, vinyl chloride, and arsenic. Kaposi's sarcoma may be found as an isolated process in the spleen. Other splenic sarcomas, including malignant fibrous histiocytoma, fibrosarcoma, and leiomyosarcoma, are extremely rare.

SPLENIC METASTASIS

Considering the large percentage of the total blood flow that supplies the spleen, it is a surprisingly rare site for metastasis. In autopsy series of cancer patients, the finding of metastasis involving the spleen ranges from 1.6% to 30%. Splenic metastasis is rarely a clinically relevant problem. Melanoma, breast, and lung cancer are the most frequently detected metastases. Splenomegaly is an unusual finding with solitary metastasis. Several small series have reported the use of splenectomy for an isolated splenic metastasis. Resection with curative intent is rarely possible with splenic metastasis, but splenectomy may be necessary for complications such as perforation, splenic vein thrombosis, and growth into adjacent viscera.

Splenectomy

SPLENECTOMY FOR HYPERSPLENISM

Anemia, neutropenia, and thrombocytopenia may occur for a number of reasons in patients with hematologic malignancies. Because only patients with excessive destruction of a blood component will benefit from a splenectomy, a careful work-up should be done to identify the etiology of the process. Patients with hypersplenism may present with a normal-sized spleen, and others may have massive splenomegaly without hypersplenism.

Infusion of the patient's or normal donor platelets tagged with [111]indium is helpful in determining whether the spleen is the site of destruction. Patients with an acquired hemolytic anemia generally have a positive Coombs' test, and the detection of the warm antibody is a good indication that splenectomy will be beneficial. Although chromium-labeled red blood cell scans may be useful in demonstrating decreases in red blood cell survival, they are not as helpful in identifying the site of sequestration. In cases of suspected splenic sequestration, a bone marrow biopsy is important to determine whether adequate precursor cells are available or whether the patient depends on the hematopoietic activity of the spleen.

Splenectomy in patients with CML has been associated with severe bleeding problems. These may be related to impaired clot formation caused by proteases and serases produced by granulocytes. CML patients with severe leukocytosis should receive chemotherapy in an attempt to decrease the WBC count to approximately 20,000 cells/ml. Experience at M. D. Anderson suggests that splenectomy is best avoided in CML patients whose WBC counts cannot be controlled with chemotherapy. Splenectomy should also be avoided in CML patients who have had splenic irradiation.

Bleeding and infection are the greatest perioperative risks. Qualitative platelet function should be evaluated rather than relying on a platelet count. The template bleeding time is currently the most widely available laboratory value for identifying adequacy of platelet function. The patient's current and recent medications should be carefully reviewed to identify any drugs that may impair coagulation. Because of potential bleeding problems associated with certain antibiotics, prophylactic coverage must be carefully chosen to avoid increasing the risk of hemorrhage.

Although splenectomy may be performed through either a midline or a subcostal approach, the midline incision is preferred when coagulation defects, thrombocytopenia, or splenomegaly is present. After the splenic pedicle is clamped, thrombocytopenic patients are transfused with fresh single-donor platelets to achieve a platelet count of more than 60,000 cells/ml. Careful hemostasis at the conclusion of the procedure is mandatory. Postoperatively, patients should be monitored closely during the first 48 hours for signs of bleeding. A blood count with differential and platelet counts should be obtained every 6 hours for the first 24 hours after the operation. Decreasing platelet and blood counts, despite adequate replacement, suggest an ongoing bleeding process.

A limited number of laparoscopic splenectomies performed in leukemia patients with hypersplenism has been reported in the literature. The role and risks of minimally invasive surgery in this subset of patients is yet to be defined.

SPLENECTOMY FOR THE MASSIVELY ENLARGED SPLEEN

Indications for splenectomy in patients with massively enlarged spleens include debilitating symptoms of splenomegaly, excessive destruction of blood components, and concerns of possible splenic rupture. These patients often complain of chronic severe upper abdominal and back pain, impaired respiration, and early satiety. Hypersplenism may be present. Depending on the size of the spleen and the body habitus, the patient may be judged to be at increased risk of splenic trauma.

Preoperatively, it is important to check quantitative and qualitative platelet function values and coagulation studies because hemorrhage is the major complication of splenectomy in this group. Portal venous contrast studies should be performed in patients with possible portal hypertension. In splenic vein thrombosis, splenectomy is appropriate, but otherwise it may deprive a patient with portal hypertension of the option of a splenorenal shunt.

Adequate blood products must be available preoperatively. The blood of these patients may be difficult to crossmatch because of numerous past transfusions, and fresh single-donor platelets may be required. Patients should undergo routine bowel preparation, and prophylactic antibiotics should be given.

A midline, rather than subcostal, incision is preferred because the rectus muscles are not severed, which limits bleeding. With increasing size, the spleen becomes more of a midline structure and lends itself to this approach. Prior to mobilization of the spleen, its vessels should be isolated. The gastrocolic omentum is divided, the lesser sac is entered, and the splenic artery is identified along the posterior-superior surface of the pancreas. The artery is doubly ligated but left intact. The splenic vein is not disturbed yet. The spleen may decrease 20–30% in size at this point and allow platelet transfusion without consumption. The splenic flexure of the colon is mobilized, the splenic ligaments are divided, and the spleen is delivered from the splenic fossa. The normally avascular splenic ligaments often contain small vessels in the presence of hematologic malignancies. Dense adhesions between the spleen and the diaphragm may complicate mobilization, and when dissection is particularly difficult, it is better to resect part of the diaphragm with the spleen than to risk hypertrophy of splenic remnants. Such adhesions are formed in areas of splenic infarction and are the most frequent sites of postoperative bleeding in this group of patients. After the spleen is mobilized, the artery and vein are suture ligated and divided. Liver biopsy may be indicated if involvement by lymphoma is suspected. If an injury to the pancreatic tail is recognized, it should be repaired and drained appropriately. Achieving hemostasis in the splenic bed is crucial and may require suture ligation, cautery, platelet transfusions, and thrombostatic agents. Drains do not reliably warn of postoperative hemorrhage or prevent infection, and except in cases of pancreatic injury, they are not routinely used. Postoperatively, patients should be closely monitored for signs of bleeding or infection.

Prophylaxis for Asplenic Sepsis

Patients with hematologic malignancies who undergo splenectomy are at greater risk for asplenic sepsis than are those who have the procedure for other indications. Some hematologic malignancy patients, especially those with CML and CLL, are at increased risk for sepsis even before splenectomy. The risk of overwhelming postsplenectomy infection (OPSI) is greatest for children. The expected death rate from OPSI in children is 1 in every 300–350 patient-years, and in adults it is 1 in every 800–1,000 patient-years. For all patients, the risk is greatest for the first few years following splenectomy, but deaths attributed to OPSI have occurred 30 or more years after splenectomy.

Following splenectomy, there is loss of the opsonins tuftsin and properdin, a decrease in immunoglobulin M production, impaired phagocytosis, and altered cellular immunity. Poorly opsonized bacteria are best cleared by the spleen, and following the spleen's removal patients are particularly susceptible to the encapsulated bacteria.

Vaccination can decrease the risk of postsplenectomy pneumococcal infection. The 23-valent form of the pneumococcal vaccine should be used. The vaccine is most effective when given several weeks preoperatively. Nevertheless, despite the diminished immunity obtained if the vaccine is given after splenectomy, adequate protection is still achieved in most patients. In patients who are not immunized preoperatively there is no benefit from delaying the immunization for several weeks after surgery, so these patients should be vaccinated without delay. Leukemic patients may not be able to develop antibodies in response to pneumococcal vaccine, but it may still be worthwhile to vaccinate this group. Booster immunizations with the pneumococcal vaccine have no proven benefit, although reimmunization at 3–5 years may be required if a drop in specific antibody levels is documented. Certain subsets of patients are at increased risk of infection with *Haemophilus influenzae* and *Neisseria meningitidis* and should receive the appropriate vaccinations.

Long-term use of prophylactic oral antibiotics is often recommended in the pediatric population or in patients who may have difficulty reaching a physician. Penicillin is commonly prescribed to these patients. Data have shown benefit of prophylactic penicillin in preventing pneumococcal infection in children with sickle cell disease, but the benefit of this practice has never been proved for other subsets of asplenic patients.

Selected References

Bouroncle BA. Thirty-five years in the progress of hairy cell leukemia. *Leuk Lymphoma* 14:1, 1994.

Bouvet M, Babiera GV, Termuhlen PM, et al. Splenectomy in the accelerated or blastic phase of chronic myelogenous leukemia: A single institution, 25-year experience. *Surgery* 122:20, 1997.

Brenner B, Nagler A, Tatarsky I, et al. Splenectomy in agnogenic myeloid metaplasia and postpolycythemic myeloid metaplasia. *Arch Intern Med* 148:2501, 1988.

Canady MR, Welling RE, Strobel SL. Splenic rupture in leukemia. *J Surg Oncol* 41:194, 1989.

Carde P, Hagenbeek A, Hayat M, et al. Clinical staging versus laparotomy and combined modality with MOPP versus ABVD in early-stage Hodgkin's disease: The H6 twin randomized trials from the European Organization for Research and Treatment of Cancer Lymphoma Cooperative group. *J Clin Oncol* 11:2258, 1993.

Coad JE, Matutes E, Catovsky D. Splenectomy in lymphoproliferative disorders: A report on 70 cases and review of the literature. *Leuk Lymphoma* 10:245, 1993.

Cortes J, Talpaz M, Kantarjian H. Chronic myelogenous leukemia: A review. *Am J Med* 100:555, 1996.

Cusack JC, Seymour JF, Lerner S, et al. The role of splenectomy in chronic lymphocytic leukemia. *J Am Coll Surg* 185:237, 1997.

Dawes LG, Malangoni MA. Cystic masses of the spleen. *Am Surg* 52:333, 1986.

Edwards MJ, Balch CM. Surgical aspects of lymphoma. *Adv Surg* 22:225, 1989.

Farrar WB, Kim JA. Biopsy techniques to establish diagnosis and type of malignant lymphoma. *Surg Oncol Clin North Am* 2:159, 1993.

Feldman EJ, Arlin ZA. Modern management of chronic myelogenous leukemia (CML). *Cancer Invest* 6:737, 1988.

Fielding AK. Prophylaxis against late infection following splenectomy and bone marrow transplant. *Blood Rev* 8:179, 1994.

Flexner JM, Stein RS, Greer JP. Outline of treatment of lymphoma based on hematologic and clinical stage with expected end results. *Surg Oncol Clin North Am* 2:283, 1993.

Hagemeister FB, Fuller LM, Martin RG. Staging laparotomy: Findings and applications to treatment decisions. In L Fuller (ed.), *Hodgkin's Disease and Non-Hodgkin's Lymphoma in Adults and Children*. New York: Raven, 1988.

Harris NL. The pathology of lymphomas: A practical approach to diagnosis and classification. *Surg Oncol Clin North Am* 2:167, 1993.

Hubbard SM, Longo DL. Treatment-related morbidity in patients with lymphoma. *Curr Opin Oncol* 3:852, 1991.

Johnson HA, Deterling RA. Massive splenomegaly. *Surg Gynecol Obstet* 168:131, 1989.

Kalhs P, Schwarzinger I, Anderson G, et al. A retrospective analysis of the long term effect of splenectomy on late infections, graft-versus-host disease, relapse, and survival after allogenic marrow transplantation for chronic myelogenous leukemia. *Blood* 86:2028, 1995.

Kantarjian HM, Smith TL, O'Brien S, et al. Prolonged survival in chronic myelogenous leukemia after cytogenetic response to interferon-a therapy. *Ann Intern Med* 122:254, 1995.

Klein B, Stein M, Kuten A, et al. Splenomegaly and solitary spleen metastasis in solid tumors. *Cancer* 60:100, 1987.

Kluin-Nelemans HC, Noordijk EM. Staging of patients with Hodgkin's disease: What should be done? *Leukemia* 4:132, 1991.

Kurzrock R, Talpaz M, Gutterman JU. Hairy cell leukaemia: Review of treatment. *Br J Haematol* 79(Suppl 1):17, 1991.

McBride CM, Hester JP. Chronic myelogenous leukemia: Management of splenectomy in a high-risk population. *Cancer* 39:653, 1977.

Morgenstern L, Rosenberg J, Geller SA. Tumors of the spleen. *World J Surg* 9:468, 1985.

Mower WR, Hawkins JA, Nelson EW. Postsplenectomy infection in patients with chronic leukemia. *Am J Surg* 152:583, 1986.

Noordijk EM, Carde P, Mandard AM, et al. Preliminary results of the EORTC-GPMC controlled clinical trial H7 in early stage Hodgkin's disease. *Ann Oncol* 5(Suppl 2):107, 1994.

Parker SL, Tong T, Bolden S, Wingo PA. Cancer statistics 1997. *CA* 47:5, 1997.

Pittaluga S, Bijnens L. Teodorovic A, et al. Clinical analysis of 670 cases in two trials of the European Organization for the Research and Treatment of Cancer Lymphoma Cooperative Group subtyped according to the Revised European-American Classification of lymphoid neoplasms: A comparison with the Working Formulation. *Blood* 10:4358, 1996.

Pollock R, Hohn D. Splenectomy. In MS Roh, FC Ames (eds.), *Advanced Oncologic Surgery*. New York: Mosby-Wolfe, 1994.

Shaw JHF, Print CG. Postsplenectomy sepsis. *Br J Surg* 76:1074, 1989.

Schrenk P, Wayand W. Value of diagnostic laparoscopy in abdominal malignancies. *Int Surg* 80:353, 1995.

Styrt B. Infection associated with asplenia: Risks, mechanisms, and prevention. *Am J Med* 88:33N, 1990.

Tefferi A, Silverstein MN, Noel P. Agnogenic myeloid metaplasia. *Semin Oncol* 22:327, 1995.

Wiernik PH, Rader M, Becker NH, et al. Inflammatory pseudotumor of spleen. *Cancer* 66:597, 1990.

Metastatic Cancer
of Unknown Primary Site

Barry J. Roseman

Patients with metastatic cancer of unknown primary site comprise less than 5% of patients with newly diagnosed cancer. The diagnostic evaluation and treatment of these patients can be challenging, and although care of these patients is largely coordinated by the medical oncologist, the surgeon may also play an important role in these patients' management. In particular, a surgeon is often asked to evaluate a patient with cancer that has spread to a lymph node, the liver, or the peritoneal cavity. This chapter will define the problem of metastatic cancer of unknown primary site, outline a logical and practical approach to the diagnostic evaluation of these patients, and discuss the role of surgery in several clinical scenarios.

Definition and General Considerations

The syndrome of metastatic cancer of unknown primary site has multiple synonyms in the clinical literature (Table 18-1). These tumors are often grouped according to histologic subtype. The major subtypes include squamous cell cancer, adenocarcinoma, and undifferentiated neoplasms, the name given to a heterogeneous group of tumors of various cell origin.

In large series, the most common locations of metastases of unknown primary site are the lymph nodes, bones, lungs, and liver. Other metastatic sites include the brain, meninges, pleura, subcutaneous tissues, adrenals, peritoneum, kidney, and pancreas.

In most patients, the site of origin of the metastatic disease is never discerned. However, in others, the primary site from which the metastases are derived is ultimately identified—through exhaustive search while the patient is living, at surgery, or at autopsy. From this body of data it is clear that metastases from squamous cell cancers normally originate in the head and neck region or the lungs, whereas metastatic adenocarcinomas most frequently originate in the lungs, breasts, or thyroid in the case of metastases above the diaphragm or from the pancreas, liver, stomach, colon, or rectum in the case of metastasis below the diaphragm.

It is important to define the therapeutic goals when treating a patient with metastatic cancer of unknown primary site. This is particularly true for patients with metastatic adenocarcinoma or undifferentiated carcinoma, whose median survival is less than 6 months. However, specific subgroups of patients with metastatic cancer of unknown primary site have a considerably better prognosis than the group as a whole, when given appropriate therapy. This includes patients with squamous cell cancer metastatic to cervical lymph nodes, women with metastatic adenocarcinoma in axillary lymph nodes, men with undifferentiated

Table 18-1. Metastatic cancer of unknown primary

Synonyms in literature

Metastasis of unknown origin
Tumors of unknown origin
Metastasis from undetected primary cancers
Cancer of unknown primary
Metastatic carcinoma of (with) unknown primary
Metastatic cancer without detectable primary site
Carcinoma of unknown primary (site)
Metastatic adenocarcinoma of unknown primary site

cancer and elevated beta human chorionic gonadotropin or alpha-fetoprotein levels, women with peritoneal carcinomatosis, and patients with neuroendocrine cancer of unknown primary site. These specific subgroups will be discussed later in more detail.

The goals in evaluating patients with metastatic cancer of unknown primary should therefore be (1) to identify those tumor types in which a cure or good disease control is possible, (2) to determine if the tumor is locally confined or broadly metastatic, and (3) to identify any symptoms for which local therapy may be effective.

History and Physical Examination

In patients with metastatic cancer of unknown primary site, as with all cancer patients, a careful history and physical examination is essential in establishing several important facts that will have an impact on therapy. The history of a prior malignancy or a family history of cancer may guide the surgeon in establishing the site of an occult primary tumor. A complete systems review may help to determine the degree of symptoms and extent of the patient's disease. The general functional status of the patient is also a crucial factor, one that must be clarified before an individualized treatment decision can be made.

In the physical examination several areas warrant particular attention. The head and neck should be thoroughly examined, particularly when a diagnosis of squamous cell cancer has been made. This includes examination of the oropharynx, hypopharynx, and nasopharynx as well as the larynx, typically assisted by indirect or fiber-optic laryngoscopy. The thyroids should be examined for enlargement or asymmetry. All nodal basins, including those of the head and neck and the supraclavicular, axillary, and inguinal regions, should be examined for palpable or enlarged lymph nodes.

In women, a careful breast examination should be performed, and a thorough bimanual pelvic examination, including a rectal exam, is essential. For men, the testicular and prostate examinations are particularly important, as is a careful rectal examination. All patients should have a careful skin examination.

Laboratory and Radiographic Evaluation

Routine complete blood count, blood chemistry studies, liver function tests, and urinalysis should be performed in all patients, and stool should be checked for occult blood. Beyond these basic tests, the clinical laboratory has limited usefulness in the diagnostic evaluation of the patient with cancer of unknown primary site.

Radiographic studies in patients with cancer of unknown primary site should focus on identifying the primary tumor and delineating the extent of metastatic disease. A chest radiograph is indicated in all patients to assess the presence of pulmonary metastases and for preoperative evaluation. Women of childbearing age or older, particularly those with metastatic adenocarcinoma, should undergo mammography. Unfortunately, it is difficult to identify subtle radiographic abnormalities in younger women, who often have extremely dense breast tissue. Directed computed tomographic scans may be helpful. These include a neck CT scan for patients with squamous cell cancer and a chest, abdominal, and pelvic CT scan for patients with metastatic adenocarcinoma.

In general, it is not helpful to exhaustively pursue the primary site in these patients using radiography. This endeavor can be expensive, inconvenient, and traumatic for patients and often has no significant impact on patients' therapy or the ultimate course of the disease.

Biopsy and Pathologic Evaluation

The next step in evaluating the patient with metastatic cancer of unknown primary site is to perform a tissue biopsy. This is particularly true for patients who present with lymphadenopathy. Fine-needle aspiration has largely replaced core biopsy as a first technique. In some instances, such as for subtyping of lymphoma, open biopsies are needed to obtain larger tissue specimens that exhibit tissue architecture. One can start with fine-needle aspiration and proceed to core biopsy, incisional biopsy, or excisional biopsy as needed for specific cases. In patients from whom a tissue specimen has been obtained, fresh, unfixed tissue is sent to the pathology laboratory for routine microscopy (hematoxylin and eosin staining), electron microscopy, immunohistochemical, and hormone receptor studies.

Light microscopy is ordinarily insufficient to determine the cell of origin, although for difficult cases electron microscopy may be helpful, as different tumor types have characteristic electron-microscopic findings. For example, desmosomes and intracellular bridges are associated with squamous cell cancer, whereas tight junctions, microvilli, and presence of acinar spaces are associated with adenocarcinoma. Premelanosomes are associated with melanoma, and neurosecretory granules are associated with small cell or neuroendocrine tumors. In lymphoma, one typically finds an absence of junctions between the cells under electron microscopy.

Immunohistochemical studies are sometimes useful as an adjunct to microscopy and have become a routine histologic technique. Several markers can be stained by monoclonal antibodies and then visualized through a secondary labeling technique. For example, prostatic acid phosphatase and prostate-specific antigen are associated with prostate cancer, whereas neuron-specific enolase and chromogranin are associated with small cell lung cancer and carcinoid tumors. Germ cell tumors often stain for human chorionic gonadotropin and alpha-fetoprotein. Alpha-fetoprotein is also seen in association with hepatocellular carcinoma. Monoclonal immunoglobulins are indicative of lymphoma or plasmacytoma, and the presence of estrogen receptor or progesterone receptor is associated with breast and ovarian cancers.

Several tumor-derived mucins can purportedly help identify the source of the cancer in patients with cancer of unknown primary site. The most well known of these are CA-125 in ovarian and uterine cancer; CA 15-3 in breast, ovarian, and pancreatic cancer; and CA 19-9 in pancreatic and gastrointestinal tract tumors. Table 18-2 lists several such proteins and other tumor markers used in helping to identify the source of metastases from an unknown primary site.

Unfortunately, patients with carcinoma of unknown primary site typically have a nonspecific overexpression of many of these tumor markers, and routine screening for elevation in serum tumor marker levels does not offer any diagnostic or prognostic assistance. None of these markers has been found to have adequate specificity or sensitivity to consistently identify a primary tumor, nor predictive value for either response to chemotherapy or survival.

Another recent tool is genetic analysis of the biopsy specimen to look for specific oncogenes that are erroneously expressed or found at abnormally high levels in human cancer cells. Examples of these include the HER-2/*neu* oncogene, which is associated with breast cancer, the *bcr/abl* oncogene, which is associated with chronic myelogenous leukemia and B-cell lymphoma, and various other oncogenes that are related to specific cancers. It is not yet known if using such sophisticated molecular techniques will be beneficial in evaluating patients with metastatic cancer of unknown primary site.

Specific Disease Sites

METASTATIC CANCER TO CERVICAL LYMPH NODES

The presence of an enlarged cervical lymph node often leads to a biopsy demonstrating metastatic cancer. The group of patients with metastatic squamous cell cancer to cervical lymph nodes and unknown primary have a better prognosis than the unknown primary group as a whole.

The neck is comprised of more than 25 nodal basins. These nodes have been grouped into six specific levels, to standardize the pathologic evaluation of patients. The classification of cervical lymph nodes is shown in Table 18-3. The most common site of

Table 18-2. Clinical role of selected tumor markers

Tumor marker	Role in differential diagnosis	Role in staging and prognosis
AFP	Identification of hepatocellular carcinoma or germ cell tumors	Serum levels correlate with tumor burden and response to therapy
B-HCG	Identification of trophoblastic and germ cell tumors	Serum levels correlate with tumor burden and response to therapy
B2-microglobulin	Not very useful	Serum levels correlate with response to therapy for myeloma and lymphoma
CA 15-3	Identification of possible breast carcinoma but elevated serum levels also noted in ovarian, lung, and gastrointestinal carcinoma	High serum levels associated with metastatic carcinoma
CA 19-9	Identification of possible pancreatic cancer or other gastrointestinal cancer	High serum levels helpful in determining response to treatment and detecting recurrence
CA 125	Identification of possible ovarian or uterine cancer but elevated serum levels may be noted in breast, lung, or GI cancers	Serum levels helpful in determining response to treatment and detecting recurrence
Calcitonin	Screening and diagnosis of medullary carcinoma of thyroid	Minimal role
CEA	Distinction of carcinoma from mesothelioma	High serum levels correlate with liver metastasis
Cytokeratin	Distinction of carcinoma from lymphoma or melanoma by immunohistochemistry	Minimal role
Epithelial membrane antigen	Distinction of carcinoma from melanoma by membrane immunohistochemistry	Minimal role
LCA	Identification of lymphoma or leukemia by immunohistochemistry	Minimal role
PSA	Identification of prostate carcinoma	Serum levels correlate with stage and response to therapy

Table 18-3.   Classification of cervical lymph nodes

Level	Nodes
I	Submental nodes
II	Upper internal jugular chain nodes
III	Middle internal jugular chain nodes
IV	Lower internal jugular chain nodes
V	Spinal accessory nodes Transverse cervical nodes
VI	Tracheoesophageal groove nodes

metastasis in patients with head and neck squamous cell cancer is the jugulodigastric or level II, upper internal jugular chain nodes, followed by the mid-jugular nodes. Metastasis to the other cervical nodal groups occurs with less frequency.

In those patients with cervical lymph nodes from an occult squamous cell cancer primary, it is particularly important to perform a careful head and neck exam. Adequate lighting and mirrors must be utilized to visualize the entire oropharynx, hypopharynx, nasopharynx, and larynx. A chest x-ray is always indicated and a CT scan of the head and neck is usually indicated in these patients, to determine the primary site and to obtain complete staging information.

If no primary tumor is found with the physical examination and radiographic studies, it is common to proceed with panendoscopy. This is normally done in the operating room under general anesthesia. Esophagoscopy, laryngoscopy, bronchoscopy, and nasopharyngoscopy are performed in an attempt to visualize and biopsy the most common sites of occult squamous cell cancer in the head and neck region. Random biopsies of the most probable tumor site locations are performed, based on the location of the adenopathy.

Typical occult primary sites in squamous cell cancer are the nasopharynx, the mid-base of the tongue, the pyriform sinus, and the tonsils. Table 18-4 shows the common pattern of cervical metastasis from different squamous cell tumors in the head and neck region. Based on the location of the nodal metastases, one is often able to extrapolate the likely source of the occult primary, and the endoscopic examination can be focused on these locations.

Following this evaluation, there is still a subgroup of patients in which the primary site is not identified. The standard approach to these patients is a combination of lymphadenectomy and radiation therapy directed to the most likely primary sites. Based on large series, expected 5-year survival in this group of patients is from 32% to 55%, and overall control of neck disease is 75–85% with this combined therapy. Patients with extra-nodal extension and/or lymph nodes greater than 6 cm (N3 disease) have a higher rate of both local recurrence and distant metastases.

Patients with metastatic adenocarcinoma in cervical lymph nodes from an occult primary have a less favorable outcome. Retrospective series have shown that attempts to treat these patients

Table 18-4. Probable site of the primary tumor according to the location of the cervical metastases

Location of nodes	Primary tumor site
Submental	Floor of the mouth, lips, and anterior tongue
Submaxillary	Retromolar trigone and glossopalatine pillar
Jugulodigastric	Hypopharynx, base of the tongue, tonsil, nasopharynx, and larynx
Midjugular	Hypopharynx, oropharynx, base of the tongue, tonsil, nasopharynx, and larynx
Low jugular	Thyroid, hypopharynx, and nasopharynx
Supraclavicular	Lung 40%, thyroid 20%, GI 12%, GU 8%
Posterior triangle	Nasopharynx

with lymphadenectomy and radiation therapy, as with squamous cell cancer, are much less effective, with nearly 100% local recurrence and 0–10% 5-year survival.

Of particular interest in surgical patients is the presence of an enlarged Virchow's (supraclavicular) node, common in patients with metastatic adenocarcinoma. One study retrospectively reviewed 152 FNA biopsies of supraclavicular lymph nodes, comparing the site of primary when the metastasis was in the right versus the left supraclavicular node. Sixteen of 19 primary pelvic tumors metastasized to the left supraclavicular node, and six of six primary abdominal malignancies metastasized to the left supraclavicular node. However, thoracic, breast, and head and neck malignancies showed no differences in metastatic patterns to the right and left supraclavicular nodes. Based on this information, the investigation for the source of primary in patients who present with adenocarcinoma found in a left-sided Virchow's node should focus on an abdominal or pelvic primary.

METASTATIC CANCER TO AXILLARY LYMPH NODES

The evaluation of patients with cancer metastatic to axillary lymph nodes should be guided by the histologic type of the tumor. For example, when a biopsy of axillary lymph nodes yields lymphoma, a complete staging evaluation should be performed to determine whether systemic chemotherapy or radiation therapy will be the appropriate treatment. Melanoma patients should be examined carefully for a primary site in the ipsilateral extremity. Patients with squamous cell cancer metastatic to the axillary lymph nodes should have a careful skin examination, a chest radiograph to rule out a lung primary tumor, a detailed head and neck examination, and a CT scan of the head and neck and the chest to look for an occult squamous cell primary tumor.

Men with adenocarcinoma metastatic to an axillary lymph node and an unknown primary source should be evaluated for lung, gastrointestinal, or genitourinary primary tumors. Women with adenocarcinoma metastatic to the axillary lymph nodes should be evaluated similarly, although in this specific subset of patients there is a high likelihood of an occult breast primary tumor. These patients should be carefully examined for a breast tumor, and every woman should have a mammogram. Ultrasonography of the breast can be utilized if the mammogram does not identify a lesion.

The biopsy specimen from the lymph node should be subjected to routine histologic and immunohistochemical evaluation for estrogen and progesterone receptors. Although neither highly sensitive nor highly specific, the presence of estrogen or progesterone receptors in this clinical scenario strongly suggests a breast primary tumor.

Several large studies demonstrate that if no extramammary primary tumor or systemic metastases are found, the most likely diagnosis is cancer of the ipsilateral breast. Occult breast cancer presenting with axillary metastases occurs in approximately 0.5% of all women with breast cancer. When large numbers of such patients are treated with a presumptive diagnosis of breast cancer, the recurrence and survival results are similar to those of patients with a similar stage of breast cancer and a known primary tumor. Retrospective review of the mastectomy specimens from patients with occult primary tumors shows that in 50–65% of cases, a primary tumor can ultimately be identified in the surgical specimen. The remainder of the tumors are probably too small to be seen by the standard sampling techniques that pathologists use to study breast specimens.

The treatment for women with adenocarcinoma metastatic to axillary lymph nodes has evolved dramatically over the past several years. There are three general approaches: immediate mastectomy, watchful waiting, and radiation therapy. Immediate mastectomy has been the traditional therapy for women with isolated metastatic adenocarcinoma in axillary lymph nodes and is associated with good long-term survival rates and low risk of local recurrence. A large series by Ashikari et al. in 1976 showed a 10-year survival rate of 79% in these patients.

Watchful waiting is another option. The principal drawback of this approach is that 25–75% of patients will have a recurrence in the breast, requiring further therapy. Although salvage treatment with mastectomy is successful in most of these patients, a small subgroup of patients may develop metastases in the interval that might have been prevented by more aggressive local therapy.

The third approach to women with axillary metastases from an unknown primary site is breast conservation therapy. This approach has been studied at the University of Texas M. D. Anderson Cancer Center, and the results are encouraging. In patients who have undergone axillary lymph node dissection alone, the incidence of local recurrence is 65% at 10 years, whereas a combination of axillary lymph node dissection and radiation therapy reduces the local recurrence rate to 25%. With this treatment, the overall survival was no different from that of patients with the same nodal stage who underwent mastectomy. Addition of adjuvant chemotherapy to surgery and radiation therapy increased the survival rate from 60% to 85% at 10 years.

Several studies have confirmed that survival rates associated with breast conservation therapy are equivalent to those associated with mastectomy in patients with occult primary breast cancer. Most patients who initially present with clinically evident positive nodes need both local and regional lymph node irradiation, and should be given the same treatment options as those given patients with known breast cancer of similar nodal stage.

METASTATIC CANCER TO THE INGUINAL NODES FROM AN UNKNOWN PRIMARY SITE

A relatively infrequent presentation of metastatic cancer of unknown primary site is metastases to the inguinal lymph nodes. Excluding melanoma, which will be discussed separately, the most common histologic type is unclassified carcinoma. The second most common type is squamous cell carcinoma, and a small number of patients will have adenocarcinoma. In evaluating patients with inguinal metastases, a thorough investigation for the primary tumor should include a skin examination of the lower extremities, perineum, and buttocks and an examination for a primary tumor of the perineal or pelvic region. After evaluation for other metastatic disease, inguinal lymph node dissection is typically performed to obtain additional pathology specimens and for regional disease control. Patients are then considered for treatment with systemic therapy on the basis of the tissue diagnosis.

Metastatic Melanoma of Unknown Primary Site

One area of clear interest to the surgical oncologist is metastatic melanoma of unknown primary site. Approximately 5% of melanoma patients present with metastatic disease of the lymph nodes from an unknown primary tumor. Several studies have compared these patients with similar cohorts of patients with equivalent nodal status and a known primary site, in terms of recurrence and survival. Although historically patients with unknown primary tumors were thought to have a worse prognosis, several recent large studies have contradicted these early findings.

Patients with metastatic melanoma and an unknown primary tumor must be examined carefully from scalp to toes for a potential primary site. For the purpose of studying this subgroup of melanoma patients, strict criteria have been established in the course of retrospective analysis to exclude patients with potential sites of an occult primary tumor that may have been missed (Table 18-5).

In an important study from Memorial Sloan-Kettering Cancer Center by Chang and Knapper in 1982, 166 patients with metastatic melanoma of unknown primary site were retrospectively reviewed. This group comprised 4.4% of all the melanoma patients followed during the review period. Several parameters were used to compare this group of patients with a control group with known primary tumors. All patients had clinical stage II disease, according to the older staging criteria in which patients with suspicious palpable lymph nodes were defined as clinical stage II.

The distribution of metastases in patients with unknown primary tumors was similar to that in patients with known primary tumors. Most tumors were found in the axillary lymph nodes,

Table 18-5.   Metastatic melanoma of unknown primary stringent definition of patient population

Exclude patient's with:
1. Past history of having had a mole, birthmark, freckle, chronic paronychia, or skin blemish previously excised, electrodesiccated, or cauterized
2. Metastatic melanoma in one of the node-bearing areas who presented with a scar of previous local treatment in the skin area drained by this lymphatic basin
3. No recorded physical examination of anus and genitalia
4. Previous orbital enucleaion or exenteration

followed by the groin and cervical regions. Patients with clinical stage II disease had a 46% 5-year survival rate and a 41% 10-year survival rate, a finding similar for men and women. Patients who had residual disease in the lymphadenectomy specimen, indicating the presence of more extensive lymph node involvement, did worse. Finally, patients who had prompt lymphadenectomy had a substantially better prognosis than those who had a delay in treatment, with a threefold improvement in the 5- and 10-year survival rates.

A second large series from the John Wayne Cancer Center reviewed 188 patients with lymph node metastases from unknown primary melanoma and compared these with a group of patients with a known primary tumor. Several variables—such as age, sex, anatomic site, and treatment with adjuvant immunotherapy—were similar in the two groups. In this group of patients with clinical stage II melanoma, patients with lymph node metastases from an unknown primary melanoma had a nonsignificant improvement in 5- and 10-year survival, compared with patients with a known primary melanoma.

Because patients with melanoma metastatic to the lymph nodes from an unknown primary tumor have as favorable an outlook as patients with a known primary melanoma, the nodal basin in patients with unknown primary tumors should be approached in a standard fashion. Patients should be offered radical lymph node dissection, followed by adjuvant immunotherapy for patients with disease localized to the nodal basin.

PERITONEAL CARCINOMATOSIS OF UNKNOWN PRIMARY SITE IN WOMEN

Another subgroup of patients with a particularly favorable prognosis consists of women with peritoneal carcinomatosis of unknown primary site. Several studies have shown that women who present with peritoneal carcinomatosis should be treated in a similar fashion to those with known advanced ovarian cancer. This would include maximal surgical cytoreduction at initial laparotomy followed by platinum-based combination chemotherapy. These patients are characterized by an indolent disease course, high rates of response to systemic therapy, and a chance for long-term, disease-free survival.

UNKNOWN PRIMARY TUMOR WITH METASTATIC LIVER DISEASE

The surgeon will occasionally be involved in the evaluation of a patient who presents with metastatic liver disease from an unknown primary tumor. The liver tumor may be discovered when the patient presents with symptoms on routine physical examination, or incidentally on a radiologic study such as an abdominal sonogram or CT scan.

When patients present with metastatic liver disease from an unknown primary tumor, the cell type is most often adenocarcinoma. However, anaplastic or poorly differentiated carcinoma, small cell carcinoma, squamous cell carcinoma, gastrinoma, insulinoma, and sarcomas such as hemangiosarcoma and leiomyosarcoma are also found. When the diagnosis is adenocarcinoma of unknown primary site metastatic to the liver, the most likely primary tumor is a gastrointestinal tract malignancy, followed by a lung or breast primary tumor.

Patients with adenocarcinoma of unknown primary site metastatic to the liver should be evaluated with a comprehensive history and physical examination, as discussed earlier in this chapter, with particular attention paid to the breast and gynecologic examination in women and the genital and rectal examination in men. A chest radiograph, mammogram, and barium study of the colon and rectum or colonoscopy are indicated to look for the most likely sources of the primary tumor. CT scan of the abdomen is useful to quantify the liver disease and may help identify the primary tumor. An exhaustive search for the primary tumor with thyroid scan, upper endoscopy, upper gastrointestinal series with small bowel follow-through, intravenous pyelogram, or other such studies is usually not productive unless the patient has significant symptoms, such as pain or gastrointestinal tract bleeding or obstruction.

Patients with suspected liver metastases and an unknown primary tumor should have a liver biopsy so that a specific tissue diagnosis can be obtained. Most of these patients will be found to have metastatic adenocarcinoma from the gastrointestinal tract, which does not respond dramatically to chemotherapy. However, several chemotherapy-sensitive tumors, such as breast, ovarian, prostate, or germ cell tumors, may be found and subsequently treated. In the remainder of patients with adenocarcinoma metastatic to the liver, the impact of chemotherapy on survival is limited.

Chemotherapy for Metastatic Cancer of Unknown Primary Site

In studying the effects of chemotherapy on patients with cancer of unknown primary site, several uncontrolled factors limit comparison of patients within and between series. Among these factors are variation in clinical and pathologic evaluation, inclusion of patients with the primary site identified, presence of visceral versus nodal metastases, age, performance status, and whether the studies were performed in a single-institution or multi-institutional fashion.

When chemotherapy is given to unselected groups of patients with metastatic cancer of unknown primary site, one can anticipate a 5–10% 5-year survival rate. There is no effective therapy for metastatic adenocarcinoma or poorly differentiated carcinoma. Several cisplatin-based regimens have produced complete response rates of 10–25%, but these regimens produce 5-year disease-free survival rates of only 5–15%. Patients with squamous cell cancer and neuroendocrine cancer have a significantly better response to chemotherapeutic agents.

Given the poor results of chemotherapy in patients with poorly differentiated carcinoma or adenocarcinoma metastatic to lymph nodes or viscera, it is important to keep a perspective on the overall disease process while treating such patients. One must compare the benefits of therapy with the toxic effects of a given chemotherapy regimen.

Although cure is an unrealistic goal for many patients with metastatic cancer of unknown primary, the surgeon is often involved in the palliative care of such patients. Examples of palliation in such patients include debulking of tumors causing pain or obstruction, thoracentesis for patients with respiratory compromise from pleural effusions, and radiation therapy for painful bone metastases. Patients should be offered adequate analgesics to ensure that they are comfortable, and both patients and their families should be provided adequate emotional support and access to resources that optimize their quality of life.

Selected References

Albers CA, Johnson RH, Mansberger AR. The management of patients with metastatic cancer from an unknown primary site. *Am Surg* 47:162, 1981.

Cervin JR, Silverman JF, Loggie BW, et al. Virchow's node revisited. *Arch Pathol Lab Med* 119:727, 1995.

Chang P, Knapper WH. Metastatic melanoma of unknown primary. *Cancer* 49:1106, 1982.

deBraud F, Al-Sarraf M. Diagnosis and management of squamous cell carcinoma of unknown primary tumor site of the neck. *Semin Oncol* 20:273, 1993.

Ellerbroek N, Holmes F, Singletary E, et al. Treatment of patients with isolated axillary nodal metastases from an occult primary carcinoma consistent with breast origin. *Cancer* 66:1461, 1990.

Glynne-Jones RG, Anand AK, Young TE, et al. Metastatic adenocarcinoma in the cervical lymph nodes from and occult primary. *Clin Oncol* 1:19, 1989.

Greco FA, Vaughn WK, Hainsworth JD. Advanced poorly differentiated carcinoma of unknown primary site: Recognition of a treatable syndrome. *Ann Intern Med* 104:547, 1986.

Greenberg BR, Lawrence HJ. Metastatic cancer with unknown primary. *Med Clin North Am* 72:1055, 1988.

Haupt HM, Rosen PP, Kinne DW. Breast carcinoma presenting with axillary lymph node metastases. *Am J Surg Pathol* 9:165, 1985.

Holmes FF, Fouts TL. Metastatic cancer of unknown primary site. *Cancer* 4:816, 1970.

Jackson B, Scott-Conner C, Moulder J. Axillary metastasis from occult breast carcinoma: Diagnosis and management. *Am Surg* 61:431, 1995.

Jakobsen J, Aschenfeldt P, Johansen J, et al. Lymph node metastases in the neck from unknown primary tumour. *Acta Oncol* 31:653, 1992.

Kambhu SA, Kelsen DP, Fiore J, et al. Metastatic adenocarcinomas of unknown primary site. *Am J Clin Oncol* 13:55, 1990.

Le Chevalier TL, Cvitkovic E, Caille P, et al. Early metastatic cancer of unknown primary origin at presentation. *Arch Intern Med* 148:2035, 1988.

Lenzi R, Hess KR, Abbruzzese MC, et al. Poorly differentiated carcinoma and poorly differentiated adenocarcinoma of unknown origin: Favorable subsets of patients with unknown-primary carcinoma? *J Clin Oncol* 15:1, 1997.

Leonard RJ, Nystrom JS. Diagnostic evaluation of patients with carcinoma of unknown primary tumor site. *Semin Oncol* 20:244, 1993.

Lleander VC, Goldstein G, Horsley JS. Chemotherapy in the management of metastatic cancer of unknown primary site. *Oncology* 26:265, 1972.

McCunniff AJ, Raben M. Metastatic carcinoma of the neck from an unknown primary. *Int J Radiat Oncol Biol Phys* 12:1849, 1986.

Muggia FM, Baranda J. Management of peritoneal carcinomatosis of unknown primary tumor site. *Semin Oncol* 20:268, 1993.

Nesbit RA, Tattersall MH, Fox RM, et al. Presentation of unknown primary cancer with metastatic liver disease: Management and natural history. *Aust N Z J Med* 11:16, 1981.

Pacini P, Olmi P, Cellai E, et al. Cervical lymph node metastases from an unknown primary tumour. *Acta Radiol Oncol* 20:311, 1981.

Pavlidis N, Kalef-Ezra J, Braissoulis E, et al. Evaluation of six tumor markers carcinoma of unknown primary. *Med Pediatr Oncol* 22:162, 1994.

Read, NE, Strom EA, McNeese MD. Carcinoma in axillary nodes in women with unknown primary site: Results of breast-conserving therapy. *Breast J* 2:403, 1996.

Reintgen DS, McCarty KS, Woodard B, et al. Metastatic malignant melanoma with an unknown primary. *Surgery, Gynecology, and Obstetrics* 156:335, 1983.

Roseman BJ, Clark O. Common clinical problems: Evaluation of the patient with a neck mass. In DW Wilmore, LY Cheung, AH Harken, et al. *Scientific American Surgery*, vol. II. New York: Scientific American, 1996.

Ruddon RW, Norton SE. Use of biological markers in the diagnosis of cancers of unknown primary tumor. *Semin Oncol* 20:251, 1993.

Schwarz D, Hamberger AD, Jesse RH. The management of squamous cell carcinoma in cervical lymph nodes in the clinical absence of a primary lesion by combined surgery and irradiation. *Cancer* 48:1746, 1981.

Steckel RJ, Kagan AR. Diagnostic persistence in working up metastatic cancer with an unknown primary site. *Radiology* 134:367, 1980.

Stewart JF, Tattersall MH, Woods RL, et al. Unknown primary adenocarcinoma: Incidence of overinvestigation and natural history. *Br Med J* 1:1530, 1979.

Strnad CM, Grosh WW, Baxter J, et al. Peritoneal carcinomatosis of unknown primary site in women. *Ann Intern Med* 11:213, 1989.

Wallack MK, Reynolds B. Cancer to the inguinal nodes from an unknown primary site. *J Surg Oncol* 17:39, 1981.

Wong JH, Cagle LA, Morton DL. Surgical treatment of lymph nodes with metastatic melanoma from unknown primary site. *Arch Surg* 122:1380, 1987.

Yang ZY, Hu YH, Yan JH, et al. Lymph node metastases in the neck from an unknown primary. *Acta Radiol Oncol* 22:17, 1983.

Genitourinary Cancer

Mark G. Delworth and Colin P.N. Dinney

Genitourinary cancers account for 16% of malignancies in humans. Prostate cancer is now the most common malignancy in American males. As the incidence of genitourinary cancers continues to increase, a clear understanding of the diagnosis and treatment of these diseases is essential. In this chapter we review the current management of prostate, bladder, renal, and testicular neoplasms.

Prostate Cancer

EPIDEMIOLOGY AND ETIOLOGY

Prostate cancer is the most common malignancy of men. From 1973 to 1988 the incidence of prostate cancer increased by an estimated 2.8% per year to a rate of 102 cases per 100,000 males in 1988. The incidence continues to climb and is higher for blacks than whites. Prostate cancer rarely occurs before age 50 years; incidence increases through the ninth decade of life. Some of this increased incidence may be attributed to the increase in prostate cancer screening using prostate-specific antigen (PSA) and transrectal ultrasound (TRUS). Carcinoma of the prostate is the second leading cause of solid cancer mortality in men, with rates of 47 per 100,000 black males and 23 per 100,000 white males. Thirty percent of men older than 50 years with no clinical evidence of prostate cancer will have a focus of cancer within the prostate on autopsy.

Many factors have been proposed as associated with the development of prostate cancer. The presence of an intact hypothalamic-pituitary-gonadal axis and advanced age are the most universally accepted risk factors. The relatively low rate of prostate cancer in the Orient is thought to be partially due to low-fat diets. It is unclear whether the increased mortality of prostate cancer in blacks is due to unique racial biologic factors or differences in health care delivery. Other factors that have been implicated (but not proved) in the development of prostate cancer include increased physical activity, increased sexual activity, cadmium exposure, increased zinc intake, and estrogen intake.

Evidence has shown that a man with one, two, or three first-degree relatives affected with prostate cancer has a two times, five times, or 11 times greater risk, respectively, for the development of prostate cancer. A Mendelian pattern of autosomal dominant transmission of prostate cancer accounts for 43% of disease occurring before age 55 years and 9% of all prostate cancers occurring by age 85 years.

ANATOMY

The normal prostate weighs 15–20 g and is divided into three major glandular zones. The *peripheral zone* constitutes 70% of the prostate and is the area palpated during digital rectal examination (DRE). The area around the ejaculatory ducts is called the *central zone* and accounts for 25% of the gland. The *transitional zone* makes up the 5% of the prostate gland around the urethra. In a pathologic review of 104 prostates from patients who underwent radical prostatectomy, 68% of the cancers were located in the peripheral zone, 24% in the transitional zone, and only 8% in the central zone. Almost all stage A (nonpalpable) cancers in that study were found in the transitional zone, the area most susceptible to benign prostatic hyperplasia.

SCREENING

Although there are good screening methods for prostate cancer, controversy surrounds the concept of screening for this disease. First, there is no consensus as to the optimal management of early-stage disease. Second, the cost of a national screening effort for all men over age 50 years would be high and possibly not cost-effective.

DIAGNOSIS

Patients with low-volume clinically localized prostate cancer are typically asymptomatic; abnormalities are detected by DRE or elevated serum PSA level. Advanced prostate cancer can be asymptomatic; present as local symptoms of urinary hesitancy, frequency, and urgency; or present as systemic symptoms of weight loss, fatigue, and bone pain.

Prostatic acid phosphatase (PAP) levels were widely used in the past as markers of prostate cancer; however, their use has been supplanted by PSA. PAP remains useful in the detection of metastatic disease and is a part of the staging system for prostate cancer, although it exhibits greater specificity but less sensitivity than PSA in the detection of metastatic disease.

PSA is a serine protease produced by the epithelium of the prostate. PSA is not specific for prostate cancer and can be elevated in such benign conditions of the prostate as prostatitis, prostatic infarction, and prostatic hyperplasia. Transurethral resection of the prostate (TURP) and prostatic needle biopsy have been shown to increase significantly the serum PSA level above baseline for up to 8 weeks. DRE, cystoscopy, and TRUS do not alter serum PSA to a clinically significant degree. Only 4% of men with a PSA <4 ng/ml have prostate cancer detectable by biopsy, whereas 58% with a PSA >10 ng/ml have prostate cancer. A palpable abnormality on DRE is associated with a 36% incidence of prostate cancer, compared with a 5% incidence of prostate cancer in patients with a normal DRE.

TRUS is performed using real-time imaging with a 7-MHz transducer, which allows both transverse and sagittal imaging of the prostate. Prostate cancer typically appears as a hypoechoic region within the prostate. TRUS can also be used to measure the dimensions of the prostate to calculate the glandular volume.

Lymphatic metastases can be detected by computed tomography (CT), lymphangiography, and magnetic resonance imaging (MRI). However, the only reliable method for staging pelvic lymph nodes is staging pelvic lymphadenectomy.

Radionuclide bone scan remains the most sensitive test to detect skeletal metastases. However, Chybowski et al. reviewed the medical records of 521 patients and found that only one patient with a PSA level below 20 ng/ml had evidence of skeletal metastasis. Therefore, based on these data, radionuclide bone scans may not be necessary for staging prostate cancer patients who have a low serum PSA level and no skeletal symptoms. When bone metastases are present, 80% are osteoblastic, 15% are mixed osteoblastic-osteolytic, and 5% are osteolytic. A chest radiograph is performed to detect the presence of pulmonary metastases.

The diagnosis of prostate cancer is made by the histologic finding of prostate cancer in a prostatic biopsy, in a prostatic needle aspiration, or in tissue obtained from prostatectomy for benign disease. Adenocarcinoma is the predominant cell type of prostate cancer and is the only type discussed in this chapter.

GRADING AND STAGING

The University of Texas M. D. Anderson Cancer Center grading system is based on the percentage of glandular formation by the tumor cells. Grade I carcinoma has greater than 75% gland formation, grade 2 has 51–75%, grade 3 has 26–50%, and grade 4 has less than 25% gland formation. The M. D. Anderson grading system has been shown to correlate with survival. The Gleason grading system is the other major grading system and recognizes five histologic patterns of prostate cancer. The scores of the predominant and secondary patterns are added to yield a range of tumor grades from 2 to 10.

The biologic behavior of the tumor can be further categorized by stage, which accounts for tumor volume and location. Prostate cancer typically spreads to the pelvic lymph nodes, bone, and lungs. The Organ Systems Coordinating Center and Hopkins (modified Jewett) staging systems are shown in Table 19-1.

MANAGEMENT OF LOCAL DISEASE

In 1987 the National Cancer Institute published a consensus statement on the treatment of early-stage prostate cancer. The report concluded, "Radical prostatectomy and radiation therapy are clearly effective forms of treatment in the attempt to cure tumors limited to the prostate for appropriately selected patients. . . . What remains unclear is the relative merit of each in producing lifelong freedom from cancer recurrence. . . . Properly designed and completed randomized trials that evaluate both disease control and quality of life after modern radiation therapy compared with radical prostatectomy are essential."

Surgery

The surgical excision of prostate cancer by complete removal of the prostate, seminal vesicles, and ampullae of the vasa deferentia was first performed in the early 1900s. This procedure, known

Table 19-1. Staging systems for prostate cancer

	Hopkins	OSCC
Primary tumor		
Anatomic relationship indefinable		TX
Digitally unrecognizable cancer		TA
<5% total surgical specimen, low or medium grade	A1	TA1
>5% total surgical specimen, any grade	A2	TA2
TA, but not A1 or A2		TAX
Digitally palpable cancer, organ-confined	B	TB
< half of one lobe, regardless of location	B1	TB1
> half lobe but <1 lobe	B1	TB2
>1 lobe or bilaterally palpable cancer	B2	TB3
Palpable cancer extending beyond prostate	C	TC
Extension beyond margin unilaterally		TC1
Extension beyond margin bilaterally		TC2
Extension into bladder, rectum, levator muscles, or pelvic side walls		TC3
Nodal status		
No regional lymph node metastases		N0
Microscopic regional lymph node metastasis, proven histologically	D1	N1
Gross regional lymph node metastases	D1	N2
Extraregional lymph node metastases		N3
Minimal requirements have not been met		NX
Distant metastases		
No evidence of metastases		M0
Elevated acid phosphatase only	D0	M1
Visceral and/or bone metastases	D2	M2
Minimal requirements not met		MX

OSCC = Organ Systems Coordinating Center.

as a *radical prostatectomy,* can be performed using a perineal or retropubic approach.

Gibbons et al. reviewed their experience of total prostatectomy in 215 patients and found that overall and disease-free survival rates, respectively, were 94% and 86% at 5 years, 75% and 67% at 10 years, and 55% and 48% at 15 years. Morbidity has decreased significantly over the past several decades. Leandri et al. reported on 620 patients and found a 6.9% early complication rate, 1.3% late complication rate, and 0.2% mortality rate. Sexual potency was maintained in 71% in whom a nerve-sparing technique was used, and 5% experienced stress incontinence after 1 year.

Radiotherapy

External-beam radiotherapy has been used for the definitive treatment of localized and regionally extensive prostatic adenocarcinoma. At M. D. Anderson, 60–70 Gy was given to 114 patients with localized prostate cancer as primary therapy. The 5- and 10-year uncorrected survival rates are comparable to radical surgery (89% and 68%, respectively). In this series there was no difference in survival between patients with stages A and B disease. Skeletal metastases were the major site of relapse. Serious complications developed in only 1.8% of treated patients. At M. D. Anderson we currently recommend radical prostatectomy for the treatment of early-stage prostate cancer. Primary radiotherapy is reserved for patients with significant comorbid medical illnesses.

Stage C Disease

Stage C prostate cancer involves areas outside the prostatic capsule, such as fat, seminal vesicles, levator muscles, or other adjacent structures. This stage of prostate cancer is associated with a 53% incidence of lymph node metastases and decreased overall survival rate. At M. D. Anderson, stage C disease is treated with primary radiotherapy with 5-, 10-, and 15-year uncorrected actuarial survival rates of 72%, 47%, and 17%, respectively. The local control rate in our experience with stage C disease is 75% at 15 years of follow-up.

Treatment modalities, other than radiotherapy, used for stage C disease include radical prostatectomy, TURP, and hormonal therapy. Tumor grade, stage, bulk of tumor, and seminal vesicle involvement in stage C disease are associated with the interval between radical prostatectomy and disease progression. The actuarial 5-year survival rate for patients with stage C disease who have undergone TURP in stage C disease is 64%, making TURP an option for patients with short life expectancies, such as the very elderly and those with serious coexisting medical problems. Currently, several groups are investigating the use of hormonal therapy in an attempt to downstage B2/C tumors before extirpative surgery.

Stage D Disease

Approximately 20% of patients present with stage D1 prostate cancer, and 75% of these patients develop bone metastases. As with other stages of prostate cancer, there appears to be a great deal of variability within D1 disease. Barzell et al. found that patients with low-volume nodal disease had a 71% 5-year metastasis-free survival with treatment. However, a similar population of patients followed for 10 years had a 14% disease-free survival rate. The optimal treatment for D1 disease is controversial. Observation, hormonal treatment, radiation, cytoreductive surgery, and combinations of these have been used with various degrees of success. For patients with low-volume nodal disease, cytoreductive surgery combined with hormonal treatment appears to yield the best 5-year disease-free survival rate: 65–95%.

Stage D2 represents systemic disease. Patients have a median survival of 30 months, with an estimated 5-year survival rate of 20%. The treatment of metastatic prostate cancer is androgen ablation therapy. The hypothalamus produces luteinizing hormone-releasing hormone (LHRH) and corticotropin-releasing factor (CRF), which stimulate the anterior pituitary to release adrenocorticotropic hormone (ACTH) and luteinizing hormone

(LH). LH stimulates testosterone production by the testes, and ACTH stimulates the adrenals to produce androstenedione and dehydroepiandrosterone, precursors of testosterone and dihydrotestosterone (DHT). Although the testes are the major source of testosterone, the adrenals can supply up to 20% of the DHT found in the prostate.

Early androgen ablation therapy consisted of either estrogen supplementation or bilateral orchiectomy. More recently, LHRH agonists have been developed that chronically stimulate the pituitary, resulting in a decrease in LH release. This, in turn, leads to castrate levels of testosterone production by the testes. Flutamide, an antiandrogen, works by blocking uptake or binding of androgen in target tissues.

Bilateral orchiectomy, estrogens, and LHRH agonists appear to have equal efficacy when used as monotherapy for metastatic prostate cancer. Total androgen ablation with an LHRH agonist plus an antiandrogen may be more effective than any form of monotherapy. Despite effective initial therapy, the eventual emergence of androgen-insensitive tumor cells leads to the demise of the patient.

Bladder Cancer

EPIDEMIOLOGY AND ETIOLOGY

Bladder cancer is the second most common genitourinary malignancy. It is the fourth most common cancer in males and the eleventh most common cancer in females. The incidence is lowest in black females (6 per 100,000) and highest in white males (33 per 100,000). White males also have the highest mortality rate—6 deaths per 100,000.

The etiology of urothelial cancers, of which bladder cancer is the most common, is well established. Cigarette smoking has been linked to 30–40% of all cases of bladder cancer. The chemicals 1-naphthylamine, 2-naphthylamine, benzidine, and 4-aminobiphenyl have been shown to promote urothelial carcinogenesis. Workers in the textile, leather, aluminum refining, rubber, and chemical industries who are exposed to high levels of these chemicals have an increased incidence of bladder cancer. Other chemicals that have been linked to urothelial cancer are MBUCCA (plastics industry), phenacetin, and the antineoplastic agent cyclophosphamide. In addition, recurrent bladder infections, as well as infections with the parasite *Schistosoma haematobium,* have been associated with squamous cell carcinoma of the bladder.

PATHOLOGY

The urinary bladder is a hollow viscus that functions in both the storage and evacuation of urine. Histologically, the bladder is composed of mucosa, lamina propria, muscularis, and serosa (limited to the dome). Localized bladder cancer is classified as *superficial disease,* which is limited to the mucosa and lamina propria, or *inva-*

sive disease, which extends into the muscularis and beyond. About 70% of newly diagnosed bladder cancer is superficial, whereas the remaining 30% is invasive or metastatic. Once a bladder cancer extends through the basal layer of the mucosa, it may invade blood vessels and lymphatics, thereby providing a route of metastasis. Carcinoma *in situ,* an aggressive form of superficial disease, is composed of anaplastic cells limited to the mucosal layer.

The World Health Organization (WHO) classifies epithelial tumors of the bladder into four histologic types: transitional cell carcinoma (TCC) (91%), squamous cell carcinoma (7%), adenocarcinoma (2%), and undifferentiated carcinoma (<1%). However, up to 20% of TCCs contain areas of squamous differentiation, and up to 7% contain areas of adenomatous differentiation. The remainder of this section discusses TCC.

CLINICAL PRESENTATION

Eighty percent of all patients who present with bladder carcinoma have gross or microscopic hematuria, typically painless and intermittent. About 20% of patients complain of symptoms of vesical irritability, including urinary frequency, urgency, and dysuria. Other symptoms include pelvic pain, flank pain (from ureteral obstruction), and lower-extremity edema. Patients with systemic disease may present with anemia, weight loss, and bone pain.

DIAGNOSIS

A patient who presents with hematuria or other symptoms of bladder cancer should undergo a thorough urologic evaluation consisting of a history, physical examination, urinalysis, intravenous urogram, and cystoscopic examination of the urinary bladder with barbotage of urine for cytologic examination. The most useful of these steps is the examination of the bladder using a rigid or flexible cystoscope. Papillary and sessile tumors are easily visualized through the cystoscope; carcinoma *in situ,* however, can appear as normal mucosa. Fewer than 60% of bladder tumors can be seen on an intravenous urogram, but this examination will also identify other abnormalities that may be present in the genitourinary tract. Results of barbotage of urine can be expected to be positive in 10% of patients with grade 1 tumors, 50% of patients with grade 2 tumors, and up to 90% of patients with grade 3 tumors or carcinoma *in situ.* Flow cytometric examination of urine can detect hyperdiploid cell lines with a high degree of sensitivity. Quantitative fluorescent image analysis, a relatively new method of detection that combines quantification of DNA and morphometric analysis, is reported to be both sensitive (76%) and specific (94%).

GRADING AND STAGING

The WHO uses a grading system based on the cytologic features of the tumor. Grade 1 represents a well-differentiated tumor; grade 2, a moderately differentiated tumor; and grade 3, a poorly differentiated bladder cancer.

Once a bladder tumor is diagnosed, the urologist must accurately stage the tumor. The initial transurethral resection of the bladder tumor (TURBT) will determine the histologic depth of

Table 19-2. Staging systems for bladder cancer

	Jewett-Strong-Marshall stage	TNM stage	
		Clinical	Pathologic
No tumor in specimen	O	T0	Po
Carcinoma *in situ*	O	Tis	Pis
Noninvasive papillary tumor	O	TA	PA
Lamina propria invasion	A	T1	P1
Superficial muscle invasion	B1	T2	P2
Deep muscle invasion	B2	T3A	P3
Invasion of perivesical fat	C	T3B	P3
Invasion of contiguous organ	D1	T4	P4
Regional lymph node metastases	D1		
Single homolateral node			N1
Bilateral regional or contralateral nodes			N2
Fixed regional nodes			N3
Juxtaregional lymph node metastases	D2		N4
Distant metastases	D2	M1	M1

invasion of the tumor as well as the presence or absence of dysplasia or carcinoma *in situ*. A bimanual examination should be performed at the time of resection to determine whether a mass is present and, if so, whether it is fixed or mobile.

Further work-up for detecting metastasis consists of a CT scan, liver function tests, a chest radiograph, and a bone scan (if the alkaline phosphatase level is elevated or the patient's symptoms suggest systemic disease). The Jewett-Strong-Marshall and International Union Against Cancer (TNM) staging systems are listed in Table 19-2.

MANAGEMENT

Superficial Bladder Cancer

Most bladder cancers present as superficial disease. Approximately 70% of these superficial cancers are papillary, 10% are nodular, and 20% are mixed. After the initial treatment of superficial bladder cancer, the cancer can be cured, can recur with the same stage and grade, or can recur with progression of stage or grade. Risk factors associated with both disease recurrence and progression include a high tumor grade, lamina propria invasion, dysplasia elsewhere in the bladder, positive urinary cytology findings, and tumor diameter larger than 5 cm.

Initial treatment of superficial bladder cancer focuses on eradication of the existing disease and prophylaxis against disease recurrence or progression. TURBT has been the standard treatment for existing stage TA and T1 tumors as well as visible stage Tis tumors. Other treatment modalities for the eradication of superficial disease include laser fulguration and photodynamic therapy. The advantage of transurethral resection over the other modalities is that it provides tissue for histologic examination.

Patients with high-grade TA or T1 lesions, multiple tumors, recurrent tumors, tumors associated with Tis, aneuploid tumors, tumors larger than 5 cm, and persistently positive cytology findings may be candidates for adjuvant intravesical therapy. Intravesical agents can be used as therapeutic, adjuvant, or prophylactic treatment for bladder cancer. Thiotepa, mitomycin C, doxorubicin, and etoglucid are the chemotherapeutic agents used most frequently. Bacillus Calmette-Guérin (BCG), a live attenuated tuberculosis organism, has become the most widely used intravesical agent in superficial bladder cancer. BCG enhances the patient's own immune response against the tumor, providing resistance to disease recurrence and progression. Although specific dose scheduling varies, most treatment regimens include intravesical treatment weekly for a period of 4–8 weeks, followed by an optional series of maintenance treatments administered over many months.

Invasive Bladder Cancer

Tumors that have penetrated the muscularis propria are considered invasive. There are several options for treatment of patients with invasive tumors. A small subset of patients may be eligible for bladder-sparing therapy. With aggressive transurethral re-resection of invasive bladder tumors, a 67% survival rate can be obtained for those retaining their bladder (median follow-up was 5 years). Patients with a muscle invasive tumor that is primary and solitary, does not have surrounding urothelial atypia, and allows for a 2-cm surgical margin may be candidates for partial cystectomy. At M. D. Anderson, data have shown that approximately 5% of patients are actually suitable for bladder-sparing surgery; 5-year survival rates have been comparable to those achieved with radical cystectomy.

Primary external beam radiotherapy has been used to treat invasive bladder cancer. Treatment protocols advocate doses of 65–70 Gy. Five-year survival rates range from 21% to 52% for stage B2 and from 18% to 30% for stage C. Local recurrence occurs in 50–70% of these patients. Stage T4 lesions fare worse, with 5-year survival rates consistently below 10%. Thus external beam radiotherapy may be useful in patients who do not wish to have surgery or for whom radical surgery is medically contraindicated; however, the survival rate for radiotherapy is below that for radical surgery.

Radical cystectomy with pelvic lymphadenectomy is performed with the intent of removing all localized and lymphatic disease present. At M. D. Anderson, the 5-year actuarial survival rate for patients with invasive bladder carcinoma after radical cystectomy alone is 79% for stage B, 46% for stage C, 54% for stage D with nodal spread, and 32% for stage D with visceral metastases. The local recurrence rate is 7% and the operative mortality rate is 1.1%. Fourteen percent of patients undergoing cystectomy with lymphadenectomy are found to have unsuspected metastases to the pelvic lymph nodes. The majority of these cases involve one or two nodes limited to an area below the bifurcation of the common iliac arteries and medial to the external iliac artery.

Once a patient undergoes cystectomy, the ureters must be diverted into an alternate drainage system. The most common urinary diversion used today is the cutaneous ureteroileal diversion popularized by Bricker in the 1950s. This form of urinary diversion involves the anastomosis of each ureter to the proximal end of an isolated piece of ileum; the distal end is brought out as a cutaneous stoma for drainage into a urinary appliance.

Metastatic Disease

Cisplatin appears to be the single agent with the greatest activity against TCC of the bladder; however, single-agent therapy response rates are only in the range of 10–30%. The highest response rates documented to date have been with regimens that include cisplatin, methotrexate, vinblastine, and doxorubicin (M-VAC). In the M. D. Anderson trial of M-VAC, a complete response rate of 35% and a partial response rate of 30% were observed. Other trials have documented similar response rates, with median survival of approximately 1 year. Many groups have proposed the use of M-VAC in both a neoadjuvant and adjuvant setting. Data from prospective randomized trials are needed to clarify the role M-VAC should play in each of these areas.

Renal Cancer

EPIDEMIOLOGY AND ETIOLOGY

Tumors of the renal and perirenal tissues comprise 2–3% of all adult visceral tumors. Renal cell carcinoma (RCC) represents 85% of all renal parenchymal tumors and is the only renal tumor discussed in this chapter. In 1994, an estimated 27,600 people will be diagnosed with renal cancer and 11,300 people will die of this disease. Males are affected twice as often as females. RCC most frequently occurs in the fifth to sixth decade of life.

In contrast with the known causes of bladder cancer, the etiology of RCC is unknown. It has been speculated that smoking, industrial contamination, asbestos, petroleum by-products, and viruses may play roles in the development of RCC. RCC may occur either sporadically or genetically as part of von Hippel-Lindau disease, which is characterized by cerebellar hemangioblastoma, retinal angiomata, bilateral RCC, and islet cell tumors of the pancreas. Both disease types have a common genetic mechanism that includes loss of a region of chromosome 3. RCC is also associated with polycystic kidney disease, "horseshoe kidneys," and acquired renal cystic disease.

PATHOLOGY

Most RCCs originate in the proximal tubular cell of the kidney. The tumor is multicentric in up to 7% of cases. Local extension of the tumor is limited by the renal capsule and Gerota's fascia surrounding the kidney. The predominant cell type is clear cell, but granular and spindle-shaped cells also may be present. The tumor cells are typically rich in glycogen and lipid, giving the tumor a clear cell appearance microscopically and a characteristic yellow appearance grossly.

CLINICAL PRESENTATION

RCC has often been called the "internist's tumor" because of its subtle presentation. Gross or microscopic hematuria, the most common presenting symptom, is present in more than half of patients with RCC. The classic triad of hematuria, abdominal mass, and flank pain occurs in about 19% of patients. Paraneoplastic syndromes occur in 10–40% of cases and consist of pyrexia, anemia, erythrocytosis, hypercalcemia, liver dysfunction (Stauffer's syndrome), and hypertension. Other symptoms can include bone pain and central nervous system abnormalities, as up to 30% of patients present with bone and brain metastases.

DIAGNOSIS

The work-up of a patient with the preceding symptoms should include a history, physical examination, complete blood count, serum chemistry panel, urinalysis, urine culture, and IV urogram. Typically, the IV urogram will show a renal mass (if present), which can be categorized as solid, cystic, or indeterminate. Cystic masses should undergo renal ultrasound, which will confirm the characteristics of a simple renal cyst (through transmission, smooth wall, posterior enhancement). A patient with a solid or indeterminate mass or complex cyst should have a contrast-enhanced CT scan. In most cases, the CT scan will define the nature of the mass. A renal angiogram can be used to demonstrate hypervascularity, which is present in 90% of RCCs, as well as to provide useful information for planning an operative procedure, especially when a partial nephrectomy is considered. If any of the studies obtained suggests involvement of the renal vein or vena cava, an abdominal ultrasound, color Doppler, or MRI study should be obtained to assess the extent of the tumor thrombus. In contrast to the management of other renal tumors, a surgeon may perform a radical nephrectomy for RCC without preoperative histologic diagnosis of the tumor.

If a mass suggests RCC, a metastatic work-up consisting of a chest radiograph, CT scan (if not already obtained), and liver function tests should be performed. The most common sites of metastases of RCC in decreasing order are the lung, bone, and regional lymph nodes. If the patient does not have an elevated alkaline phosphatase level or skeletal pain, a bone scan is usually not required. A CT scan of the brain can be performed if there is any suspicion of brain metastases; however, this is not done routinely.

GRADING AND STAGING

There is no universal grading system for RCC. Patients with the sarcomatoid variant seem to fare slightly worse than those

Table 19-3. Staging systems for renal cell cancer

	Robson	TNM
Tumor confined by renal capsule	I	
Small tumor, minimal calyceal distortion		T1
Large tumor, calyceal deformity		T2
Tumor extension to perirenal fat or ipsilateral adrenal, confined by Gerota's fascia	II	T3a
Renal vein involvement	IIIa	T3b
Renal vein and vena caval involvement below the diaphragm	IIIa	T3c
Vena caval involvement above the diaphragm	IIIa	T4b
Lymphatic involvement	IIIb	
Single homolateral regional node		N1
Multiple regional, contralateral, or bilateral nodes		N2
Fixed regional nodes		N3
Juxtaregional nodes involved		N4
Combination of IIIa and IIIb	IIIc	
Spread to contiguous organs except ipsilateral adrenal	IVa	T4a
Distant metastases	IVb	M1

with the granular or clear cell type, and it is generally agreed that the sarcomatoid cell type is found in more aggressive tumors.

The Robson and TNM staging systems, the most commonly used in the United States, are shown in Table 19-3.

MANAGEMENT

Localized Renal Cell Carcinoma

Surgical excision is the only effective treatment of localized RCC. In a radical nephrectomy, the kidney, ipsilateral adrenal, and surrounding Gerota's fascia are all resected en bloc. Although no randomized study has proved its benefit over simple nephrectomy, radical nephrectomy has the theoretic advantage of removing the lymphatics within the perinephric fat. Up to 20% of patients have evidence of regional lymphatic metastases without distant disease. The 5-year survival rates for patients with positive lymph nodes range from 8% to 35%. Extended lymphadenectomy has never been proved to be of benefit in patients who undergo radical nephrectomy, and many surgeons prefer to do a limited node dissection, which has limited morbidity, for prognostic information.

The surgical approach to radical nephrectomy is determined by the size and location of the tumor as well as the surgeon's preference. A modified flank, midline, or subcostal (chevron) incision can be used. Large upper-pole tumors may be approached through a thoracoabdominal incision for greater exposure. Because the incidence of ipsilateral adrenal metastasis in lower-pole tumors is rare, it is acceptable not to remove the adrenal at the time of nephrectomy for a lower-pole lesion.

Approximately 15–20% of RCCs invade the renal vein and 8–15% invade the vena cava. Involvement of RCC in the renal vein usually does not pose a significant problem. Vena caval involvement, however, may require additional extensive procedures. Vena caval thrombi have been divided by many authors into three groups. Type 1 thrombi (50%) are completely infrahepatic, type 2 (40%) are intrahepatic, and type 3 (10%) extend up into the right atrium of the heart. In cases with vena caval involvement it is imperative that the surgeon be familiar with techniques of vascular surgery, and consideration should be given to consulting with a cardiothoracic surgeon, especially for type 3 thrombi.

There are situations in which radical nephrectomy may not be the best option for the patient. For example, in cases of bilateral tumor involvement, renal insufficiency, a solitary kidney, or von Hippel-Lindau disease, a parenchyma-sparing procedure may be indicated. In this procedure, the renal artery is temporarily occluded, the kidney cooled down, and partial nephrectomy or wedge resection performed. Frozen sections of the surgical margins are typically analyzed to ensure adequacy of resection. After restoration of arterial blood flow, the renal capsule is closed or, alternatively, omentum or perirenal fat is sutured to the defect to promote healing. Five-year survival rates after partial nephrectomy for patients with stage I and II disease are approximately 70% and 60%, respectively.

Advanced Renal Cell Carcinoma

Approximately 10% of patients present with locally advanced disease that has invaded adjacent structures. In general, the 3-year survival rate for these patients after surgery is less than 10%. Nephrectomy in this situation is done to improve the quality of life for symptomatic patients rather than to prolong survival. Recently, however, nephrectomy has also been performed in the presence of metastatic disease to satisfy clinical protocols that require removal of the primary lesion.

Distant metastatic disease can be categorized as a solitary metastasis or bulky metastatic disease. Several studies have shown improved 3-year survival rates, ranging from 20% to 60%, after radical nephrectomy with removal of a solitary metastasis. Solitary lung metastases appear to be associated with better survival rates than metastases to other organ sites.

Cytotoxic chemotherapy is ineffective in RCC; the highest objective response rate for single-agent therapy is only 16%. Thus medical treatment for metastatic RCC has focused on the use of immunotherapy. The combination of alpha-interferon (IFN-α) and interleukin-2 (IL-2) has yielded response rates of 21–50% in various trials. In addition, it has been shown that both IFN-α and IL-2 can be given subcutaneously on an outpatient basis with side effects that are well tolerated. Currently, it is unclear whether nephrectomy will augment this response.

Testicular Cancer

EPIDEMIOLOGY AND ETIOLOGY

Malignant tumors of the testis are rare. It is estimated that 6,800 cases of testis cancer will be diagnosed in 1994, but only 325 men will die of this disease. Ninety-five percent of these tumors are of germ cell origin. Although testis tumors can occur at any age, specific tumor types tend to occur at different ages. Choriocarcinomas tend to occur between 24 and 28 years of age, embryonal carcinomas from 26 to 34 years of age, seminomas from 32 to 42 years of age, and lymphomas and spermatocytic seminomas after the age of 50 years.

The most well-known etiologic factor in the development of testis cancer is cryptorchidism. Between 3% and 11% of all cases of testis cancer occur in cryptorchid testes. Although trauma to the testis has been linked to testis cancer, there is no evidence of a definite relationship.

CLINICAL PRESENTATION

Testicular cancer typically presents as a painless testicular enlargement. Advanced disease can present as back pain, flank pain, or systemic symptoms. The differential diagnosis includes varicocele, hydrocele, hematoma, epididymitis, orchitis, and inguinal hernia.

DIAGNOSIS

Although the diagnosis is usually evident at physical examination to an experienced clinician, scrotal ultrasound can be useful in establishing the diagnosis. Any solid testicular mass is considered a testicular tumor until proved otherwise. Once a testicular tumor is suspected, the patient's levels of the tumor markers alpha-fetoprotein (AFP) and human chorionic gonadotropin (HCG) should be tested. Following this, he should undergo a radical (inguinal) orchiectomy. There is no role for fine-needle aspiration or Tru-cut biopsy in the work-up of this disease.

After radical orchiectomy, a CT scan of the chest, abdomen, and pelvis should be performed. If they were initially elevated, tumor markers should be reanalyzed following orchiectomy, after allowing the appropriate time for each marker to return to baseline.

STAGING

The M. D. Anderson staging system for testicular cancer is outlined in Table 19-4. In terms of biologic behavior and therapy, testicular tumors can be categorized as seminomatous or non-seminomatous germ cell tumors (NSGCT). Seminomas are radio-sensitive and chemosensitive tumors that undergo lymphatic spread in an orderly fashion. In contrast, NSGCT are less radio-sensitive and have a higher metastatic rate than seminomas.

Table 19-4.   M. D. Anderson Cancer Center staging systems for testicular cancer

	Stage
Seminoma	
Confined to testicle	I
Retroperitoneal disease only, mass < 10 cm	IIA
Retroperitoneal disease only, mass > 10 cm	IIB
Supradiaphragmatic nodal disease	IIIA
Visceral disease	IIIB
Nonseminomatous germ cell tumor	
Confined to testicle	I
Negative clinical, positive surgical RPLND or elevated markers postorchiectomy	IIA
RPLND mass < 2 cm	IIB
RPLND mass < 5 cm	IIC
RPLND mass < 10 cm	IID
Supraclavicular nodal disease	IIIA
Elevated marker(s) post-RPLND dissection	IIIB1
Pulmonary disease (minimal or advanced)	IIIB2
Advanced abdominal disease (mass > 10 cm)	IIIB3
Visceral disease other than lung	IIIB4
β-hCG > 50,000 IU, ± IIIB2, − IIIB4	IIIB5

RPLND = retroperitoneal lymph node dissection; β-hCG = human chorionic gonadotropin (beta subunit).

MANAGEMENT

Seminomatous Germ Cell Tumors

Stage I and IIA seminomas are typically treated with radiotherapy to the ipsilateral iliac and periaortic areas up to the level of the diaphragm after radical orchiectomy. Using radiotherapy, the cure rate for stage I disease approaches 100%. Although 10–15% of patients with stage IIA disease have relapses, more than half of these respond successfully to salvage therapy, yielding a survival rate of 95% for patients with stage IIa disease.

Stage IIB or III disease is usually treated with cisplatin- or carboplatin-based chemotherapy. Surgery is generally reserved for lymphatic disease that does not respond to chemotherapy or radiotherapy. Using this approach, 5-year disease-free survival rates of 86% and 92% have been obtained for patients with stages IIB and III disease, respectively.

Nonseminomatous Germ Cell Tumors

The optimal therapy for stage I disease is controversial; options include surveillance, retroperitoneal lymph node dissection (RPLND), and primary systemic chemotherapy. Overall, about 20–30% of stage I patients who undergo surveillance relapse. Wishnow et al. at M. D. Anderson Cancer Center found that patients with vascular invasion in their tumor, AFP levels greater than 80 ng/ml, or more than 80% embryonal elements in their tumor were at high risk for relapse. Twenty to thirty percent of patients who undergo RPLND are upstaged to stage II, allowing rational use of adjuvant chemotherapy. In addition, RPLND offers excellent local control for stage I tumors. After treatment with RPLND (and chemotherapy, if needed), survival rates are 99% for stage I and 95% for those upstaged to stage IIA.

The recurrence rate after RPLND for stage IIA disease is less than 20%. Thus both RPLND and primary systemic chemotherapy have been used to treat low-volume retroperitoneal disease. Survival rates of 97% or better have been associated with both forms of therapy.

Because of the high recurrence rates associated with RPLND for stage IIB and III NSGCTs, primary systemic chemotherapy is the treatment of choice for this disease. RPLND is used to remove any residual disease that may be present after primary chemotherapy and to determine the need for further therapy. Recent experience with chemotherapy for advanced NSGCT at M. D. Anderson has shown survival rates of 96% and 76% for low- and high-volume stage III disease, respectively.

Because a majority of NCGCTs produce either AFP or β-hCG, these markers are helpful in monitoring the patient for treatment response and recurrent disease.

Despite the relatively early age of onset of testis cancer, this disease remains one of the most curable cancers in humans.

Selected References

PROSTATE CANCER

Barzell W, Bean MA, Hilaris BS, Whitmore WF Jr. Prostatic adenocarcinoma: Relationship of grade and local extent to the pattern of metastases. *J Urol* 118:278, 1977.

Brawn PN, Ayala AG, von Eschenbach AC, et al. Histologic grading study of prostate adenocarcinoma: The development of a new system and comparison of other methods—a preliminary study. *Cancer* 49:525, 1982.

Chybowski FM, Keller JJ, Bergstralh EJ, Oesterling JE. Predicting radionuclide bone scan findings in patients with newly diagnosed untreated prostate cancer: Prostate specific antigen is superior to all other clinical parameters. *J Urol* 145:313, 1991.

Cooner WH, Mosley BR, Rutherford JR, et al. Prostate cancer detection in a clinical urological practice by ultrasonography, digital rectal examination and prostate specific antigen. *J Urol* 143:1146, 1990.

Crawford ED, Nabors WL. Total androgen ablation: American experience. *Urol Clin North Am* 18:55, 1991.

Gibbons RP, Correa RJ Jr, Brannen GE, et al. Total prostatectomy for localized prostate cancer. *J Urol* 131:73, 1984.

Kazlowski JM, Grayhack JT. Carcinoma of the Prostate. In JY Gillenwater, JT Grayhack, SS Howards, et al. (eds), *Adult and Pediatric Urology*. Chicago: Year Book, 1987.

Leandri P, Rossignol G, Gautier JR, et al. Radical retropubic prostatectomy: Morbidity and quality of life. Experience with 620 consecutive cases. *J Urol* 147:883, 1992.

McNeal JE, Redwine EA, Freiha FS, et al. Zonal distribution of prostatic adenocarcinoma. *Am J Surg Pathol* 12:897, 1988.

National Institutes of Health. Consensus development conference on
the management of clinically localized prostate cancer (1987:
Bethesda, MD). NCI monograph no. 7, NIH publication no. 88-3005.
Washington, DC: U.S. Government Printing Office. Pp. 3–6, 1988.

Scardino PT, Frankel JM, Wheeler TM, et al. The prognostic significance of post-irradiation biopsy results in patients with prostate
cancer. *J Urol* 135:510, 1986.

Stamey TA, McNeal JE. Adenocarcinoma of the prostate. In PC
Walsh, AB Retik, TA Stamey, et al. (eds.), *Campbell's Urology* (6th
ed). Philadelphia: Saunders, 1992.

Wynder EL, Mabuchi K, Whitmore WF. Epidemiology of cancer of the
prostate. *Cancer* 28:344, 1971.

Zagars GK, von Eschenbach AC, Johnson DE, et al. The role of radiation therapy in stages A2 and B adenocarcinoma of the prostate.
Int J Radiat Oncol Biol Phys 14:701, 1988.

BLADDER CANCER

Catalona WJ. Bladder Cancer. In JY Gillenwater, JT Grayhack, SS
Howards, et al. (eds.), *Adult and Pediatric Urology*. Chicago: Year
Book, 1987.

Cummings KB, Barone JG, Ward WS. Diagnosis and staging of bladder cancer. *Urol Clin North Am* 19:429, 1992.

Heney NM, Ahmad S, Flanagan MJ, et al. Superficial bladder cancer:
Progression and recurrence. *J Urol* 130:1083, 1983.

Lamm DL. Long term results of intravesical therapy for superficial
bladder cancer. *Urol Clin North Am* 19:573, 1992.

Logothetis CJ, Dexeus FH, Finn L, et al. A prospective randomized
trial comparing MVAC and CISCA chemotherapy for patients with
metastatic urothelial tumors. *J Clin Oncol* 8:1050, 1990.

RENAL CANCER

Couillard DR, deVere White RW. Surgery of renal cell carcinoma.
Urol Clin North Am 20:263, 1993.

Williams RD. Renal, Perirenal, and Ureteral Neoplasms. In JY
Gillenwater, JT Grayhack, SS Howards, et al. (eds.), *Adult and
Pediatric Urology*. Chicago: Year Book, 1987.

Wirth MP. Immunotherapy for metastatic renal cell carcinoma. *Urol
Clin North Am* 20:283, 1993.

TESTIS CANCER

Logothetis CJ. The case for relevant staging of germ cell tumors.
Cancer 65:709, 1990.

Sternberg CN. Role of primary chemotherapy in stage I and low-
volume stage II nonseminomatous germ-cell testis tumors. *Urol
Clin North Am* 20:93, 1993.

Wishnow KI, Johnson DE, Swanson DA, et al. Identifying patients
with low-risk clinical stage I nonseminomatous testicular tumors
who should be treated by surveillance. *Urology* 34:339, 1989.

Gynecologic Cancers

Michael W. Bevers, Diane C. Bodurka Bevers, and Judith K. Wolf

The surgical oncologist and the gynecologic oncologist share a common territory—the abdomen. The surgical oncologist must at a minimum maintain a familiarity with all oncologic processes affecting the abdominal cavity. Unfortunately, the subspecialization of medicine not only challenges physicians to keep pace with advances in their own fields, but also makes learning about advances and trends in other fields a Herculean task. This chapter discusses the basics of gynecologic oncology so that these disease processes are considered when examining patients and appropriate management occurs when encountering these neoplasms unexpectedly. Emphasis is placed on diagnosis, staging, and surgical management.

Vulvar Cancer

INCIDENCE

Vulvar cancer accounts for 3–5% of all female genital malignancies and 1% of all malignancies in women. Between 2,000 and 3,000 new cases are diagnosed annually. The average age at diagnosis is 65, with the trend moving toward younger age at time of diagnosis.

RISK FACTORS

The cause of vulvar cancer appears to be multifactorial; this disease is not as strongly associated with human papillomavirus as is cervical cancer. Risk factors include advanced age, low socioeconomic status, hypertension, diabetes, prior lower genital tract malignancy (cervical cancer), and immunosuppressed status.

PATHOLOGY

Eighty-five percent of vulvar malignancies are squamous cell carcinomas; 6% of cases are malignant melanomas.

ROUTES OF SPREAD

Vulvar cancer spreads by direct extension, embolization to regional lymphatics (groin), and hematogenous spread to distant sites.

CLINICAL FEATURES

Symptoms
Chronic pruritis, ulceration, and the presence of nodules are symptoms of this disease.

Physical Findings

Lesions arise from the labia majora (40%), labia minora (20%), periclitoral area (10%), and perineum/posterior fourchette (15%). Lesions may appear as a dominant mass, warty area, ulcerated area, or thickened white epithelium.

DIAGNOSIS

Five percent of cases are multifocal. It is critical to biopsy any suspicious area. Use a Keye's punch biopsy and lidocaine without epinephrine for anesthesia. Most patients tolerate mild discomfort well.

PRETREATMENT WORK-UP

Careful physical examination, including pelvic examination and measurement of the lesion, is required. Other components of the pretreatment work-up include complete blood count, serum glucose, blood urea nitrogen, creatinine, and liver function tests; chest x-ray; mammogram; and cystoscopy and/or proctoscopy, depending on site and extent of lesion. Barium enema, computed tomography (CT), or magnetic resonance imaging (MRI) should be performed if indicated. Preoperative medical clearance is necessary for patients with chronic disease or other appropriate indications.

STAGING

Since 1988, vulvar cancer has been surgically staged using a system that incorporates the TNM (tumor, node, metastasis) classification; modifications to the TNM system were added in 1995 (Table 20-1).

Treatment of Vulvar Cancer by Stage

Stage I
Wide local excision should be performed if the lesion is microinvasive (<1 mm invasion). Radical wide excision with a traditional 2-cm gross margin (measured with ruler) and superficial dissection of the ipsilateral groin is appropriate for all other stage I lesions. Bilateral superficial groin dissection should be performed if the lesion is within 1 cm of the midline.

Stage II
Radical vulvectomy with bilateral node dissection, including superficial and deep inguinal nodes, is the standard approach to stage II disease. A more conservative approach used at M. D. Anderson Cancer Center is radical wide excision instead of radical vulvectomy; local recurrence rates are similar. Adjuvant radiotherapy may be indicated if the tumor-free margin of resection is <8 mm, tumor thickness is >5 mm, or lymphovascular space invasion is present.

Stage III
Treatment must be individualized for each patient with stage III disease. Options include surgery, radiation, and/or a combination of treatment modalities, again depending on each patient's case. A

Table 20-1. Surgical staging of vulvar cancer

Stage	Classification	Description
IA	T1N0M0	Tumor confined to the vulva and/or perineum; lesion is 2 cm or smaller in diameter with stromal invasion no greater than 1 mm; negative nodes.
IB	T1N0M0	Tumor confined to the vulva and/or perineum; lesion is 2 cm or less in diameter with stromal invasion greater than 1 mm; negative nodes.
II	T2N0M0	Tumor confined to the vulva and/or perineum; lesion is larger than 2 cm in diameter; negative nodes.
III	T3N0M0 T3N1M0 T1N1M0 T2N1M0	Tumor of any size with adjacent spread to the lower urethra and/or vagina, the anus, or unilateral regional lymph node metastasis.
IVA	T1N2M0 T2N2M0 T3N2M0 T4, any N, M0	Tumor invades the upper urethra, bladder mucosa, rectal mucosa, pelvic bone, and/or bilateral regional metastasis.
IVB	Any T or N, M1	Any distant metastasis, including pelvic nodes.

modified radical vulvectomy (radical wide local excision is used in some institutions) with inguinal and femoral node dissection can be performed; pelvic and groin radiotherapy are administered with positive groin nodes. Preoperative radiotherapy (with or without radiosensitizing chemotherapy) can be given to increase the operability and decrease the extent of resection. This is followed by radical excision with bilateral superficial and deep groin node dissection. Radiotherapy alone is an option if the patient or extent of lesion is deemed unsuitable for radical surgery.

Stage IV

Treatment of stage IV disease must also be individualized for each patient. Options include radical vulvectomy and pelvic exenteration, radical vulvectomy followed by radiotherapy, preoperative radiotherapy (with or without radiosensitizing chemotherapy) followed by radical surgical excision, and radiotherapy (with or without radiosensitizing chemotherapy) if the patient is not eligible for surgery or the lesion is deemed inoperable.

RECURRENT DISEASE

Treatment of recurrent disease depends on the site and extent of the recurrence. Options include radical wide excision with or without radiotherapy (depending on prior treatment and extent of recurrence), groin node debulking followed by radiotherapy

Table 20-2. Five-year survival rate (by stage)

Stage I	95%
Stage II	75–85%
Stage III	5%
Stage IVA	20%
Stage IVB	5%

(depends on prior treatment), and pelvic exenteration. Patients with regional or distant metastasis are more difficult to treat; often palliative therapy is the only option.

PROGNOSTIC FACTORS

There are a variety of prognostic factors for vulvar carcinoma. Inguinal node metastasis appears to be the single most important prognostic variable (Table 20-2). Other factors include lymphovascular space invasion, stage, including lesion size, site of lesion, histologic grade, and depth of invasion.

RECOMMENDED SURVEILLANCE

Physical and pelvic examinations should be performed every 3 months the first year, every 4 months in years 2 and 3, every 6 months in years 4 and 5, and once a year thereafter. A PAP smear should be performed annually.

Vaginal Cancer

INCIDENCE

Primary vaginal cancer represents 1–2% of malignancies of the female genital tract. The average age at diagnosis is 60 years. Most vaginal neoplasms represent metastases from another primary source.

RISK FACTORS

A variety of risk factors are associated with vaginal cancer, including low socioeconomic status, history of human papillomavirus infection, chronic vaginal irritation, and prior abnormal PAP smear with cervical intraepithelial neoplasia. Other factors are prior hysterectomy (59% of patients with primary vaginal cancer), prior treatment for cervical cancer, and *in utero* exposure to diethylstilbestrol during the first half of pregnancy. Diethylstilbestrol was used to prevent complications of pregnancy such as threatened abortion and prematurity from 1940 to 1971; about 1 in 1,000 women exposed to diethylstilbestrol *in utero* develop clear cell carcinoma of the vagina. The peak age at diagnosis is 19 years.

PATHOLOGY

Eighty-five percent of vaginal cancers are squamous cell neoplasms. Other histologic subtypes include adenocarcinomas (9%), sarcomas (6%), melanomas, clear cell carcinoma, and other rare histologies.

ROUTES OF SPREAD

Vaginal cancer metastasizes via direct extension to adjacent structures. It can also spread through a well-established lymphatic drainage distribution. Lesions of the upper two-thirds of the vagina metastasize directly to pelvic lymph nodes. Lesions of the lower one-third of the vagina metastasize primarily to the inguinofemoral nodes and secondarily to pelvic nodes. Hematogenous spread represents late occurrence, as disease is confined primarily to the pelvis in the majority of cases.

CLINICAL FEATURES

Symptoms

Painless vaginal bleeding and vaginal discharge are the primary symptoms associated with vaginal cancer. Bladder symptoms, tenesmus, and pelvic pain, which is usually indicative of locally advanced disease, are less commonly seen.

Physical Findings

Lesions are located primarily in the upper one-third of the vagina, usually on the posterior wall. The appearance of lesions varies, ranging from exophytic to endophytic. Surface ulceration is usually not present except in advanced cases.

Visualization of lesions identified by PAP smear may require colposcopy.

PRETREATMENT WORK-UP

Careful physical examination, including pelvic examination with colposcopy, is required, unless the lesion is visible. Other components of the pretreatment work-up include complete blood count, serum glucose, blood urea nitrogen, creatinine, and liver function tests; chest x-ray; mammogram; and cystoscopy and/or proctoscopy, depending on site and extent of lesion. Barium enema, CT, or MRI should be performed if indicated. Preoperative medical clearance is necessary for patients with chronic disease or other appropriate indications.

STAGING

The clinical staging scheme for vaginal cancers is outlined in Table 20-3.

Treatment of Vaginal Cancer by Stage

Stage 0

Stage 0 disease may be treated by surgical excision, laser ablation, and, in some cases, topical 5-fluorouracil.

Table 20-3.   Clinical staging of vaginal cancer

Stage	Description
0	Carcinoma *in situ,* intraepithelial carcinoma
I	Carcinoma limited to vaginal wall
II	Carcinoma involves subvaginal tissue but does not extend to pelvic wall
III	Extension to pelvic wall
IV	Extension beyond the true pelvis or involvement of bladder or rectal mucosa
IVA	Spread to adjacent organs and/or direct extension beyond the pelvis
IVB	Spread to distant organs

Stage I

Lesions of the upper vaginal fornices may be treated with radical hysterectomy and lymphadenectomy or radiotherapy alone. All stage I lesions (including lesions of the upper vaginal fornices) may be treated with radiotherapy, usually in the form of an intracavitary cylinder.

Stages II–IV

External-beam radiotherapy and intracavitary and/or interstitial therapy are utilized for stage II–IV disease. The groin should be treated if the lower one-third of the vagina is involved with tumor.

RECURRENT DISEASE

Treatment of recurrent disease depends on the extent of recurrence. Options include wide local excision, partial vaginectomy, and exenteration. Chemotherapy may be given for distant metastatic disease; however, the role of chemotherapy is unclear because of the rarity of the disease.

PROGNOSTIC FACTORS

The most important prognostic factor for vaginal cancer is the stage of disease (Table 20-4).

Table 20-4.   Five-year survival rate (by stage)

Stage I	80%
Stage II	45%
Stage III	35%
Stage IV	10%

RECOMMENDED SURVEILLANCE

Physical and pelvic examinations should be performed every 3 months the first year, every 4 months in years 2 and 3, every 6 months in years 4 and 5, and once a year thereafter. A PAP smear should be performed annually.

Cervical Cancer

INCIDENCE

Approximately 15,000 new cases of cervical cancer are reported annually, and there are approximately 4,000–5,000 annual associated deaths.

RISK FACTORS

Cervical cancer is a sexually transmitted disease, and the first solid tumor to be linked to a virus. Infection with human papillomavirus, specifically types 16 and 18, is associated with the development of this disease. Other risk factors include early age at first intercourse, multiple sexual partners, multiparity, sexual contact with men at high risk for penile cancers or men who have had partners with cervical cancer, and smoking. One-half of the women with newly diagnosed invasive cervical cancer have never had a PAP smear, and another 10% have not had a PAP smear in the past 5 years.

PATHOLOGY

Eighty-five percent of cervical cancers are squamous cell carcinomas, and 10–15% are adenocarcinomas, including the less common adenosquamous type. The remainder of cases are rarer histologies, including small cell tumors, sarcomas, lymphomas, and melanomas.

ROUTES OF SPREAD

Cervical cancer spreads by a variety of mechanisms. It can directly invade surrounding structures, including the parametria, corpus, and vagina. Lymphatic metastases are relatively ordered and predictable, sequentially involving parametrial, pelvic, iliac, and para-aortic nodes. Hematogenous metastases and intraperitoneal implantation can also occur.

CLINICAL FEATURES

Symptoms

Discharge and abnormal bleeding—including postcoital, intermenstrual, and postmenopausal bleeding, and menorrhagia—are often the first signs of cervical cancer. Urinary frequency and pain can also occur and may indicate advanced disease.

Physical Findings

Examination varies, depending on the site of the lesion (endocervix or ectocervix). Careful inspection and palpation, including bimanual and rectovaginal examinations, are required to identify the size and extent of the lesion.

PRETREATMENT WORK-UP

Careful physical examination must be performed, including pelvic examination and biopsy of the lesion. Other components of the pretreatment work-up include complete blood count, serum glucose, blood urea nitrogen, creatinine, and liver function tests; chest x-ray; and mammogram. The following additional studies should be performed for patients with symptoms and disease stages IB2-IV: cystoscopy, proctoscopy, barium enema (as indicated), and CT scan. MRI may be useful, especially when attempting to delineate endometrial lesions from endocervical lesions. According to the guidelines established by the International Federation of Gynecology and Obstetrics (FIGO), staging procedures are limited to physical examination, cervical conization, intravenous pyelogram, barium enema, cystoscopy, proctoscopy, and chest x-ray.

STAGING

The clinical staging scheme for classifying cervical cancer is outlined in Table 20-5. The term *microinvasive cervical cancer* is sometimes applied to stage IA lesions. This diagnosis must be made from either a cone biopsy or a hysterectomy specimen. The following definitions have been derived by two different medical associations and are referred to when considering therapy:

FIGO definition. See the definition under FIGO stage IA, Table 20-5.

Society of Gynecologic Oncologists (SGO) definition. Microinvasion with depth of invasion in one or more foci of <3 and no lymphovascular space involvement (LVSI).

Treatment of Cervical Cancer by Stage

Stage IA

Lesions that satisfy the SGO definition of microinvasion may be treated conservatively with any of the following modalities: simple hysterectomy, cervical conization in cases where maintenance of fertility is an issue, and intracavitary radiotherapy for patients who do not qualify for surgery.

Lesions that do not satisfy the SGO definition of microinvasion (lymphovascularspace invasion or invasion >3 mm) are significantly more likely to recur when treated conservatively; therefore radical hysterectomy and lymph node dissection or radiotherapy should be performed.

Stages IB, IIA

Surgery and radiotherapy result in similar cure rates when patients are carefully selected; squamous lesions <4–5 cm and adenocarcinomas <3 cm are potential surgical candidates. The standard treatment options are radical hysterectomy and pelvic lymph node dissection and radiotherapy with 40–45 Gy external-beam irradiation and two intracavitary systems. Patients with

Table 20-5. Clinical staging of cervical cancer

Stage	Description
I	In general, lesions are confined to the cervix; uterine involvement is disregarded.
	IA Preclinical cervical cancers diagnosed by microscopy alone
	IA1 Stromal invasion ≤3 mm deep and ≤7 mm wide
	IA2 Stromal invasion >3 mm but ≤5 mm deep and ≤7 mm wide
	IB Lesions larger than stage IA lesions, whether seen clinically or not
	IB1 Clinical lesions ≤4 cm
	IB2 Clinical lesions >4 cm
II	Extension beyond the cervix, but no extension to the pelvic sidewall or the lower one-third of the vagina
	IIA No obvious parametrial involvement
	IIB Parametrial involvement
III	Extension to the pelvic wall with no cancer-free space between the tumor and the pelvic wall; tumor involves the lower one-third of the vagina. All cases of hydronephrosis or nonfunctioning kidney, unless secondary to unrelated cause.
	IIIA Involvement of the lower one-third of the vagina; no extension to the pelvic sidewall
	IIIB Extension to the pelvic wall, hydronephrosis or nonfunctioning kidney
IV	Extension beyond the true pelvis or clinical involvement of the mucosa of the bladder or rectum
	IVA Spread to adjacent organs
	IVB Spread to distant organs

risk factors for recurrence on pathologic evaluation (i.e., two or more positive nodes) also receive adjuvant radiotherapy. Simple hysterectomy after pelvic radiotherapy is indicated primarily in a patient whose tumor responds slowly to radiotherapy or when vaginal anatomy precludes optimal intracavitary placement.

Stages IIB–IVA

Radiotherapy is the treatment of choice for locally advanced disease. Surgery may be used as adjuvant therapy for stage IVA disease without parametrial involvement and in cases of persistent central disease following radiotherapy.

Stage IVB

Stage IVB disease is primarily treated with chemotherapy, as the disease is disseminated. Radiotherapy can be used for local control and palliation of symptoms. Cisplatin is the most studied active agent; other options include ifosfamide and mitomycin C. Current clinical trials using vinorelbine (Navelbine) have also demonstrated some activity in cervix cancer.

Table 20-6.   Incidence of nodal metastasis by stage

Stage	Positive pelvic nodes (%)	Positive para-aortic nodes (%)
IA1	0	0
IA2 (1–3 mm)	0.6	0
IA2 (3–5 mm)	4.8	<1
IB	15.9	2.2
IIA	24.5	11
IIB	31.4	19
III	44.8	30
IVA	55	40

RECURRENT DISEASE

The treatment of recurrent disease depends upon disease location and original treatment modality. Central recurrence may be managed with pelvic exenteration if no contraindicating factors are present. Patients who have had prior radiotherapy and extensive pelvic recurrence or distant metastatic disease are treated similarly to those patients with stage IVB disease.

PROGNOSTIC FACTORS

The most important prognostic factors for stage I disease include lymphovascular space involvement, tumor size, depth of invasion, and presence of lymph node metastases (Table 20-6). For stages II–IV disease, stage, presence of lymph node metastases, tumor volume, age, and the patient's performance status are key prognostic factors. The overall survival rates for cervical cancer are highlighted in Table 20-7.

RECOMMENDED SURVEILLANCE

Greater than 50% of all recurrences are diagnosed in the first year following treatment. Seventy-five percent are diagnosed by year 2 following treatment, and 95% within 5 years of treatment.

Table 20-7.   Five-year survival rate (by stage and histology)

Stage I	Squamous, 65–90%
	Adenocarcinoma, 70–75%
Stage II	Squamous, 45–80%
	Adenocarcinoma, 30–40%
Stage III	Squamous up to 60%
	Adenocarcinoma, 20–30%
Stage IV	Squamous and adenocarcinoma, <15%

Endometrial Cancer

INCIDENCE

Endometrial cancer is the most common malignancy of the female genital tract and the fourth most common malignancy in women (following breast, lung, and colon cancers). Approximately 35,000 new cases are diagnosed annually, and approximately 6,000 women die yearly from this disease. The median age at onset is 63 years; however, up to 25% of patients are premenopausal.

RISK FACTORS

Risk factors for endometrial cancer reflect a chronic estrogenized state. These factors include nulliparity, early menarche, late menopause, obesity, unopposed estrogen therapy, and chronic disease (i.e., diabetes and hypertension).

PATHOLOGY

Ninety percent of endometrial cancers are adenocarcinomas (70% grade 1, 15% grade 2, and 15% grade 3), 5–7% are papillary serous carcinomas, and the remaining 2–3% are clear cell carcinomas. The latter two cell types represent a more aggressive histology.

ROUTES OF SPREAD

Endometrial cancer metastasizes by myometrial invasion and direct extension to adjacent structures. Transtubal passage of exfoliated cells, lymphatic embolization, and hematogenous dissemination can also occur.

CLINICAL FEATURES

Symptoms

Ninety percent of patient present to their physicians complaining of abnormal uterine bleeding or postmenopausal bleeding; approximately 15% of patients with postmenopausal bleeding have uterine cancer. Patients may also experience pelvic pressure and pelvic pain. Associated findings include pyometria, hematometria, an abnormal PAP smear (the presence of atypical glandular cells on a PAP smear requires that an endometrial biopsy be performed to rule out malignancy), heavy menses, and intermenstrual bleeding.

PRETREATMENT WORK-UP

Careful physical examination, including pelvic examination, is required. Pathologic confirmation of disease by endometrial biopsy or dilatation and curettage is essential. Other components of the pretreatment work-up include complete blood count, serum glucose, blood urea nitrogen, creatinine, and CA-125; chest x-ray; and mammogram. Diagnostic tests—including CT, barium enema, intravenous pyelogram, proctosigmoidoscopy, cystoscopy, and, in some cases, MRI—should be performed as indicated by symptoms or examination findings.

Table 20-8.   Surgical staging of endometrial cancer

Stage	Description
I	Carcinoma confined to the uterine corpus IA: Tumor limited to the endometrium B: Invasion of one-half or less of the myometrium IC: Invasion of more than one-half of the myometrium
II	Extension of cancer to cervix but not outside uterus IIA: Endocervical glandular involvement only IIB: Cervical stromal invasion
III	Extension of the tumor outside the uterus but confined to the true pelvis or para-aortic area IIIA: Tumor invades serosa and/or adnexa, with or without positive cytology IIIB: Vaginal metastases IIIC: Metastases to pelvic and/or para-aortic lymph nodes
IV	Distant metastases or involvement of adjacent pelvic organs IVA: Tumor invasion of the bowel or bladder mucosa IVB: Distant metastases including intra-abdominal and/or inguinal lymph nodes

STAGING

The staging schema for endometrial cancer is described in Tables 20-8 and 20-9.

TREATMENT

The most active chemotherapeutic agents in the treatment of endometrial cancer are cisplatin, doxorubicin, and taxol. Alone these agents produce a 30% response rate; when combined, the response rate is about 50%. Progestin therapy may be used to treat metastatic tumors with progesterone receptors; response is seen in 25–30% of cases. Hormone therapy with tamoxifen produces a response in about 20% of cases.

PROGNOSTIC FACTORS

Surgical stage is the most important prognostic variable (Table 20-10). Other prognostic factors are myometrial invasion,

Table 20-9.   FIGO definitions for tumor grading

Grade	Definition
1	5% or less of a nonsquamous or nonmorular solid growth pattern
2	6–50% of a nonsquamous or nonmorular solid growth pattern
3	More than 50% of a nonsquamous or nonmorular solid growth pattern

Table 20-10.   Five-year survival rate (by stage)

Stage I	90%
Stage II	75%
Stage III	40%
Stage IV	10%

lymphovascular space invasion, nuclear grade, histologic type, tumor size, patient age, positive peritoneal cytology, hormone receptor status, and type of primary treatment used (surgery versus radiotherapy).

Uterine Sarcomas

INCIDENCE

Uterine sarcomas account for approximately 3–5% of uterine cancers.

RISK FACTORS

Most patients have no known risk factors. A small number of patients have a history of pelvic irradiation.

PATHOLOGY

The disease arises from mesodermal derivatives that include uterine smooth muscle, endometrial stroma, and blood and lymphatic vessel walls. The number of mitoses per 10 high-power fields, degree of cytologic atypia, and presence of coagulative necrosis are the most reliable predictors of biologic behavior. Uterine sarcomas are classified according to the types of elements involved (pure [only mesodermal elements present] or mixed [both mesodermal and epithelial elements present]) and whether malignant mesodermal elements are normally present in the uterus (homologous [only smooth muscle and stroma present] or heterologous [striated muscle and cartilage present]) (Table 20-11).

ROUTES OF SPREAD

Sarcomas demonstrate a propensity for early hematogenous dissemination and lymphatic spread (one-third of patients).

HISTOLOGIC FREQUENCIES

One-half of endometrial sarcomas are malignant mixed mullerian tumors. Other histologies include leiomyosarcomas (40%), endometrial stromal sarcomas (8%), adenosarcomas, pure heterologous sarcomas, and other variants (1–2%).

Table 20-11.   Classifications of uterine sarcomas

Type	Homologous	Heterologous
Pure	Leiomyosarcoma Stromal sarcoma	Rhabdomyosarcoma Chondrosarcoma Osteosarcoma Liposarcoma
Mixed	Mixed mesodermal (mullerian) sarcoma or malignant mixed mesodermal (mullerian) tumors with homologous components (also called carcinosarcomas)	Mixed mesodermal (mullerian) sarcomas or malignant mixed mesodermal (mullerian) tumors with heterologous components

PRETREATMENT WORK-UP

Careful physical examination, including pelvic examination, is required (Table 20-12). Endometrial biopsy, dilatation and curettage, or both are essential to provide pathologic confirmation of disease. Other components of the pretreatment work-up include complete blood count, serum glucose, blood urea nitrogen, creatinine, and liver function tests; chest x-ray; mammogram; and cystoscopy and/or proctoscopy, depending on site and extent of lesion. Preoperative medical clearance is necessary for patients with chronic disease or other appropriate indications.

STAGING

No official staging system exists for sarcomas; therefore the FIGO staging system for uterine corpus carcinoma is used. (See Table 20-8.)

TREATMENT

Surgical excision is the only treatment of curative value. Pelvic radiotherapy has a role in local control of tumor; however, because of the propensity for early hematogenous spread, this treatment does not affect outcome. Leiomyosarcomas generally do not respond to radiotherapy. Cisplatin, doxorubicin, and ifosfamide have shown some activity against uterine sarcomas; leiomyosarcomas are more sensitive to doxorubicin. There may be some benefit to hormonal therapy with megestrol acetate; tamoxifen is recommended in cases where hormone receptors have been identified. Hormonal therapy is the treatment of choice for low-grade endometrial stromal sarcoma.

PROGNOSTIC FACTORS

The most important prognostic factor is surgical stage of disease (Table 20-13). The presence of sarcomatous overgrowth and deep myometrial invasion must be considered in cases of adenosarcoma because it adds to an adverse prognosis.

Table 20-12. Clinical features of uterine sarcomas

Cell type	Patient's age (years)	Signs and symptoms	Diagnosis
Endometrial stromal sarcoma	42–53	Vaginal bleeding Uterine enlargement Lower abdominal pain or pressure	EMB or D&C
Leiomyosarcoma	45–55	Vaginal bleeding Rapid uterine enlargement Lower abdominal pain or pressure	Difficult preoperative diagnosis; only 15% diagnosed by EMB or D&C
Malignant mixed mesodermal tumors	65–75	Several factors in common with endometrial cancer (nulliparity, obesity, and diabetes) Vaginal bleeding Enlarged uterus	EMB or D&C (In up to 50% of cases, the tumor protrudes through the cervix.)
Adenosarcoma	Any age; most common in the 5th decade of life	Vaginal bleeding Uterine enlargement	EMB or D&C (In up to 50% of cases, the tumor protrudes through the cervix.)

EMB = endometrial biopsy; D&C = dilatation and curettage.

Table 20-13.   Five-year survival rate (by stage)

Stage I	50%
Stages II–IV	15% or less

RECOMMENDED SURVEILLANCE

Physical and pelvic examinations should be performed every 3 months the first year, every 4 months in years 2 and 3, every 6 months in years 4 and 5, and once a year thereafter. A PAP smear and CXR should be performed annually.

Epithelial Ovarian Cancer

INCIDENCE

Epithelial ovarian cancer occurs in 1 in 70 women. Approximately 27,000 new cases are diagnosed annually, and approximately 15,000 women will die each year from this disease. Epithelial ovarian cancer comprises 90% of all ovarian cancers. The median age at diagnosis is 61 years. Less than 10% of cases are due to transmission of an autosomal dominant gene. Three hereditary forms of ovarian cancer have been identified: site-specific familial ovarian cancer, breast–ovarian familial cancer syndrome (associated with an abnormality in *BRCA-1*, or *BRCA-2*, the breast-ovarian cancer susceptibility genes), and Lynch II syndrome (nonpolyposis colon cancer, endometrial cancer, breast cancer, and ovarian cancer clusters in first- and second-degree relatives).

RISK FACTORS

A variety of factors are thought to increase the risk of developing ovarian cancer. These include increased age (peak age is 70 years), nulliparity, early menarche, late menopause, delayed childbearing, and Ashkenazi Jewish descent. There may be an association with use of fertility drugs, but this has not been conclusively demonstrated. The use of oral contraceptives appears to have a protective effect against the development of epithelial ovarian cancer; this effect may last up to 10 years.

PATHOLOGY

There is a 15–30% incidence of concomitant endometrial carcinoma in cases of endometrioid ovarian carcinoma. Cases of synchronous appendiceal and ovarian mucinous tumors have also been reported; however, it is not unusual for appendiceal cancer to spread to the ovaries, and this often makes it difficult to determine the site of the primary disease (Table 20-14).

Table 20-14. Major histologic types of epithelial ovarian carcinomas

Histologic type	Percent of ovarian tumors	Percent bilaterality
Serous	46	73
Mucinous	36	47
Endometrioid	8	33
Clear cell	3	13
Transitional	2	–
Mixed	3	–
Undifferentiated	<2	53
Unclassified	<1	–

ROUTES OF SPREAD

The most common route of spread is transcoelomic, as exfoliated cells tend to assume the circulatory path of the peritoneal fluid and implant along this path. Ovarian cancer may also metastasize to the lymph nodes, but hematogenous spread is uncommon.

CLINICAL FEATURES

General

The interval from onset of disease to diagnosis is often prolonged because of a lack of specific symptoms during the early stages; therefore diagnosis is often not made until patients have disseminated disease. Approximately 65% of cases are stage III or stage IV disease at time of diagnosis.

Symptoms

Symptoms that may be suggestive of ovarian cancer include abdominal fullness, early satiety, dyspepsia, urinary frequency, constipation, unexplained pelvic pain, and increased flatulence.

Physical Findings

An adnexal mass noted on routine pelvic examination and a palpable fluid wave are often found in patients with ovarian cancer. Five percent of patients with presumed ovarian cancer have another primary that has metastasized to the ovary. The most common primary sites that metastasize to the ovary are the breast, gastrointestinal tract, and pelvic organs.

PRETREATMENT WORK-UP

Careful physical examination, including pelvic examination, is required. Other components of the pretreatment work-up include complete blood count, serum glucose, blood urea nitrogen, creatinine, liver function tests, serum albumin, CA-125 (elevated in approximately 80% of cases), chest x-ray, and mammogram. Imaging studies may be helpful but most often do not change the planned staging procedure. CT may help determine the extent of disease.

Barium enema is useful in examination of the colon. In older patients, barium enema can be particularly helpful in diagnosing a colonic primary, which may present similarly to ovarian cancer. Intravenous pyelogram is also helpful in certain clinical situations.

STAGING

The staging schema for epithelial ovarian cancer is outlined in Table 20-15.

TREATMENT

The initial step in treatment is surgical cytoreduction with appropriate intraoperative staging procedures, including abdo-

Table 20-15. Surgical staging of epithelial ovarian cancer

Stage	Description
I	Growth limited to the ovaries
	IA Growth limited to one ovary, no ascites, no tumor on the external surfaces, capsules intact
	IB Growth in both ovaries, no ascites, no tumors on external surfaces, capsule intact
	IC Stage IA or IB characteristics, but with tumor on the surface of one or both ovaries, ruptured capsule(s), or malignant ascites with positive peritoneal cytology
II	Growth involving one or both ovaries with pelvic extension
	IIA Extension and/or metastases to the uterus and/or tubes
	IIB Extension to other pelvic tissues
	IIC Stage IIA or IIB characteristics, but with tumor on the surface of one or both ovaries, ruptured capsule(s), or malignant ascites with positive peritoneal cytology
III	Growth involving one or both ovaries with peritoneal implants outside the pelvis and/or positive retroperitoneal or inguinal nodes; superficial liver metastasis equals stage III; tumor limited to the true pelvis but with histologically proved malignant extension to small bowel or omentum
	IIIA Tumor grossly limited to the true pelvis with negative nodes but histologically confirmed microscopic seeding of abdominal peritoneal surfaces
	IIIB Tumor involving one or both ovaries with histologically confirmed implants of abdominal peritoneal surfaces, none exceeding 2 cm in diameter; nodes are negative
	IIIC Abdominal implants greater than 2 cm in diameter and/or positive retroperitoneal or inguinal nodes
IV	Growth involving one or both ovaries with distant metastases; positive cytology from pleural effusion or pathologic confirmation of parenchymal liver metastases

minal and pelvic cytology, careful exploration of all abdominal and pelvic structures and surfaces, total abdominal hysterectomy and bilateral salpingo-oophorectomy (exceptions include concern about fertility and early-stage disease), infracolic omentectomy with or without appendectomy, and selective pelvic and para-aortic lymph node sampling. Primary cytoreduction is a key component in advanced cases; survival is directly correlated to the amount of residual tumor remaining. Optimal tumor reductive surgery is loosely defined as the diameter of the largest residual tumor implant being <2 cm. If the residual mass is greater in size, the cytoreduction is deemed suboptimal. At the M. D. Anderson Cancer Center, routine "second-look" operations are no longer performed. A "second-look" operation may be included as part of an investigational trial. There are certain exceptions to the use of surgical exploration and cytoreduction as initial treatment. Primary chemotherapy may be used, followed by interval debulking, in certain subsets of patients such as those with advanced disease (i.e., patients with pleural effusions that reaccumulate rapidly after thoracentesis), those with bulky disease, and those who did not undergo appropriate primary cytoreductive surgery. The impact this approach has on survival, however, is unproven in those patients with advanced and bulky disease.

PROGNOSTIC FACTORS

Prognostic histopathologic factors include histologic type, histologic grade, and DNA ploidy (Table 20-16). Clinical factors that are of prognostic significance include surgicopathologic stage, extent of residual disease remaining following primary cytoreduction, volume of ascites, patient age, and patient performance status.

Survival Based on Performance Status

Patients with poor performance status before treatment (Karnofsky status <70%) have significantly shorter survival.

Ovarian Tumors of Low Malignant Potential

INCIDENCE

These tumors comprise as many as 5–15% of all ovarian malignancies. The highest incidence is among white women, with a mean age at diagnosis of 39–45 years (approximately 10 years younger than the mean age at diagnosis of epithelial ovarian cancer).

RISK FACTORS

No significant risk factors have been identified, and there does not appear to be a protective effect associated with pregnancy or

Table 20-16.   Five-year survival rate

Stage	Serous carcinoma by stage and grade			
	All grades(%)	Grade 1(%)	Grade 2(%)	Grade 3(%)
IA	85	92.5	86	63
IB	69	85	90	79
IC	59	78	49	51
IIA	62	64	65	39
IIB	51	79	43	42
IIC	43	68	46	20
IIIA	31	58	38	20
IIIB	38	73	42	21
IIIC	18	46	22	14
IV	8	14	8	6

Residual disease, all stages, following primary cytoreductive surgery	
Amount of residual disease	Survival (%)
Microscopic (residual disease)	40–75
Macroscopic (optimal debulking)	30–5
Macroscopic (suboptimal debulking)	5

Status at second look, all stages by disease status	
Disease status	Survival (%)
No evidence of disease	50
Microscopic disease	35
Macroscopic disease	5

exogenous hormones. There is no apparent association with family history.

PATHOLOGY

The main histologic categories are serous and mucinous. Secondary categories include transitional, endometrioid, clear cell, and mixed. Diagnosis of tumors of low malignant potential requires the absence of frank stromal invasion (there is a subcategory for microinvasive tumor implants) and the presence of any two of the following factors: nuclear atypia, mitotic activity, multilayering of epithelium, and epithelial budding.

ROUTES OF SPREAD

As with epithelial ovarian cancer, low malignant potential tumors spread via a transcoelomic route. Lymphatic metastases may also occur.

CLINICAL FEATURES

Ovarian tumors of low malignant potential present in a manner similar to that of epithelial ovarian cancer. The most common symptoms are low abdominal pain or discomfort, early satiety, dyspepsia, sense of abdominal enlargement, and discovery of an adnexal mass on routine pelvic examination. The CA-125 may be elevated in serous tumors.

PRETREATMENT WORK-UP

Careful physical examination, including pelvic examination, is required. Other components of the pretreatment work-up include complete blood count, serum glucose, blood urea nitrogen, creatinine, liver function tests, serum albumin, CA-125 (may be elevated), chest x-ray, and mammogram. Imaging studies may be helpful but most often do not change the planned staging procedure. CT may help determine the extent of disease. Barium enema is useful in examination of the colon. In older patients, barium enema can be particularly helpful in diagnosing a colonic primary, which may present similarly to ovarian cancer. Intravenous pyelogram is also helpful in certain clinical situations.

STAGING

The surgical staging scheme for ovarian tumors of low malignant potential is identical to that used for epithelial ovarian cancer (see Table 20-15). Their distribution is outlined in Table 20-17.

TREATMENT

Recommended treatment for all patients is primary surgery; fertility-sparing procedures should be performed if fertility is a factor in patients with stage I disease.

Stages I and II

Surgical cytoreduction is the key element with close surveillance postoperatively.

No role for adjuvant chemotherapy or radiotherapy has been documented.

Table 20-17. Distribution of ovarian tumors of low malignant potential by stage

	Histologic type	
Stage	Serous (%)	Mucinous (%)
I	65	89.5
II	14	1
III	20	9
IV	1	0.5

Table 20-18.   Five-year survival rate (by stage)

Stage I	95%
Stage II	75–80%
Stage III	65–70%

Stages III and IV

Surgical cytoreduction is the key element. Platinum-based chemotherapy may be of benefit for residual disease following cytoreduction, but adjuvant therapy is unproven to date.

RECURRENT DISEASE

Tumors of low malignant potential typically have an indolent clinical course and may recur late. Cytoreduction as outlined for stages III and IV can be considered in select patients.

PROPOSED PROGNOSTIC FACTORS

Proposed prognostic factors include stage at diagnosis, residual tumor volume, and presence of invasive implants (Table 20-18).

Sex Cord Stromal Tumors

INCIDENCE

Sex cord stromal tumors account for 5–8% of all ovarian malignancies and represent 5% of childhood malignancies. These tumors are uncommon before menarche; occurrence before menarche is associated with precocious puberty.

PATHOLOGY

As their name suggests, these tumors are derived from sex cords and/or stroma. Derivatives include granulosa cells, theca cells, stromal cells, Sertoli cells, Leydig cells, and/or cells resembling embryonic precursors of these cell types (Table 20-19). These tumors are also referred to as "functioning tumors" because as many as 85% synthesize steroids (estrogen, progesterone, testosterone, and corticosteroids).

ROUTES OF SPREAD

The pattern of metastatic spread is analogous to epithelial ovarian cancers (see page 393).

CLINICAL FEATURES

Granulosa Cell Tumors

Granulosa cell tumors comprise 1–2% of all ovarian tumors. Adult-type tumors (95% of all granulosa cell tumors) are character-

Table 20-19. Major classifications

Granulosa cell tumors
    Adult
    Juvenile
Thecomas and fibromas
    Thecomas
        Fibromas-fibrosarcomas
Stromal tumors with minor sex cord elements
Sertoli stromal cell tumors
    Sertoli cell
    Leydig cell
    Sertoli-Leydig cell tumors
Gynandroblastomas
Sex cord tumors with annular tubules
Unclassified

ized by secretion of excess estrogen. Patients may experience menstrual irregularities or postmenopausal bleeding. Five percent of patients present with an acute abdomen caused by tumor hemorrhage. Patients with juvenile-type granulosa cell tumors (5% of granulosa cell tumors) can also present with menstrual abnormalities, abdominal pain, and, rarely, postmenopausal bleeding. Associated pathology includes coexisting endometrial hyperplasia (5%), coexisting endometrial carcinoma (6–30%), leiomyomata, and virilizing features in rare tumors producing testosterone. Granulosa cell tumors produce estrogen and rarely may also produce testosterone.

Thecomas

Thecomas are responsible for 1% of all ovarian tumors and are one-third as common as granulosa cell tumors. The mean age at diagnosis is 53 years, and 2–3% of these tumors are bilateral. Menstrual abnormalities and postmenopausal bleeding are the most common presenting symptoms. Associated pathology includes leiomyomata, endometrial hyperplasia, and coexisting endometrial cancer. Thecomas produce estrogen.

Fibromas and Fibrosarcoma

Fibromas and fibrosarcoma are the most common sex cord stromal tumors and comprise 4% of all ovarian neoplasms. The mean age at diagnosis is 46 years; 10% of these lesions are bilateral. Symptoms include ascites in 50% of patients with tumors >6 cm, increased abdominal girth, Meig's syndrome (right pleural effusion and ascites), and Gorlin's syndrome with basal nevi. These tumors are primarily inert but may secrete small amounts of estrogen.

Sertoli Cell Tumors

The average age of women with sertoli cell tumors is 27 years, but these tumors can occur at any age. Sertoli cell tumors are unilateral. Seventy percent of patients have symptoms related to excess estrogen, whereas 20% exhibit signs of virilization. Rarely, patients may develop hyperaldosteronemia manifested as hypertension and hyperkalemia. Seventy percent of these tumors produce both estrogen and androgens, whereas 20% produce androgens alone.

Leydig Cell Tumors

Leydig cell tumors occur at an average age of 50–70 years but can occur at any age.

Tumors are unilateral, and patients experience symptoms related to the peripheral effects of hormone products. Thyroid disease and familial occurrence are associated with these tumors. Eighty percent of Leydig cell tumors produce androgens, 10% produce estrogen, and 10% are inert.

Sertoli-Leydig Cell Tumors

Sertoli-Leydig cell tumors occur at an average age of 25–40 years but can occur at any age. These tumors are rarely bilateral. Symptoms include virilization in one-third to one-half of patients and amenorrhea. Most of these tumors produce testosterone, and some may produce alpha-fetoprotein.

Gynandroblastomas

Gynandroblastomas are unilateral tumors that can occur at any age. Patients may experience either estrogenic effects or virilization secondary to the hormone products of these tumors. Histologically, both granulosa cell and Sertoli-Leydig cell components may be present in these tumors. These tumors may produce androgens, may produce estrogen, or may be inert.

Sex Cord Tumors with Annular Tubules

The average age of patients with sex cord tumors with annular tubules is 25–35 years. Sixty-six percent of the tumors associated with Peutz-Jeghers syndrome are bilateral; the remaining are predominantly unilateral. Patients exhibit symptoms of excess estrogen when these tumors are associated with Peutz-Jeghers syndrome. Excess estrogen is present in only 40% of those without Peutz-Jeghers syndrome. Associated pathology includes Peutz-Jeghers syndrome and endocervical adenocarcinoma. Sex cord tumors with annular tubules produce estrogen.

PRETREATMENT WORK-UP

Careful physical examination, including pelvic examination, is required. Other components of the pretreatment work-up include complete blood count, serum glucose, blood urea nitrogen, creatinine, liver function tests, serum albumin, CA-125, chest x-ray, and mammogram. Evaluation of levels of serum estradiol, dehydroepiandrosterone, testosterone, 17-OH-progesterone, and hydrocortisone may be helpful in diagnosis. CT and ultrasound should be performed to evaluate the adrenal glands and ovaries. Imaging studies may be helpful but most often do not change the planned staging procedure.

STAGING

In general, surgical staging can be accomplished by unilateral salpingo-oophorectomy if there is a desire to maintain fertility,

Table 20-20. Five-year survival rate (by tumor type)

Granulosa cell tumors
  85–90% for tumors confined to the ovary
  55–60% for tumors with extraovarian extension

Sertoli or Leydig cell tumors with poor differentiation have a
  poor prognosis.

Other tumors of sex cord stromal origin have survival rates consistent
  with benign processes and low-grade malignancies.

peritoneal cytology, infracolic omentectomy, selective biopsies of
nodes and abdominal structures, and appropriately targeted biopsies. Dilatation and curettage, and endocervical curettage should
be performed to evaluate any coexistent pathologic process. These
tumors are surgically staged according to the staging scheme for
epithelial ovarian cancer (see Table 20-15).

TREATMENT

Tumors of stromal origin (thecomas, fibromas) and Leydig cell
tumors generally follow a benign course; surgery is the only treatment. Sertoli or granulosa types are generally of low malignant
potential, tend to recur late, and rarely metastasize. Chemotherapy should be considered for advanced disease. Postoperative
adjunctive therapy with bleomycin, etoposide, and cisplatin or
other platinum-based chemotherapy should be considered in
patients with Sertoli or Leydig cell tumors with poor differentiation and heterologous components and in patients with advanced
or recurrent stromal tumors; pelvic radiotherapy can also play a
role in treatment of these patients. Survival rates are described
in Table 20-20.

Ovarian Germ Cell Tumors

INCIDENCE

Germ cell tumors comprise 15–20% of all ovarian neoplasms
and are the second most common type of ovarian tumor. In the
first two decades of life, 70% of ovarian tumors are of germ cell
origin and one-third are malignant. The mean age at diagnosis is
19 years; germ cell tumors rarely occur after the third decade of
life. Sixty to seventy-five percent of cases are stage I at time of
diagnosis.

PATHOLOGY

The seven types of germ cell tumors and the percentage of
occurrence are

Dysgerminoma (40%)
Endodermal sinus tumor (yolk sac tumor; 22%)
Immature teratoma (20%)

Table 20-21.   Clinical Features of Ovarian Germ Cell Tumors

Tumor	Bilaterality	Tumor markers		
		HCG	AFP	LDH
Dysgerminoma	10–15%	±	−	+
Endodermal sinus tumor	Rare; dermoids common in contralateral ovary	−	+	±
Immature teratoma	Rare; dermoids common in contralateral ovary	−	±	±
Embryonal carcinoma	Rare	+	+	±
Choriocarcinoma	Rare	+	−	−
Polyembryoma	Rare	±	±	±

hCG = human chorionic gonadotropin; AFP = alpha-fetoprotein; LDH = lactate dehydrogenase

Embryonal carcinoma (rare)
Choriocarcinoma (rare)
Polyembryoma (rare)
Mixed forms (10–15%)

ROUTES OF SPREAD

See the discussion of epithelial ovarian cancer, page 393.

CLINICAL FEATURES

Germ cell malignancies grow rapidly and are often characterized by pain secondary to torsion, hemorrhage, or necrosis (Table 20-21). Germ cell malignancies may also cause bladder, rectal, or menstrual abnormalities. Dysgerminomas account for 20–30% of malignant ovarian tumors diagnosed during pregnancy. Embryonal carcinomas may produce estrogen and cause precocious puberty.

PRETREATMENT WORK-UP

Careful physical examination, including pelvic examination, is required. Other components of the pretreatment work-up include complete blood count, serum glucose, blood urea nitrogen, creatinine, liver function tests, serum albumin, and chest x-ray. Serum markers, including alpha-fetoprotein, human chorionic gonadotropin, and lactic dehydrogenase, should be drawn. It is important to check the karyotype in premenopausal women with ovarian masses due to an increased incidence of dysgenic gonads in patients with these tumors.

STAGING

In general, surgical staging can be accompanied by unilateral salpingo-oophorectomy if there is a desire to preserve fertility, peritoneal cytology, infracolic omentectomy, and selective biopsies of nodes and abdominal structures. In patients who are inadequately staged, there are two options: surgical reexploration and appropriate staging, or initiation of chemotherapy without reexploration. It is most prudent not to delay chemotherapy by reexploration and staging, as these tumors are highly chemosensitive. These tumors are surgically staged according to the staging schema for epithelial ovarian cancer (see Table 20-15).

TREATMENT

The primary treatment component is chemotherapy; this is recommended for all patients with germ cell tumors except those with stage I tumors. Chemotherapy should begin 7–10 days after surgical exploration because of rapid tumor growth. The first-line regimen is bleomycin, etoposide, and cisplatin administered for three or four cycles in 21-day intervals. Patients who experience a recurrence less than 6 weeks after chemotherapy are said to be "platinum resistant"; those who experience a recurrence more than 6 weeks after the last cycle of chemotherapy are said to be "platinum sensitive." Bleomycin, etoposide, and cisplatin may be restarted in patients who are platinum sensitive.

High-dose chemotherapy with autologous bone marrow rescue is a viable option in patients who are platinum resistant. Ifosfamide has shown some activity in patients with testicular cancer and may be useful for patients who are platinum resistant. Radiotherapy may have a limited role in treatment of dysgerminomas.

PROGNOSTIC FACTORS

Dysgerminomas >10–15 cm in diameter or with a high mitotic index and anaplasia tend to recur most often. Prognostic factors for immature teratomas include grade of lesion, extent of disease at diagnosis, and amount of residual tumor; tumor grade is determined by the presence of immature neural elements (Table 20-22).

MANAGEMENT OF THE UNSUSPECTED OVARIAN MASS FOUND AT LAPAROTOMY

The finding of an unsuspected ovarian mass at the time of exploratory laparotomy or at laparotomy for an unrelated condition can pose a therapeutic dilemma to the surgeon. Appropriate treatment depends on several factors, including the patient's age, the size and consistency of the mass, possible bilaterality, and gross involvement of other structures.

Ovarian Masses in Women of Childbearing Age

An unsuspected mass in a young patient is most likely benign. Among the most frequently found benign masses involving the adnexa are the nonneoplastic or functional cysts, which are related to the process of ovulation. These cysts are significant primarily because they cannot be easily distinguished from true neoplasms

Table 20-22.   Survival rate (by tumor type and time interval)

Dysgerminoma (5 years)	
Stage I	90–95%
All stages	60–90%
Endodermal sinus tumors (2 years)	
Stages I and II	90%
Stages III and IV	50%
Immature teratoma (5 years)	
Stage I	90–95%
All stages	70–80%
Grade 1	82%
Grade 2	62%
Grade 3	30%
Embryonal carcinoma (5 years)	
All stages	39%

Choriocarcinoma has a poor prognosis. Polyembryoma has a poor prognosis.
Mixed tumor has a variable survival and is dependent on the tumor composition.

on clinical grounds alone. If ovulation does not occur, a clear, fluid-filled follicular cyst up to 10 cm in diameter may develop. This functional cyst usually resolves spontaneously within several days to 2 weeks. When a patient ovulates, a corpus luteum is formed that may become abnormally large because of hemorrhage within the corpus luteum or cyst formation. A patient with a hemorrhagic corpus luteum may present with an acute abdomen necessitating laparotomy. Often the bleeding area may be oversewn without performing a cystectomy or salpingo-oophorectomy. It is critical to check a pregnancy test in a premenopausal woman who presents with an acute abdomen, because surgery may result in loss of function of the corpus luteum, which sustains pregnancy during the first trimester. In pregnant patients, postoperative support with progesterone therapy can be used to help carry the pregnancy through the critical period.

Ovulating patients can also present with functional ovarian cysts. These are usually asymptomatic but can cause lower abdominal or pelvic pain; however, signs of an acute abdomen are rare. A simple cyst up to 5 cm in diameter found incidentally at the time of surgery in an ovulating patient can be safely followed. If it is only a functional cyst, it should disappear after the patient's next menstrual period. Resolution can be evaluated with physical examination alone or in conjunction with pelvic ultrasound. Functional cysts are more common in patients who have anovulatory cycles, such as patients with polycystic ovarian syndrome or obese patients.

Dermoid cysts, or benign cystic teratomas, are the most common ovarian tumors in women in the second and third decades of life. These cystic masses may be of any size, and up to 15% are bilateral. Torsion is the most frequent complication and commonly occurs in children, young women, and pregnant women. Severe acute abdominal pain is usually the initial symptom, and this condition is considered to be an emergency. Treatment is cystectomy, with close inspection of the other ovary. A cystectomy can usually be performed even for large lesions. The remainder of the ovary should be reapproximated with an absorbable suture; it will usually continue to function normally.

Other common benign neoplasms that occur in young patients include serous and mucinous cystadenomas. These are treated with unilateral salpingo-oophorectomy if the other ovary appears normal. Endometriomas, or the so-called chocolate cysts of endometriosis, can also occur in young women. These patients may have a history of endometriosis and/or chronic pelvic pain. Often other endometriotic implants may be seen in the pelvis or abdominal cavity, which may be helpful in establishing the diagnosis. The treatment of endometriomas may be cystectomy or unilateral oophorectomy, again depending upon the degree of normal-appearing ovarian tissue that remains. Every effort should be made to salvage the normal-appearing portion of ovary.

If, upon opening the abdomen, ascites is present, the ascites should be evacuated and submitted for cytologic analysis. After careful inspection and palpation, if the tumor appears to be confined to one ovary and malignancy is suspected, unilateral salpingo-oophorectomy is appropriate in most circumstances. If the ovarian mass is thought to be benign, ovarian cystectomy may be preferable. The ovarian capsule should be inspected for any evidence of rupture, adherence, or excrescence. Once removed, the ovarian specimen should be sent for frozen-section examination. If malignancy is diagnosed, surgical staging is appropriate, with biopsy of the omentum, peritoneal surfaces of the pelvis and upper abdomen, and retroperitoneal lymph nodes (including both the para-aortic and bilateral pelvic regions).

If the contralateral ovary appears normal, existing information suggests that random biopsy or wedge resection is not indicated because of the potential for future infertility caused by peritoneal adhesions or ovarian failure. One should also not rely too heavily on frozen-section diagnosis in making the decision to perform hysterectomy and bilateral salpingo-oophorectomy in a young patient. If the histologic diagnosis is questionable, it is always preferable to wait for permanent section results. General criteria for conservative management include the following:

1. Young patient desirous of future childbearing.
2. Patient and family consent and agree to close follow-up.
3. No evidence of dysgenetic gonads.
4. Any unilateral malignant germ cell tumor.
5. Any unilateral stromal tumor.
6. Any unilateral borderline tumor.
7. Stage Ia invasive epithelial tumor.

The advent of *in vitro* fertilization technology should also have an impact on intraoperative management. Convention has dictated that, if a bilateral salpingo-oophorectomy is indicated, a hysterectomy should also be performed. However, current technology for donor oocyte transfer and hormonal support allows a woman without ovaries to sustain a normal intrauterine pregnancy. Similarly, if the uterus and one tube and ovary are resected because of tumor involvement, current techniques allow for retrieval of oocytes from the patient's remaining ovary, *in vitro* fertilization with sperm from her partner, and implantation of the embryo into a surrogate's uterus.

To summarize, in any patient for whom the diagnosis is unclear by examination and/or after consultation with a gynecologic oncologist, the most prudent procedure is removal of the involved ovary with frozen-section diagnosis to rule out malignancy. Again, this assumes that the operator does not feel the mass is benign. The most frequently seen malignant tumors in young women and girls are those of germ cell or stromal origin. These are usually unilateral, may be multicystic, or may contain solid components. Treatment of these tumors has been described earlier. Malignant epithelial tumors are particularly uncommon in young women; however, if a multiseptated or solid mass is found at laparotomy, suggesting an epithelial tumor, the involved ovary should be removed and frozen-section diagnosis obtained. Management of epithelial ovarian cancer has been addressed previously.

Ovarian Masses in Postmenopausal Women

The risk of an ovarian mass being malignant begins to increase at 40 years of age and rises steadily thereafter. Therefore the finding of an unsuspected ovarian mass in a postmenopausal woman is a more ominous sign. The most common malignant neoplasms in this age group are malignant epithelial tumors; germ cell and stromal cell tumors rarely occur. Note that benign lesions, such as epithelial cystadenomas and dermoid cysts, can still occur in this population, although at a much less frequent rate than in younger patients. Treatment of an unanticipated ovarian mass in a postmenopausal patient includes salpingo-oophorectomy and frozen-section diagnosis. Appropriate staging biopsies should also be performed. A gynecologic oncologist should be consulted if at all possible.

Conclusions

An unsuspected mass on the ovary at the time of surgery should be considered a significant finding, and appropriate consultation and/or removal of the tumor with frozen-section diagnosis should be undertaken in all cases except for simple functional cysts in young premenopausal patients. If frozen-section analysis is not immediately available, the lesion should still be removed and sent for permanent section pathologic diagnosis (assuming the remainder of the pelvic and abdominal organs are normal). It must be understood that the patient may need additional definitive surgery at a later time if the lesion is ultimately found to be malignant (Fig. 20-1).

Fallopian Tube Cancer

INCIDENCE

Fallopian tube cancer accounts for 0.1–0.5% of all gynecologic malignancies. The average age at diagnosis is 55 years.

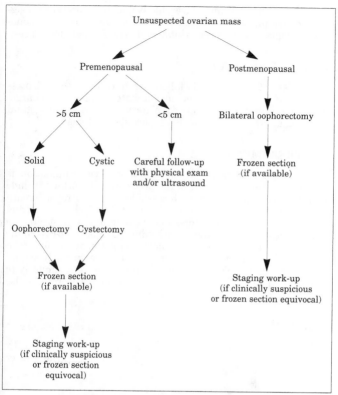

Fig. 20-1. Management of the unsuspected
ovarian mass found at the time of laparotomy.

RISK FACTORS

No known risk factors exist for developing this disease.

PATHOLOGY

The most common histology is adenocarcinoma, and the most
common tumors of the fallopian tube are metastatic lesions from
other sites. To establish a diagnosis of primary fallopian tube cancer, the following criteria (Hu's criteria) must be met: the main
tumor must be in the tube; the mucosa should be involved microscopically and should exhibit a papillary pattern; the transition
between benign and malignant tubal epithelium should be demonstrated if the tubal wall is significantly involved with tumor.

ROUTES OF SPREAD

Fallopian tube cancer metastasizes in a manner similar to that
of epithelial ovarian cancer. Lymphatic spread tends to play more

of a role in fallopian tube cancer, likely due to the presence of significant lymphatics in the fallopian tubes. One-third of patients with fallopian tube cancer exhibit evidence of nodal metastases.

CLINICAL FEATURES

The classic triad of primary fallopian tube cancer, although present in <15% of patients, includes a watery vaginal discharge, pelvic pain, and a pelvic mass. Watery discharge and vaginal bleeding are the most commonly reported symptoms.

PRETREATMENT WORK-UP

Careful physical examination, including pelvic examination, is required. Other components of the pretreatment work-up include complete blood count, serum glucose, blood urea nitrogen, creatinine, liver function tests, serum albumin, CA-125, chest x-ray, and mammogram. Imaging studies may be helpful but most often do not change the planned staging procedure. CT may help determine the extent of disease. Barium enema is useful in examination of the colon. In older patients, barium enema can be particularly helpful in diagnosing a colonic primary, which may present similarly to ovarian and fallopian tube cancers. Intravenous pyelogram is also helpful in certain clinical situations.

STAGING

There is no official FIGO staging for fallopian tube cancer; by convention, the staging criteria used for epithelial ovarian cancer are used (see Table 20-15).

TREATMENT

Treatment of fallopian tube cancer is analogous to that of epithelial ovarian cancer (see page 394).

PROGNOSTIC FACTORS

Although prognostic factors are unclear because of the rarity of this tumor, they are most likely similar to those of epithelial ovarian cancer. Overall survival is estimated to be 40%, which is higher than the 5-year survival rate for patients with epithelial ovarian cancer. This survival rate is likely related to diagnosis at earlier stages (Table 20-23).

Table 20-23. Five-year survival rate (by stage)

Stage I	72%
Stage II	38%
Stage III	18%
Stage IV	0%

Gestational Trophoblastic Disease

DEFINITION

Gestational trophoblastic disease (GTD) is characterized by an abnormal proliferation of trophoblastic tissue; all forms develop in association with pregnancy. Malignant gestational trophoblastic disease can be subdivided into two categories: nonmetastatic or locally invasive gestational trophoblastic disease and metastatic gestational trophoblastic disease.

INCIDENCE

Because this category of interrelated diseases is associated with a gestational event, the age of occurrence spans the entire reproductive spectrum. Hydatidiform moles occur in 1/600 therapeutic abortions and in 1/1,000 to 1/2,000 pregnancies in the United States; of these, approximately 20% develop malignant sequelae, including invasive moles, placental site trophoblastic tumors, and gestational choriocarcinoma. Choriocarcinoma is estimated to occur in 1 in 20–40,000 pregnancies, with half of the cases following term gestations, 25% following molar gestations, and 25% following other gestational events.

PATHOLOGY

Gestational trophoblastic disease is divided into the following categories: hydatidiform mole (Table 20-24), invasive mole, choriocarcinoma, and placental site trophoblastic tumor. Nonmetastatic disease following molar evacuation may histologically be that of hydatidiform (invasive) mole or choriocarcinoma. Persistent gestational trophoblastic disease following a nonmolar pregnancy is predominantly choriocarcinoma and in rare instances may be placental site trophoblastic tumor. Metastatic gestational trophoblastic disease diagnosed in the early months after molar evacuation may be hydatidiform mole or choriocarcinoma. When gestational trophoblastic disease is found remote from a gestational event, it is most characteristically choriocarcinoma.

RISK FACTORS FOR HYDATIDIFORM MOLE

Various well-established risk factors are associated with hydatidiform mole (Table 20-25). These include age (increased risk is associated with age <20 years and >40 years); previous molar pregnancy (women who have had one molar pregnancy have a 0.5–2.5% risk of a second occurrence; women who have had two molar pregnancies have a 33% risk of a third occurrence); previous spontaneous abortion (risk of a molar gestation increases with each subsequent spontaneous abortion), and race (increased incidence among Asian women; decreased risk among black women).

ROUTES OF SPREAD

Malignant gestational trophoblastic disease spreads primarily by a hematogenous route.

Table 20-24.   Classifications of hydatidiform mole

Feature	Partial mole	Complete mole
Hydatidiform swelling of villi	Diffuse	Focal
Trophoblast	Cyto- and syncytial hyperplasia	Syncytial hyperplasia
Embryo	Absent	Present
Villous capillaries	No fetal RBCs	Many fetal RBCs
Gestational age at diagnosis	8–16 weeks	10–22 weeks
β-hCG	Usually >50,000 mIU/ml	Usually <50,000 mIU/ml
Malignant potential	15–25%	5–10%
Karyotype	46XX (95%) 46XY(5%)	Triploid (80%)
Size for dates:		
Small	33%	65%
Large	33%	10%

RBCs = red blood cells; β-hCG = β-human chorionic gonadotropin.

Table 20-25.   Clinical features of molar pregnancy and the associated risk for development of malignant gestational trophoblastic disease

Clinical feature	Percent malignant GTD
Delayed postmolar evacuation hemorrhage	75
Theca lutein cyst > 5 cm	60
Acute pulmonary insufficiency following mole evacuation	58
Uterus large for dates	45
Serum β-hCG > 100,000 mIU/ml	45
Second molar gestation	40
Maternal age > 40 years	25

GTD = gestational trophoblastic disease; β-human chorionic gonadotropin.

CLINICAL FEATURES

Hydatidiform Mole

Vaginal bleeding, uterine size larger than dates, and presence of prominent theca-lutein ovarian cysts are all characteristic clinical features of hydatidiform mole. Other associated findings include toxemia, hyperemesis, hyperthyroidism, and respiratory symptoms such as dyspnea, respiratory distress, and oral pain.

Partial Mole

Patients with partial moles may present in the same manner as those with missed or incomplete abortions, exhibiting vaginal bleeding and the passage of tissue per vagina.

PRETREATMENT WORK-UP FOR MOLAR PREGNANCY

Careful physical examination, including pelvic examination, is required. Other components of the pretreatment work-up include complete blood count, serum glucose, blood urea nitrogen, creatinine, liver function tests, serum albumin, thyroid function tests, β-human chorionic gonadotropin (serum) and chest x-ray.

METASTATIC WORK-UP FOR MALIGNANT/ PERSISTENT GESTATIONAL TROPHOBLASTIC DISEASE

Metastatic work-up for malignant/persistent gestational trophoblastic disease consists of all the preceding tests described for molar pregnancy, as well as pelvic sonogram, CT scan of abdomen/ pelvis, CT scan and/or MRI of brain, and CT scan of chest. Measurement of cerebrospinal β-human chorionic gonadotropin by lumbar puncture should be performed if any metastatic disease is present and CT scan and/or MRI of the brain is negative. The plasma-to-cerebrospinal fluid β-human chorionic gonadotropin ratio is usually <60 in cases with cerebral metastases. Metastatic lesion should not be biopsied (i.e., a vaginal nodule), as these lesions are very vascular, and patients have exsanguinated from such biopsies.

COMMON METASTATIC SITES

Malignant gestational trophoblastic disease may metastasize to a wide variety of sites, including the lungs (80%); vagina (30%); pelvis (20%); brain (10%); liver (10%); bowel, kidney, spleen (<5%); and other locations (<5%). In less than 5% of cases, the β-hCG titer may remain elevated without clinical or radiographic evidence of disease. The staging of this disease progression is outlined in Table 20-26.

TREATMENT

Molar Pregnancy

Dilation and curettage is the standard treatment of molar pregnancy. Hysterectomy may be performed if fertility is not an issue.

Table 20-26.   FIGO staging

Stage I: Confined to the uterine corpus

Stage II: Metastasis to pelvis and vagina

Stage III: Metastasis to the lung

Stage IV: Distant metastasis to the brain, liver, kidneys, or gastrointestinal tract

Nonmetastatic Gestational Trophoblastic Disease (FIGO Stage I)

If preservation of fertility is not desired, hysterectomy is recommended for stage I disease. If preservation of fertility is desired, adjuvant single-agent chemotherapy with methotrexate or dactinomycin should be administered for at least one menstrual cycle past a normal β-human chorionic gonadotropin level. If there is resistance (demonstrated β-human chorionic gonadotropin level that rises or remains at a plateau), the patient should be crossed over to the agent that was not initially administered. If resistance persists, combination chemotherapy with EMA-CO (etoposide, methotrexate, dactinomycin, cyclophosphamide, and vincristine) or MAC (methotrexate, actinomycin, and cyclophosphamide) should be administered.

Metastatic Gestational Trophoblastic Disease (FIGO Stages II–IV)

Low-Risk Gestational Trophoblastic Disease (World Health Organization Risk Score of 0–4)

As initial treatment, patients should receive methotrexate or dactinomycin. If there is resistance, the patient should be crossed over to the agent that was not initially administered. If resistance persists, combination chemotherapy with EMA-CO or MAC should be administered. If there is resistance to EMA-CO and MAC, salvage therapy includes the combination of cisplatin, bleomycin, and vinblastine. Ifosfamide also may have a role in refractory cases.

Intermediate Risk (World Health Organization Risk Score of 5–7)

Variable treatment regimens exist for intermediate-risk GTD. Single agents can be given, but the failure rate is 20%. Combination chemotherapy is often administered as first-line therapy.

High Risk (World Health Organization Risk Score of 8 or More)

Combination chemotherapy is treatment of choice for high-risk disease. EMA-CO is the initial chemotherapeutic regimen, with cisplatin, bleomycin, and vinblastine used as salvage treatment.

SPECIAL CONSIDERATIONS

Patients with brain metastases may be treated with radiotherapy for local control and prophylaxis against hemorrhage. Patients with residual solitary liver or lung lesions may be candidates for surgical resection.

PROGNOSTIC FACTORS

Factors that may affect a patient's prognosis and response to treatment are outlined in Table 20-27.

SURVIVAL

The cure rate for stage I–III disease is greater than 80%. The cure rate for stage IV disease is approximately 50%.

Table 20-27. Factors affecting prognosis and response to therapy based on World Health Organization Prognostic Index Score

Factor	World Health Organization Index Score			
	0	1	2	4
Age (years)	<39	>39		
Antecedent pregnancy	Hyd mole	Abortion	Term	—
Interval between antecedent pregnancy and start of chemotherapy (mon)	<4	4–6	7–12	>12
β-hCG (mIU/ml)	<10³	10³–10⁴	10⁴–10⁵	>10⁵
ABO blood groups (female × male)		O×A A×O	B, AB	—
Largest tumor (cm)		3–5	>5	—
Site of metastasis	Lung, vagina, pelvis	Spleen, kidney	GI tract, liver	Brain
Number of metastases identified	0	1–4	4–8	>8
Prior chemotherapy			Single drug	≥2 drugs

Hyd = hydatidiform; β-hCG = β-human chorionic gonadotropin; GI = gastrointestinal.

RECOMMENDED SURVEILLANCE

Post-treatment surveillance is essentially the same for all cases of gestational trophoblastic disease, with the exception of patients with stage IV disease, because they require a longer period of surveillance. Weekly measurements of β-human chorionic gonadotropin levels are drawn until levels are normal for 3 consecutive weeks. Monthly β-human chorionic gonadotropin values are then drawn until levels are normal for 12 consecutive months, except with stage IV disease, which requires 24 months of surveillance. Contraception is mandatory throughout the follow-up period.

GENE THERAPY

During the last decade, advances in molecular biology and technology have opened the door to novel treatment strategies. The ability to modify genetic material and transfer it into cells to either replace a missing or malfunctioning gene or provide a new function to a cell has opened a new spectrum of potential therapeutic possibilities in the treatment of gynecologic malignancies.

In broad, general terms, gene therapy involves the production of genetic material (DNA or RNA) and subsequent injection into the host via a delivery system followed by integration into the host genome and its subsequent effect. Currently, the gene transfer systems under study utilize liposomes, retroviruses, or adenoviruses as delivery vehicles to integrate the gene sequences into the host genome and exert one of the following antitumor or protective effects:

1. Immunoregulatory gene alteration and antitumor vaccines. This approach may involve the manipulation of cytokine and immunosuppressive expression, redirection of tumor infiltrating lymphocytes, or stimulation of dendritic cells.
2. Antioncogene and tumor suppressor gene alterations. These include the oncogenes *erbB-2*, *c-myc*, *jun*, *fos*, *k-ras*, and the suppressor gene *p-53*.
3. Pro-drug therapy that utilizes cancer cells transfected with a gene that encodes an enzyme capable of converting a normally nontoxic substance into a toxic metabolite. Upon presentation of the substrate, the toxic metabolite produced in the transgene expressing tumor cells induces its death. A current example of this approach is the HSV-TK/ganciclovir system.

Another unique approach to gene therapy involves the *MDR1* gene which is known to confer immunity from certain chemotherapeutic agents. Research is currently evaluating the transfer of the *MDR1* gene to the host's bone marrow to theoretically allow higher doses of chemotherapy to be given with less bone marrow suppression.

At present there are ongoing phase I trials, primarily in ovarian cancer, that have shown that the genetic modification of cancer cells and subsequent expression of transgenes is feasible. The current clinical trials are promising and indicate that gene therapy may be further refined as our knowledge of immunomodulatory factors, cancer genetics, and improvement of delivery systems evolves. At present, gene therapy is still in its infancy, but one day it may be a truly effective treatment alternative for patients.

Selected References

VULVAR CANCER REFERENCES

Anderson JM, Cassady JR, Shimm DS, et al. Vulvar carcinoma. *Int J Radiat Oncol Biol Phys* 32:1351, 1995.

Berek JS, Heaps JM, Fu YS, et al. Concurrent cisplatin and 5-fluorouracil chemotherapy and radiation therapy for advanced-stage squamous carcinoma of the vulva. *Gynecol Oncol* 42:197, 1991.

Binder SW, Huang I, Fu YS, et al. Risk factors for the development of lymph node metastasis in vulvar squamous cell carcinoma. *Gynecol Oncol* 37:9, 1990.

Boyce J, Fruchter RG, Kasambilides E, et al. Prognostic factors in carcinoma of the vulva. *Gynecol Oncol* 20:364, 1985.

Burke TW, Stringer CA, Gershenson DM, et al. Radical wide excision and selective inguinal node dissection for squamous cell carcinoma of the vulva. *Gynecol Oncol* 38:328, 1990.

Chung AF, Woodruff JW, Lewis JL, Jr. Malignant melanoma of the vulva: A report of 44 cases. *Obstet Gynecol* 45:638, 1975.

Creasman WT. New gynecologic cancer staging. *Gynecol Oncol* 58:157, 1995.

Hacker NF, Van der Velden J. Conservative management of early vulvar cancer. *Cancer* 71(Suppl):1673, 1993.

Heaps JM, Fu YS, Montz FJ, et al. Surgical-pathologic variables predictive of local recurrence in squamous cell carcinoma of the vulva. *Gynecol Oncol* 38:309, 1990.

Homesley HD, Bundy BN, Sedlis A, et al. Assessment of current International Federation of Gynecology and Obstetrics staging of vulvar carcinoma relative to prognostic factors for survival (a Gynecologic Oncology Group study). *Am J Obstet Gynecol* 164:997, 1991.

Homesley HD, Bundy BN, Sedlis A, et al. Prognostic factors for groin node metastasis in squamous cell carcinoma of the vulva (a Gynecologic Oncology Group study). *Gynecol Oncol* 49:279, 1993.

Hopkins MP, Reid GC, Morley GW. The surgical management of recurrent squamous cell carcinoma of the vulva. *Obstet Gynecol* 75:1001, 1990.

Keys H. Gynecologic Oncology Group randomized trials of combined technique therapy for vulvar cancer. *Cancer* 71(Suppl):1691, 1993.

Malfetano JH, Piver MS, Tsukada Y, et al. Univariate and multivariate analyses of 5-year survival, recurrence, and inguinal node metastases in stage I and II vulvar carcinoma. *J Surg Oncol* 30:124, 1985.

Perez CA, Grigsby PW, Galakatos A, et al. Radiation therapy in management of carcinoma of the vulva with emphasis on conservation therapy. *Cancer* 71:3707, 1993.

Podratz KC, Symmonds RE, Taylor WF, et al. Carcinoma of the vulva: Analysis of treatment and survival. *Obstet Gynecol* 61:63, 1983.

Russell AH, Mesic JB, Scudder SA, et al. Synchronous radiation and cytotoxic chemotherapy for locally advanced or recurrent squamous cancer of the vulva. *Gynecol Oncol* 47:14, 1992.

Sedlis A, Homesley H, Bundy BN, et al. Positive groin lymph nodes in superficial squamous cell vulvar cancer: A Gynecologic Oncology Group study. *Am J Obstet Gynecol* 156:1159, 1987.

Shimm DS, Fuller AF, Orlow EL, et al. Prognostic variables in the treatment of squamous cell carcinoma of the vulva. *Gynecol Oncol* 24:343, 1986.

Stehman FB, Bundy BN, Dvoretsky PM, et al. Early stage I carcinoma of the vulva treated with ipsilateral superficial inguinal lymphadenectomy and modified radical hemivulvectomy: A prospective study of the Gynecologic Oncology Group. *Obstet Gynecol* 79:490, 1992.

Thomas GM, Dembo AJ, Bryson SC, et al. Changing concepts in the management of vulvar cancer. *Gynecol Oncol* 42:9, 1991.

VAGINAL CANCER REFERENCES

Berek JS, Hacker NF. *Practical Gynecologic Oncology* (2nd ed.). Baltimore: Williams and Wilkins, 1994.

Delclos L, Wharton JT, Rutledge FN. Tumors of the vagina and female urethra. In GH Fletcher (ed.), *Textbook of Radiotherapy* (3rd ed.). Philadelphia: Lea and Febiger, 1980.

Herbst AL, Robboy SJ, Scully RE, et al. Clear cell adenocarcinoma of the vagina and cervix in girls: Analysis of 170 registry cases. *Am J Obstet Gynecol* 119:713, 1974.

Kucera H, Vavra N. Primary carcinoma of the vagina: Clinical and histopathological variables associated with survival. *Gynecol Oncol* 40:12, 1991.

Kucera H, Vavra N. Radiation management of primary carcinoma of the vagina: Clinical and histopathological variables associated with survival. *Gynecol Oncol* 40:12, 1991.

Morrow CP, Curtin JP, Townsend DE. *Synopsis of Gynecologic Oncology* (4th ed.). New York: Churchill Livingstone, 1993.

Perez CA, Camel HM, Galakatos AE, et al. Definitive irradiation in carcinoma of the vagina: Long-term evaluation of results. *Int J Radiat Oncol Biol Phys* 15:1283, 1988.

Stock RG, Chen AS, Seski J. A 30-year experience in the management of primary carcinoma of the vagina: Analysis of prognostic factors and treatment modalities. *Gynecol Oncol* 56:45, 1995.

CERVICAL CANCER REFERENCES

Alberts DS, Kronmal R, Baker LH, et al. Phase II randomized trial of cisplatin chemotherapy regimens in the treatment of recurrent or metastatic squamous cell cancer of the cervix: A Southwest Oncology Group study. *J Clin Oncol* 5:1791, 1987.

American Cancer Society. Cancer Facts and Figures. Atlanta: American Cancer Society, 1995.

Artman LE, Hoskins WJ, Bibro MC, et al. Radical hysterectomy and pelvic lymphadenectomy for stage IB carcinoma of the cervix: 21 years' experience. *Gynecol Oncol* 28:8, 1987.

Coia L, Won M, Lanciano R, et al. The patterns of care outcome study for cancer of the uterine cervix: Results of the Second National Practice Survey. *Cancer* 66:2451, 1990.

Coleman RE, Harper PG, Gallagher C, et al. A phase II study of ifosfamide in advanced and relapsed carcinoma of the cervix. *Cancer Chemother Pharmacol* 18:280, 1986.

Creasman WT. New gynecologic cancer staging. *Gynecol Oncol* 58:157, 1995.

Creasman WF, Fetter BF, Clarke-Pearson DL, et al. Management of stage IA carcinoma of the cervix. *Am J Obstet Gynecol* 153:164, 1985.

Dembo AJ, Balogh JM. Advances in radiotherapy in the gynecologic malignancies. *Semin Surg Oncol* 6:323, 1990.

Eifel PJ, Burke TW, Delclos L, et al. Early stage I adenocarcinoma of the uterine cervix: Treatment results in patients with tumors ≤4 cm in diameter. *Gynecol Oncol* 41:199, 1991.

Fletcher GH, Rutledge FN. Overall results in radiotherapy for carcinoma of the cervix. *Clin Obstet Gynecol* 10:958, 1967.

Grigsby PW, Perez CA. Radiotherapy alone for medically inoperable carcinoma of the cervix: Stage IA and carcinoma *in situ*. *Int J Radiat Oncol Biol Phys* 21:375, 1991.

Hopkins MP, Morley GW. Squamous cell cancer of the cervix: Prognostic factors related to survival. *Int J Gynecol Cancer* 1:173, 1991.

Morrow CP, Curtin JP, Townsend DE. *Synopsis of Gynecologic Oncology* (4th ed.). New York: Churchill Livingstone, 1993.

Perez CA, Grigsby PW, Nene SM, et al. Effect of tumor size on the prognosis of carcinoma of the uterine cervix treated with irradiation alone. *Cancer* 69:2796, 1992.

Rutledge FN, Smith JP, Wharton JT, O'Quinn AG. Pelvic exenteration: Analysis of 296 patients. *Am J Obstet Gynecol* 129:881, 1977.

Sevin BU, Nadji M, Averette HE, et al. Microinvasive carcinoma of the cervix. *Cancer* 70:2121, 1992.

Stehman FB, Bundy BN, DiSaia PJ, et al. Carcinoma of the cervix treated with radiation therapy: A multivariate analysis of prognostic variables in the Gynecologic Oncology Group. *Cancer* 67:2776, 1991.

Thomas G, Dembo A, Fyles A, et al. Concurrent chemoradiation in advanced cervical cancer. *Gynecol Oncol* 38:446, 1990.

Vermorken JB. The role of chemotherapy in squamous cell carcinoma of the uterine cervix: A review. *Int J Gynecol Cancer* 3:129, 1993.

ENDOMETRIAL CANCER REFERENCES

American Cancer Society. *Cancer Facts and Figures*. Atlanta: American Cancer Society, 1995.

Axelrod JH, Gynecologic Oncology Group. Phase II study of whole-abdominal radiotherapy in patients with papillary serous carcinoma and clear cell carcinoma of the endometrium or with maximally debulked advanced endometrial carcinoma (summary last modified 05/91), GOG-94, clinical trial, closed, 02/24/92.

Boring CC, Squires TS, Tong T. Cancer statistics, 1991. *Cancer* 41:19, 1991.

Burke TW, Munkarah A, Kavanagh JJ, et al. Treatment of advanced or recurrent endometrial carcinoma with single-agent carboplatin. *Gynecol Oncol* 51:397, 1993.

Burke TW, Stringer CL, Morris M, et al. Prospective treatment of advanced or recurrent endometrial carcinoma with cisplatin, doxorubicin, and cyclophosphamide. *Gynecol Oncol* 40:264, 1991.

Creasman WT. New gynecologic cancer staging. *Obstet Gynecol* 75:287, 1990.

Creasman WT, Morrow CP, Bundy BN, et al. Surgical pathologic spread patterns of endometrial cancer: A Gynecologic Oncology Group study. *Cancer* 60:2035, 1987.

Gusberg SB. Virulence factors in endometrial cancer. *Cancer* 71(Suppl): 1464, 1993.

Hancock KC, Freedman RS, Edwards CL, et al. Use of cisplatin, doxorubicin, and cyclophosphamide to treat advanced and recurrent adenocarcinoma of the endometrium. *Cancer Treat Rep* 70:789, 1986.

Homesley HD, Zaino R. Endometrial cancer: Prognostic factors. *Semin Oncol* 21:71, 1994.

Lanciano RM, Corn BW, Schultz DJ, et al. The justification for a surgical staging system in endometrial carcinoma. *Radiother Oncol* 28:189, 1993.

Lentz SS. Advanced and recurrent endometrial carcinoma: Hormonal therapy. *Semin Oncol* 21:100, 1994.

Marchetti DL, Caglar H, Driscoll DL, et al. Pelvic radiation in stage I endometrial adenocarcinoma with high-risk attributes. *Gynecol Oncol* 37:51, 1990.

Morrow CP, Bundy BN, Kurman RJ, et al. Relationship between surgical-pathological risk factors and outcome in clinical stage I and II carcinoma of the endometrium: A Gynecologic Oncology Group study. *Gynecol Oncol* 40:55, 1991.

Morrow CP, Curtin JP, Townsend DE. *Synopsis of Gynecologic Oncology* (4th ed.). New York: Churchill Livingstone, 1993.

Nori D, Hilaris BS, Tome M, et al. Combined surgery and radiation in endometrial carcinoma: An analysis of prognostic factors. *Int J Radiat Oncol Biol Phys* 13:489, 1987.

Piver MS, Hempling RE. A prospective trial of postoperative vaginal radium/cesium for grade 1–2 less than 50% myometrial invasion and pelvic radiation therapy for grade 3 or deep myometrial invasion in surgical stage I endometrial adenocarcinoma. *Cancer* 66:1133, 1990.

Potish RA, Twiggs LB, Adcock LL, Prem KA. Role of whole abdominal radiation therapy in the management of endometrial cancer: Prognostic importance of factors indicating peritoneal metastases. *Gynecol Oncol* 21:80, 1985.

Quinn MA, Campbell JJ. Tamoxifen therapy in advanced/recurrent endometrial carcinoma. *Gynecol Oncol* 32:1, 1989.

Roberts JA, Gynecologic Oncology Group. Phase III Randomized Evaluation of Adjuvant Postoperative Pelvic Radiotherapy vs No Adjuvant Therapy for Surgical Stage I and Occult Stage II Intermediate-Risk Endometrial Carcinoma (Summary Last Modified 08/95), GOG-99, clinical trial, closed, 07/03/95.

Rutledge F. The role of radical hysterectomy in adenocarcinoma of the endometrium. *Gynecol Oncol* 2:331, 1974.

Seski JC, Edwards CL, Herson J, et al. Cisplatin chemotherapy for disseminated endometrial cancer. *Obstet Gynecol* 59:225, 1982.

UTERINE SARCOMAS REFERENCES

Berek JS, Hacker NF. *Practical Gynecologic Oncology* (2nd ed.). Baltimore: Williams and Wilkins, 1994.

Gershenson DM, Kavanagh JJ, Copeland LJ, et al. Cisplatin therapy for disseminated mixed mesodermal sarcoma of the uterus. *J Clin Oncol* 5:618, 1987.

Harlow BL, Weiss NS, Lofton S. The epidemiology of sarcomas of the uterus. *J Natl Cancer Inst* 76:399, 1986.

Hornback NB, Omura G, Major FJ. Observations on the use of adjuvant radiation therapy in patients with stage I and II uterine sarcoma. *Int J Radiat Oncol Biol Phys* 12:2127, 1986.

Major FJ, Blessing JA, Silverberg SG, et al. Prognostic factors in early-stage uterine sarcoma: A Gynecologic Oncology Group study. *Cancer* 71(Suppl):1702, 1993.

Morrow CP, Curtin JP, Townsend DE. *Synopsis of Gynecologic Oncology* (4th ed.). New York: Churchill Livingstone, 1993.

Norris HJ, Taylor HB. Postirradiation sarcomas of the uterus. *Obstet Gynecol* 26:689, 1965.

Olah KS, Dunn JA, Gee H. Leiomyosarcomas have a poorer prognosis than mixed mesodermal tumours when adjusting for known prognostic factors: The result of a retrospective study of 423 cases of uterine sarcoma. *Br J Obstet Gynaecol* 99:590, 1992.

Omura GA, Blessing JA, Lifshitz S, et al. A randomized clinical trial of adjuvant adriamycin in uterine sarcomas: A Gynecologic Oncology Group study. *J Clin Oncol* 3:1240, 1985.

Omura GA, Blessing JA, Major F, et al. A randomized clinical trial of adjuvant adriamycin in uterine sarcomas: A Gynecologic Oncology Group study. *J Clin Oncol* 3:1240, 1985.

Silverberg SG, Major FJ, Blessing JA, et al. Carcinosarcoma (malignant mixed mesodermal tumor) of the uterus: A Gynecologic Oncology Group pathologic study of 203 cases. *Int J Gynecol Pathol* 9:1, 1990.

Sutton GP, Blessing JA, Barrett RJ, et al. Phase II trial of ifosfamide and mesna in leiomyosarcoma of the uterus: A Gynecologic Oncology Group study. *Am J Obstet Gynecol* 166:556, 1992.

Sutton GP, Gynecologic Oncology Group. Phase II Master protocol study of chemotherapeutic agents in the treatment of recurrent or advanced uterine sarcomas—IFF plus Mesna (summary last modified 04/93), GOG-87B, clinical trial, completed, 12/28/94.

Sutton GP, Gynecologic Oncology Group. Phase III study of IFF and the uroprotector mesna administered alone or with CDDP in patients with advanced or recurrent mixed mesodermal tumors of the uterus (summary last modified 08/95), GOG-108, clinical trial, active, 02/15/89.

Wheelock JB, Krebs H-B, Schneider V, Goplerud DR. Uterine sarcoma: Analysis of prognostic variables in 71 cases. *Am J Obstet Gynecol* 151:1016, 1985.

EPITHELIAL OVARIAN CANCER REFERENCES

Berek JS, Hacker NF. *Practical Gynecologic Oncology* (2nd ed.). Baltimore: Williams and Wilkins, 1994.

Cannistra SA. Cancer of the ovary. *N Engl J Med* 329:1550, 1993.

Dembo AJ, Davy M, Stenwig AE. Prognostic factors in patients with stage I epithelial ovarian cancer. *Obstet Gynecol* 75:263, 1990.

Einzig AI, Wiernik PH, Sasloff J, et al. Phase II study and long-term follow-up of patients treated with taxol for advanced ovarian adenocarcinoma. *J Clin Oncol* 10:1748, 1992.

Eisenhauer EA, ten Bokkel Huinink WW, Swenerton KD, et al. European-Canadian randomized trial of paclitaxel in relapsed ovarian cancer: High-dose versus low-dose and long versus short infusion. *J Clin Oncol* 12:2654, 1994.

Flam F, Einhorn N, Sjovall K. Symptomatology of ovarian cancer. *Eur J Obstet Gynecol Reprod Biol* 27:53, 1988.

Gershenson DM, Mitchell MF, Atkinson N, et al. The effect of prolonged cisplatin-based chemotherapy on progression-free survival in patients with optimal epithelial ovarian cancer: "Maintenance" therapy reconsidered. *Gynecol Oncol* 47:7, 1992.

Goodman HM, Harlow BL, Sheets EE, et al. The role of cytoreductive surgery in the management of stage IV epithelial ovarian carcinoma. *Gynecol Oncol* 46:367, 1992.

Hakes TB, Chalas E, Hoskins WJ, et al. Randomized prospective trial of 5 versus 10 cycles of cyclophosphamide, doxorubicin, and cisplatin in advanced ovarian carcinoma. *Gynecol Oncol* 45:284, 1992.

Heintz APM, Hacker NF, Lagasse LD. Epidemiology and etiology of ovarian cancer: A review. *Obstet Gynecol* 66:127, 1985.

Hogberg T, Kagedal B. Long-term follow-up of ovarian cancer with monthly determinations of serum CA 125. *Gynecol Oncol* 46:191, 1992.

Hoskins WJ. Surgical staging and cytoreductive surgery of epithelial ovarian cancer. *Cancer* 71(Suppl):1534, 1993.

Hoskins WJ, Bundy BN, Thigpen JT, et al. The influence of cytoreductive surgery on recurrence-free interval and survival in small-volume stage III epithelial ovarian cancer: A Gynecologic Oncology Group study. *Gynecol Oncol* 47:159, 1992.

Hoskins WJ, McGuire WP, Brady MF, et al. The effect of diameter of largest residual disease on survival after primary cytoreductive surgery in patients with suboptimal residual epithelial ovarian carcinoma. *Am J Obstet Gynecol* 170:974, 1994.

Kohn EC, Sarosy G, Bicher A, et al. Dose-intense taxol: High response rate in patients with platinum-resistant recurrent ovarian cancer. *J Natl Cancer Inst* 86:18, 1994.

Krag KJ, Canellos GP, Griffiths CT, et al. Predictive factors for long term survival in patients with advanced ovarian cancer. *Gynecol Oncol* 34:88, 1989.

Lynch HT, Watson P, Lynch JF, et al. Hereditary ovarian cancer: Heterogeneity in age at onset. *Cancer* 71(Suppl):573, 1993.

Martinez A, Schray MF, Howes AE, et al. Postoperative radiation therapy for epithelial ovarian cancer: The curative role based on a 24-year experience. *J Clin Oncol* 3:901, 1985.

McGuire WP, Hoskins WJ, Brady MF, et al. Cyclophosphamide and cisplatin compared with paclitaxel and cisplatin in patients with stage III and stage IV ovarian cancer. *N Engl J Med* 334:1, 1996.

Morris M, Gershenson DM, Wharton JT, et al. Secondary cytoreductive surgery for recurrent epithelial ovarian cancer. *Gynecol Oncol* 34:334, 1989.

NIH Consensus Conference. Ovarian cancer: Screening treatment, and follow-up. *JAMA* 273:491, 1995.

Omura GA, Brady MF, Homesley HD, et al. Long-term follow-up and prognostic factor analysis in advanced ovarian carcinoma: The Gynecologic Oncology Group experience. *J Clin Oncol* 9:1138, 1991.

Omura GA, Bundy BN, Berek JS, et al. Randomized trial of cyclophosphamide plus cisplatin with or without doxorubicin in ovarian carcinoma: A Gynecologic Oncology Group study. *J Clin Oncol* 7:457, 1989.

Pecorelli S, Bolis G, Colombo N, et al. Adjuvant therapy in early ovarian cancer: Results of two randomized trials. *Gynecol Oncol* 52:102, 1994.

Pettersson F. *Annual Report of the Results of Treatment in Gynecologic Cancer.* International Federation of Gynecology and Obstetrics (FIGO), vol. 20. Stockholm: Panoramic Press, 1988.

Piver MS, Baker TR, Jishi MF, et al. Familial ovarian cancer: A report of 658 families from the Gilda Radner Familial Ovarian Cancer Registry 1981–1991. *Cancer* 71(Suppl):582, 1993.

Piver MS, Malfetano J, Baker TR, et al. Five-year survival for stage IC or stage I, grade 3 epithelial ovarian cancer treated with cisplatin-based chemotherapy. *Gynecol Oncol* 46:357, 1992.

Potter ME, Partridge EE, Hatch KD, et al. Primary surgical therapy of ovarian cancer: How much and when? *Gynecol Oncol* 40:195, 1991.

Sigurdsson K, Alm P, Gullberg B. Prognostic factors in malignant ovarian tumors. *Gynecol Oncol* 15:370, 1983.

Trimble EL, Arbuck SG, McGuire WP. Options for primary chemotherapy of epithelial ovarian cancer: Taxanes. *Gynecol Oncol* 55:S114, 1994.

van der Burg ME, van Lent M, Buyse M, et al. The effect of debulking surgery after induction chemotherapy on the prognosis in advanced epithelial ovarian cancer. *N Engl J Med* 332:629, 1995.

Williams L. The role of secondary cytoreductive surgery in epithelial ovarian malignancies. *Oncology* 6:25, 1992.

Young RC, Gynecologic Oncology Group. Phase III randomized study of CBDCA/TAX administered for 3 vs 6 courses for selected stages IA-C and stages IIA-C ovarian epithelial cancer (summary last modified 10/95), GOG-157, clinical trial, active, 03/20/95.

Young RC, Walton LA, Ellenberg SS, et al. Adjuvant therapy in stage I and stage II epithelial ovarian cancer: Results of two prospective randomized trials. *N Engl J Med* 322:1021, 1990.

Zaino RJ, Unger ER, Whitney C. Synchronous carcinomas of the uterine corpus and ovary. *Gynecol Oncol* 19:329, 1984.

OVARIAN TUMORS OF LOW MALIGNANT POTENTIAL REFERENCES

Bell DA, Scully RE. Serous borderline tumors of the peritoneum. *Am J Surg Pathol* 14:230, 1990.

Casey AC, Bell DA, Lage JM, et al. Epithelial ovarian tumors of borderline malignancy: Long-term follow-up. *Gynecol Oncol* 50:316, 1993.

de Nictolis M, Montironi R, Tommasoni S, et al. Serous borderline tumors of the ovary. *Cancer* 70:152, 1992.

Fort MG, Pierce VK, Saigo PE, et al. Evidence for the efficacy of adjuvant therapy in epithelial ovarian tumors of low malignant potential. *Gynecol Oncol* 32:269, 1989.

Gershenson DM, Silva EG. Serous ovarian tumors of low malignant potential with peritoneal implants. *Cancer* 65:578, 1990.

Hopkins MP, Kumar NB, Morley GW. An assessment of pathologic features and treatment modalities in ovarian tumors of low malignant potential. *Obstet Gynecol* 70:293, 1987.

Koern J, Trope CG, Abeler VM. A retrospective study of 370 borderline tumors of the ovary treated at the Norwegian Radium Hospital from 1970 to 1982. *Cancer* 71:1810, 1993.

Kurman RJ, Trimble CL. The behavior of serous tumors of low malignant potential: Are they ever malignant? *Int J Gynecol Pathol* 12:120, 1993.

Leake JF, Currie JL, Rosenshein NB, et al. Long-term follow-up of serous ovarian tumors of low malignant potential. *Gynecol Oncol* 47:150, 1992.

Michael H, Roth LM. Invasive and noninvasive implants in ovarian serous tumors of low malignant potential. *Cancer* 57:1240, 1986.

Rice LW, Berkowitz RS, Mark SD, et al. Epithelial ovarian tumors of borderline malignancy. *Gynecol Oncol* 39:195, 1990.

Sutton GP, Bundy BN, Omura GA, et al. Stage III ovarian tumors of low malignant potential treated with cisplatin combination therapy (a Gynecologic Oncology Group study). *Gynecol Oncol* 41:230, 1991.

Trimble EL, Trimble CL. Epithelial ovarian tumors of low malignant potential. In M Markman, WJ Hoskins (eds.), *Cancer of the Ovary*. New York: Raven Press, 1993.

Trope C, Kaern J, Vergote IB, et al. Are borderline tumors of the ovary overtreated both surgically and systematically? A review of four prospective randomized trials including 253 patients with borderline tumors. *Gynecol Oncol* 51:236, 1993.

Yazigi R, Sandstad J, Munoz AK. Primary staging in ovarian tumors of low malignant potential. *Gynecol Oncol* 31:402, 1988.

SEX CORD STROMAL TUMORS REFERENCES

Berek JS, Hacker NF. *Practical Gynecologic Oncology* (2nd ed.). Baltimore: Williams and Wilkins, 1994.

Bjorkholm E, Silversward C. Prognostic factors in granulosa-cell tumors. *Gynecol Oncol* 11:261, 1981.

Bjorkholm E, Silversward C. Theca cell tumors. Clinical features and prognosis. *Acta Radiol* 19:241, 1980.

Evans AT III, Gaffey TA, Malkasian GD, Jr. Clinicopathologic review of 118 granulosa and 82 theca cell tumors. *Obstet Gynecol* 55:231, 1980.

Fox H, Agarical K, Langley FA. A clinicopathologic study of 92 cases of granulosa cell tumors of the ovary with special reference to the factors influencing prognosis. *Cancer* 35:231, 1975.

Gershenson DM. Management of early ovarian cancer: Germ cell and sex cord-stromal tumors. *Gynecol Oncol* 55:S62, 1994.

Lappohn RE, Burger HG, Bouma J, Bangah M, Krans M, deBruijn HW. Inhibin as a marker for granulosa-cell tumors. *N Engl J Med* 321:790, 1989.

Meigs JV, Armstrong SH, Hamilton HH. A further contribution to the syndrome of fibroma of the ovary with fluid in the abdomen and chest, Meig's syndrome. *Am J Obstet Gynecol* 46:19, 1943.

Norris HJ, Taylor HB. Prognosis of granulosa-theca tumors of the ovary. *Cancer* 21:255, 1968.

Roth LM, Anderson MC, Govan AD, et al. Sertoli-Leydig cell tumors: A clinicopathologic study of 34 cases. *Cancer* 48:187, 1981.

Scully RE. Ovarian tumors: A review. *Am J Pathol* 87:686, 1977.

Young RH, Scully RE. Ovarian sex cord-stromal tumors: Recent progress. *Int J Gynecol Pathol* 1:101, 1982.

Young RH, Scully RE. Ovarian sex cord stromal and steroid cell tumors. In: LM Roth, B Czernobilsky (eds.), *Tumors and Tumorlike Conditions of the Ovary*. New York: Churchill Livingstone, 1985.

Young RH, Welch WR, Dickersin GR, Scully RE. Ovarian sex cord tumor with annular tubules. Review of 74 cases including 27 with Peutz-Jeghers syndrome and four with adenoma malignum of the cervix. *Cancer* 50:1384, 1982.

OVARIAN GERM CELL TUMORS REFERENCES

Gershenson DM. Update on malignant ovarian germ cell tumors. *Cancer* 71(Suppl):1581, 1993.

Gershenson DM, Morris M, Cangir A, et al. Treatment of malignant germ cell tumors of the ovary with bleomycin, etoposide, and cisplatin. *J Clin Oncol* 8:715, 1990.

Kurman RJ, Norris HJ. Malignant germ cell tumors of the ovary. *Hum Pathol* 8:551, 1977.

Morrow CP, Curtin JP, Townsend DE. *Synopsis of Gynecologic Oncology* (4th ed.). New York: Churchill Livingstone, 1993.

Munshi NC, Loehrer PJ, Roth BJ, et al. Vinblastine, ifosfamide and cisplatin (VeIP) as second line chemotherapy in metastatic germ cell tumors (GCT). *Proceed Am Soc Clin Oncol* 9:134, 1990.

Romero R, Schwartz PE. Alpha-fetoprotein determinations in the management of endodermal sinus tumors and mixed germ cell tumors of the ovary. *Am J Obstet Gynecol* 141:126, 1981.

Schwartz PE, Morris JM. Serum lactic dehydrogenase: A tumor marker for dysgerminoma. *Obstet Gynecol* 72:511, 1988.

Serov SF, Scully RE, Robin IH. *International Histologic Classification of Tumours*, no. 9. *Histological Typing of Ovarian Tumours.* Geneva: World Health Organization, 1973.

Slayton RE, Park RC, Silverberg SG, et al. Vincristine, dactinomycin, and cyclophosphamide in the treatment of malignant germ cell tumors of the ovary. *Cancer* 56:243, 1985.

Williams SD, Birch R, Einhorn LH, et al. Treatment of disseminated germ-cell tumors with cisplatin, bleomycin, and either vinblastine or etoposide. *N Engl J Med* 316:1435, 1987.

Williams SD, Blessing JA, Hatch KD, et al. Chemotherapy of advanced dysgerminoma: Trials of the Gynecologic Oncology Group. *J Clin Oncol* 9:1950, 1991.

Williams S, Blessing JA, Liao SY, et al. Adjuvant therapy of ovarian germ cell tumors with cisplatin, etoposide, and bleomycin: A trial of the Gynecologic Oncology Group. *J Clin Oncol* 12:701, 1994.

Williams SD, Blessing JA, Moore DH, et al. Cisplatin, vinblastine, and bleomycin in advanced and recurrent ovarian germ-cell tumors: A trial of the Gynecologic Oncology Group. *Ann Intern Med* 111:22, 1989.

Williams SD, Gershenson DM. Management of germ cell tumors of the ovary. In M Markman, WJ Hoskins (eds.), *Cancer of the Ovary.* New York: Raven Press, 1993.

Williams SD, Gynecologic Oncology Group. Phase II combination chemotherapy with BEP (CDDP/VP-16/BLEO) as induction followed by VAC (VCR/DACT/CTX) as consolidation in patients with incompletely resected malignant ovarian germ cell tumors (summary last modified 10/95), GOG-90, clinical trial, active, 09/15/86.

FALLOPIAN TUBE CANCER REFERENCES

Eddy GL, Copeland LJ, Gershenson DM, et al. Fallopian tube carcinoma. *Obstet Gynecol* 64:156, 1984.

Hu CY, Taymor ML, Hertig AT. Primary carcinoma of the fallopian tube. *Am J Obstet Gynecol* 59:58, 1950.

Morris M, Gershenson DM, Burke TW, et al. Treatment of fallopian tube carcinoma with cisplatin, doxorubicin and cyclophosphamide. *Obstet Gynecol* 76:1020, 1990.

Rose PG, Piver MS, Tsukada Y. Fallopian tube cancer. *Cancer* 66: 2661, 1990.

Sedlis A. Carcinoma of the fallopian tube. *Surg Clin North Am* 58:121, 1978.

GESTATIONAL TROPHOBLASTIC DISEASE REFERENCES

Azab M, Droz JP, Theodore C, et al. Cisplatin, vinblastine, and bleomycin combination in the treatment of resistant high-risk gestational trophoblastic tumors. *Cancer* 64:1829, 1989.

Bagshawe KD. High-risk metastatic trophoblastic disease. *Obstet Gynecol Clin North Am* 15:531, 1988.

Berek JS, Hacker NF. *Practical Gynecologic Oncology* (2nd ed.). Baltimore: Williams and Wilkins, 1994.

Lurain JR. Gestational trophoblastic tumors. *Semin Surg Oncol* 6:347, 1990.

Morrow CP, Curtin JP, Townsend DE. *Synopsis of Gynecologic Oncology* (4th ed.). New York: Churchill Livingstone, 1993.

Mutch DG, Soper JT, Babcock CJ, et al. Recurrent gestational trophoblastic disease: Experience of the Southeastern Regional Trophoblastic Disease Center. *Cancer* 66:978, 1990.

Newlands ES, Bagshawe KD, Begent RH, et al. Results with the EMA/CO (etoposide, methotrexate, actinomycin D, cyclophosphamide, vincristine) regimen in high risk gestational trophoblastic tumours, 1979 to 1989. *Br J Obstet Gynaecol* 98:550, 1991.

Surwit EA. Management of high-risk gestational trophoblastic disease. *J Reprod Med* 32:657, 1987.

World Health Organization Scientific Group. Gestational trophoblastic diseases. World Health Organization Technical Report Series 692:1, 1983.

GENE THERAPY REFERENCES

Dorigo O, Berek JS. Gene therapy for ovarian cancer: Development of novel treatment strategies. *Int J Gynecol Cancer* 7:2, 1997.

Sobol RE, Shawler DL, Dorigo O, Gold D, Royston I, Fakhrai H. Immunogene therapy of cancer. In RE Sobol, KJ Scanlon (eds.), *The Internet Book of Gene Therapy*. Norwalk: Appleton and Lange, 1995.

Vile R, Russell SJ. Gene transfer technologies for the gene therapy of cancer. *Gene Therapy* 1:88, 1995.

Oncologic Emergencies

Richard J. Bold

The spectrum of emergencies that may occur in patients with cancer is too extensive to cover in the present forum. Therefore this chapter will focus on some of the more common problems that may require emergency treatment in the cancer patient. Most of these problems are unique to patients with a known malignancy, and subsequent treatment should also be individualized to the patient, with specific thought regarding comorbid disease, overall prognosis, and the patient's wishes for possibly prolonged medical treatment.

The emergencies that may be encountered in the cancer patient can be generally divided into those complications related to the tumor itself and those complications related to the treatment of the neoplasm. The cancer may cause symptoms related to compression and/or obstruction of adjacent structures (e.g., intestinal obstruction, superior vena cava syndrome, spinal cord compression). The tumor may also secrete various chemicals (termed *paraneoplastic syndromes*) that may alter homeostasis and subsequently induce symptoms related to chemical imbalances. Finally, therapy directed at tumor ablation may produce several conditions necessitating emergency care (e.g., tumor lysis syndrome, neutropenic enterocolitis, opportunistic infections). Overall, most acute events with which the cancer patient will present do not require emergency surgical intervention.

Intestinal Obstruction

Bowel obstruction continues to be a considerable source of morbidity and mortality in the cancer patient. The decisions regarding timing of operation and the extent of operation continue to be difficult, and few studies offer much guidance. Approximately two-thirds of patients with ovarian cancer will present with at least one episode of bowel obstruction, and nearly all patients with carcinomatosis will suffer some sort of intestinal complication. In all patients with a history of cancer presenting with a bowel obstruction, the etiology of the obstruction will be from a benign cause in up to one-third (e.g., adhesions, hernias, radiation enteritis). The remainder of these patients will have either primary or metastatic disease as the source of their intestinal obstruction. Intra-abdominal malignancies most often associated with obstruction of the gastrointestinal tract include carcinoma of the ovary, colon, and stomach. Extra-abdominal malignancies may metastasize to the peritoneal cavity and cause obstruction; the most common sources are carcinoma of the lung or breast as well as melanoma.

Functional obstruction without a mechanical cause ("pseudo-obstruction") is a common problem in cancer patients. Narcotic analgesics, electrolyte abnormalities, radiation therapy, malnutrition, and prolonged bedrest may all contribute to delayed intestinal motility. The treatment lies in correction of the underlying cause in combination with bowel decompression, often with either a nasogastric tube or colonoscopic evacuation. Surgery is only indicated when the degree of intestinal dilatation has progressed to the point of impending perforation, usually of the cecum. Therapy consists of placement of a tube cecostomy.

The evaluation of the cancer patient with intestinal obstruction should be similar to that for patients with benign disease. After a complete history, physical examination, evaluation of laboratory and radiologic data, the degree and site of obstruction should be delineated. Immediate laparotomy is indicated for those patients who have signs or symptoms of intestinal ischemia, necrosis, or frank perforation (abdominal tenderness, leukocytosis, fever, or tachycardia). Nearly 10% of patients will have concurrent small- and large-bowel obstruction; a hypaque enema may be useful to exclude colonic obstruction prior to laparotomy, particularly in patients with multiple sites of intra-abdominal tumor. An upper GI series is useful to determine the degree and site of obstruction, especially in those patients with recurrent partial small-bowel obstructions. Finally, a CAT scan of the abdomen and pelvis using triple contrast (intravenous, oral, and rectal) may help identify the location as well as the etiology of the obstruction. All patients should undergo fluid administration, correction of electrolyte abnormalities, and placement of a nasogastric tube.

Medical management is certainly worthwhile in those patients with a partial small-bowel obstruction. Up to 50% of patients will respond to conservative treatment, which may require up to 2 weeks of intestinal decompression. Surgery is only advocated for those who do not respond to medical management or who progress to complete obstruction. Medical management is rarely successful in patients with a complete obstruction at any level, and these patients should undergo exploration. At surgery, relief of the obstruction is the goal, although this cannot always be accomplished, and symptomatic relief may be all that can be attained.

The surgeon should fully explore the abdomen and attempt to identify the cause of the obstruction. Lysis of benign adhesions will certainly benefit the patient and usually allow full recovery to the preoperative functional status. In cases of radiation enteritis, gentle handling of the bowel is essential. Resection of short segments of intestine may be adequate; however, long segments are best treated by internal bypass. A similar approach should be taken in bowel obstruction from malignant causes, although occasionally none of these options are applicable because of the extent of the malignant disease. In such cases, placement of a venting gastrostomy for symptomatic relief is all that is usually indicated. Such a gastrostomy provides significant relief from continued emesis and avoids the need for prolonged nasogastric tube placement.

The associated morbidity and mortality from exploration related to a malignant bowel obstruction are significant. Almost 10% of patients will die as a result of surgery, and another 30% will suffer operative complications. Furthermore, patients have a mean survival of approximately 6 months following laparotomy for a malignant bowel obstruction. Finally, bowel obstruction from benign disease is rare in patients with known residual or recurrent intra-abdominal tumor. Therefore bowel obstruction in patients with documented intra-abdominal disease can be interpreted as a pre-morbid event, with prolonged survival unlikely despite any method of management. This should certainly be discussed with the patient preoperatively, and nonsurgical options (e.g., percutaneous endoscopic gastrostomy tube placement) should be pursued, depending on the patient's wishes.

Intestinal Perforation

Perforation of the gastrointestinal tract in the cancer patient may occur at nearly any time in the course of the patient's disease. It may be the presenting sign due to perforation of a primary colonic carcinoma, it may occur during treatment (either chemo- or radiotherapy), or it may be the result of metastatic tumor much later in the course of the patient's disease. Certainly most perforations of the gastrointestinal tract in the cancer patient are from benign causes (e.g., peptic ulcer disease, diverticulitis, appendicitis) and should be treated according to standard surgical principles. Surgical therapy carries a significant morbidity and mortality, although this is often the only therapeutic option available in this life-threatening complication of cancer. Therefore the patient must be well informed of the serious risks of surgery, as well as understand that an ostomy is a possibility prior to an emergency laparotomy. Nonsurgical treatment and/or comfort care may be appropriate, depending on the patient's wishes and overall medical status.

Intestinal perforation accounts for the presentation of a small group of patients with undiagnosed colorectal carcinoma. However, on further questioning, these patients will usually relate some symptoms attributable to the tumor, whether related to obstruction or bleeding. The perforation may be the result of full-thickness colonic involvement with tumor and subsequent necrosis of a region of the intestinal wall. A nearly or completely obstructing carcinoma may also present with perforation proximal in the intestinal tract, usually the cecum. In general, patients who present with either perforated or obstructing colorectal cancer have a poorer overall prognosis, stage for stage, than patients without these presentations. Furthermore, the operative mortality of emergency laparotomy for a perforated colorectal cancer approaches 30%. Certainly, colorectal cancer must be considered a possible cause in the differential diagnosis when evaluating elderly patients with evidence of peritonitis, without evidence of other etiologies for perforation, and the possibility of colostomy must be discussed with the patient preoperatively.

Perforation of the gastrointestinal tract following chemotherapy for metastatic solid tumors is a potentially life-threatening complication. Operative mortality has been reported to be as high as 80% for an emergency laparotomy in patients with metastatic cancer receiving chemotherapy. Factors associated with a high rate of complication include chemotherapy-induced myeloid toxicity, protein malnutrition, and immunosuppression. Furthermore, traditional signs of an acute surgical abdomen may be masked in these patients, leading to a delay in diagnosis to the point of frank septic shock or even going unrecognized until autopsy. Finally, the prognosis of these patients is poor, given the underlying malignancy; therefore the decision to proceed with exploratory laparotomy is difficult and often made late in the clinical course.

In several series examining gastrointestinal perforation from malignant disease, hematologic malignancies constitute most cases, with ovarian carcinoma being an extremely uncommon cause. Intestinal involvement by lymphoma is the malignancy most likely to lead to gastrointestinal perforation following systemic chemotherapy. This is most likely related to the transmural intestinal involvement, resulting in full-thickness necrosis following chemotherapy. Furthermore, the extensive involvement of the gastrointestinal tract by lymphoma and the relative chemosensitivity of this neoplasm make perforation not uncommon following chemotherapy. On the other hand, metastases from solid organ tumors are often limited to the serosal surface and therefore will not lead to full-thickness necrosis following chemotherapy.

Radiation therapy directed at the abdomen may damage the gastrointestinal tract. The extent of injury depends on the dose of radiation delivered, the radiation fields utilized, the energy of the ionizing radiation, and the use of adjunctive methods (such as "belly boards") to shield the intestines. Immediate effects include damage and subsequent sloughing of the mucosal layer of the intestinal tract. Most of the immediate effects lead to significant although temporary symptoms of nausea and vomiting. Most patients can be managed as outpatients with oral and rectal pharmacologic agents to control the symptoms. However, a small but significant fraction of patients will require hospitalization for intravenous fluid and medication administration. Finally, in its severest form, radiation injury may lead to full-thickness injury to the intestinal tract with subsequent perforation. This usually happens later in the course of the radiotherapy or following the completion of treatment. The management is similar to the management of any intestinal perforation once the diagnosis is accurately made.

Upon abdominal exploration, the area of perforation should be resected if possible. A conservative approach toward reestablishing gastrointestinal continuity should be used, especially in the face of poor nutritional status, altered host immune response, or impending shock. Ostomies should be used liberally and are easily reversed at a subsequent procedure when appropriate; in contrast, anastomotic leaks may have dire consequences. Furthermore, gastrostomy and feeding jejunostomy tubes should similarly be used liberally. Such devices eliminate the need for prolonged nasogastric intubation and may allow the institution of early enteral feeding. Copious irrigation of the abdominal cavity and debridement of any devitalized tissue are essential. Retention sutures should also be considered, as these patients have a significant risk of fascial dehiscence and evisceration.

Superior Vena Cava Syndrome

Obstruction of the superior vena cava results in a constellation of signs and symptoms collectively known as the superior vena cava syndrome (SVCS). Impedance to caval outflow may result from external compression by neoplastic disease, fibrosis secondary to inflammation, or thrombosis. At one time, common etiologies of SVCS included granulomatous disease and syphilitic aortitis. With improvements in antimicrobial therapy, these diseases are now rare, and malignant disease is present in 87–97% of patients with SVCS; lung cancer and lymphoma are the most frequent causes. An increasingly common etiology of SVCS is thrombosis secondary to indwelling central venous catheters and cardiac pacemakers. Treatment of SVCS is predicated on establishing the underlying cause of caval obstruction, as this guides therapy and determines prognosis. It is no longer acceptable to begin empiric treatment such as mediastinal radiation without a pathologic diagnosis. In the past, patients with SVCS were treated with mediastinal radiation on an emergent basis. This often frustrated later attempts at tissue diagnosis, as radiation-induced tissue necrosis begins within 72 hours of treatment. Appropriate therapy directed at a specific tumor type can result in meaningful palliation and even cure for patients presenting with SVCS.

The superior vena cava is the primary conduit for venous drainage of the head, neck, upper extremities, and upper thorax. It is a thin-walled, compliant vessel surrounded by more rigid structures, including the mediastinal and paratracheal lymph nodes, trachea and right mainstem bronchus, pulmonary artery, and aorta. As such, the superior vena cava is susceptible to external compression by any space-occupying lesion. Obstruction of caval outflow results in venous hypertension of the head, neck, and upper extremities, which in turn is responsible for the characteristic clinical presentation of SVCS. In most cases, obstruction of the superior vena cava does not occur acutely, and the signs and symptoms of SVCS develop gradually. The most common symptoms include dyspnea and feelings of facial fullness, which are present in 63% and 50% of patients, respectively. The common physical findings include facial edema, venous engorgement of the neck and chest wall, cyanosis, and plethora. Symptoms worsen when the patient bends forward or reclines. Obstruction of the superior vena cava becomes a true emergency when associated laryngeal edema results in significant airway compromise or in cases of severely elevated intracranial pressure.

In the absence of airway compromise or elevated intracranial pressure, the patient with SVCS should be thoroughly evaluated, beginning with a careful history and physical examination. A prior history of malignancy, heavy smoking, or symptoms such as cough, fever, and night sweats should be noted. On physical examination it is important to carefully examine all lymph node basins and to note the presence of a pacemaker or central venous catheter. A chest radiograph will reveal an abnormality in 84% of patients with SVCS, although the findings are often nonspecific.

A computed tomography (CT) scan of the chest is the test of choice and will readily define the etiology of the obstruction (external compression versus thrombosis). It also provides anatomic detail regarding the presence of a tumor mass and can be used to guide a percutaneous biopsy. Magnetic resonance imaging (MRI) is an excellent alternative for the patient with renal insufficiency or contrast allergy. Minimally invasive techniques for tissue diagnosis include sputum cytology, CT-guided percutaneous biopsy, bronchoscopy, lymph node biopsy, and bone marrow biopsy. Invasive procedures such as mediastinoscopy and thoracotomy should be considered if all initial measures are inadequate for diagnosis. Such invasive procedures can be performed safely in most patients with SVCS and are preferable to proceeding with non-specific therapy.

When the etiology of SVCS is due to malignant disease, treatment is based on tumor type. It is now recognized that the symptoms of SVCS may be temporized by using diuretics and head elevation. Steroids have been used to reduce inflammation, although their effectiveness has never been adequately demonstrated. Only those patients with impending airway obstruction or severely elevated intracranial pressure should be considered for emergent radiation therapy. Even in such cases, intubation, mechanical ventilation, and osmotic diuretics can provide time for a tissue diagnosis to be obtained. When a tissue diagnosis is secured, tumor-specific therapy is begun. Small cell lung cancer and lymphoma are best treated with combination chemotherapy; radiation may be used for consolidation. In a series of 56 patients with small cell lung cancer, SVCS resolved in all 23 patients treated with chemotherapy alone, 64% of those treated with radiation therapy alone, and 83% of those treated with combination therapy. Non–small cell lung cancer is most often treated with radiation therapy. One commonly used fractionation schedule provides high-dose (3–4 Gy/day) treatment for 3 days followed by conventional dose fractionation (1.8–2.0 Gy/day) to a total of 50–60 Gy. On such a treatment schedule, 70% of patients will respond within 2 weeks.

Patients with SVCS secondary to catheter-induced thrombosis may be successfully treated with thrombolytic agents followed by systemic anticoagulation. Thrombolytic agents are most effective when patients are treated within 5 days of the onset of symptoms. Alternatively, systemic anticoagulation followed by catheter removal often results in gradual recanalization of the vessel and resolution of symptoms. Balloon angioplasty and expandable stents are palliative modalities for SVCS refractory to more standard therapy. Surgical intervention consisting of innominate vein–right atrial bypass is generally reserved for patients with benign causes of superior vena cava obstruction.

Spinal Cord Compression

Spinal cord compression is the second most common neurologic complication of cancer. Autopsy studies suggest that 5% of patients with malignancies have evidence of spinal cord involvement, with the annual incidence estimated at 18,000 new cases in the United States this year. Spinal cord compression can produce paralysis and loss of sphincter control if left untreated. Early recognition and diagnosis are essential. Patients who present early with minimal neurologic deficits have a more favorable prognosis. Unfortunately, close to 80% of patients are unable to walk at the time of presentation.

The mechanism of spinal cord compression usually involves extradural metastatic lesions of the vertebral body or neural arch. Tumor expansion occurs posteriorly, resulting in anterior compression of the dural sac. Rarely, metastasis can occur in intradural locations without bony involvement. Paraspinal tumors can also cause cord compression by penetrating through the intervertebral foramen.

Most of the data regarding spinal cord compression in malignancy are extrapolated from animal models. If spinal cord compression develops gradually, decompression can be delayed without impairing the return of neurologic function; however, rapid cord compression requires immediate therapeutic intervention to avoid irreversible neurologic deficits.

Spinal cord edema plays a significant role in the development of neurologic injury. Siegal et al. demonstrated in a rat model that edema in the compressed spinal cord segment was associated with a consistent elevation of prostaglandin estradiol (PGE_2), a mediator of inflammation and edema.

Although spinal cord compression can occur as the initial manifestation of disease, most patients who develop malignant spinal cord involvement have been previously diagnosed with cancer. The interval from primary diagnosis to epidural cord compression varies with the type of tumor involved. Lung cancer has an aggressive presentation, with epidural cord compression developing within a few months after diagnosis of the primary lesion. In contrast to lung cancer, patients with carcinoma of the breast have been reported to manifest spinal cord compression as long as 20 years after their initial presentation.

The distribution of spinal cord segments involved—cervical, 10%; thoracic, 70%; lumbosacral, 20%—reflects the number of vertebrae in each anatomic segment. More than 90% of patients present with localized back pain, which may be exacerbated by movement, recumbency, coughing, sneezing, or straining. The pain due to cord compression can be radicular in distribution. Pain is usually present for several weeks before neurologic symptoms develop. Left untreated, weakness and numbness occur, usually beginning in the toes and ascending to the level of the lesion. Autonomic dysfunction usually occurs late in the disease process. The onset of urinary retention and constipation represents an ominous sign, indicating possible progression to irreversible paraplegia if left untreated.

Physical examination may reveal tenderness to palpation over the involved vertebrae. Straight leg raise and neck flexion may produce pain at the level of the involved vertebrae. Weakness, spasticity, abnormal reflexes, and extensor plantar response (Babinski's sign) may be evident on physical examination. A palpable urinary bladder or decreased anal sphincter tone suggests autonomic involvement and an advanced stage of disease.

Patients with signs of impending neurologic deficits and of impending paralysis should undergo emergency evaluation and treatment. Based on the history and physical examination, dexamethasone should be given (10 mg IV followed by 4 mg every 6 hours). Rapid radiographic assessment should then take place. More than two-thirds of patients with cord compression have radiographic evidence of bony abnormalities on plain films of the spine. Radiographic findings suggestive of a spine metastasis include erosion and loss of vertebral pedicles, partial or complete collapse of vertebral bodies, and paraspinal soft-tissue masses. The finding of normal spine radiographs does not exclude the possibility of epidural metastases. For instance, patients with lymphoma typically have normal spine radiographs even in the presence of epidural tumors.

Currently, MRI is the initial study of choice in evaluating patients with suspected spinal cord compression after plain radiographs have been obtained. The MRI has several advantages over the standard myelogram. Lumbar puncture, which is required for a myelogram, is associated with significant morbidity in the presence of a space-occupying lesion and potential bleeding complications in patients with coagulopathies. This procedure is eliminated with the use of MRI. Also, MRI is less invasive and requires less time to perform than myelography. MRI is useful in defining the extent of tumor involvement and designing portals for radiation therapy or for planning operative intervention.

MRI gives excellent delineation of extradural versus intradural lesions. Gadolinium (Gd-DPTA) contrast is usually not required for extradural lesions, but optimal imaging of extramedullary and intramedullary intradural lesions requires the use of this agent. If the MRI results in equivocal or negative findings, then myelography with or without CT scan should be performed.

Early intervention is essential in the management of malignant spinal cord compression. There is a clear correlation between the functional status at the time of presentation and the post-treatment outcome. Fewer than 10% of patients who present with paraplegia become ambulatory after treatment. Radiotherapy and/or surgical intervention are the standard treatment modalities. Typically, 3,000 cGy is given in 300- to 500-cGy-dose fractions, with excellent resolution of pain and neurologic symptoms. Laminectomy is effective in managing patients with epidural masses but has limited use if the pathologic process is anterior to the spinal cord. In select cases surgical resection may provide symptomatic relief, but careful patient selection is essential. Chemotherapy may play a role in managing patients with epidural cord compression from lesions that are sensitive to certain agents; however, the role of chemotherapy in an adjuvant setting or as primary treatment has not clearly been defined.

Biliary Obstruction

Biliary obstruction by tumors metastatic to the hilum of the liver or portal lymph nodes is an uncommon but troublesome problem in the cancer patient. A variety of tumor types—including lymphoma, melanoma, and carcinoma of the breast, colon, stomach, lung, and ovary—may cause such obstruction. Obstruction of the biliary tree due to primary carcinomas of the common bile duct and pancreas is discussed in Chapter 12. Evaluation is best performed with CT scan, which provides information on the site of obstruction, degree of biliary obstruction, evaluation of the remainder of the abdomen, and often clues as to the cause of obstruction. When necessary, CT-guided FNA can be performed in this region to obtain a tissue diagnosis.

In a series of 12 patients with biliary obstruction from metastases, 11 patients had disease either in other intra-abdominal sites or in extra-abdominal locations. Thus the prognosis for patients with biliary obstruction from metastatic disease is poor. The 60-day mortality in this group has been reported to be as high as 67%. Thus treatment should be directed at the palliation of jaundice and the prevention of cholangitis. Drainage of the biliary tree is best accomplished by endoscopic retrograde cholangiopancreatography (ERCP) and biliary stenting. If this approach is unsuccessful, percutaneous transhepatic drainage is indicated. External-beam irradiation, with or without chemotherapy, may also provide a significant palliation. This is especially true of obstruction due to primary biliary or pancreatic carcinomas. Surgery should be reserved for low-risk patients in whom the suspicion of metastatic disease is low and expected long-term survival is high.

Pericardial Tamponade

Pericardial tamponade in the cancer patient most often results from malignant obstruction of pericardial lymphatics, leading to the accumulation of pericardial fluid. Both primary neoplasms of the heart and metastatic lesions may incite development of pericardial effusions. Metastatic disease to the pericardium is the prevailing etiology of pericardial effusion and tamponade. Carcinoma of the lung and breast, lymphoma, leukemia, and melanoma are the most commonly associated malignancies. Radiation-induced effusions may also occur in the cancer patient.

The pericardial sac normally contains 20 ml of fluid at a mean pressure below that of right and left ventricular end-diastolic pressure. With the gradual accumulation of pericardial fluid, this pressure will rise until the intrapericardial pressure equals or surpasses that of ventricular end-diastolic pressure. At this point, diastolic filling is compromised and cardiac output falls. The development of pericardial tamponade depends on the rate and volume of pericardial fluid accumulation, as well as the compliance of the pericardial sac. A pericardial effusion as small as 150 ml may induce tamponade. In cases of more gradual accumulation, effusions may reach 1–2 liters.

The symptoms of pericardial tamponade are often vague. Frequent complaints include chest pain, anxiety, and dyspnea. Clinical signs include tachycardia, diminished heart sounds, jugular venous distention, pulsus paradoxus, and ultimately shock. The electrocardiogram reveals low voltage throughout all leads, with sinus tachycardia. Two-dimensional echocardiography will best demonstrate the presence of pericardial fluid and is the test of choice for the stable patient with suspected pericardial tamponade.

The treatment of pericardial tamponade is removal of the pericardial effusion, which may be accomplished in the emergent setting at the bedside via needle pericardiocentesis. A drainage catheter may then be inserted into the pericardial space over a guidewire. If the patient is stable, pericardiocentesis under echocardiographic guidance will help minimize complications. Removal of a small amount of fluid results in dramatic and immediate improvement for the patient in extremis. Without additional treatment, malignant pericardial effusions will often recur. Thus the drainage catheter should be left in place to assess the rate of fluid accumulation. The options for preventing reaccumulation include tetracycline sclerosis, surgery, and radiation therapy. The instillation of 500–1,000 mg of tetracycline into the pericardial sac induces an inflammatory response, with subsequent fibrosis and obliteration of the pericardial space. Multiple instillations are usually necessary. Treatment should be repeated until the drainage is less than 25 ml in 24 hours to achieve optimal results. Successful control of effusions with this technique is obtained in 86% of treated patients. Surgical options include subxiphoid pericardiotomy, window pericardiectomy, and complete pericardiectomy. In most cases, the subxiphoid approach is preferred. It avoids thoracotomy and can be performed under local anesthesia. Multiple series have documented a recurrence rate of 7% using this technique. Complete pericardiectomy should be reserved for patients with radiation-induced effusions. Radiation therapy is useful in the stable patient with a malignant effusion secondary to lymphoma. Treatment is given in 2- to 3-Gy fractions to a total dose of 20–40 Gy.

Outcome after treatment of pericardial tamponade is related to tumor type. The median survival ranges from 3.5 months for patients with lung cancer to as long as 18.5 months in patients with breast cancer. Thus the presence of a malignant pericardial effusion does not preclude meaningful survival.

Paraneoplastic Crises

Some tumors retain the biochemical characteristics of the cell type of origin with respect to the ability to secrete biologically active substances. Other tumors develop the ability to synthesize and produce hormones that have a wide range of biologic effects. Homeostasis is often disrupted, as the secretion of these substances is unregulated; this has been termed *paraneoplastic syndromes*. A cancer patient may develop severe symptoms from these syndromes that require emergency treatment. The spectrum of paraneoplastic syndromes is too extensive to cover and therefore this section will comment on the more common syndromes, physiologic manifestations, pathophysiology, and treatment.

HYPERCALCEMIA

Hypercalcemia is the most common metabolic complication of malignancy, occurring in approximately 10% of cancer patients. Tumors most commonly associated with hypercalcemia include carcinomas of the breast, lung, and kidney, and multiple myeloma. Patients with parathyroid carcinoma characteristically present with intractable hypercalcemia. Although more than 80% of patients with hypercalcemia have bone metastasis, there is no correlation between the extent of bony involvement and the degree of hypercalcemia. Nor is there any correlation between the presence of bony metastasis and the development of hypercalcemia. Current data suggest that the hypercalcemia is mediated by tumor-induced humoral factors. Parathyroid hormone-related protein (PTHRP), osteoclast-activating factor (OAF), prostaglandins, and numerous other cytokines may play a role in the development of hypercalcemia in patients with malignancies.

Calcium homeostasis is normally a tightly regulated process. Serum calcium level is primarily controlled by parathyroid hormone (PTH), 1,25-dihydroxyvitamin D_3, and calcitonin. The effect of these hormones on bone, intestine, and kidneys is primarily to ensure that the net absorption of calcium by the GI tract is balanced with the amount excreted by the kidney. Under normal conditions the serum calcium level is maintained between 8.5 mg/dl and 10.5 mg/dl. Approximately 45% of calcium exists in the ionized, metabolically active form, with the remaining calcium being protein bound. Most cases of hormonally mediated hypercalcemia in cancer patients result from the activity of PTHRP, which affects the kidney and bone in a manner similar to PTH (enhancement of renal tubular resorption of calcium). In contrast to hyperparathyroidism, patients with hypercalcemia secondary to PTHRP have impaired production of 1,25-dihydroxyvitamin D_3 and show no evidence of renal bicarbonate wasting. This mechanism is particularly prevalent in solid tumors, especially epidermoid carcinomas.

OAF is responsible for hypercalcemia in patients with multiple myeloma and lymphoma. This osteolytic polypeptide stimulates osteoclast proliferation and the release of lysosomal enzymes and collagenase. Despite the potent osteolytic activity of OAF *in vitro*, patients with elevated OAF levels do not always develop hypercalcemia unless there is associated renal insufficiency. Transforming growth factor, epidermal growth factor, interleukin-1, platelet-derived growth factor, tumor-derived hematopoietic colony-stimulating factors, tumor necrosis factor (TNF) (particularly TNF-β), and lymphotoxin are all potent inducers of bone resorption *in vitro* and may have a role in the hypercalcemia of malignancy.

Multiple organ systems are involved in the constellation of symptoms caused by hypercalcemia. These symptoms are nonspecific, with the severity being directly related to the degree of calcium elevation. Neuromuscular symptoms often predominate, with the initial manifestations of fatigue, weakness, lethargy, and apathy progressing to profound mental status changes and psychotic behavior if left untreated. Nausea, vomiting, anorexia, obstipation, ileus, and abdominal pain are among the GI symptoms that may occur with hypercalcemia. Renal tubular dysfunction can occur secondary to hypercalcemia and is manifested by the development of polydipsia, polyuria, and nocturia. Polydipsia and polyuria are among the earliest symptoms of hypercalcemia and are due to a reversible defect in renal tubular concentrating ability, similar to nephrogenic diabetes insipidus. Severe volume contraction occurs, potentiating serum calcium elevation. If untreated, prolonged hypercalcemia may progress to permanent renal tubular damage.

The role of calcium as a neurotransmitter makes the myocardium particularly prone to hypercalcemia-induced toxicity. Acute hypercalcemia can slow the heart rate and shorten ventricular systole. With moderate elevation of the calcium level, the QT interval is shortened, and atrial and ventricular arrhythmias may occur. Electrocardiographic changes seen with elevated serum calcium levels include bradycardia, prolonged PR interval, shortened QT interval, and widened T waves. Under extreme circumstances, sudden death from cardiac arrhythmias can occur when the serum calcium rises acutely.

Critical laboratory studies in the work-up of patients with hypercalcemia include serum calcium, phosphate, alkaline phosphatase, PTH, electrolytes, blood urea nitrogen (BUN), total protein, albumin, and creatinine levels. In patients with severe hypoalbuminemia, the ionized calcium level is a more accurate measure of the effective calcium level. Severely malnourished, protein-depleted patients may show an elevated ionized calcium level without an increase in total calcium. Also, abnormal calcium binding to paraprotein without an elevation in the ionized calcium can be seen in patients with multiple myeloma. Elevated immunoreactive PTH levels in association with hypophosphatemia suggest ectopic PTH secretion. Hypercalcemia secondary to malignancy usually has an acute onset, high serum calcium level (>14 mg/dl), low serum chloride level, and elevated or normal serum phosphate and bicarbonate levels. These laboratory findings help differentiate hypercalcemia caused by cancer from that secondary to hyperparathyroidism, which is associated with an elevated serum calcium in the presence of decreased serum phosphate and bicarbonate levels.

Prompt identification and treatment of hypercalcemia are essential. Symptomatic patients with hypercalcemia and/or those patients with a serum calcium level of 12 mg/dl or greater need emergency medical treatment. IV hydration with restoration of intravascular volume increases glomerular filtration rate and is the mainstay of hypercalcemia management. Diuretics that block calcium resorption in the ascending loop of Henle and augment renal calcium excretion (e.g., furosemide) may be helpful after intravascular volume repletion has taken place. The initial dose of furosemide in patients without renal impairment is 40 mg given as an IV bolus, followed by 40–80 mg every 2–4 hours as needed. Ethacrynic acid (50 mg IV or 0.5–1.0 mg/kg) can occasionally serve as an alternative to furosemide; however, thiazide diuretics may potentiate hypercalcemia and should never be used.

Biphosphonates block osteoclastic bone resorption with significant reduction of serum calcium levels. Etidronate disodium is the only diphosphonate approved for use in the United States. A typical dose regimen is 7.5 mg kg^{-1} day^{-1} IV for several days followed by 20 mg kg^{-1} day^{-1} PO. Pamidronate is a "second-generation" biphosphonate and has been shown to be more effective than etidronate. Pamidronate has the advantage of inhibiting bone resorption by osteoclast activity while not impairing bone mineralization. Furthermore, the effect of pamidronate seems to have a faster onset, a longer effect, and a more durable response. The dose of pamidronate is either 60 mg intravenously over 4 hours or 90 mg intravenously over 24 hours for moderate to severe hypercalcemia. Patients will usually begin to notice relief of symptoms within hours, and the effect will usually last for 2–3 weeks. Maintenance therapy can be achieved by either intermittent intravenous infusions or continuous oral administration. Oral doses of between 400 and 1,200 mg/day in divided doses have been used with a fairly good response.

Plicamycin (Mithracin) is an effective inhibitor of bone resorption that generally induces a decline in serum calcium within 6–48 hours. Plicamycin is an antitumor antibiotic with limited antineoplastic activity but excellent reduction in bone resorption when used at doses of 25 mg kg^{-1} day^{-1} by IV infusion. The toxicities of plicamycin include thrombocytopenia, hypotension, and hepatic and renal insufficiency. These toxicities are rare when the dose is restricted to less than 30 mg kg^{-1} day^{-1}.

Ralston et al. evaluated 39 patients with hypercalcemia of malignancy (serum calcium >11.2 mg/dl). All patients evaluated underwent aggressive saline diuresis along with randomly assigned treatment with diphosphonate, plicamycin, or corticosteroids and calcitonin. All three therapeutic regimens produced significant decreases in serum calcium. The regimen containing corticosteroids produced the most rapid reduction in serum calcium level; however, the calcium level rarely decreased to the normal range. Diphosphonates produced a more sustained and complete reduction in the serum calcium level, although the onset of action was slower. Plicamycin effectively lowered the serum calcium level, but this effect was transient, with approximately half of the patients studied showing an increase in the serum calcium level by day 9 of treatment.

Gallium nitrate, a new agent used in the treatment of hypercalcemia, is a potent inhibitor of bone resorption, with profound effects in reducing serum calcium in patients with malignant disease and hyperparathyroidism. Hydroxyapatite is rendered less soluble and more resistant to cell-mediated resorption when gallium nitrate is incorporated into bone. Gallium nitrate causes impairment in osteoclast acidification of bone matrix by decreasing transmembrane proton transport. This agent may also enhance bone formation by stimulating bone collagen synthesis and increasing calcium incorporation into bone. These actions result in a net reduction of serum calcium. The dose of gallium nitrate is 100–200 mg kg^{-1} day^{-1} via continuous IV infusion given for a total of 5–7 days. Normal serum calcium levels are seen in 80–90% of patients. Nephrotoxicity, the dose-limiting factor, may be minimized by pretreatment IV hydration.

HYPONATREMIA/SYNDROME OF INAPPROPRIATE ANTIDIURETIC HORMONE

Significant neurologic dysfunction can occur when the serum sodium level falls abruptly or when it decreases to levels below 115–125 mg/dl. Mental status changes, seizures, coma, and ultimately death may result if therapeutic intervention is not urgently instituted. The syndrome of inappropriate antidiuretic hormone (SIADH) may be associated with cancers of the prostate, adrenal glands, esophagus, pancreas, colon, and head and neck; carcinoid tumors; and mesotheliomas. Small cell carcinoma of the lung is the most common malignancy associated with SIADH.

Dilutional hyponatremia occurs due to excessive water resorption in the collecting ducts. This increase in intravascular volume leads to increased renal perfusion along with a significant decrease in proximal tubular absorption of sodium. In the presence of renal insufficiency, there is increased ADH secretion and excessive water reabsorption from the collecting ducts, resulting in a significant dilutional hyponatremia.

Patients with mild hyponatremia frequently complain of anorexia, nausea, myalgia, headaches, and subtle neurologic symptoms. When the onset of hyponatremia is rapid or the absolute serum sodium level falls below 115 mg/dl, patients develop more severe neurologic dysfunction. Alterations in mental status can range from lethargy to confusion and coma. Seizures and psychotic behavior can occur at critically low serum sodium levels. Physical findings in patients with profound hyponatremia include alterations in mental status, pathologic reflexes, papilledema, and, occasionally, focal neurologic signs.

Laboratory data and diagnostic studies should aid the clinician in determining the etiology of hyponatremia. Pseudo-hyponatremia, or dilutional hyponatremia, due to hyperproteinemia, hyperglycemia, or hyperlipidemia can be ruled out by serum protein electrophoresis, serum glucose, and serum lipid determinations. The possibility of drug-induced hyponatremia should also be considered. Chemotherapeutic agents such as vincristine and cyclophosphamide, as well as mannitol, morphine, diuretics, and abrupt withdrawal of steroids, may contribute to hyponatremia.

A detailed history and physical examination along with meticulous evaluation of the patient's intake and output will aid in determining whether the patient's intravascular volume is adequate and will eliminate the possibility of water toxicity as the cause of hyponatremia. Laboratory investigation should include measurement of serum and urine electrolytes and creatinine. A typical finding in patients with SIADH is that the urine sodium concentration is inappropriately high for the level of hyponatremia. Also, the urine osmolality is greater than plasma osmolality, and the urine is never maximally diluted. Other significant findings might include a low BUN, hypouricemia, and hypophosphatemia resulting from a decreased proximal tubular resorption of these compounds. Chest radiograph and brain CT scan should be done if pathology of the pulmonary or central nervous system (CNS) is suspected.

Ideally, therapy for SIADH should be directed toward the underlying cause. In the case of small cell lung cancer, effective multidrug chemotherapy usually results in resolution of hyponatremia. SIADH resulting from CNS metastasis may improve with the use of corticosteroids and radiation therapy. If the etiology of SIADH cannot be identified, then the therapy for patients with severe hyponatremia is water restriction. A restriction of free water to 500–1,000 ml/day should correct the hyponatremia within 5–10 days. If no improvement is seen in the serum sodium level with restriction of free water after this time period, then demeclocycline should be used. Demeclocycline is an ADH antagonist that produces a dose-dependent, reversible nephrogenic diabetes insipidus. The recommended initial dose of demeclocycline is 600 mg daily (given in two or three divided doses). The potential adverse effect of nephrotoxicity with demeclocycline is usually seen only when extremely high doses are used (1,200 mg/day). Because this agent is secreted in urine and bile, dose adjustments must be made in patients with renal or hepatic insufficiencies.

When severe hyponatremia produces seizures or coma, 3% hypertonic saline or normal saline infusion with IV furosemide should be used. The rate of serum sodium correction should be limited to 0.5–1.0 mEq liter^{-1} hour^{-1} to minimize the risk of CNS toxicity.

HYPOGLYCEMIA

Insulin-producing islet cell tumors are the prototypical lesions associated with hypoglycemia. The non–islet cell tumors most often associated with hypoglycemia include hepatomas, adrenocortical tumors, and tumors of mesenchymal origin. Mesenchymal tumors comprise more than 50% of non–islet cell neoplasms seen in association with hypoglycemia. Of these, mesothelioma, fibrosarcoma, neurofibrosarcoma, and hemangiopericytoma are most commonly associated with hypoglycemia.

The mechanism of hypoglycemia resulting from insulin-secreting islet cell tumors involves the unregulated and inappropriate excess secretion of insulin. In contrast, the serum insulin level is normal with non–islet cell tumors. Substances with nonsuppressible insulin-like activities (NSILAs) have been detected in patients with malignancy-associated hypoglycemia. Two classes of compounds have been isolated based on molecular weight and ethanol solubility. The low-molecular-weight compounds consist of IGF-I, IGF-II, somatomedin A, and somatomedin C. IGF-I and IGF-II share similar amino acid sequences with proinsulin; however, they do not react with anti-insulin antibodies. The metabolic activity of these compounds is only 1–2% that of insulin. Approximately 40% of cancer patients with symptomatic hypoglycemia have elevated plasma levels of NSILAs. This supports the role of NSILA in hypoglycemia of malignancy.

Increased glucose use may account for the hypoglycemia seen in association with large tumors. Hepatic glucose production (700 g/day) may fall short of daily glucose requirements in the presence of tumors weighing more than 1 kg (which use 50–200 g/day of glucose). Defects in the usual counterregulatory mechanism of glucose control may also account for malignancy-induced hypoglycemia. Cancer-related hypoglycemia usually develops gradually. It does not allow the usual increase in counterregulatory hormones seen with hypoglycemia from other etiologies.

Symptoms of hypoglycemia include excessive fatigue, weakness, dizziness, and confusion. In malignancy-associated hypoglycemia, neurologic symptoms usually predominate and may progress to seizures and coma if left untreated. These more severe neurologic complications are usually associated with serum glucose levels below 40–45 mg/dl.

Before concluding that cancer is the etiology of hypoglycemia, all other potential causes must be excluded. Exogenous insulin or oral hypoglycemic agents, adrenal insufficiency, pituitary insufficiency, ethanol abuse, and malnutrition are among the common causes of hypoglycemia. Measurement of fasting and late-afternoon serum glucose levels will aid in determining if hypoglycemia is due to an islet cell or non–islet cell tumor. Patients with insulinomas have increased insulin levels, with fasting glucose levels below 50 mg/dl. This finding is quite different from that of non–islet cell tumors, in which there is a normal or low insulin level associated with hypoglycemia. Also, because insulinomas produce large amounts of proinsulin, they tend to have an elevated proinsulin-to-insulin ratio.

Under ideal circumstances, complete extirpation of the tumor is the optimal therapeutic intervention for hypoglycemia secondary to solid tumors. In the case of an insulinoma, simple enucleation or subtotal pancreatectomy will frequently provide cure. These tumors are usually benign, with excellent results from simple tumor resection. Diazoxide may be beneficial in patients with insulin-secreting tumors by inhibiting insulin secretion. For the same reason, this drug is not effective in the treatment of non–islet cell tumors. Radiation therapy may at times reduce tumor bulk and provide palliation of hypoglycemia. Diet modification should be the second line of therapy when resection is impossible. Frequent feedings between meals and nightly can reduce hypoglycemic attacks. Corticosteroids and growth hormone may provide temporary relief. Glucagon injections subcutaneously can also be used as an aid in glucose regulation.

Tumor Lysis Syndrome

Tumor lysis syndrome is a critical complication of cytotoxic therapy that requires a team approach in the intensive care unit to prevent the sequelae of permanent renal failure and death. Tumor lysis syndrome occurs when there is rapid cell turnover and increased release of intracellular contents into the bloodstream. This syndrome is characterized by hyperuricemia, hyperkalemia, hyperphosphatemia, and hypocalcemia. Occasionally, this syndrome occurs spontaneously in patients with lymphomas and leukemia; however, it is more common after cytotoxic chemotherapy-induced rapid cell lysis. The rapid release of intracellular contents can overwhelm the excretory ability of the kidneys, and electrolyte levels can become dangerously elevated. Patients with large, bulky tumors that are sensitive to cytotoxic chemotherapy are particularly prone to this syndrome, as are patients undergoing treatment for Burkitt's and non-Hodgkin's lymphoma, acute lymphoblastic leukemia, acute nonlymphoblastic leukemia, and chronic myelogenous leukemia in blast crisis. Although rare, tumor lysis syndrome can occur after treatment of small cell lung cancer, metastatic breast cancer, and metastatic medulloblastoma. Tumor lysis syndrome occurs not only with cytotoxic chemotherapy but also following radiation and hormonal therapy (e.g., tamoxifen, steroids, interferon).

As mentioned earlier, the metabolic abnormalities associated with tumor lysis syndrome include hyperuricemia, hyperkalemia, and hyperphosphatemia with hypocalcemia. The pathologic processes seen with this syndrome are due to the propensity of uric acid, xanthine, and phosphate to precipitate in the renal tubules. This can impair renal excretory function and cause further serum elevation of these metabolites. Renal insufficiency usually does not develop from the metabolic derangements alone; a combination of low urine flow rates and elevated serum metabolites is usually required to precipitate renal dysfunction. Thus oliguric patients are at significantly higher risk of developing renal failure during rapid cellular lysis.

Hyperkalemia results from the release of intracellular contents and is further perpetuated by renal insufficiency. The potential toxicities of potassium elevation are life-threatening and require urgent intervention. Signs of cardiac toxicity are evident by the characteristic electrocardiographic changes seen with potassium levels above 6 mEq/liter. Loss of P waves, peaked T waves, widened QRS complex, and depressed ST segments indicate severe hyperkalemia effects that may progress to heart block and diastolic cardiac arrest if left untreated.

Hyperphosphatemia can also result from rapid tumor lysis and is usually accompanied by hypocalcemia. The mechanism of hypocalcemia in tumor lysis syndrome is thought to be due to the formation of calcium-phosphate salts that precipitate in the soft tissues. Hyperphosphatemia is further exacerbated by the formation of these calcium-phosphate complexes in renal tubules, causing progressive renal insufficiency.

Preventive measures can be taken to minimize the toxicities of tumor lysis. Patients should undergo vigorous IV hydration before initiating potentially toxic chemotherapeutic agents. Another important preventive measure is to alkalinize the urine during the first 1–2 days of cytotoxic treatment. These measures counteract hyperuricemia by increasing the solubility of uric acid. Allopurinol has also been shown to effectively decrease the formation of uric acid and to reduce the incidence of uric acid nephropathy. In patients with large, bulky tumors that are known to have a high growth fraction, allopurinol should be administered before chemotherapeutic intervention.

An electrocardiogram should be obtained in patients with hyperkalemia or hypocalcemia, and continuous cardiac monitoring should be instituted. Hyperkalemia should be treated with the standard measures for acutely lowering the serum potassium level. These include IV administration of insulin and glucose, loop diuretics, and/or bicarbonate. Calcium should be used to acutely counteract cardiac toxicities if the patient is not on digitalis. Regardless of the measures used to acutely lower the serum potassium, an oral or rectal sodium-potassium exchange resin should be given to lower the total body potassium load (15 g sodium polystyrene sulfonate [Kayexalate] PO every 6 hours).

If there is evidence of worsening renal function with poor resolution of the metabolic abnormalities, hemodialysis should be considered.

Neutropenic Enterocolitis

The terms *neutropenic enterocolitis, typhlitis, necrotizing enteropathy*, and *ileocecal syndrome* have all been used to describe a clinical entity characterized by febrile neutropenia, abdominal distension, right-sided abdominal pain, tenderness, and diarrhea. The syndrome most often occurs in patients undergoing chemotherapy for hematologic malignancy, although it may also be seen in patients with solid tumors. Signs and symptoms characteristically develop after prolonged neutropenia (7 days or more). The initial presentation—consisting of right-sided abdominal pain, tenderness, and fever—often suggests appendicitis. The presence of significant watery diarrhea may mimic pseudomembranous colitis, but all conditions associated with acute abdominal pain must be considered in the differential diagnosis. The diagnosis is made clinically, often by exclusion of other pathologic causes. Serial examinations by the same examiner are critical to proper diagnosis and treatment. Abdominal films characteristically reveal an ileus pattern with some dilation of the cecum. Pneumatosis is an inconsistent finding. The CT findings in neutropenic enterocolitis are nonspecific, consisting mainly of bowel wall thickening and edema. The CT scan is often more valuable in ruling out other pathologic conditions. Complete work-up should include stool cultures for bacteria, fungus, and *Clostridium difficile* toxin.

The severity of neutropenic enterocolitis varies, and therapy must be individualized. Medical treatment—including bowel rest, nasogastric suction, broad-spectrum antibiotics, and IV hyperalimentation—is successful in many cases. Although granulocyte transfusion has never been proven to be effective, granulocyte colony-stimulating factors, which shorten the neutropenic period, will likely improve outcome. Surgical intervention is indicated in cases of perforation, uncontrolled hemorrhage, sepsis, and progression of symptoms on medical therapy. Right hemicolectomy with ileostomy is the operation of choice in most cases.

Central Venous Catheter Sepsis

The use of indwelling vascular access catheters is now standard practice in cancer care. Catheter-based infection is a major source of morbidity. When catheter infection is suspected, a careful examination of the access site should be performed. Erythema, induration, and suppuration are signs of site infection requiring immediate catheter removal. Bacteremia and sepsis from catheter infection should be documented by blood cultures drawn from both the catheter and peripheral sites. Coagulase-negative staphylococci are the most common pathogen isolated in catheter-based infection, although numerous gram-positive, gram-negative, and fungal species may also be responsible. More than 80% of catheter-based infections can be treated effectively with a 10- to 14-day course of IV antibiotics. Antibiotic therapy should be given through the infected catheter and rotated between ports when multilumen catheters are present. Persistence of positive blood cultures or signs of systemic sepsis, particularly in the neutropenic patient, necessitates immediate catheter removal. Patients with vascular grafts or implanted prostheses should not be treated initially with antibiotics; immediate catheter removal is indicated in these patients once an infection has been documented.

Hemorrhage

Tumors are rarely the source of intra-abdominal hemorrhage even in the known cancer patient. More frequent scenarios include bleeding because of severe thrombocytopenia and coagulopathy or as a complication of an invasive procedure. Peptic ulcer disease and gastritis, the most common causes of bleeding in unselected series, are the leading culprits in 54–75% of patients with cancer. GI lymphomas and metastatic tumors are the most common lesions to initiate massive hemorrhage. Because tumors are responsible for spontaneous hemorrhage in a minority of patients, the same systematic approach to diagnosis and treatment should be undertaken as in those patients without malignant disease. While resuscitation with crystalloid and blood products is under way, the diagnostic work-up to define the site and etiology of bleeding should begin. Bleeding proximal to the ligament of Treitz is marked clinically by hematemesis or blood per nasogastric aspirate. Such signs should be followed by prompt upper endoscopy.

Bright red blood per rectum should initiate investigation of a colonic or rectal source. In such cases, proctoscopy or sigmoidoscopy is an expedient initial diagnostic maneuver. Angiography and nuclear red cell scans are often needed to localize colonic and small bowel bleeding sites. Mild blood loss from a colonic neoplasm can usually be treated endoscopically with electrocautery or placement of topical hemostatic agents if the lesion is within the rectum. Some patients may require urgent surgical resection of the colonic neoplasm for continuing bleeding, but this can usually be delayed until the bowel has been mechanically cleansed to allow for a primary anastomosis, if appropriate. When the bleeding cannot be localized and the hemorrhage is massive, immediate exploration with intraoperative endoscopy should be considered. The exploration and/or the endoscopy may allow localization of the bleeding site so that surgical resection may be directed; however, total abdominal colectomy may be needed if the hemorrhage cannot be localized exactly. Small-bowel tumors rarely present with massive gastrointestinal hemorrhage, although gastric carcinoma may occasionally present with acute bleeding. The evaluation and treatment are nearly identical to those of a colonic source, with endoscopy as the first line of treatment and surgical resection reserved for a more elective setting.

Extraluminal, intra-abdominal hemorrhage should be suspected when there is significant blood loss without hematemesis, melena, or hematochezia. The retroperitoneum is the most frequent site of occult intra-abdominal hemorrhage. If suspected, it is best evaluated with a CT scan. Therapy for intra-abdominal hemorrhage is initially directed at resuscitation and correction of any existing coagulopathy. A history of aspirin or nonsteroidal anti-inflammatory use within 1 week must raise suspicion of platelet dysfunction, and a bleeding time should be obtained. When the site and source of bleeding are identified, specific therapy is instituted. Under controlled conditions, invasive therapies such as endoscopic coagulation and angiographic embolization may be attempted. The timing of surgical intervention is based on the rate and volume of blood loss, the underlying pathology, and the patient's overall health status.

Selected References

Aabo K, Pedersen H, Bach F, Knudsen J. Surgical management of intestinal obstruction in the late course of malignant disease. *Acta Chir Scand* 150:173, 1984.

Alt B, Glass NR, Sollinger H. Neutropenic enterocolitis in adults. Review of the literature and assessment of surgical intervention. *Am J Surg* 149:405, 1985.

Annest LS, Jolly PC. The results of surgical treatment of bowel obstruction caused by peritoneal carcinomatosis. *Am Surg* 45:718, 1979.

Armstrong BA, Perez CA, Simpson J, et al. Role of irradiation in the management of superior vena cava syndrome. *Int J Radiol Oncol Biol Phys* 13:531, 1987.

Arrambide K, Toto RD. Tumor lysis syndrome. *Semin Nephrol* 13:273; 1993.

Baker GL, Barnes HJ. Superior vena cava syndrome: Etiology, diagnosis and treatment. *Am J Crit Care* 1:54; 1992.

Bear HD, Turner MA, Parker GA, et al. Treatment of biliary obstruction caused by metastatic cancer. *Am J Surg* 157:381, 1989.

Besarob A, Caro JF. Mechanism of hypercalcemia in malignancy. *Cancer* 41:2276, 1978.

Boss GR, Seegimiller JE. Hyperuricemia and gout: Classification complications and management. *N Engl J Med* 300:1459, 1979.

Castaldo TW, Petrelli ES, Ballon SC, Lagasse LD. Intestinal operations in patients with ovarian carcinoma. *Am J Obstet Gynecol* 139:80, 1981.

Chisolm MA, Mulloy AL, Taylor AT. Acute management of cancer-related hypercalcemia. *Ann Pharmacother* 30:507; 1996.

Clark-Pearson DL, Chin NO, DeLong ER, Rice R, Creasman WT. Surgical management of intestinal obstruction in ovarian cancer: Clinical features, postoperative complications and survival. *Gynecol Oncol* 26:11, 1987.

Delaney TF, Oldfield EH. Spinal Cord Compression. In VT DeVita, S Hellman, SA Rosenberg (eds.), *Cancer: Principles and Practice of Oncology* (4th ed). Philadelphia: Lippincott, 1993.

Einzig AI. Hypercalcemia in Malignancies. In JP Dutcher, PH Wiesnik (eds.), *Handbook of Hematologic and Oncologic Emergencies.* New York: Plenum, 1987.

Escalante CP. Causes and management of superior vena cava syndrome. *Oncology* 7:61, 1993.

Ferrara JJ, Martin EW Jr, Carey LC. Morbidity of emergency operations in patients with metastatic cancer receiving chemotherapy. *Surgery* 92:605, 1982.

Fukuya T, Hawes DR, Lu CC, Chang PJ, Barloon TJ. CT diagnosis of small-bowel obstruction: Efficacy in 60 patients. *Am J Roentgenol* 158:765, 1992.

Gallick HL, Weaver DW, Sachs RJ, et al. Intestinal obstruction in cancer patients: An assessment of risk factors and outcome. *Am Surg* 8:434, 1986.

Gray BH, Olin JW, Graor RA, et al. Safety and efficacy of thrombolytic therapy for superior vena cava syndrome. *Chest* 99:54, 1991.

Gregory JR, McMurtrey MJ, Mountain CF. A surgical approach to the treatment of pericardial effusion in cancer patients. *Am J Clin Oncol* 8:319, 1985.

Helms SR, Carlson MD. Cardiovascular emergencies. *Semin Oncol* 16:463, 1989.

Henderson JE, Shustic C, Kremer R, et al. Circulating concentrations of parathyroid hormone-like peptide in malignancy and hyperparathyroidism. *J Bone Miner Res* 5:105, 1990.

Kahn CR. The riddle of tumour hypoglycemia revised. *Clin Endocrinol Metab* 9:335, 1980.

Kemeny N, Brennan MF. The surgical complications of chemotherapy in the cancer patient. *Curr Probl Surg* 24:607, 1987.

Kim RY, Spenser SA, Meredith RF, et al. Extradural spinal cord compression: Analysis of factors determining functional prognosis. *Radiology* 176:279, 1990.

Krebs H-B, Goplerud DR. Surgical management of bowel obstruction in advanced ovarian carcinoma. *Obstet Gynecol* 61:327, 1983.

Lightdale CJ, Kurtz RC, Boyle CC, et al. Cancer and upper gastrointestinal tract hemorrhage: Benign causes of bleeding demonstrated by endoscopy. *JAMA* 226:139, 1973.

Maddox AM, Valdivieso M, Lukeman J, et al. Superior vena cava obstruction in small cell bronchogenic carcinoma: Clinical parameters and survival. *Cancer* 52:2165, 1983.

Makris A, Kunkler IH. Controversies in the management of metastatic spinal cord compression. *Clin Oncol* 7:77; 1995.

Massaferri EL, O'Dorisio TM, LoBuglio AF. Treatment of hypercalcemia associated with malignancy. *Semin Oncol* 5:141, 1978.

Millard PR, Jerrome DW, Millward-Sadler GH. Spindle-cell tumours and hypoglycaemia. *J Clin Pathol* 29:520, 1976.

Mundy GR. The hypercalcemia of malignancy revised. *J Clin Invest* 82:1, 1988.

Mundy GR, Martin JT. The hypercalcemia of malignancy: Pathogenesis and management. *Metabolism* 31:1247, 1982.

Novak JM, Collins JT, Donowitz M, Farman J, Sheahan DG, Spiro HM. Effects of radiation on the human gastrointestinal tract. *J Clin Gastroenterol* 1:9; 1979.

Osteen RT, Guyton S, Steele G, et al. Malignant intestinal obstruction. *Surgery* 87:611, 1980.

Press OW, Livingston R. Management of malignant pericardial effusion and tamponade. *JAMA* 257:1088, 1987.

Ralston SH, Gardner MD, Drybrugh FJ, et al. Comparison of amino-hydroxypylidene diphosphonate, mithramycin, and corticosteroids/calcitonin in treatment of cancer associated hypercalcemia. *Lancet* 2:907, 1985.

Ricci JL, Turnbull DM. Spontaneous gastroduodenal perforation in cancer patients receiving cytotoxic therapy. *J Surg Oncol* 41:219; 1989.

Rinkevich D, Borovik R, Bendett M, Markiewicz W. Malignant pericardial tamponade. *Med Pediatr Oncol* 18:287; 1990.

Schwartz EE, Goodman LR, Haskin ME. Role of CT scanning in the superior vena cava syndrome. *Am J Clin Oncol* 9:71, 1986.

Sheperd FA, Morgan C, Evans WK, et al. Medical management of malignant pericardial effusion by tetracycline sclerosis. *Am J Cardiol* 60:1161, 1987.

Siegal T, Shohami E, Siegal TG. Indomethacin and dexamethasone treatment in experimental spinal cord compression. Part II. Effect on edema and prostaglandin synthesis. *Neurosurgery* 22:334, 1988.

Silverman P, Distelhorst CW. Metabolic emergencies in clinical oncology. *Semin Oncol* 16:504, 1989.

Steinberg SM, Barkin JS, Kaplan RS, Stablein DM. Prognostic indicators of colon tumors. The Gastrointestinal Study Group experience. *Cancer* 57:1866; 1986.

Stellato TA, Shenk RR. Gastrointestinal emergencies in the oncology patient. *Semin Oncol* 16:521, 1989.

Stellato TA, Zollinger RM Jr, Shuck JM. Metastatic malignant biliary obstruction. *Am Surg* 53:385, 1987.

Tang E, Davis D, Silberman H. Bowel obstruction in cancer patients. *Arch Surg* 130:832, 1995

Theologides A. Neoplastic cardiac tamponade. *Semin Oncol* 5:181, 1978.

Theriault RL. Hypercalcemia of malignancy: Pathophysiology and implications for treatment. *Oncology* 7:47, 1993.

Torosian MH, Turnbull ADM. Emergency laparotomy for spontaneous intestinal and colonic perforations in cancer patients receiving corticosteroids and chemotherapy. *J Clin Oncol* 6:291, 1988.

Tunca JC, Buchler DA, Mack EA, Ruzicka FF, Crowley JJ, Carr WF. The management of ovarian-cancer-caused bowel obstruction. *Gynecol Oncol* 12:186, 1981.

Ushio Y, Posner R, Posner JB, Shapiro WR. Experimental spinal cord compression by epidural neoplasms. *Neurology* 27:422, 1977.

Wade DS, Nava HR, Douglass Ho Jr. Neutropenic enterocolitis. *Cancer* 69:17; 1992.

Warrell RP Jr, Bockman RS, Coonley CJ, et al. Gallium nitrate inhibits calcium resorption from bone and is effective treatment for cancer-related hypercalcemia. *J Clin Invest* 73:1487, 1984.

Weiss SM, Skibber JM, Rosato FE. Bowel obstruction in cancer patients: performance status as a predictor of survival. *J Surg Oncol* 25:15, 1984

Yoachim J. Superior vena cava syndrome. In VT DeVita, S Hellman, SA Rosenberg (eds.), *Cancer: Principles and Practice of Oncology* (4th ed). Philadelphia: Lippincott, 1993.

22

Biologic Cancer Therapy

George E. Peoples and Alexander R. Miller

Surgery, radiation, and chemotherapy have long been the mainstays to traditional cancer therapy; however, in recent years, biologic cancer therapy has emerged as a fourth arm to cancer treatment. This form of therapy induces, utilizes, and/or modifies the host immune system to more efficiently recognize and destroy cancer cells. The basic components, the mechanisms of action, and the communications of the immune system must be understood to fully appreciate biologic cancer therapies; therefore these facets will be reviewed briefly in this chapter. Basic science research into many aspects of the immune system has produced immunotherapeutics such as cytokines, monoclonal antibodies, cellular therapies, vaccines, and gene therapies that are currently under investigation in clinical trials. The review of these new alternative forms of therapy is the fundamental purpose of this chapter.

The Immune System

The immune system is made up of a wide array of cell types, but lymphocytes provide the specificity of the immune response. The immune system can largely be divided into the humoral branch and the cellular branch. These branches differ in both effector cell type and mechanism of antigen recognition. The T lymphocyte is responsible for many of the functions of the cellular branch such as delayed type hypersensitivity (DTH) and rejection of grafts and tumors. The humoral branch is largely associated with B lymphocytes and the production of antibodies (Abs).

CELLULAR IMMUNITY

Thymus-derived lymphocytes, or T cells, are all $CD3^+$ cells that recognize antigens via the T-cell receptor (TCR). This receptor has a specificity that is analogous to the immunoglobulins. T cells can be divided into two major types: $CD8^+$ cytotoxic T lymphocytes (CTL), which are capable of direct cellular killing, and $CD4^+$ T helper (Th) lymphocytes, which produce cytokines. $CD8^+$ T cells interact with target cells expressing human leukocyte antigen (HLA) class I molecules on their cell surface. The HLA class I molecule is ubiquitously expressed on all cells and presents short 8- to 10–amino acid peptides that have been processed from degraded endogenous self proteins or viral proteins. The $CD8^+$ T cell's TCR/CD3 complex specifically recognizes a single peptide/HLA complex and then is triggered to destroy that cell by granule exocytosis. This process involves the release of cytolysin (perforin) and granzymes (serine protease-containing granules) that lead to target apoptosis.

The $CD4^+$ T cell interacts with specialized antigen-presenting cells (APC) such as macrophages, dendritic cells, and B lymphocytes that express HLA class II molecules. HLA class II molecules present longer 12- to 20–amino acid peptides processed from exogenous proteins that have been taken up and processed by the APC. When a CD4$^+$ T cell's specific TCR has been activated, the cell begins to produce cytokines that enhance B-cell antibody production, support T-cell responses, and activate other immune cells. T helper cells can be further divided into subtypes based on their pattern of cytokine production, as well as the antigens that stimulate them and the immune responses they support. Th1 cells promote cytotoxic cellular responses, DTH, and macrophage activation by secreting interleukin (IL)-2, interferon (IFN)-γ, and tumor necrosis factor (TNF)-β. Th2 cells support B-cell responses and the production of IgG, IgA, and IgE Abs by secreting IL-4, IL-5, IL-6, and IL-10. Both subsets of CD4$^+$ cells produce TNF-α, IL-3, and granulocyte, macrophage-colony stimulating factor (GM-CSF). Th1 cells are usually stimulated by infectious agents such as viruses and bacteria, whereas Th2 cells respond to allergens and parasites.

Natural killer (NK) cells are large, granular cytotoxic lymphocytes that are distinct from T and B cells. NK cells participate in the host's first line of defense and are nonspecific. These cells are CD3$^-$ and do not express TCR. NK cells express the CD56 molecule, which promotes cellular adhesion and the receptor for immunoglobulins (FcR). These cells participate in antibody-dependent cellular cytotoxicity (ADCC). NK cells are not target cell specific but demonstrate target cell selectivity by unknown mechanisms. Clearly, these cells are more cytotoxic for tumor cells and virally infected cells than for normal cells.

HUMORAL IMMUNITY

"Bursa-equivalent" lymphocytes, B cells, are the major cell type of the humoral branch of the immune system. Although T cells are restricted to recognizing processed antigens from only protein sources and presented in the context of "self" HLA molecules, B cells can recognize unprocessed antigens and, without the context, other molecules. Moreover, these antigens may be polysaccharides, nucleic acids, or proteins. Abs form tight, noncovalent complexes with specific antigens and act first as cell surface receptors. Once a B cell becomes activated by the binding of a cell surface Ab to its specific target antigen, the cell undergoes maturation to a plasma cell, producing the specific immunoglobulin bound. The Abs are then soluble, secreted molecules that bind the target fixing complement, marking it for phagocytosis or initiating ADCC.

All Abs are composed of two identical heavy and light chains that are covalently bound by disulfide bonds, forming a Y-shaped molecule. There are five major classes of Abs that differ in structure and function. IgG Abs are monomers with a γ-heavy chain and four subclasses. IgG Abs fix complement, cross the placenta, bind monocytes and neutrophils, and are the predominant Abs in secondary immune responses. IgM Abs are pentamers with a μ-heavy chain and two subclasses. IgM Abs fix complement, are involved in primary immune responses, and function as lymphocyte surface receptors and as accessory secretory Abs. IgA Abs are monomers with an α-heavy chain and two subclasses. IgA

Abs predominate in secretions. IgD Abs are monomers with a δ-heavy chain. IgD Abs are thought to act as lymphocyte receptors. IgE Abs are monomers with ε-heavy chains. IgE Abs bind basophils and mast cells, and are effectors of allergic and anaphylactic reactions.

The specificity of an Ab is determined by gene rearrangement in the variable domains of the heavy and light chains. Within these variable regions are three distinct widely separated areas that are hypervariable. These segments are called collectively the complementary determining regions (CDR). When the polypeptide is folded, these CDRs are brought together to form the antigen binding site. The diversity of Abs is generated by gene rearrangements within the variable region genes, as well as in the D and J joining genes, of both the heavy and light chains in addition to the CDRs. The diversity and specificity of the TCR are similarly determined.

CYTOKINES

Cytokines may be defined as immunobiologically active molecules produced by defined cell populations that either enhance or suppress specific immunologic functions. Certain cytokines enhance the expression of target antigens, major histocompatibility complex (MHC) molecules (e.g., IFN-γ), or antigen-presenting cells (GM-CSF). Other biologicals may facilitate antigen presentation by providing accessory signals that enhance the ability of lymphocytes to respond to mitogenic stimuli (IL-1, TNF, IL-6, IL-7, IL-12). The absence of such accessory signals can lead to immunologic anergy. The cytokines IL-2 and IL-4 may augment T-cell proliferation and overcome the requirement for cellular cooperation in the generation of cytotoxic T-cell responses. Finally, lymphocytes and some tumors may produce molecules, such as transforming growth factor (TGF)-β and IL-10, that suppress immune responses.

Biologic Cancer Therapy

Several factors suggest the presence of host immune influences on cancer, such as spontaneous regression, the latency period prior to metastasis or recurrence, and metastatic spread without known primary. These observations have prompted much interest in immunotherapies, and these interests have led to the foundation of an ever-expanding field of research. Currently, biologic therapies attempt by many different strategies to induce specific immune responses against a cancer and provide long-term protective immunity. Prior to the recent accumulation of an enormous amount of information regarding the specifics of antitumor immune responses, investigators attempted nonspecific induction of the immune system and were encouraged by occasional tumor regression and even complete, durable responses in animal studies. These findings and the recent advances in our understanding of the immune system have led to many clinical trials of biologic therapies, both specific and nonspecific.

CYTOKINES

The use of cytokines known to have accessory function in the generation of T-cell-mediated immunity (e.g., TNF, IL-1, IL-6, IL-7, IL-12) is a logical approach to cancer immunotherapy that has been studied in some detail. The hypothesis is that such signals could be lacking or deficient in the tumor-bearing host. Because T-cell recognition of antigen in the absence of accessory signals can lead to immunologic anergy, this pathway is of extreme importance. Systemic administration or, more elegantly, vaccination with cells expressing such cytokines would be expected to be beneficial. In addition to modifying the *in vivo* inflammatory environment, cytokine transduction may cause other phenotypic changes in tumors. An autocrine action of cytokines may be linked to cell growth, secondary cytokine production, and the secreted extracellular matrix.

Inflammatory/T-Cell Reactive Cytokines

IL-2

IL-2 is the most extensively studied cytokine to date. It is a lymphocyte-secreted, 15-kDa glycoprotein produced in response to several stimuli. In addition to stimulating the proliferation of T cells, it activates T and B cells, NK cells, and macrophages, and induces the production of other cytokines such as TNF, IFN-γ, and GM-CSF. Systemic administration of IL-2 alone and in combination with other cytokines has been studied in several trials, principally for patients with melanoma and renal cell carcinoma. Because it has been studied for the longest period of time of any of the cytokines, data regarding the consistency of IL-2 responses are substantial. Most protocols involve high-dose bolus regimens of 720,000 international units (IU)/kg every 8 hours for days 1–5 and 15–19, repeated every 4–6 weeks. Other trials have involved lower doses (72,000 IU/kg) or continuous infusion therapy and have demonstrated results similar to those for high-dose treatment schemes. The lower dosing schedules substantially reduce the toxicity associated with higher-dose therapy, which includes capillary leak syndrome, hypotension, azotemia, and metabolic acidosis. Toxicity seems related to induction of TNF-α, and the magnitude of this response appears to be genetically determined, resulting in individual variation in the clinical significance of the toxic response.

Overall response rates of approximately 20% (approximately 20% of these are complete) have been achieved, evaluating a variety of dosing levels and schedules. Meta-analyses reveal that a survival advantage may be conferred to patients with excellent performance status, compared with standard nonbiologic therapy. Combinations of IL-2 and IFN-α have been used in the treatment of renal cell carcinoma and melanoma and have demonstrated responses similar to IL-2 alone. Adding cisplatin to the IL-2 and IFN-α regimen may well enhance the antitumor response in patients with metastatic melanoma. The use of this combination produced a 54% response rate in a recent trial. IL-2 has been tested in the treatment of a variety of hematologic malignancies, with occasional responses documented. The combination of IL-2 and melatonin has been evaluated in several clinical trials involving patients with hepatocellular carcinoma, non–small cell lung cancer, and renal cell cancer. Objective responses have occurred in all disease types, some of which were improved, compared with the use of IL-2 alone, and were associated with less toxicity.

IL-4

IL-4 is a lymphocyte-derived cytokine. Originally termed *B-cell stimulatory factor*, this 20-kDa glycoprotein was identified as a potent activator of B and T lymphocytes, including $CD4^+$ and $CD8^+$ populations, as well as macrophages, mast cells, and hematopoietic progenitors. In several reports, IL-4 demonstrated stronger stimulatory effects than IL-2 on primed murine cytotoxic T lymphocytes. IL-4 induces the proliferation and differentiation of lymphocytes and up-regulates MHC class II and immunoglobulin expression by stimulated macrophages and B cells. IL-4 inhibits the expression of several inflammatory cytokines (IL-1, IFN-γ, TNF, IL-6) and enhances the antiproliferative effects of TNF in many tumor lines. IL-4 has been shown to induce cytotoxic T cells in peripheral blood lymphocytes (PBL) and tumor-infiltrating lymphocyte (TIL) populations that preferentially kill autologous tumors. IL-4 is currently being investigated in clinical protocols involving patients with renal cell carcinoma and melanoma, and appears less effective in inducing antitumor responses than IL-2 in solid tumors, but may have more activity against hematologic malignancies, specifically B-cell lymphomas and myelomas. Combinations of IL-2 and IL-4 have also been evaluated without significant responses to date.

TNF-α

TNF-α is a 17-kDa protein first described as a serum component responsible for inducing hemorrhagic necrosis of certain tumors *in vivo*. TNF-α is produced by several cell types, including T and B lymphocytes, macrophages, neutrophils, endothelial cells, and some tumors. This cytokine up-regulates IL-1, IL-6, GM-CSF, and intercellular adhesion molecule (ICAM)-1 production; acts as a costimulus for T-cell proliferation; and increases the expression of MHC class I antigens.

Systemically administered TNF-α will alter the growth of some tumor cell lines *in vitro* and *in vivo*, perhaps by acting on tumor microvasculature. However, high systemic levels of TNF-α induce a septic shock-like syndrome associated with tissue injury, organ failure, and cachexia. Clinical cancer trials have been largely disappointing; however, TNF alone or with IFN-α in hyperthermic isolated limb perfusion protocols for patients with melanoma and sarcoma have been associated with significant tumor responses and have obviated the need for amputation in some patients. Regional toxicity has also been reported and has resulted in ischemic compartment syndromes in affected limbs.

IFN-γ

IFN-γ is a 20-kDa glycoprotein produced by activated lymphocytes in response to various stimuli and induces the development of cytotoxic T cells, NK cells, and macrophages. This cytokine possesses direct cytotoxic effects as well as an ability to up-regulate MHC antigens and adhesion molecules. IFN-γ has demonstrated divergent properties in different tumor models. This cytokine has been reported to promote tumorigenicity and metastatic potential in certain murine systems, whereas it has demonstrated anti-neoplastic activity in other models. Clinically, the most encouraging data have come from studies involving patients with malignant mesothelioma who demonstrated approximately 15% response rates to intrapleural therapy.

IFN-α

IFN-α is another member of the IFN family and is a leukocyte-secreted cytokine possessing tumoricidal effects. It also increases the activity of cytotoxic effectors, including NK cells and macrophages. Systemic administration of IFN-α has been associated with up-regulation of MHC class I antigen expression to a greater degree than administration of IFN-γ. IFN-α also increases expression of tumor antigens capable of eliciting monoclonal antibody (MAb) recognition. The treatment of several human malignancies by IFN-α has been evaluated, particularly renal cell carcinoma, melanoma, and hematologic malignancies.

IFN-α is currently recommended as an initial treatment for patients with hairy cell and chronic myelogenous leukemias, and is capable of inducing hematologic and karyotypic remissions in treated patients.

Recently, Kirkwood et al. from the Eastern Cooperative Oncology Group (ECOG) published the most compelling evidence to date regarding the efficacy of systemically administered IFN-α2b in patients with malignant melanoma. In a multicenter randomized trial comparing adjuvant high-dose interferon for 52 weeks with observation for the same period, a significant prolongation of relapse-free and overall survival was observed. The patients most likely to benefit from this therapy were those with regional lymph node metastases. The associated toxicity was significant, however, and a substantial proportion of patients could not tolerate full treatment dosing schedules and/or experienced significant or life-threatening toxicity, including myelosuppression, hepatotoxicity, and neurologic symptoms.

Combinations of IFN-α and standard chemotherapy agents have been evaluated in the treatment of several solid tumor types. Though occasional responses have been observed, the addition of IFN-α to established chemotherapy regimens has not produced dramatic changes in response rates, but it does appear to alter the pharmacokinetics and toxicity profiles of many therapies, some adversely.

IL-1

IL-1 is a 17-kDa cytokine initially recognized for its effect as an endogenous pyrogen. It is produced by cells of the monocyte/macrophage lineage in response to perceived host stress or enhanced metabolic activity. Subsequently, IL-1 was found to be produced by NK cells, fibroblasts, T-cell lines, and some tumor cell lines. Properties attributed to IL-1 include participation in inflammatory responses, septic shock, T-helper cell responses, and induction of other cytokines and adhesion molecules such as TNF, GM-CSF, IL-2, IL-2 receptor, IL-3, IL-4, IL-6, IL-7, and ICAM-1. IL-1 expression is stimulated by endotoxin, exotoxins,

TNF-α, and GM-CSF. This cytokine has been observed to induce cytotoxic effects in certain tumors, but its significant toxic side effects have limited its clinical utility. Antitumor effects of IL-1 administration have been disappointing, but combinations of IL-2 and IL-1 have suggested activity in phase II trials of patients with a variety of metastatic solid tumor malignancies. Furthermore, IL-1 may play a role in enhancing platelet recovery following chemotherapy and has been studied in this capacity.

IL-6

IL-6 is a 25-kDa glycoprotein that functions as a growth factor and is capable of augmenting the *in vitro* cytotoxic capacity of T-cell subsets. Its release by various cell types—including T and B cells, platelets, macrophages, and fibroblasts—may be induced by TNF, IL-2, IL-3, GM-CSF, and IL-7. IL-6 has been shown to exert variable influences on the growth of tumor cells *in vitro* and when systemically administered. This cytokine demonstrated significant antineoplastic activity in tumor-bearing mice, the effect of which was abrogated by sublethal irradiation of the animals. In a melanoma model, IL-6 differentially regulated the growth of metastatic and nonmetastatic cells. IL-6 has been clinically evaluated both as a platelet growth factor and as an antineoplastic agent. It appears to function more effectively in the former role than in the latter. Results of current studies have been mixed in a variety of tumor types, though anecdotal reports of response by melanoma patients are encouraging. Toxicity of therapy includes anemia, neurologic symptoms, cardiac arrhythmias, and constitutional symptoms.

IL-7

IL-7 is a 25-kDa glycoprotein secreted by keratinocytes, dendritic cells, and certain T-cell populations. IL-7 acts as a costimulator of lymphocyte growth and differentiation independently, and in concert with IL-2. It up-regulates the expression of IL-6 and down-regulates the potent immunosuppressant TGF-β. In a direct comparison with IL-2, IL-7 was a more potent generator of antitumor cytotoxic T cells in a murine model. Additionally, intratumoral injection of high doses of IL-7 resulted in decreased tumor growth and rejection in a proportion of animals treated. Mice that rejected tumors after IL-7 administration were found to be specifically immune to subsequent tumor challenge. Currently, there are no specific clinical protocols involving direct administration of IL-7. There is one phase I protocol evaluating IL-7 in a gene therapy tumor vaccine model for melanoma, however, that will be discussed later in gene therapy.

IL-12

IL-12 was purified and cloned after its identification as a stimulatory factor of several cytotoxic lymphocyte populations, particularly NK cells. This cytokine is normally produced by B lymphocytes and cells of the monocyte/macrophage lineage. The molecule exists as a disulfide-linked heterodimer composed of 40- and 35-kDa subunits, both of which are required for biologic activity. Because of this unique structure, IL-12 has a longer half-life (measured in hours) than other cytokines, and its longer duration of action may allow less frequent dosing schedules and possibly less associated toxicity. IL-12 has been observed to up-regulate and induce IFN-γ in cultured T and NK cells, act synergistically with IL-2, and block the production of IL-4. IL-12 may also induce TNF, GM-CSF, and IL-3 in lymphocyte populations. Recently, IL-12 was shown to stimulate T-helper subpopulation Th1 cells, which characteristically secrete IL-2, IFN-γ, and TNF-β. Cells of the Th2 lineage are less affected by IL-12. Systemic and intratumoral administration of recombinant IL-12 to tumor-bearing animals caused growth inhibition of established primary and metastatic lesions that was at least partially dependent on CD8[+] cells. Mice were specifically immune to tumor rechallenge in certain systems. Clinical trials have recently been initiated, and responses in patients with metastatic renal cell cancer have been suggested.

Colony Stimulating Factors

IL-3

IL-3 is a T-cell-derived pleuripotent hematopoietic growth factor of approximate 28 kDa molecular weight. In a comparison with several other cytokines, exogenous IL-3 administration was found to enhance the immunogenicity of irradiated tumor cells significantly, including a nonimmunogenic tumor. Clinical use has primarily involved bone marrow rescue, with principal responses involving leukocytes and platelets. Combinations of IL-3 and other colony stimulating factors are also ongoing.

G-CSF

G-CSF is an approximately 20-kDa glycoprotein required for the growth and differentiation of hematopoietic precursors of the granulocyte lineage. Cells of the monocyte/macrophage lineage are the primary producers of G-CSF, which is not species specific and therefore demonstrates biologic activity in human and murine models. Clinical trials using this cytokine have demonstrated its efficacy in reducing the period of myelosuppression after chemotherapy for solid and hematologic malignancies, as well as in the setting of bone marrow transplantation.

GM-CSF

GM-CSF is a 22-kDa glycoprotein secreted by stimulated T lymphocytes. It is integral to the development of hematopoietic progenitor cells as well as mature neutrophils, eosinophils, and macrophages, in bone marrow and peripheral circulation. This cytokine is involved in the generation of bone marrow-derived dendritic cells participating in antigen presentation to unprimed CD4[+] and CD8[+] T cells. GM-CSF may also induce the expression of TNF and prostaglandin E2 in activated macrophages and may synergize with G-CSF in certain systems. GM-CSF-treated monocytes display enhanced antibody-directed cytotoxicity and phagocytosis *in vitro*. Clinical trials using this cytokine have reported increased peripheral granulocyte counts after myelosuppressive treatment in cytopenic patients. GM-CSF may also act to enhance cytokine levels in treated patients, thereby promoting antineoplastic inflammatory responses.

MONOCLONAL ANTIBODIES

Whereas a number of investigations have focused on immunotherapy protocols designed to alter or enhance cell-mediated antitumor activity, manipulation of the humoral immune system represents a relatively underutilized area of inquiry. For decades it has been known that tumors possess antigens that, although relatively weak immunogenically, may be recognized as foreign by the immunocompetent host. For certain tumors, Abs to these antigens have been identified that have been useful in clinical determinations of disease presence or recurrence as in the case of carcinoembryonic antigen (CEA) for assessing colorectal cancer, alpha-fetoprotein for testicular tumors and hepatocellular carcinoma, and prostate specific antigen for prostate carcinoma.

MAb Production

MAbs are generated by fusing B lymphocytes to a murine myeloma cell line, resulting in a hybridoma that may produce large quantities of single Ab type, each with unique specificity. MAbs have been evaluated as therapeutic as well as diagnostic tools in cancer therapy with varying degrees of success. MAb therapy is limited by physical characteristics of tumors, including variations in tumor vascularity and cellular density that often inhibits the ability of Mabs to sufficiently penetrate bulky tumors. Construction of Abs that only recognize tumor tissue and ignore nonneoplastic cells is difficult also. Furthermore, tumor antigen heterogeneity also impedes the ability of Mabs to generate clinically significant tumoricidal effects. Probably the most significant obstacle to MAb efficacy is the reaction to the murine component of the antibody that is recognized as foreign by human hosts, resulting in the generation of human antimouse Ab (HAMA) reactions that destroy circulating MAbs and enhance their serum clearance. Attempts to reduce the immunogenicity of Mabs have included the use of antibody fragments that lack the Fc domain (the portion binding the effector cell). However, reduced binding affinity typically accompanies the loss of this portion of the antibody. Humanized MAbs have also been attempted.

MAb / Immunotoxins

One strategy used to enhance the clinical efficacy of monoclonal antibodies has been to combine antibodies with known cellular toxins to create immunotoxins. Several clinical trials have evaluated the use of various forms of ricin immunotoxins. Although antitumor responses have occurred in a minority of patients and have been transient, these immunotoxins have been associated with consistent toxic effects in patients that include fatigue/myalgias, capillary leak syndromes, elevation of hepatic transaminases, and bone marrow suppression. In two studies involving breast carcinoma patients, substantial neurotoxicity was observed, the etiology of which was attributed to cross-reactivity to antigens contained within neural tissue.

Bispecific MAb

Another strategy involves the construction of bispecific MAbs that target additional effectors of the immune system as well as tumor antigens. For example, some MAbs have dual specificity for tumor antigens and the CD3/TCR or the CD16/FcRIII receptor on NK cells. This technology has been used in clinical trials directed toward B-cell neoplasms in certain patients, but disappointing results have been obtained thus far.

MAb / Conjugates

Other MAb models have employed drug immunoconjugates in which the antibody is fused to a chemotherapeutic drug such as doxorubicin. Radioimmunoconjugates have also been created in which radioactive sources such as I^{125} and I^{131} have been combined with MAbs to elicit antineoplastic responses. Limitations common to all these manipulations continue to be HAMA responses and host toxicity induced by cross-reactivity with rapidly dividing normal cells (e.g., bone marrow).

Clinical Results

Results of clinical trials of MAbs have been disappointing overall, but a few responses have been noted. A murine IgM MAb JD118 specific for neoplastic B cells has been constructed and found to destroy human leukemia and lymphoma cells in the presence of human complement. An anti-CD19 MAb HD37 induced cell cycle arrest in several Burkitt's lymphoma cell lines *in vitro* and in a xenograft model. Also, treatment with an anti-ganglioside MAb caused objective antitumor responses in patients with metastatic melanoma as well as neuroblastoma. Finally, a large randomized trial demonstrated that adjuvant therapy with a murine MAb 17-1A recognizing a 37-kDa cell surface glycoprotein induced improved remission durations and extended overall survival in patients with resected, locally metastatic colorectal carcinomas.

Although MAb therapy remains a theoretically intriguing focus of attention, it has yet to overcome the problem of significant toxicity and host inactivation.

CELLULAR THERAPY

With the discovery of IL-2 and the ability to efficiently expand T cells in culture, the idea of cellular therapies became a true possibility. As has been previously discussed, systemic IL-2 induces an anticancer response but with high levels of toxicity. These findings stimulated interest in adoptive immunotherapy that involves the transfer of specific immune cells with antitumor activity to the tumor-bearing host with less anticipated toxicity. The vast majority of clinical experience has been gained from IL-2-generated lymphokine-activated killer (LAK) cells and more recently from tumor-infiltrating lymphocytes (TIL).

LAK Cell Therapy

LAK cells are a heterogeneous population of cells made up of T cells and NK cells harvested from the peripheral blood that develop antitumor activity after being incubated in high doses of IL-2. The mechanism of selective cellular killing is unknown; however, these cells maintain their antitumor activity *in vivo* with exogenous IL-2 administration. LAK cells were first described in

1980, and clinical studies to determine the safety of infusional therapies were initiated shortly thereafter at the NCI. The first series was published in 1985 of 25 patients demonstrating the effectiveness of the therapy with regression of metastatic cancer of several histologies in some patients. The follow-up series of 178 consecutive patients treated with LAK cells at the NCI revealed a 14% complete response (CR) and 30% partial response (PR), with the best results seen in renal cell carcinoma (35% CR+PR), melanoma (21% CR + PR), and non-Hodgkin's lymphoma (57% CR + PR). Other institutions have reported variable results with response rates for melanoma (0–56%, composite = 18%), renal cell (0–50%, composite = 27%), lymphoma (0–100%, composite = 50%), and colorectal (0–100%, composite = 9%). The composite results are from pooled data from nine studies. The variability of results between institutions was likely due to differences in the numbers of infused LAK cells, the length of time cells were incubated in IL-2, and the dose and method of systemic IL-2 administration. The duration of response was usually less than 6 months; however, long-term CRs have been reported. Significant toxicity was reported in most studies related to the systemic IL-2. In a prospective randomized study between IL-2 alone and IL-2 with LAK, the latter resulted in an improved response rate, but only a trend toward improved overall survival.

With the sentinel report in 1986 describing the enhanced antitumor activity of tumor-infiltrating lymphocytes (TIL), most of the clinical attention has shifted away from LAK cells. However, some recent reports have looked at new ways to develop LAK cells in IL-12 instead of IL-2 and new ways to use LAK cells, such as in the treatment of myelodysplastic syndrome. The regional use of LAK cells has also been reported, such as intraperitoneal or intrapleural administration and even intralesional therapy in neurologic malignancies.

TIL Therapy

TIL are reported to be 50–100 times more potent on a cell-to-cell basis than LAK cells in antitumor activity, as demonstrated in animal models. TIL are derived from an individual's surgically resected tumor by cell separation. These T cells have been shown to be cytotoxic for the tumor cells, and this killing has been demonstrated to be limited to the individual's tumor, suggesting HLA restriction. In fact, it is now widely accepted that TIL recognize and lyse tumor cells by CD3/TCR interaction with HLA class I/peptide complexes on the tumor cell surface. Many of the involved TCRs, HLA class I molecules, and even peptides in this specific recognition are now known, and the latter are being investigated in vaccine trials.

In 1988 the NCI reported the first clinical trial with TIL demonstrating complete and partial regression of melanoma in some patients. The follow-up series of 86 melanoma patients revealed a 34% CR + PR. This response rate is almost twice the composite response rate for LAK cells in melanoma and has been confirmed at other institutions with some variation in results. Similar to the LAK cell trials, variable results appear to be related to IL-2 dose and administration, TIL number, and most important, TIL culture characteristics. Better results are seen with cultures grown over shorter periods of time, which are predominantly CD8$^+$ and demonstrate *in vitro* antitumor activity.

In renal cell carcinoma, there does not appear to be a significantly improved response rate between TIL and LAK cells. Some response has been seen with TIL therapy in both the treatment of primary lung cancer and the often associated malignant effusions. Several groups have utilized TIL in ovarian cancer with and without chemotherapy with some success. Intraperitoneal TIL infusions and IL-2 resulted in some marginal clinical activity; however, the results with combination therapy are very promising with TIL and cyclophosphamide (14% CR and 57% PR) and TIL with cisplatinum (70% CR and 20% PR). TIL studies in other malignancies are currently under way.

Some limitations to TIL therapies include the need for surgically resected tumor and 4–6 weeks to grow TIL cultures. Some groups have overcome the necessity of surgery by isolating tumor-associated lymphocytes from malignant ascites and/or effusions. The culture expansion time can be decreased with nonspecific stimulation and cytokines but often at the expense of the tumor-specific cytotoxicity of the TIL. Because the latter is the best predictor of clinical response, the goal is efficient culture conditions with improved tumor reactivity. Current advances have included repeat *in vitro* stimulation with tumor cells and most recently with newly identified, HLA-presented, immunodominant peptides. *In vitro* peptide stimulation has resulted in TIL 50–100 times more potent than TIL grown conventionally. This enhanced efficiency may allow for clinically effective peripheral blood lymphocyte (PBL) cultures, obviating the need for surgically resected tumor. Other attempts to improve adoptive immunotherapy include *in vivo* stimulation with tumor immunization and subsequent harvest of the draining lymph nodes as the source of TIL. This method has been preliminarily studied in clinical trials without apparent improvement in response. Some other groups have modified the TIL with transduced cytokine genes to enhance their potency; others are experimenting with combination therapies with other immunomodulators or chemotherapies. Clinical studies investigating these methods are being performed.

VACCINES

The notion of vaccinations against cancer analogous to antiviral vaccines has been intriguing researchers since the conception of the field of biologic cancer therapy. Recent advances in the understanding of the immune response to tumors have brought this notion to clinical trial in many forms. All types of cancer vaccines have as a common denominator the need to induce a host immunologic response against specific antigens in order to rid or protect the host from the malignancy. The first step in vaccine development is to determine the specific antigens of concern. Optimally, these antigens efficiently stimulate a tumor-specific, tumor-protective immune response. The discovery of tumor-specific antigens (TSA), expressed exclusively on tumors, and tumor-associated antigens (TAA), expressed preferentially on tumors, has accelerated in the 1990s, leading to new candidate antigens for vaccines. Some groups argue that the exact antigens need not be known and favor whole tumor cell vaccines (WTCV) or viral oncolysates to induce an immune response against many tumor antigens, thus addressing the issue of heterogeneous antigen expression in the tumor. Despite these differences, all vaccine regimens require stimulation of the host with nonspecific immunoadjuvants to enhance the vaccine efficiency.

Immune Adjuvants and Immunomodulators

Immune adjuvants are substances that nonspecifically enhance the immune response to antigens. These substances can generally be classified as bacterial products, polysaccharides (glucans), immunogenic proteins (Keyhole limpet hemocyanin, KLH), haptens, or synthetic products. The bacterial products are either cell wall components or intact organisms such as viable BCG, viable/Pen-G-inactivated Grp A streptococcus (OK-432), or nonviable *Cryptosporidium parvum*. Haptens such as dinitrophenyl (DNP) or Trinitrophenyl (TNP) either supply helper determinants or act as neoantigens. Purified or synthetic products such as muramyl dipeptides, trehalose, or endotoxins (lipid A) have also been studied. These substances can also be utilized in combination.

Immunomodulators are substances (e.g., the interleukins, the colony-stimulating factors, and the interferons) that have already been described. This group also includes levamisole and the thymic hormones. Levamisole is a synthetic antihelminthic with immunostimulatory abilities. This drug stimulates monocytes, macrophages, and neutrophils in both chemotaxis and phagocytosis. It also augments IL-2-induced T-cell proliferation and demonstrates Fc receptor activity. Levamisole has been studied as a single anticancer agent with variable results but has been most extensively used in combination with 5-FU for the treatment of Duke's C colon cancer.

The thymic hormones include thymosins (α and β), thymosin fraction 5 (TF-5), and thymopoietin pentapeptide (TP-5). These substances have been shown to promote the proliferation/maturation of T-cell precursors. Most of the research utilizing the thymic hormones has been in the area of restoration of the immune system after immunosuppression with chemotherapy or radiotherapy, and some survival advantage has been seen in non–small cell lung, breast, and ovarian cancers.

The therapeutic benefit of most immune adjuvants and immunomodulators is dependent on their use in combination with other biologic therapies or chemotherapies, with the notable exceptions of BCG in bladder cancer and IFN-α in hairy cell leukemia.

Whole Tumor Cell Vaccines (WTCV)

Most clinical data on anticancer vaccines have been generated in WTCV studies, and all other vaccines are compared against this information. The theoretical advantage of WTCV is that individual antigens do not need to be known. The latter require an enormous amount of work and, theoretically, must be individualized in each cancer. Because the whole tumor cell is utilized, it should express all the possibly important antigens, and the tumor cell itself can act as an APC. The tumor cell can also be genetically altered to enhance its ability to express and present antigens. The theoretical disadvantages include safety issues of introducing tumor cells into a patient. This concern is obviously less for patients who already have cancer but would be more of an issue in preventive vaccines, as would the source of tumor cells for the latter vaccine. Any alterations in the tumor cell to decrease its virulence for safety purposes may diminish its effectiveness as a vaccine. The whole tumor cell also expresses many irrelevant antigens, and the expression of the relevant antigens may be low. The tumor cell may also be an inefficient APC. For these and other concerns, it is not surprising that early clinical trials in melanoma with unaltered, irradiated, autologous WTCV were disappointing (1 CR in 64 patients in four studies). The introduction of immunoadjuvants such as BCG and microbial antigens with the WTCVs enhanced their performance (10–20% overall response rates). In one study of advanced melanoma by Seigler et al. utilizing a complicated regimen of BCG sensitization followed by vaccination with BCG and then finally autologous and allogenic WTCs, the disease-free survival (DFS) was 32% at 2 years. The results of this study are difficult to assess fully because of a high dropout rate and lack of controls.

Several studies have looked at combination therapy with WTCV and chemotherapy in metastatic melanoma. Only one randomized study has shown an improvement in response rates in the biochemotherapy group, but this study had many protocol problems, and many of the partial responders had mixed responses, with progression of disease at other sites. Survival was not improved. The failure of these WTCVs is possibly related to overall tumor burden; therefore several studies were designed to vaccinate patients rendered surgically free of disease but at a high risk of recurrence. The results of these studies have been mixed, with two of the studies being halted because the biochemotherapy group appeared to be recurring more frequently than the control chemotherapy group. This observation did not prove to be true on subsequent follow-up, however. Morton et al. reported a 45% recurrence rate in a group randomized to surgery with WTCV, as compared with 59% in a surgery-alone group. Survival was not affected, though, in these 95 patients. Other studies have likewise found no survival benefit to WTCV as compared with chemotherapy alone in advanced melanoma.

Some other tumor histologies have also been studied, such as colorectal, renal cell, and non–small cell lung cancer. Though it has been difficult to demonstrate an endogenous immune response in colorectal cancer except for its responsiveness to the immune stimulator levamisole, several groups have attempted WTCVs after surgical resection for advanced disease. Hoover et al. reported a significant increase in 10-year DFS in patients vaccinated with BCG and autologous WTC in colon cancer but not in rectal cancer. This finding had not been confirmed in the multi-institutional, randomized ECOG trial at the time of the interim analysis; however, this study had many design and accrual difficulties. The studies in renal cell carcinoma to date show a few significant objective responders, though tumor regression was rare. Perlin et al. showed a strong trend toward better DFS in non–small cell lung cancer vaccinated with BCG and allogeneic WTC after surgery, but this was not yet significant.

Other attempts to improve WTCV have included the addition of the immunopotentiating cyclophosphamide to overcome immunologic tolerance and the modification of WTCV to make them more antigenic. Cyclophosphamide in low doses augments both humoral and cellular immunity, as has been shown in many clinical studies demonstrating enhanced Ab and DTH responses to WTCV. However, this improvement in immune parameters has not translated into improved disease response rates. The xenogenization of tumor cells with animal proteins or viruses is thought to enhance the immune response to a tumor cell by adding T-helper determinants or new immunogens. This form of WTCV modification has been studied with goat and rabbit globulins, as well as the Newcastle virus, without significant improvement in disease response rates over unmodified WTCVs, although some impressive durable responses have been seen. Berd et al. (1993) have reported that hap-tenization with DNP has shown a significantly improved DFS at 33 months as compared with their earlier results with an unmodified WTCV, although this is a nonrandomized study. Other clinical studies are under way with genetically modified WTCV and will be discussed later in gene therapy.

Viral Oncolysates Vaccines

The oncolytic property of viruses has been known for many years and has been shown to induce protective immunity in animals that survived the viral oncolysis. The same protective immunity for a specific tumor could be induced if animals were injected with the oncolysates, the product of viral oncolysis, prepared from the same tumor. The mechanism by which oncolysates induce an immune response is believed to be due to haptenization of tumor antigens with viral antigens. The theoretical advantages of viral oncolysates vaccines (VOV) include not needing to identify specific antigens, less safety concern than using whole tumor cells, preserved antigen diversity, and enhancement of antigenicity with viral haptenization. The theoretical disadvantages include safety concerns over viral infection because these vaccines are inactivated when the virus is killed. Furthermore, the VOVs include mostly irrelevant antigens and are derived mostly from cultured MHC-unmatched cell lines, not from the patient's own tumor. Some of the earlier clinical studies were accomplished by *in vivo* preparation of the VOV to overcome the latter concern by intralesional injection of the virus. This technique resulted in unpredictable results secondary to the lack of standardization between studies. More recent studies have utilized *in vitro* VOV preparation and have been performed in melanoma and in colorectal and ovarian cancer. The results of early *in vitro* VOV had minimal clinical response and resulted in toxicity associated with the influenza virus used in most of the VOVs. The change to vaccinia virus decreased the toxicity and revealed the best response in melanoma. The most extensively studied VOV for melanoma is the vaccinia melanoma oncolysate (VMO) prepared from four allogeneic melanoma cell lines. It has been shown to be well tolerated and resulted in a significantly improved DFS in phase II trials. Similar results have been reported by other groups. However, in a prospective, randomized phase III trial, there was no significant improvement in DFS or overall survival; however, there were some encouraging trends toward improved survival on subset analysis.

Less information is available on VOV treatment of other tumor types. However, nine out of 40 ovarian patients had some clinical response to intraperitoneal influenza-modified allogeneic VOV, and four out of 19 CR and nine out of 19 PR were seen in sarcoma patients treated with a combination of VOV and chemotherapy.

Tumor Antigen Vaccines

Tumor antigen vaccines (TAV) may be partially purified or highly purified/synthetic in nature. The pure antigen vaccines (PAV) offer the best theoretical advantage over WTCVs by delivering the specific immunogenic antigen(s) that would induce an efficient, specific, tumor-protective immunity without the irrelevant antigens or need of autologous or allogeneic tumor material. The PAVs could be easily and reproducibly manufactured, and delivered in high volumes safely. The obvious disadvantage is that effective TAA and/or TSA must be defined. A few of these antigens are known and just beginning clinical trial. A form of vaccine intermediate between WTCVs and PAVs consists of partially purified vaccines (PPV). These offer the theoretical advantage of not needing to know specific TAA and/or TSA, but they are more selective than WTCVs, delivering less irrelevant antigens and providing safer treatment than WTCVs. PPVs have taken many forms, such as soluble membrane extracts, autologous tumor protein polymer particles, and shed antigens. Clinical studies with extracts and protein polymers in melanoma demonstrated some clinical activity, but these studies lacked controls. Melanoma-associated antigen (MAA) vaccines prepared by the collection and partial purification of shed antigens from multiple cultured melanoma cell lines have been reported by Bystryn et al. to increase the median DFS by 50% compared with pooled historical controls. Responders were accurately predicted by Ab and DTH responses, with the best results among those with both parameters. This vaccine has not been evaluated in a prospective, randomized study to date.

Potential PAV are becoming more common as more TAA and TSA are being described. Currently, in melanoma several protein products have been described as targets for cellular immunity. They include the MAGE-1 and MAGE-3 antigens presented by HLA-A1 and the HLA-A2-presented antigens derived from tyrosinase, MART-1, and gp100/pmel 17. Ab responses have been reported to the protein gp75 and the gangliosides GM2 and GD2. These antigens are all being studied as PAV in clinical trials. Preliminary studies with a MAGE-1-derived peptide vaccine have demonstrated induction of cellular and humoral responses *in vivo*; however, no clinical response data are available to date. In a prospective, randomized trial comparing vaccination of surgically disease-free stage III melanoma patients with BCG or BCG and GM2, there was no significant increase in DFS or overall survival. However, there was a significantly improved DFI and overall survival between patients with anti-GM2 antibodies and those without. In an attempt to enhance the immunogenicity of GM2, a new conjugate with KLH is currently being tested by ECOG.

Much less work has been accomplished in epithelial tumors, but Ab responses have been shown to the Thomsen-Friedenreich (TF) antigen and to sialylated Tn (sTn) overexpressed in epithelial tumors. Ab responses have also been described to *p53* in several tumor histologies. Both Ab and CTL responses have been seen to viral transformation antigens in Hodgkin's disease and nasopharyngeal cancer (EBV) and cervical cancer (HPV). MUC-1, an antigen derived from the protein core of mucin molecules on the cell surface of epithelial tumors, has been described as a CTL target recognized in an HLA-unrestricted fashion. The latter fact has made this antigen the focus of several clinical trials because it may be universally applicable in epithelial tumors, although the mechanism of recognition is poorly understood.

The oncogene product HER2/*neu* has been demonstrated to be the target of both humoral and cellular immunity in many epithelial tumors such as ovarian, breast, pancreas, and non–small lung cancer. Unlike MUC-1, the specific immunodominant peptides are presented in the context of HLA-A2 and induce a very specific, effective immune response. The PAV derived from HER2/*neu* may be very promising, because 50% of the population is HLA-A2$^+$, and the HER2/*neu* antigen appears to be widely, and differentially, expressed in epithelial tumors. Clinical studies are just beginning, but animal immunizations against *neu*-derived peptides have induced both humoral and cellular immunity.

GENE THERAPY

The concept of gene therapy focuses on the theory that the host response to tumorigenesis is deficient and might be improved, given the introduction of either novel or excess levels of existing genes. A variety of strategies have been conceived to exploit this basic concept. Most gene therapy models have focused on melanoma and renal cell carcinoma because these two tumor types are considered more immunogenic than most other solid organ malignancies and have demonstrated spontaneous regressions. Furthermore, tumor antigens and cell-mediated immune responses to these neoplasms have been demonstrated *in vitro* and *in vivo*.

As previously discussed, biologic therapies for solid tumors originally concentrated on cytokines to augment host immune responses; likewise, early gene therapies have concentrated on these substances. The large systemic doses of cytokines required to sustain biologically significant tissue levels have been associated with substantial toxicity and only modest antitumor responses. Therefore searches for alternative delivery systems have resulted in multiple strategies to deliver relatively low, continuous concentrations of cytokines directly into tumor or effector cells by inserting the gene responsible for these protein products within a biologic (typically viral) vector capable of infecting designated target cells.

The introduction of novel genetic information (DNA) into eukaryotic cells has been accomplished by chemical, physical, and biologic means. Calcium phosphate transfection and electroporation are gene transfer techniques that have been useful in the laboratory but that are limited in their clinical application.

The most widely used biologic gene transfer vehicles are modified RNA and DNA viruses. Murine retroviral vectors (RVV) have been the most extensively studied. Retroviral vectors can transduce dividing cells and allow stable integration of proviral sequences via a receptor-mediated process of endocytosis. This process is accompanied by certain limitations, however. Despite the introduction of safety features in viral and packaging systems, recombination events and the generation of wild-type virus can occur. There is also the absolute requirement for target cell replication at the time of retroviral infection to permit integration. Viral titers of moderate magnitude have been achieved.

Adeno-associated viruses (AAVs) and adenoviruses (AVs) represent two additional viral vectors that have been evaluated in gene transfer models. AAVs are single-stranded DNA (4.5 kb) parvoviruses that are not pathogenic in humans and may integrate into the host genome at specific regions in chromosome 19. Recombinant AAV vectors allow the insertion of relatively small DNA constructs of up to 4 kb. AAV vectors may not require target cell replication for integration, and multiple concatemeric copies may be integrated per cell. High AAV titers also may be achieved.

Adenovirus-based vectors are currently being used for many gene transfer efforts because they combine the characteristics of high achieved titers and infection of nondividing cells with a broad host range and a tropism for epithelial tissue. Consequently, transduction efficiencies approach 80–90% of cells, in contrast to RVVs, which transduce between 5% and 20% of targets following multiple transduction attempts at high multiplicities of infection ratios. These viruses are composed of double-stranded DNA of approximately 35 kb. Recombinant adenovirus vectors may accommodate up to 7.5 kb of inserted DNA. Limitations of adenoviral vectors include the fact that proviral DNA is not integrated but, rather, episomally inserted into target cells, resulting in transient gene expression. Furthermore, host immune reactions have been observed directed toward recognition of adenoviral proteins. These reactions have resulted in decreased gene expression and have necessitated repeated delivery of adenoviral vectors to the host.

Clearly, each vector system has advantages and disadvantages for use in different tumor models. A problem common to all vectors (although less so for adenoviral vectors) is that of low-level gene expression. Investigators have tried to optimize proviral gene expression using a variety of gene promoters and induction sequences. The cytomegalovirus (CMV) promoter has been used in a variety of systems with success in several tissue types. Regrettably, the CMV promoter also induces gene expression in nontargeted cells, and relatively low-level expression in certain *in vivo* systems. To direct gene expression more precisely, tissue-specific promoters have been developed, including the insulin promoter (for pancreatic islet cell transduction), the tyrosinase promoter (melanoma), the albumin promoter (tumors of the liver), CEA promoter (gastrointestinal tumors, tumors of the breast, and lung adenocarcinomas) and the T-cell receptor promoter (T lymphocytes). Though theoretically intriguing and logical, the use of these promoters in various viral constructs has not yet been demonstrated to be superior to nonspecific high-level promoters such as CMV in any models to date.

Target Cells for Gene Therapy

Lymphocytes

Various cells have been evaluated as targets of gene therapy. Early interest in activated lymphocytes was motivated by trials of LAK cells and TIL, demonstrating antitumor activity in adoptive immunotherapy protocols. Initial studies of genetic modification of lymphocyte populations, including PBL, seemed promising and demonstrated successful transduction and selection of cells secreting proviral genetic elements. Rosenberg et al. at the NCI pioneered early efforts to transduce TIL, and initial reports suggested high-level gene expression, particularly of TNF. However, experience has demonstrated that lymphocytes are difficult to transduce with retroviral vectors because only a small percentage of cells are dividing during transduction and repeated transduction results in significant cell death. Similar difficulties exist with AAV vectors, and lymphocytes are impossible to transduce with AV constructs. Furthermore, evidence of transcriptional silencing of gene products has tempered enthusiasm for transduction of lymphocytes. Finally, the debate continues on whether TIL selectively locate within tumors in greater numbers than PBL. Although the gene-marking studies utilized to generate these data advanced the field in terms of quantitation of gene copy number within large groups of untransduced cells, the clinical ramifications of this effort have been minimal, except to move investigators away from transduction of mature lymphocytes. Stem cell and progenitor transduction has been attempted with greater efficiency than mature lymphocyte transduction and has been clinically successful in the treatment of patients with adenosine deaminase (ADA) deficiency. Certain models involving hematologic malignancies are currently being tested in clinical protocols involving the transduction of drug resistance genes in hematologic and solid tumors utilizing retroviral vectors.

Fibroblasts

Given the recent findings that the particular properties of transduced cells do not necessarily affect antitumor effects, investigators have sought to transduce heartier cells that are easier to grow *in vitro* and *in vivo* and to maintain. Several studies (principally involving IL-2 and IL-12) have evaluated the transduction of fibroblast cell lines such as NIH 3T3 cells and reintroduced transduced cells into tumor-bearing host, either alone or in mixing experiments with tumor cells as vaccines. Transduction efficiencies have been high, and antineoplastic responses have been observed. It may well be more cost-effective and less labor intensive to maintain fibroblasts in culture than to attempt to grow tumor explants for *ex vivo* protocols.

Tumor Cells

A variety of tumor cell lines are easily maintained *in vitro* and can maintain excellent growth kinetics despite multiple transduction attempts with cytokine and other types of genes. Additionally, readministration of nondividing, irradiated tumor cells to patients has the theoretical advantage of stimulating a specific immune response in the host, as in a vaccine model. Safety concerns of tumor growth following readministration have necessitated irradiation that still allows for continued proviral gene expression, albeit for shorter periods of time and at somewhat lower levels than with nonirradiated cells. This model has been employed with varying degrees of success by many investigators and is currently being evaluated in most of tumor-directed gene therapy clinical protocols.

Cytokines in Gene Therapy

The introduction and expression of cytokine genes in tumor cells may modify their phenotype and alter the tumor–host relationship. The introduction of virtually all inflammatory cytokines into tumors has been found to decrease tumorigenicity *in vivo*. Reduced primary tumor growth is largely due to the infiltration and activation of host effector cells. The composition and activity of the cellular infiltrate depend on the cytokine used, the amount produced, the ability of the host to generate responses, and inherent properties of the tumor. It has been difficult to demonstrate regression of established lesions in certain systems, probably because murine tumors appear to outgrow cytokine-transduced cells, thus exceeding the latter's ability to generate immunity in a short time period.

The initial response to tumor inoculation involves nonspecific inflammatory immune mechanisms both in the immunocompetent and in the immunodeficient host. A major question yet to be resolved is how this initial response relates to the development of specific immunity that often follows primary tumor rejection. The mechanism of this "cross-talk" is unknown but presumably relates to the processing and presentation of antigens capable of generating target-specific tumor immunity. Gene therapy using cytokines as immunologic effectors has been attempted for virtually all known cytokines, with favorable *in vivo* and *in vitro* results in most systems. Rather than providing an exhaustive list that may be reviewed in other texts, a brief analysis of selected cytokine gene therapy models will be provided.

IL-2

Gene-modified, IL-2-secreting tumors consistently have had dose-dependent decreased tumorigenicity regardless of histology, immunogenicity, or metastatic potential without altering *in vitro* tumor growth or morphology. Nanogram levels (50–5,000 IU/10^6 cells daily) of human IL-2 were produced in several engineered tumor cell lines. IL-2-transduced cells did not demonstrate changes in MHC antigens or adhesion molecules. An important observation is that IL-2-producing cells mixed *in vitro* with autologous or allogeneic lymphocytes generate enhanced *in vitro* lymphocyte cytotoxicity at levels that could not be reproduced by the addition of recombinant IL-2 to cultures.

The growth of parental tumors is inhibited when mixed with IL-2-producing cells injected at the tumor site, an effect not observed when the modified and unmodified cells are injected at sites remote from the tumor. This local "bystander" effect has been observed by several investigators.

T cells are not required for decreased *in vivo* tumorigenicity. IL-2-modified human and murine melanomas and sarcomas have retarded or absent growth in congenitally athymic (nude) mice, with such tumors generating a mononuclear cell infiltrate. In immunologically competent animals, IL-2 induced CD8[+] T-cell-mediated tumor rejection in a murine colon cancer model. Decreased tumorigenicity was shown to depend on NK cells in a nonimmunogenic murine fibrosarcoma and was associated with granulocyte activity in a murine breast carcinoma system.

The development of specific systemic immunity was reported in syngeneic animals rejecting weakly immunogenic tumors of varying histologies. At least one group has reported that an IL-2-dose-dependent window exists in the optimal generation of protective immunity to parental tumor challenge.

The observation that tumor killing in the immunologically competent host occurred in the absence of CD4[+] cells led to a hypothesis that the T helper cell response may be insufficient (because of unfavorable antigen–MHC complex presentation) to drive cytotoxic T-cell generation against the tumor and that IL-2 could overcome this deficiency. Virtually all investigators have concluded that primary tumor rejection may be induced by nonspecific inflammatory responses (NK cells, neutrophils, or macrophages) but that T-cell-dependent systemic immunity develops in the same host.

IL-2 has been compared with several other inflammatory agents (IFN-γ, IFN-α, IL-7, GM-CSF) in tumor-directed gene therapy investigations. IL-2 was equal or superior to most other cytokines in the mediation of antitumor effects, particularly in T-cell-deprived animals. This finding, and the considerable clinical experience with this cytokine, has led to the development and approval of several clinical protocols studying the effects of IL-2-producing vectors and tumors.

IL-4

Despite the reported antiproliferative effects of IL-4, *in vitro* growth of IL-4-transduced tumors of several histologies producing 2,000–10,000 IU/10^6 cells every 48 hours was unaltered compared with parental cells. IL-4-secreting cells were rejected after injection in immunocompetent and immunodeficient mice. This effect was reversed by administration of anti-IL-4 MAb. Reduced tumorigenicity was also demonstrated for untransduced murine melanoma and plasmacytomas when mixed with IL-4 producers before injection. Significant tumor regression was also observed in established plasmacytomas after intralesional injection of exogenous IL-4 or autologous tumor cells producing this cytokine.

IL-4-producing tumors in syngeneic mice induced the infiltration of eosinophils initially and the later accumulation of macrophages in several tumor models. Tepper et al. demonstrated that tumor rejection was abolished in syngeneic immunocompetent animals by depleting the hosts of mature granulocytes. Tumors were rejected in lymphocyte-depleted mice, but protective (T-cell-dependent) immunity against parental tumor rechallenge was not observed, suggesting that nonspecific effectors were involved in primary tumor rejection, and confirming the requirement of T cells for the generation of immunologic memory.

In two reports, the induction of systemic immunity was observed in immunocompetent animals rejecting IL-4 producing tumors. Tumor-specific immunity was completely abolished by MAb depletion of CD8[+] cells and incompletely inhibited by CD4[+] cells depletion. The systemic immunity demonstrated in this model might have been due to enhanced tumor antigen presentation by the macrophage infiltrate induced by IL-4. Several clinical trials are currently in progress.

TNF-α

Several investigators have studied the properties of tumor cell lines engineered to produce TNF. TNF-transduced cells do not demonstrate altered cell growth or cell morphology *in vitro*. However, the efficiency of gene transduction of TNF-sensitive cells is low because of cell death, suggesting that TNF-resistant cells are selected in such cultures. Deleterious host effects were not observed after injection of tumor cells producing TNF at levels <100 ng/10^6 cells every 24 hours; however, tumors producing much higher levels of this cytokine did demonstrate significant host toxicity and death. Inoculation of TNF-secreting tumors into syngeneic mice resulted in dose-dependent decreased tumorigenicity that was reversed by MAbs to TNF. Parental murine sarcomas were rejected by gene-modified cells injected at the same anatomic site, but not when the two cell types were implanted at different sites. Antineoplastic effects have been inconsistently observed in nude mice in certain models but were reported in others.

The cellular infiltrate surrounding a TNF-producing murine plasmacytoma was predominantly composed of macrophages. Blankenstein et al. noted that the antitumor effect in this model was abolished by anti–type 3 complement receptor MAb that inhibited the migration of inflammatory cells such as neutrophils, NK cells, and macrophages. These findings emphasize the role of non-T-cell effectors in TNF-mediated antineoplastic responses. However, Asher et al. noted that immunologically intact animals experiencing complete regression of murine sarcomas were found to be specifically immune to subsequent tumor challenge and have a predominantly lymphocytic infiltrate. Selective depletion of CD4$^+$ or CD8$^+$ T cells completely abrogated the development of protective immunity in syngeneic mice. This finding documented the importance of T-cell-mediated immunity in this particular TNF tumor model.

Asher et al. attempted to resolve the disparity between their findings and observations regarding the role of macrophages in inducing TNF-mediated antitumor responses by suggesting that secretion of a membrane-bound form of TNF might be incapable of recruiting other effectors. A therapeutic distinction between the membrane-bound and secretory forms of TNF was later described. Although both forms of TNF demonstrated biologic activity *in vitro*, only the secretory form reduced tumorigenicity *in vivo*. The mechanisms responsible for these divergent effects of the two TNF molecules remain unclear, but clinical protocols using secretory TNF gene-modified autologous tumors are in progress.

IL-7

Tumor models using cells engineered to secrete IL-7 in the range of 1–80 ng/10^6 cells every 24 hours demonstrated significant antineoplastic effects. No alterations of *in vitro* growth or cell morphology were observed in IL-7-secreting cells. An IL-7-

producing melanoma cell line expressed lower levels of TGF-β messenger RNA and protein than did untransduced or IL-2-transduced cells. Expression of melanoma antigens MAGE-1 and MAGE-3 was not altered by cytokine gene transfer.

IL-7-transduced cell lines had decreased tumorigenicity in immunocompetent syngeneic mice. Animals rejecting these tumors were immunologically protected against tumor rechallenge. In nude mice, however, growth of gene-modified tumors was either unchanged or slightly decreased compared with parental cells. Histologic analyses of the cellular infiltrates surrounding these tumors in immunocompetent animals showed a predominance of lymphocytes, although eosinophils and basophils were also present. Specifically, increased numbers (fivefold greater) of CD4$^+$ and CD8$^+$ cells were recruited to IL-7-secreting tumor sites compared with parental tumors. Lymphocyte depletion analyses performed using MAbs to CD4$^+$, CD8$^+$, macrophages (anti-CR3$^+$), and NK cells were performed. Tumor rejection was inhibited by anti-CD4$^+$ MAbs in a plasmacytoma line, and dependence of the antitumor response on CD8$^+$ cells was demonstrated in a murine glioma model. Selective depletion of macrophages, but not NK cells, also inhibited tumor rejection, but to a lesser degree than treatment with MAbs for T cells.

Lymphocytes isolated from transduced tumors demonstrated significantly enhanced cytotoxicity toward parental tumor targets. Interestingly, allogeneic lymphocytes cocultured with IL-7-producing melanoma cell lines demonstrated increased cytotoxicity toward parental tumors compared with untransduced cells; this could not be duplicated by the addition to culture of recombinant IL-7. This stimulation of *in vitro* cytotoxicity was comparable to that produced by IL-2-transduced cells of the same tumor cell lines. It appears that IL-7 acts primarily through T-cell-mediated mechanisms in generating antineoplastic effects, although its ability to down-regulate TGF-β production may be a distinct component of its biologic activity. The relative importance of CD4$^+$ or CD8$^+$ cells in mediating tumor rejection may vary between particular tumors. Currently, Economou et al. are conducting a phase I clinical protocol involving vaccination of patients with melanomas with autologous-irradiated melanoma cells producing IL-7 contained within a retroviral construct. A few patients have been treated, but the results of therapy are as yet unreported.

IL-12

Recent reports have described the transfection of IL-12 into NIH/3T3 cells. These IL-12-producing fibroblasts were mixed with murine melanoma cells in syngeneic mice and reduced tumorigenicity in most animals treated. IL-12-transduced murine colon carcinoma cells grew in a delayed fashion compared with unmanipulated tumors and resulted in delay in the formation of pulmonary and hepatic metastases. Antitumor activity was also recently demonstrated in a murine fibrosarcoma model using a vaccinia virus vector. The question of which T-cell subsets are most responsible for IL-12's antitumor effect is as yet unclear, as CD4$^+$ and CD8$^+$ cells appear to act differently, depending on the specific model tested.

GM-CSF

Gene therapy efforts involving GM-CSF were evaluated in a murine model and compared with cytokine gene therapy involving at least nine other cytokines by Dranoff et al. The investigators used both live and irradiated genetically modified tumors producing high levels of GM-CSF (300 ng/10^6 cells every 24 hours) in syngeneic mice. This report was noteworthy in several respects. First, it demonstrated that vaccination of irradiated parental tumors alone resulted in some degree of antitumor immunity. Second, systemic murine toxicity was described, apparently induced by injection of tumor cells secreting high concentrations of this cytokine. Third, in contrast to many other investigations, systemic immunity was not conferred upon animals treated with live IL-2-producing tumors, although these cells were the only type to be rejected in this comparative analysis. However, irradiated tumors producing GM-CSF alone and live cells secreting a combination of IL-2 and GM-CSF did induce resistance to subsequent tumor challenge. Finally, MAb depletion of several effector cell subsets demonstrated dependence on both CD4+ and CD8+ T cells for the establishment of systemic immunity induced by GM-CSF-secreting murine melanoma cells.

A recent report from Johns Hopkins on renal cell carcinoma patients randomized and treated prospectively with either a GM-CSF gene-transduced autologous tumor cell vaccine or a nontransduced autologous tumor cell vaccine demonstrated only one objective partial responder in 16 evaluable patients.

Tumor Suppressor Genes

p53 has been identified as a putative tumor suppressor gene. Tumor suppressors are recessively functioning genes that must both be mutated to elicit phenotypic alterations supporting malignancy in the host. Therefore it has been hypothesized that delivering one copy of the wild-type (wt) gene could reverse a neoplastic process. *p53* is mutated in a wide variety of tumors, including head and neck squamous cell cancer, non–small cell lung cancer, colorectal carcinoma, and premalignant conditions such as Barrett's esophagitis. The *p53* gene encodes a 393–amino acid phosphoprotein that forms complexes with a series of viral proteins. Other areas within the gene interact with other proteins, allowing *p53* oligomers to form and resulting in transactivation of gene expression. Wild-type *p53* appears to regulate the cell cycle and to control cell growth and proliferation, at least in part through the mechanism of apoptosis or programmed cell death. *p53* also has a role in controlling transcriptional regulation and DNA replication. Mutated *p53* allows unregulated cell growth to occur, while restoring wt-*p53* restores cell cycle regulation and renders cells apoptotic or in G1 arrest.

A variety of viral constructs have been evaluated that contain wt-*p53* in several tumor systems. Roth et al. (1996) have demonstrated that retroviral vectors containing wt-*p53* can suppress *in vivo* and *in vitro* growth of human lung carcinoma cell lines that contain deleted or mutated *p53*. Conversely, tumor cell lines containing wt-*p53* are not significantly altered by the retroviral construct. The phenomenon of the bystander effect has also been observed in these studies as the growth of nontransduced cells was reduced following co-culture with a transduced population.

Several models involving adenoviral vectors containing wt-*p53* have also been evaluated. Apoptosis has been observed in tumor cells whose genome contained mutated or deleted *p53* following transduction with adenoviral wt-*p53*. *p53* constructs have also been shown to act synergistically with cisplatinum in inducing apoptosis in human lung tumors grown in nude mice. These results have led to several clinical gene therapy protocols involving wt-*p53* introduced through a variety of delivery systems. Clinical responses have been modest to date, although the toxicity of therapy appears minimal. Additionally, viral vectors containing related cell cycle control genes (*p21* and *p16*) are currently being evaluated and may soon be used in clinical protocols.

Suicide Gene Therapy

One gene therapy strategy that has been used with some degree of success in CNS tumor models involves so-called suicide gene therapy. This technique involves the transduction of cells with a gene that renders these cells sensitive to killing by systemic administration of a compound toxic to all cells containing the gene. Most commonly, the gene for the herpes simplex virus (HSV) driven by the thymidine kinase promoter has been introduced via both adenoviral and retroviral vectors. Following transduction, the host is administered gancyclovir, which is toxic to all HSV-containing cells. Additional cell killing has been observed in nontransduced cells in proximity to the transduced population, suggesting a "bystander effect" in this model. This strategy is currently employed in more than 20 approved clinical protocols worldwide, most of which are directed toward treatment of brain tumors.

Costimulatory Molecules—B7

B7 is the ligand for the CD28 receptor of lymphocytes. Antigen presentation to T cells and subsequent T-cell activation depend on binding to CD28, yet most tumors lack B7 molecules on their surface. Murine models of B7 tumor transfection have demonstrated antineoplastic responses and the generation of systemic immunity. Gene therapy studies involving the delivery of B7 in patients with melanoma are currently under way. B7 is commonly confused with but is structurally and functionally different from the HLA-B7 molecule that is a major histocompatibility class I haplotype also being studied in gene therapy models involving patients with melanoma and colorectal cancer. This system utilizes nonviral, liposomally delivered gene constructs involving intratumoral injection. It has demonstrated some antineoplastic responses in melanoma patients but no documented responses in studies evaluating direct injection of liver metastases from colorectal carcinoma.

Antisense Gene Therapy

Antisense gene therapy strategies involve the creation of genetic sequences that are complementary to specific regions of RNA known to be critical for gene expression and transcription. Typically, regions of interest for antisense binding involve oncogene coding regions. Oncogenes act predominantly to promote neoplastic cell growth. Antisense constructs may be directed toward oncogenes and may be composed of oligonucleotides that bind to double-stranded DNA, thereby interfering with transcription. Other alternatives include antisense RNA, which may bind to single-stranded DNA or to mRNA and interfere with transcription, splicing, and translation.

Antisense oligonucleotides have been tested in phase II clinical studies, but efficacy has been limited by rapid host-induced degradation by nuclease *in vivo*. Antioncogenic oligonucleotides have been constructed to disrupt expression of *abl, fos, kit, myc, src,* and *ras* gene families, again with limited clinical consequence.

Roth et al. (1997) described a model in which an antisense RNA construct was used to induce tumoricidal activity in a human lung cancer cell line expressing K-*ras*. The anti-K-*ras* retroviral constructs reduced tumorigenicity of a cell line with a homozygous K-*ras* mutation in nude mice. These observations have led to clinical trials involving direct intratumor injection of anti-K-*ras* retroviral particles in patients with unresectable pulmonary malignancies. Also, an adenoviral anti-K-*ras* construct has been reported recently to have potent antitumor activity in murine models involving human cancer cell lines.

Conclusion

Biologic cancer therapies hold enormous promise because many different forms of therapeutics, from cytokines to vaccines, have been shown to induce tumor regression in many human clinical trials. Although the response rates are not high, they are encouraging because the best results in trials in animals have been in small-volume disease and prevention, not in the treatment of established large cancers. Because most of these therapies rely on the induction of the host immune responses, patients with end-stage, bulky disease and poor nutritional status may not respond optimally. Therefore most biologic modalities may not have been adequately tested clinically to date. Furthermore, more specific and possibly more potent therapies are just now entering clinical trial. Advances in biotechnology offer the promise of even more sophisticated therapeutics. The next generation of biologic therapies will most likely consist of multimodality biologic treatments targeting both humoral and cellular immunity against multiple tumor antigens.

Selected References

CYTOKINES

Anderson CM, Buzaid AC, Grimm EA. Interaction of chemotherapy and biological response modifiers in the treatment of melanoma. *Cancer Treat Res* 87:357, 1996.

Brunda MJ, Luistro L, Rumennik L, et al. Antitumor activity of interleukin-12 in preclinical models. *Cancer Chemother Pharmacol* 38(Suppl):S16, 1996.

Dutcher JP. Therapeutic strategies for cytokines. *Curr Opin Oncol* 7:566, 1995.

Eggermont AMM. Treatment of melanoma in-transit metastases confined to the limb. *Cancer Surv* 26:335, 1996.

Kirkwood JM, Strawderman MH, Ernstoff MS. et al. Interferon alpha-2b adjuvant therapy of high-risk resected cutaneous melanoma: The Eastern Cooperative Oncology Group Trial EST 1684. *J Clin Oncol* 14:7, 1996.

Kopp WC, Holmlund JT. Cytokines and immunological monitoring. *Cancer Chemother Biol Response Modif* 16:189, 1996.

Mosmann TR, Coffman RL. Heterogeneity of cytokine secretion patterns and functions of helper T cells. *Adv Immunol* 46:111, 1989.

Parkinson DR. Present status of biological response modifiers in cancer. *Am J Med* 99(6A):54S, 1995.

Platanias LC. Interferons: Laboratory to clinic investigations. *Curr Opin Oncol* 7:560, 1995.

Tepper RI, Pattengale PK, Leder P, et al. Murine interleukin-4 displays potent anti-tumor activity *in vivo*. *Cell* 57:503, 1989.

Veltri S, Smith JW 2nd. Interleukin-1 trials in cancer patients: A review of the toxicity, antitumor and hematopoietic effects. *Stem Cells* 14:164, 1996.

MONOCLONAL ANTIBODIES

Greiner JW, Guadagni F, Roselli M, et al. Novel approaches to tumor detection and therapy using a combination of monoclonal antibody and cytokine. *Anticancer Res* 16:2129, 1996.

Jurcic JG, Scheinberg DA, Houghton AN. Monoclonal antibody therapy of cancer. *Cancer Chemother Biol Response Modif* 16:168, 1996.

CELLULAR THERAPY

Aoki Y, Takakuwa K, Kodama S, et al. Use of adoptive transfer of tumor-infiltrating lymphocytes alone or in combination with cisplatin-containing chemotherapy in patients with epithelial ovarian cancer. *Cancer Res* 51:1934, 1991.

Chang AE, Yoshizawa H, Sakai K, et al. Clinical observations on adoptive immunotherapy with vaccine-primed T-lymphocytes secondarily sensitized to tumor *in vitro*. *Cancer Res* 53:1043, 1993.

Goedegebuure PS, Douville LM, Li H, et al. Adoptive immunotherapy with tumor-infiltrating lymphocytes and interleukin-2 in patients with metastatic malignant melanoma and renal cell carcinoma: A pilot study. *J Clin Oncol* 13:1939, 1995.

Itoh K, Tilden AB, Balch CM. Interleukin-2 activation of cytotoxic T-lymphocytes infiltrating into human metastatic melanomas. *Cancer Res* 46:3011, 1986.

Mule JJ, Shu S, Schwarz SL, et al. Adoptive immunotherapy of established pulmonary metastases with LAK cells and recombinant interleukin-2. *Science* 225:1487, 1984.

Rivoltini L, Kawakami Y, Robbins P, et al. Efficient induction of tumor reactive CTL from peripheral blood and tumor-infiltrating lymphocytes of melanoma patients by *in vitro* stimulation with the human melanoma antigen MART-1 peptide. *J Exp Med* 184:647, 1996.

Rosenberg SA. The immunotherapy and gene therapy of cancer. *J Clin Oncol* 10:180, 1992.

Rosenberg SA, Lotze MT, Aebersold PM, et al. Prospective randomized trial of high dose interleukin-2 alone or with lymphokine activated killer cells for the treatment of patients with advanced cancer. *J Natl Cancer Inst* 85:622, 1993.

Rosenberg SA, Packard BS, Aebersold PM, et al. Use of tumor-infiltrating lymphocytes and interleukin-2 in the immunotherapy of patients with metastatic melanoma, special report. *N Engl J Med* 319:1676, 1988.

Rosenberg SA, Spiess P, Lafreniere R. A new approach to the adoptive immunotherapy of cancer with tumor-infiltrating lymphocytes. *Science* 223:1318, 1986.

Rosenberg SA, Terry WD. Passive immunotherapy of cancer in animals and man. *Adv Cancer Res* 25:323, 1977.

Rosenberg SA, Yannelli JR, Yang JC, et al. Treatment of patients with metastatic melanoma with autologous tumor-infiltrating lymphocytes and interleukin-2. *J Natl Cancer Inst* 86:1159, 1994.

Schoof DD, Gramolini BA, Davidson DL, et al. Adoptive immunotherapy of human using low-dose recombinant interleukin-2 and lymphokine-activated killer cells. *Cancer Res* 48:5007, 1988.

VACCINES

Linehan DC, Goedegebuure PS, Eberlein TJ. Vaccine therapy for cancer. *Ann Surg Oncol* 3:219, 1996.

Immunoadjuvants and immunomodulators

Akporiaye ET, Hersh EM. Immune adjuvants. In VT DeVita Jr, S Hellman, SA Rosenberg (eds.), *Biologic Therapy of Cancer* (2nd ed). Philadelphia: Lippincott, 1995.

Schultz N, Oratz R, Chen D, et al. Effect of DETOX as an adjuvant for melanoma vaccine. *Vaccine* 13:503, 1995.

WTCV

Berd D, Maguire HC Jr, McCue P, et al. Treatment of metastatic melanoma with an autologous tumor-cell vaccine: Clinical and immunologic results in 64 patients. *J Clin Oncol* 8:1858, 1990.

Berd D, Maguire HC Jr, Mastrangelo MJ. Treatment of human melanoma with a hapten-modified autologous vaccine. *Ann NY Acad Sci* 690:147, 1993.

Hoover HC Jr, Bandhorst JS, Peters LC, et al. Adjuvant active specific immunotherapy for human colorectal cancer: 6.5 year median follow-up of a phase III prospectively randomized trial. *J Clin Oncol* 11:390, 1993.

Mastrangelo MJ, Maguire HC Jr, Sato T, et al. Active specific immunization in the treatment of patients with melanoma. *Semin Oncol* 23:773, 1996.

Morton DL. Adjuvant immunotherapy of malignant melanoma: Status of clinical trials at UCLA. *Int J Immunother* 2:31, 1986.

Perlin E, Oldham RK, Weese JL, et al. Carcinoma of the lung: Immunotherapy with intradermal BCG and allogeneic tumor cells. *Int J Radiat Oncol Biol Phys* 6:1033, 1980.

Seigler HF, Buckley CE, Sheppard LB, et al. Adoptive transfer and specific active immunization of patients with malignant melanoma. *Ann NY Acad Sci* 277:522, 1977.

Schlag P, Manasterski M, gerneth T, et al. Active specific immunotherapy with Newcastle-disease-virus-modified autologous tumor
cells following resection of liver metastases in colorectal cancer.
Cancer Immunol Immunother 35:325, 1992.

VOV

Freedman RS, Edwards CL, Bowen JM, et al. Viral oncolysates in
patients with advanced ovarian cancer. *Gynecol Oncol* 29:337, 1988.
Hersey P. Active immunotherapy with viral lysates of micrometastases following surgical removal of high risk melanoma. *World J
Surg* 16:251, 1992.
Morton DL, Foshag LJ, Hoon DSB, et al. Prolongation of survival in
metastatic malignant melanoma after active specific immunotherapy with a new polyvalent melanoma vaccine. *Ann Surg* 216:463,
1992.
Sivanandham M, Scoggin S, Tanaka N, et al. Therapeutic effect of a
vaccinia colon oncolysate prepared with interleukin-2 gene encoded
vaccinia virus studied in syngeneic CC-36 murine colon hepatic
metastasis model. *Cancer Immunol Immunother* 38:259, 1994.
Wallack MK, Sivanandham M, Balch CM, et al. A phase III randomized, double-blind multi-institutional trial of vaccinia melanoma
oncolysate-active specific immunotherapy for patients with stage II
melanoma. *Cancer* 75:34, 1995.
Wallack MK, Sivanandham M, Whooley B, et al. Favorable clinical
responses in subsets of patients from a randomized, multi-institutional melanoma vaccine trial. *Ann Surg Oncol* 3:110, 1996.

TAV

Brichard V, Van Pel A, Wolfel T, et al. The tyrosinase gene codes for
an antigen recognized by autologous cytolytic T lymphocytes on
HLA-A2 melanomas. *J Exp Med* 178:48, 1993
Bystryn JC. Clinical activity of a polyvalent melanoma antigen vaccine. *Recent Results Cancer Res* 139:337, 1995.
Bystryn JC, Oratz R, Henn M, et al. Relationship between immune
response to melanoma vaccine and clinical outcome in stage II
malignant melanoma. *Cancer* 69:1157, 1992.
Cox AL, Skipper J, Chen Y, et al. Identification of a peptide recognized
by five melanoma-specific human cytotoxic T-cell lines. *Science*
264:716, 1994.
Disis ML, Gralow JR, Bernhard H, et al. Peptide-based, but not
whole protein, vaccines elicit immunity to HER2/neu, oncogenic self-
protein. *J Immunol* 156:3151, 1996.
Fisk B, Blevins TL, Wharton JT, et al. Identification of an immunodominant peptide of HER-2/neu proto-oncogene recognized by
ovarian tumor-specific CTL lines. *J Exp Med* 181:2709, 1995.
Gaugler B, Van den Eynde B, van der Bruggen P, et al. Human gene
MAGE-3 codes for an antigen recognized on a melanoma by autologous cytolytic T lymphocytes. *J Exp Med* 179:921, 1994.
Hollinshead A, Arlen M, Yonemoto R, et al. Pilot studies using
melanoma tumor-associated antigens (TAA) in specific-active
immunotherapy of malignant melanoma. *Cancer* 49:1387, 1982.
Hu X, Chakraborty NG, Sporn JR, e al. Enhancement of cytolytic
T lymphocyte precursor frequency in melanoma patients following
immunization with the MAGE-1 peptide loaded antigen presenting
cell-based vaccine. *Cancer Res* 56:2479, 1996.

Jerome KR, Barnd DL, Bendt KM, et al. Cytotoxic T-lymphocytes derived from patients with breast adenocarcinoma recognize an epitope present on the protein core of a mucin molecule preferentially expressed by malignant cells. *Cancer Res* 51:2908, 1991.

Kawakami Y, Eliyahu S, Sakaguchi K, et al. Identification of the immunodominant peptides of the MART-1 human melanoma antigen recognized by the majority of HLA-A2-restricted tumor infiltrating lymphocytes. *J Exp Med* 180:347, 1994.

Livingston PO. Approaches to augmenting the immunogenicity of melanoma gangliosides: From whole melanoma cells to ganglioside-KLH conjugate vaccines. *Immunol Rev* 145:147, 1995.

Livingston PO, Wong GY, Adluri S, et al. Improved survival in stage III melanoma patients with GM2 antibodies: A randomized trial of adjuvant vaccination with GM2 ganglioside. *J Clin Oncol* 12:1036, 1994.

Maeurer MJ, Storkus WJ, Kirkwood JM, et al. New treatment options for patients with melanoma: Review of melanoma-derived T-cell epitope-based peptide vaccines. *Melanoma Res* 6:11, 1996.

Peoples GE, Goedegebuure PS, Smith R, et al. Breast and ovarian cancer-specific cytotoxic T-lymphocytes recognize the same HER2/neu-derived peptide. *Proc Natl Acad Sci USA* 92:432, 1995.

Van der Bruggen P, Traversari C, Chomez P, et al. A gene encoding an antigen recognized by cytolytic T lymphocytes on a human melanoma. *Science* 254:1643, 1991.

GENE THERAPY

Asher AL, Mule JJ, Kasid A, et al. Murine tumor cells transduced with the gene for tumor necrosis factor-alpha. *J Immunol* 146:3227, 1991.

Blankenstein TH, Qin Z, Uberla K, et al. Tumor suppression after cell-targeted tumor necrosis factor alpha gene transfer. *J Exp Med* 173:1047, 1991.

Descamps V, Duffour M-T, Mathieu M-C, et al. Strategies for cancer gene therapy using adenoviral vectors. *J Mol Med* 74:183, 1996.

Dranoff G, Jaffee E, Lazenby A, et al. Vaccination with irradiated tumor cells engineered to secrete murine granulocyte-macrophage colony-stimulating factor stimulates potent, specific, and long-lasting anti-tumor immunity. *Proc Natl Acad Sci USA* 90:3539, 1993.

Gunzburg WH, Salmons B. Development of retroviral vectors as safe, targeted gene delivery systems. *J Mol Med* 74:171, 1996.

Mastrangelo MJ, Berd D, Nathan FE, et al. Gene therapy for human cancer: An assay for clinicians. *Semin Oncol* 23:4, 1996.

Miller AR, McBride WH, Hunt K, et al. Cytokine-mediated gene therapy for cancer. *Ann Surg Oncol* 1:436, 1994.

Rosenberg SA, Anderson WF, Blaese M, et al. The development of gene therapy for the treatment of cancer. *Ann Surg* 218:455, 1993.

Roth JA, Cristiano RJ. Gene therapy for cancer: What have we done and where are we going? *J Natl Cancer Inst* 89:21, 1997.

Roth JA, Nguyen D, Lawrence DD, et al. Retroviral-mediated wild-type p53 gene transfer to tumors of patients with lung cancer. *Nat Med* 2:985, 1996.

Simons JW, Jaffee EM, Weber CE, et al. Bioactivity of autologous irradiated renal cell carcinoma vaccines generated by *ex vivo* granulocyte-macrophage colony-stimulating factor gene transfer. *Cancer Res* 57:1537, 1997.

Toloza EM, Hunt K, Miller AR, et al. Transduction of murine and human tumors using recombinant adenovirus vectors. *Ann Surg Oncol* 4:70, 1997.

Zhang WW. Antisense oncogene and tumor suppressor gene therapy of cancer. *J Mol Med* 74:191, 1996.

Zhang Y, Mukhopadhyay T, Donehower LA. et al. Retroviral vector-mediated transduction of K-ras antisense RNA into human lung cancer cells inhibits expression of the malignant phenotype. *Hum Gene Ther* 4:451, 1993.

GENERAL

Clark JI, Weiner LM. Biologic treatment of human cancer. *Curr Probl Cancer* 19:185, 1995.

Clark JW. Biological response modifiers. *Cancer Chemother Biol Response Modif* 16:239, 1996.

Del Prete G, Maggi E, Romagnani S. Human Th1 and Th2 cells: Functional properties, mechanisms of regulation and role in disease. *Lab Invest* 70:299, 1994.

DeVita VT, Hellman S, Rosenberg SA (eds.). *Biologic Therapy of Cancer* (2nd ed.). Philadelphia: Lippincott, 1995.

Nutrition in Cancer Patients

Paula M. Termuhlen

Cancer patients face unique problems that can result in nutritional depletion during the perioperative period. For example, cancer cachexia is a well-described condition in which the abnormal metabolic priorities of the patient (host) and tumor alter the body's usual protein and energy requirements. Furthermore, tumors of the head and neck or gastrointestinal tract often compromise nutrition by interfering with ingestion, digestion, and absorption. Preoperative and postoperative chemotherapy and radiation therapy can adversely affect the integrity and function of the alimentary tract, contributing to the difficulty of maintaining adequate nutrition.

Nutrition plays a key role in the recovery and rehabilitation of cancer patients. Adequate protein, calories, and essential micronutrients help maintain a reasonable quality of life for these patients. Surgeons caring for cancer patients must be knowledgeable about the general principles of nutritional assessment and the unique nutritional problems of cancer patients if optimal recovery from treatment is to be achieved.

Cancer Cachexia

Cachexia of malignancy, a nutritional problem unique to cancer patients, is a syndrome of progressive involuntary weight loss and intractable anorexia. Without effective intervention, cancer cachexia will result in death. The physical and biochemical features of this syndrome include tissue wasting, skeletal muscle atrophy, myopathy, anergy, anemia, and glucose intolerance. In addition, patients are unable to absorb and use nutrients adequately.

Not all tumors produce the same degree of cachexia, and much variation is observed among individual patients. Greater weight loss is associated with a tumor in a visceral organ (e.g., pancreas or stomach) than with a tumor in a nonvisceral organ (e.g., breast). Based on common indices of nutritional assessment, protein-calorie malnutrition exists preoperatively in up to 50% of cancer patients. Cancer cachexia may also have prognostic significance. Patients who have no weight loss at the time of surgery demonstrate lower morbidity and higher survival rates than those who have had moderate to severe weight loss, regardless of tumor type.

ANOREXIA

The etiology of cancer cachexia is multifactorial, but the most obvious contributing factor is anorexia due to the presence of a malignancy or to its treatment. Many patients report altered taste perception that contributes to decreased food intake; however, this alteration appears to be an individual phenomenon unrelated to specific tumor types or sites. Adjuvant therapy, such as chemotherapy and radiation therapy, often causes nausea and vomiting and thus food aversion. In addition, radiotherapy can cause mucosal damage, malabsorption, and diarrhea, all of which contribute to reduced oral intake.

SUBSTRATE UTILIZATION

Aside from anorexia, other causes of cancer cachexia are abnormal host carbohydrate, protein, and lipid metabolism. Studies have shown that even with adequate caloric intake, specific substrate utilization is abnormal and insufficient for adequate nutritional support.

Glucose

Glucose intolerance and insulin resistance are often found in cancer patients, and studies have documented abnormal glucose clearance in patients with many different tumors, including lung and colorectal cancers. A diabetes-like state develops in patients with cachexia that is a result of accentuated gluconeogenesis in the liver. Tumors can augment gluconeogenesis by the increased peripheral release of metabolic substrates such as lactate. In addition, unidentified mediators cause increased gluconeogenesis in the liver by the induction of associated enzymes. The increase in gluconeogenesis contributes to nutritional depletion by causing host energy to be used inefficiently in futile metabolic cycles.

Protein

Depletion of protein in cachectic patients manifests as skeletal muscle atrophy, visceral organ atrophy, and hypoalbuminemia. Protein wasting results from altered nitrogen metabolism, which causes not only patients with cancer to be unable to adapt to decreased food intake, but also nonstressed patients suffering from simple starvation. Even when cancer patients are given supplemental nutrition, such as total parenteral nutrition, whole-body protein turnover rates remain elevated. Studies in animals suggest that tumors use nitrogen released from tissues at the expense of the malnourished host. There is evidence of decreased protein synthesis and increased protein breakdown in skeletal muscle, which contribute to tissue wasting. Hypoalbuminemia is consistently found in cancer patients and is most likely related to increased albumin turnover. Overall, hepatic production of proteins appears increased in cancer patients, but this is offset by increased turnover in the peripheral body cell mass.

Lipids

Lipid metabolism is also abnormal, resulting in depletion of lipid stores and hyperlipidemia. Increased turnover of lipid stores plays a role because glucose infusions in weight-losing patients fail to suppress lipolysis. Hyperlipidemia results from a decrease in the amount of lipoprotein lipase, which transports triglycerides from blood into adipose tissue. Abnormally high or even normal serum insulin levels appear to not promote fat storage in cancer patients and thus to contribute to hyperlipidemia.

METABOLIC RATE

The abnormal carbohydrate, protein, and lipid metabolism of the host is accompanied by an inability to adjust the metabolic rate to food intake. Although some patients with weight loss have documented hypermetabolism, this finding is inconsistent in large studies, varying among individual patients and tumor types. Host- and tumor-secreted factors have been the focus for identifying the mechanism of the metabolic changes in cancer cachexia. To date, no tumor-produced substance having a systemic effect has been isolated. However, factors secreted by the host as part of the immune response to a tumor appear to play a role in cancer cachexia.

The cytokine tumor necrosis factor (TNF) has not only local immune effects but also systemic effects that produce clinical results similar to those seen in cachexia. TNF, also known as cachectin, has a cytotoxic effect on tumors and inhibits lipoprotein lipase, resulting in hyperlipidemia. Receptors for TNF are found ubiquitously, but particularly in the liver, adipose tissue, and muscle cells, which are key sites for abnormal metabolism in cancer patients. In healthy volunteers, TNF has been shown to increase temperature and heart rate as well as peripheral protein turnover. One theory is that cytokines such as TNF released by the immune system in response to a tumor promote an acute-phase response that reroutes nutrients from the periphery to the liver. Ultimately, this response becomes unregulated, resulting in anorexia and abnormal carbohydrate, protein, and lipid metabolism.

Preoperative Assessment of Nutritional Status

Malnutrition, as commonly manifested by weight loss, exists in more than 50% of cancer patients. Traditionally, malnourished patients without cancer who have undergone major operative procedures have had higher rates of morbidity (e.g., poor wound healing, increased wound infection rates, prolonged postoperative ileus) than their well-nourished counterparts. That finding is perhaps due to the fact that underlying the malnutrition is a depressed immune system, which is often found in cancer patients as well.

Cancer patients should undergo a thorough preoperative nutritional assessment, and high-risk patients should be identified. Many nutritional assessment techniques exist. Most are based on a complete history and physical examination as well as documentation of changes in weight over time. Other studies include anthropomorphic studies, measurements of serum albumin and transferrin, tests of immune function by assessment of delayed cutaneous hypersensitivity, and estimates of energy expenditure. However, for most patients nutritional status can be adequately assessed through a comprehensive history and physical examination.

Preoperatively, malnourished patients should have a full nutritional assessment, including an estimate of the patient's basal energy expenditure (BEE), which can be calculated indirectly by the Harris-Benedict equation:

$$\text{Male: BEE} = 66.5 + 13.7(\text{wt}) + 5(\text{ht}) - 6.7(\text{age})$$
$$\text{Female: BEE} = 66.5 + 9.6(\text{wt}) + 1.8(\text{ht}) - 4.7(\text{age})$$

where wt = weight in kilograms, ht = height in centimeters, and age is in years.

The metabolic cart assessment, based on a patient's carbon dioxide production, is a clinical method of determining energy expenditure that gives a more personalized assessment but is cumbersome, time-consuming, and expensive.

Preoperative Nutritional Supplementation

It has been difficult to establish a clear benefit to short-term preoperative nutritional supplementation in terms of decreased morbidity and mortality. However, there is some evidence to suggest a benefit to severely malnourished patients if preoperative nutritional supplementation is given for at least 7–10 days. More thorough preoperative nutritional supplementation should be considered for the nutritionally high-risk patient who may be grossly underweight (<80% of standard weight for height) or grossly overweight (>120% of standard weight for height). A recent weight loss of 12% or more of usual body weight is particularly important because patients with acute-onset protein-calorie malnutrition and associated hypoalbuminemia have a higher mortality rate than those with a marasmic or adapted form of protein-calorie malnutrition that has occurred over a longer period of time. Alcoholic patients are also at high risk for being nutritionally depleted, as are patients with malabsorptive syndromes, short gut, gastrointestinal fistulas, renal failure requiring dialysis, abscesses, and large healing wounds. In addition, patients with systemic infections and associated fever have increased metabolic needs that place them at high risk for the complications associated with nutritional depletion. Stopping oral intake and providing only IV solutions perioperatively for hydration adds additional risk. Although preoperative nutritional support remains controversial except in severely malnourished patients, postoperative nutritional supplementation is a key therapeutic modality in helping patients recover.

Postoperative Nutritional Supplementation

ACUTE PHASE

Postoperative nutritional support can be divided into two phases: acute and chronic. Patients recovering from a major operative procedure will need nutritional supplementation until they demonstrate the ability to obtain full nourishment independently. Both enteral and parenteral means of support are available. It has been recognized that enteral feeding should be used whenever possible, and many patients have enteral feeding tubes placed at the time of operation so that feeding can begin early in the postoperative period. If enteral feeding cannot meet the patient's nutritional needs, then parenteral feeding should be instituted, alone or in conjunction with enteral feeding. In general, the goals for nutritional support are approximately 25 kcal and 1.5 g of protein per kilogram of body weight per day.

CHRONIC PHASE

The chronic phase of postoperative nutritional support is related to the longer-term consequences of a particular operation and adjuvant therapy. Many operative procedures produce prolonged inability to obtain adequate nutrition orally. These include pancreaticoduodenectomy with prolonged gastric emptying, esophagectomy with gastric stasis and regurgitation, and gastrectomy with dumping syndrome. Patients undergoing operations in the head and neck region are also at particular risk for inadequate oral nutrition. For most of these patients, an enteral feeding tube can be placed into the jejunum during the operation and used for long periods. Patients are often discharged with feeding tubes in place. Thus a patient's quality of life is enhanced by the ability to manage himself or herself outside a hospital. Beyond supplying sufficient protein and calories, supplementation may need to include vitamins, iron, and pancreatic enzymes.

Nutritional Complications of Adjuvant Therapy

Additional nutritional problems can arise with adjuvant therapy. Patients may receive chemotherapy or radiotherapy as part of their treatment plan before or after surgery, or both. These therapies have various adverse effects. Mucosal inflammation and pain are the initial postradiotherapy complaints that prevent patients from obtaining adequate nutrition. Such late effects as loss of taste, fibrosis, stricture formation, obstruction, and fistulization also may occur. Each chemotherapeutic agent has its own systemic side effects, although many agents produce nausea and vomiting as well as fluid and electrolyte imbalances.

Future Considerations

Studies are under way to address the unique nutritional needs and metabolic abnormalities of cancer patients. Specific amino acids such as glutamine and arginine seem to be easily utilized by the intestine and promote more efficient nitrogen retention during stress. Arginine also seems to enhance immune function and is a potentially fruitful target for research. A promising enteral product includes supplemental arginine, RNA, and omega-3 fatty acids as part of its formula. Each of these substances individually stimulates the immune system. In one clinical trial, fewer infections and wound complications, in addition to shorter hospital stays, were documented in cancer patients who underwent major operative procedures and received this product compared with those who received a common standard enteral product as part of their nutritional support.

Future nutritional research in cancer patients will continue to focus on providing optimal nutrition in a safe and efficacious fashion. In addition, therapeutic nutritional intervention with substrates that stimulate the immune system may provide yet another modality for improving the general health of cancer patients. Furthermore, advances in molecular biology may someday result in the development of highly sophisticated products that combine nutrient substrates and antineoplastic pharmacologic agents in synergistic formulations designed to control or eradicate tumor cells while maintaining adequate nutrition.

Selected References

Buzby GP, Mullen JL, Matthews DC, et al. Prognostic nutritional index in gastrointestinal surgery. *Am J Surg* 139:160, 1980.

Daly JM, Lieberman MD, Goldfine J, et al. Enteral nutrition with supplemental arginine, RNA, and omega-3 fatty acids in patients after operation: Immunologic, metabolic, and clinical outcome. *Surgery* 112:56, 1992.

Daly JM, Redmond HP, Lieberman MD, et al. Nutritional support of patients with cancer of the gastrointestinal tract. *Surg Clin North Am* 71:523, 1991.

Heys SD, Park KGM, Garlick PJ, et al. Nutrition and malignant disease: Implications for surgical practice. *Br J Surg* 79:614, 1992.

Kern KA, Norton JA. Cancer cachexia. *JPEN* 12:286, 1988.

McClave SA, Mitoraj TE, Theilmeier KA, et al. Differentiating subtypes (hypoalbuminemic vs. marasmic) of protein calorie malnutrition: Incidence and clinical significance in a university hospital setting. *JPEN* 16:337, 1992.

Meguid MM, Debonis D, Meguid V, et al. Complications of abdominal operations for malignant disease. *Am J Surg* 156:341, 1988.

Shike M, Brennan MF. Supportive care of the cancer patient. In VT DeVita, S Hellman, SA Rosenberg (eds.), *Cancer: Principles and Practice of Oncology* (3rd ed). Philadelphia: Lippincott, 1989.

Shikova SA, Blackburn GL. Nutritional consequences of major gastrointestinal surgery: Patient outcome and starvation. *Surg Clin North Am* 71:509, 1991.

Shils ME. Nutrition and diet in cancer. In ME Shils, VR Young (eds.), *Modern Nutrition in Health and Disease* (7th ed). Philadelphia: Lea & Febiger, 1987.

Tchekmedyian NS, Zahyna D, Halpert C, et al. Clinical aspects of nutrition in advanced cancer. *Oncology* 49(Suppl 2):3, 1992.

Pharmacotherapy of Cancer

Phillip B. Ley

A basic understanding of cancer pharmacotherapy and related toxicities is mandatory for the general surgeon to be fully integrated into a multidisciplinary cancer care program. To intelligently discuss surgical options with patients, knowledge of the available adjuvant treatment regimens and their potential for toxicity is essential.

This chapter includes a discussion of basic principles of chemotherapy, an overview of the mechanisms of drug action and drug resistance, and a tabular listing of the drugs available and their places in representative combination chemotherapy protocols used in the treatment of solid tumors most commonly seen by the surgical oncologist. Finally, a summary of cancer pain management and the treatment of chemotherapy-induced emesis is included.

The reader should be aware that a complete discussion of cancer chemotherapy is beyond the scope of this brief overview. The drug and dosage regimens listed have been chosen as representative examples only and do not constitute a listing of all available protocols. For specific prescribing information, the practitioner is advised to consult individual manufacturer package inserts or one of the referenced texts.

Basic Principles of Chemotherapy

Cancer chemotherapeutic agents are the result of drug design and, largely, empiricism. Their use has developed based on an understanding of tumor growth characteristics, the cell cycle, drug mechanisms of action, and drug resistance. It is hoped that new techniques and advances in molecular biology will allow improvements in drug design to extend the possibility of complete chemotherapeutic response and possibly the cure of patients currently deemed beyond salvage.

TUMOR GROWTH AND KINETICS

Kinetic aspects of tumor growth have been well described. Two concepts that underscore our knowledge of the kinetics of tumor growth are Skipper's laws and Gompertzian growth. Skipper's laws apply to cells in the proliferating compartment of a tumor. First, the doubling time of proliferating cells is constant, creating a straight line on a semilog plot. Second, cell kill by a particular drug at a given dose is constant, irrespective of body burden. In most solid tumors, however, only a portion of cells within the tumor—the growth fraction—is proliferating at any given time. This partially accounts for the refractory nature of many solid tumors to chemotherapy.

Human tumors follow a pattern of Gompertzian, rather than straight-line, growth. Gompertzian growth describes a cell population decreasing as a result of cell death and increasing because of proliferation. Also, cell subpopulations may have ceased to proliferate but have not died, further swaying the growth curve from a straight semilog plot. The normal Gompertzian growth curve is sigmoid in shape. Maximum tumor growth rate occurs at about 30% of maximum tumor volume, where nutrient and oxygen supply to the greatest number of tumor cells is optimized. This portion of the curve is also where drug efficacy against a particular tumor may best be estimated.

The cell cycle is an important fundamental concept to understand when designing chemotherapeutic agents and treatment regimens. The cell cycle is divided into five components. The resting or nonproliferating cell is in the G0 phase, entering the active portion of the cycle following stimulation. DNA synthesis occurs during the S phase and is followed by the postsynthetic G2 phase. Mitosis occurs during the M phase and precedes the postmitotic G1 phase.

The cell cycle becomes important in drug selection because the cells in the growth fraction are more susceptible to certain agents. In a broad sense, antineoplastic agents may be classified on the basis of their activity in relation to the cell cycle. Most antimetabolites, etoposide, hydroxyurea, vinca alkaloids, and bleomycin are cell cycle–specific agents that are most effective against tumors with a high growth fraction. In contrast, alkylating agents, antineoplastic antibiotics, fluorouracil, floxuridine, and procarbazine exert their effect independent of the cell cycle and generally show more activity against slow-growing tumors.

DRUG MECHANISMS AND THERAPEUTICS

Knowledge of the basic action mechanisms of chemotherapeutic agents is critical in selecting drugs for an effective chemotherapy combination regimen, minimizing toxicity and drug interactions, and preventing emergence of drug-resistant clones. Agents may damage the DNA template by alkylation, cross-linking, double-strand cleavage by topoisomerase II, intercalation, and blockage of RNA synthesis. Mitosis may be arrested by spindle poisons. Antimetabolites block enzymes necessary for DNA synthesis. Hormonal agents and their antagonists may influence cellular signal transduction, and biologic response modifiers may influence the host's immune response to the tumor alone or in the context of concomitantly administered drugs.

Combination chemotherapy frequently is used in an effort to forestall the development of drug resistance to antineoplastic agents and to achieve synergism with reduced toxicity. The Goldie-Coldman hypothesis assumes that at the time of diagnosis, most tumors possess resistant clones. Multiple mechanisms of drug resistance develop during cancer progression. The most well studied of these involves the *mdr* gene, which codes for membrane-bound P-glycoprotein. P-glycoprotein serves as a channel through which cellular toxins (i.e., chemotherapeutic agents) may be excreted from the cell. Additional mechanisms of drug resistance are decreased drug transport into cells, reduction of drug activation, drug metabolism enhancement, development of alternative metabolic pathways, drug inhibition of enzyme targets overcome by gene amplification, and impairment of drug binding to target. A single drug may be subject to one or more mechanisms.

Interestingly, normal human cells never develop drug resistance. As a result, several caveats of combination chemotherapy have emerged. Drugs shown to be active as single agents should be chosen, and drugs selected for combined use should have different mechanisms of action. Ideally, drugs with different dose-limiting toxicities should be administered together, although toxicity overlap may necessitate dose reduction, as with myelo-suppression. Finally, drug combinations with similar patterns of resistance should be avoided.

Different patterns of chemotherapy administration are used in particular settings with specific goals. Induction chemotherapy is usually high dose and given in combination to induce complete remission. Consolidation is a repetition of an induction regimen in a complete responder to prolong remission or increase the cure rate. Chemotherapy given with an intent similar to that of consolidation but with higher doses than induction or with different agents at high doses is known as intensification. Maintenance regimens are low-dose, long-term protocols intended to delay tumor cell regrowth after complete remission. Induction, consolidation, intensification, and maintenance usually apply to hematologic malignancies but also may describe solid tumor regimens as well.

Neoadjuvant treatment in the preoperative or perioperative period is used more commonly with solid tumors, such as locally advanced breast carcinoma, soft-tissue sarcomas of the extremities, and, more recently, rectal carcinoma and squamous cell carcinoma of the head and neck. It is often given in combination with radiotherapy to improve survival, resectability, and organ preservation.

Palliative chemotherapy may be given to control symptoms or, if the toxicity profile is favorable, prolong life for incurable patients. Salvage chemotherapy involves the use of a potentially curative, high-dose protocol in patients failing or recurring after different standard treatment plans have been attempted.

Adjuvant chemotherapy is administered following curative surgery or radiotherapy as a short-course, high-dose regimen to destroy a low number of residual tumor cells. Several factors determine the effectiveness of adjuvant regimens, including tumor burden, drug dose and schedule, combination chemotherapy, and drug resistance. The drug(s) must be active locally against residual cells as well as distantly against clinically occult metastatic deposits. Extensive literature supports the use of adjuvant chemotherapy for breast, colon, rectal, and anal carcinomas and for ovarian germ cell tumors, osteosarcoma, and pediatric solid tumors. No definitive benefit has been reported yet for pancreatic, gastric, and testicular carcinomas or for cervical cancer and melanoma, although investigative adjuvant therapy protocols are ongoing and open for patient enrollment.

Most chemotherapeutic agents exhibit very steep dose–response profiles and have low therapeutic indices, making a high-dose, short-term administration desirable. This can be accomplished through regional dose intensification. One example is intraperitoneal chemotherapy of ovarian or gastric cancer with high risk of peritoneal recurrence, or low-volume intraperitoneal disease, pseudomyxoma peritonei, and peritoneal mesothelioma. Another type of regional dose intensification is intra-arterial therapy, which requires regional tumor confinement and a unique tumor blood supply and is most commonly used in hepatic artery infusion for primary or metastatic liver tumors that are surgically unresectable for cure. Intra-arterial chemotherapy also has been used for brain gliomas and some head and neck tumors. Isolated perfusion of a specific anatomic site, usually the extremities, is one more type of regional dose intensification that allows for the delivery of very high doses to the involved site with little systemic toxicity; it is often combined with hyperthermia. The largest body of literature discusses its use in all stages of melanoma, although limb perfusion for extremity sarcoma has been reported.

Chemotherapeutic Agents

Fundamental knowledge of the drugs available for cancer treatment, their mechanisms of action, general dose ranges, dominant toxicities, and indications for use is important to the general surgeon caring for cancer patients. Table 24-1 lists the available agents and their mechanisms, doses, and toxicities. Specific solid tumors germane to the practice of general surgery and representative chemotherapy combination protocols established for their treatment can be found in Table 24-2.

Management of Cancer Pain

The vast majority of patients with advanced cancer and as many as 60% of patients with any stage of disease experience significant pain. However, cancer pain frequently is undertreated for a multitude of reasons and fears that are largely unfounded. Effective management of cancer pain is achieved best with a multidisciplinary approach, including pain specialists, oncologists, nurses, pharmacists, physiatrists, physical and occupational therapists, psychologists, psychiatrists, primary care physicians, social workers, clergy, and hospice caregivers. Open lines of communication are of paramount importance to the successful management of cancer pain.

Cancer pain may be due to direct tumor involvement of bone, nerves, viscera, blood vessels, or mucous membranes and can be postoperative, postradiotherapy, or postchemotherapy. Narcotic use should follow the basic principles of cancer pain management, beginning with an agent that has the potential to provide relief; individualization of the agent, route, dose, and schedule; titration to efficacy; and provision of relief for breakthrough pain. Side effects should be anticipated and treated. Change from one route of administration to another should be done with equianalgesic doses, and the oral route should be used whenever possible. The practitioner should be aware of various adjuncts to pain management, including steroids, antidepressants, anxiolytics,

(text continues on page 494)

Table 24-1.   Cancer chemotherapeutic agents: Mechanisms, doses, and toxicities

Drug	Dose and schedule	Toxicity
Alkylating agents		
Busulfan	2–6 mg PO daily	Myelosuppression, pulmonary infiltrates pulmonary fibrosis, hemorrhagic cystitis alopecia, nausea and vomiting
Chlorambucil	4–10 mg PO daily	
Cyclophosphamide	1.0–1.5 g/m^2 IV; 50–200 mg PO daily	
Ifosfamide	1.2 g/m^2 IV daily × 5	
Mechlorethamine	16 mg/m^2 IV	
Melphalan	6–10 mg PO daily; 2–4 mg PO daily maintenance	
Thiotepa	16–32 mg/m^2 IV	
Antimetabolites		
Cytarabine	200 mg/m^2 IV daily × 5, continuous infusion	Stomatitis, GI tract injury, myelosuppression, alopecia
Fludarabine	30 mg/m^2 IV daily × 5	
Floxuridine	16–24 mg/m^2 IV or IA, daily continuous infusion	
Fluorouracil	500 mg/m^2 IV daily × 3	
6-Mercaptopurine	100 mg/m^2 PO daily	
Methotrexate	2.5–5.0 mg PO daily; 25–50 mg IV weekly; 200 mg–10 g IM with leucovorin	
6-Thioguanine	80 mg/m^2 PO daily	
Antibiotics		
Bleomycin	10 units/m^2 IV or SC daily × 5–7	Nausea, vomiting, alopecia, ulceration, pulmonary fibrosis
Dactinomycin	2.5 mg/m^2 IV	Stomatitis, GI injury, myelosuppression, alopecia

Table 24-1. *Continued*

Drug	Dose and schedule	Toxicity
Daunorubicin	90–180 mg/m² IV q3wk. Not to exceed 600 mg/m²	Stomatitis, alopecia, myelosuppression; cardiotoxicity at doses >600 mg/m²
Doxorubicin	50–75 mg/m² IV q3wk. Continuous infusion reduces cardiac toxicity	Stomatitis, alopecia, myelosuppression; cardiotoxicity at doses >500 mg/m²
Idarubicin	45–60 mg/m² PO q2-4wk; 20–25 mg/m² PO daily × 3. May be given IV.	GI toxicity, alopecia, cardiotoxicty
Mitomycin C	20 mg/m² IV q6-8wk	Myelosuppression, GI injury, hypercalcemia
Mitoxantrone	12 mg/m² IV daily × 3	Myelosuppression, alopecia, cardiotoxicty
Plicamycin	1 mg/m² IV qod × 3	Myelosuppression, hypocalcemia, hepatotoxicity
Mitotic inhibitors		
Etoposide (VP-16)	50–150 mg/m² IV daily × 3–5 q3-4wk; 50 mg/m² PO daily × 21	Myelosuppression, alopecia, GI toxicity, blisters, neuropathy, anaphylaxis
Taxol*	250 mg/m² IV daily × 5	Myelosuppression, stomatitis, neuropathy, anaphylaxis
Vinblastine	2.5–3.7 mg/m² IV weekly (not to exceed 18.5 mg/m² in adults or 12.5 mg/m² in pediatric patients)	Myelosuppression, GI toxicity, neuropathy, blisters, alopecia, hypertension, pulmonary toxicity
Vincristine	1.4 mg/m² IV weekly in adults; 2 mg/m² IV weekly in pediatric patients	Peripheral neuropathy, GI toxicity, paralytic ileus, SIADH, rash, alopecia, bladder atony
Hormonal agents		
Corticosteroids		Fluid retention, hyperglycemia, hypertension, infection
Dexamethasone	0.5–4.0 mg PO daily. Also available for IV and IM use	

continued

Table 24-1.   Cancer chemotherapeutic agents: Mechanisms, doses, and toxicities   *Continued*

Drug	Dose and schedule	Toxicity
Prednisone	15–100 mg PO daily	
Methyl-prednisolone	10–125 mg IV daily	
Androgens		Fluid retention, masculinization
Fluoxy-mesterone	10–40 mg PO daily	
Methyl-testosterone	50–200 mg PO daily	
Estrogens		Fluid retention, feminization, uterine bleeding, nausea and vomiting
Diethyl-stilbestrol	5 mg PO tid (breast); 1 mg PO daily (prostate)	
Antiestrogens		Hot flashes, nausea and vomiting
Tamoxifen	10 mg PO bid	
LHRH analogues Leuprolide	1 mg SC daily	
Antiandrogens		Decreased libido, impotence
Flutamide	250 mg PO tid	
Miscellaneous		
Amino-glutethimide	250–500 mg PO qid	Adrenal insufficiency
Megestrol acetate	40 mg PO qid	
Medroxy-progesterone	100–200 PO daily; 200–600 mg IM twice weekly	
Miscellaneous		
Asparaginase	8,000 IU/m^2 3–7 times weekly for 28 days	GI toxicity, somnolence, confusion, fatty liver
Carmustine	200 mg/m^2 IV	Myelosuppression, emesis
Lomustine	130 mg/m^2 PO	Myelosuppression, emesis
Hydroxyurea	800–1,600 mg/m^2 PO daily	Myelosuppression
Hexamethyl-melamine	100–300 mg/m^2 IV daily	Anorexia, myelosuppression, peripheral neuropathy

Table 24-1. *Continued*

Drug	Dose and schedule	Toxicity
Dacarbazine	80–160 mg/m² IV daily × 10	Myelosuppression, emesis
Procarbazine	50–200 mg/m² PO daily for 10–20 days	Myelosuppression, emesis, neuropathy
Mitotane	2–10 g PO daily	Adrenal insufficiency, emesis, diarrhea, tremors
Streptozocin	500 mg IV daily × 5 q6wk	Hypoglycemia
Cisplatin	40–120 mg/m² IV q1-4wk; 20–33 mg/m² IV daily × 3–5	Nausea and vomiting, nephrotoxicity, low magnesium, neuro-toxicity
Carboplatin	240–500 mg/m² IV q28d	Myelosuppression, emesis
Levamisole	50 mg PO q8h for 3 days q2wk with fluorouracil	Rash, arthralgia, myalgia, fever, neutropenia
Leucovorin	10 mg/m² PO with fluorouracil	Allergy

GI = gastrointestinal; SIADH = syndrome of inappropriate antidiuretic hormone; LHRH = luteinizing hormone-releasing hormone.
*Taxol is approved for investigational use only in the United States.

Table 24-2. **Specific solid tumors with combination chemotherapy regimens**

Tumor Type	Regimen	Agents
Breast	CMF	Cyclophosphamide Methotrexate Fluorouracil
	CMFVP	CMF Vincristine Prednisone
	FAC	Fluorouracil Doxorubicin Cyclophosphamide
Breast, ER-positive		Tamoxifen
Colorectal, adjuvant		Fluorouracil Levamisole
Colorectal, metastatic		Fluorouracil Leucovorin

continued

Table 24-2. Specific solid tumors with combination chemotherapy regimens *Continued*

Tumor Type	Regimen	Agents
Gastric	EAP	Etoposide Doxorubicin Cisplatin
	EFP	Etoposide Fluorouracil Cisplatin
	FAM	Fluorouracil Doxorubicin Mitomycin C
Pancreatic	SMF	Streptozocin Mitomycin C Fluorouracil
Head and neck	PFL	Cisplatin Fluorouracil Leucovorin
	CF	Cisplatin Fluorouracil
Lung, small cell	ACE	Doxorubicin Cyclophosphamide Etoposide
	CAV	Cyclophosphamide Doxorubicin Vincristine
	PACE	Cisplatin Doxorubicin Cyclophosphamide Etoposide
Lung, non-small cell	CAMP	Cyclophosphamide Doxorubicin Methotrexate Procarbazine
	DOXO/CIS	Doxorubicin Cisplatin
	MVP	Mitomycin C Vinblastine Cisplatin
Melanoma, metastatic	VBD	Vinblastine Bleomycin Cisplatin
	VDP	Vinblastine Dacarbazine Cisplatin Dacarbazine
Sarcoma, Ewing's	CAV	Cyclophosphamide Doxorubicin Vincristine
Sarcoma, osteogenic	T-10	Preoperative: methotrexate

Table 24-2.   *Continued*

Tumor Type	Regimen	Agents
Sarcoma, osteogenic		Postoperative: bleomycin, cyclophosphamide, and dactinomycin (BCD)
		Follow-up: methotrexate and doxorubicin
		Maintenance: doxorubicin, cisplatin, BCD
Sarcoma, soft tissue	MAID	Mesna Doxorubicin Ifosfamide DTIC
	CyVADiC	Cyclophosphamide Vincristine Doxorubicin DTIC
	VAC	Vincristine Dactinomycin Cyclophosphamide
Adrenocortical carcinoma		Mitotane
Neuroendocrine carcinoma		Doxorubicin Streptozocin
Neuroblastoma		Doxorubicin Cyclophosphamide Cisplatin
Liver		Doxorubicin Fluorouracil
Wilms' tumor		Dactinomycin Vincristine Doxorubicin Cyclophosphamide
Uterine cervix	BIP	Bleomycin Ifosfamide Cisplatin Mesna
Gestational trophoblastic	DMC	Dactinomycin Methotrexate Cyclophosphamide
Ovarian	CHAD	Cyclophosphamide Hexamethylmelamine Doxorubicin Cisplatin

continued

Table 24-2.   Specific solid tumors with combination chemotherapy regimens *Continued*

Tumor Type	Regimen	Agents
Testicular	BEP	Bleomycin Etoposide Cisplatin
Urinary bladder	MVAC	Methotrexate Vinblastine Doxorubicin Cisplatin
Prostate		Leuprolide Flutamide
Renal cell		Aldesleukin Interferon-alpha
Lymphoma, non-Hodgkin's	BACOP	Bleomycin Doxorubicin Cyclophosphamide Vincristine Prednisone
	CHOP	Cyclophosphamide Doxorubicin Vincristine Prednisone
	COPP	Cyclophosphamide Vincristine Prednisone
Lymphoma, Hodgkin's	MOPP	Nitrogen mustard Vincristine Procarbazine Prednisone
	ABVD	Doxorubicin Bleomycin Vinblastine Dacarbazine

ER = estrogen receptor

and neuroleptics, as well as neuroablative, neurostimulatory, and anesthetic procedures.

Table 24-3 is a compilation of various nonnarcotic and narcotic analgesic agents for treating cancer pain and includes dose ranges and expected toxicities.

Management of Chemotherapy-Induced Emesis

Because many surgical patients receive neoadjuvant and adjuvant chemotherapy, the general surgeon may be called on to treat chemotherapy-induced emesis, which is often a dose-limiting tox-

Table 24-3. Nonnarcotic and narcotic analgesic agents for treating cancer pain: dose ranges and expected toxicities*

Drug	Dose and Schedule	Equianalgesic Dose to 10 mg Morphine	Toxicity
Indomethacin	50–75 mg q6h PO	NA	Dyspepsia, allergy, antiplatelet
Diflunisal	500–1,000 mg q12h PO	NA	Dyspepsia, allergy, antiplatelet
Ibuprofen	200–800 mg q6-8h PO	NA	Dyspepsia, allergy, antiplatelet
Codeine	32–65 mg q3-4h PO	NA	Constipation, nausea, sedation
Propoxyphene	65–130 mg q3-4h	NA	Constipation, nausea, sedation
Hydrocodone	5–20 mg q4h	NA	Constipation, nausea, sedation; acetaminophen limits dosing interval
Oxycodone	2.5 mg q4h PO	NA	Constipation, nausea, sedation; acetaminophen and aspirin limit dosing
Morphine	10 mg IM q2-4h; 20–60 mg q2-4h PO	10 mg; 20–60 mg	Constipation, nausea, sedation, respiratory depression
Morphine, slow release	15–60 mg q8-12h PO	20–60 mg	Constipation, nausea, sedation, respiratory depression
Hydromorphone	1.5 mg IM q3-4h; 7.5 mg q3-4h PO	1.5 mg IM; 7.5 mg PO	Constipation, nausea, sedation, respiratory depression
Meperidine	50–125 mg q3-4h IM; 50–300 mg q3-4h PO	75 mg IM; 300 mg PO	Normeperidine accumulation limits chronic use
Levorphanol	1–4 mg IM q3-6h; 2–4 mg q3-6h PO	2 mg IM; 4 mg PO	Long half-life limits use
Methadone	5–15 mg IM q4-6h; 10–20 mg q4-6h PO	10 mg IM; 20 mg PO	Delayed toxicity accumulation
Fentanyl	25–100 mg/hr transdermal q3d	100 mg	

*Narcotic agonist/antagonists such as pentazocine, nalbuphine, and butorphanol generally are avoided for cancer pain therapy.

Table 24-4.   Available and commonly used antiemetic agents for chemotherapy-induced emesis

Drug	Dose and schedule	Toxicity
Ondansetron	8–32 mg IV daily; 4–8 mg PO q8h	Headache, constipation
Metoclopramide	2–3 mg/kg IV q2–3h; 10–20 mg PO q8h	Dystonia, akathisia, sedation, diarrhea, extrapyramidal effects
Haloperidol	1–3 mg IV q2-6h; 1–2 mg PO q3-6h	Dystonia, akathisia, hypotension, sedation
Droperidol	0.5–2.0 mg IV q4h	Extrapyramidal effect
Prochlorperazine	5–10 mg PO q3-4h; 25 mg PR q4-6h; 10–20 mg IM q3-6h	Extrapyramidal effect, sedation, dystonia, anticholinergic effects
Chlorpromazine	25–50 mg PO q3-6h	Same as prochlorperazine
Dexamethasone	10–20 mg IV daily; 4 mg PO q6-12	Hyperglycemia, euphoria, insomnia, rectal pain
Methylpred-nisolone	250–500 mg IV daily	Hyperglycemia, euphoria, insomnia, rectal pain
Lorazepam	0.025 mg/kg IV q4-8h; 1–2 mg PO q4-8h	Sedation, amnesia, confusion, hypotension
Diphenhydramine	25–50 mg IV or PO q6h	Anticholinergic effect, sedation
Dronabinol	5–10 mg/m2 PO q3-4h	Dysphoria, confusion, ataxia, hypotension, hallucination

icity that may lead patients to refuse further therapy. Three physiologic areas are included in the pathogenesis of chemotherapy-induced emesis (CIE): (1) the emetic center in the lateral reticular formation of the medulla, (2) vagal and splanchnic afferents from the gastrointestinal tract to the central nervous system, and (3) the chemoreceptor trigger zone in the area postrema of the medulla. Chemotherapeutic agents and their metabolites may trigger the latter two directly.

Three patterns of emesis tend to occur in association with chemotherapy. Acute emesis occurs within 24 hours of chemotherapy. Delayed emesis occurs more than 24 hours after the cessation of chemotherapy administration and is predisposed by female gender, high-dose cisplatin, and prior episodes of acute emesis. Anticipatory emesis may occur prior to retreatment in patients whose prior episodes of emesis were poorly controlled, occurring in up to

25% of patients who received prior chemotherapy. Younger age and history of motion sickness also predispose to CIE. Cisplatin, dacarabazine, mechlorethamine, and high-dose melphalan tend to have a very high incidence of inducing CIE. Carmustine, cyclophosphamide, procarbazine, and high-dose etoposide have a 60–90% incidence rate of causing CIE. Vincristine and chlorambucil, in contrast, have a low incidence of causing CIE.

The treatment of CIE underwent a veritable revolution with the introduction of the first selective serotonin antagonist, ondansetron. IV administration is not necessary in most cases of noncisplatin-induced emesis, because efficacy by oral administration is comparable. High-dose IV metoclopramide has been found effective in treating CIE, although less so than ondansetron, but its extrapyramidal side effects are a major problem. Standard phenothiazines are less effective but serve as useful adjuncts in the treatment of CIE. Corticosteroids, especially dexamethasone and methylprednisolone, act via a mechanism that is still unclear. In combination with other agents, corticosteroids dramatically improve antiemetic efficacy and may reduce the incidence of unwanted side effects by permitting dosage reduction. Lorazepam, a benzodiazepine, is useful in the prevention of anticipatory emesis and may reduce the incidence of dystonic reactions to metoclopramide. Most important, combinations of these agents, specifically ondansetron, dexamethasone, lorazepam, and metoclopramide, increase antiemetic efficacy and reduce troublesome side effects through presumed synergistic activity. Table 24-4 lists available and commonly used antiemetic agents with their dose ranges and the known major side effects.

Selected References

Abramowicz M (ed). Drugs of choice for cancer chemotherapy. *Med Lett Drugs Ther* 35:43, 1993.

DeVita V, Hellman S, Rosenberg S (eds.). *Cancer: Principles and Practice of Oncology* (4th ed). Philadelphia: Lippincott, 1993.

Krakoff I. Cancer chemotherapeutic and biologic agents. *CA Cancer J Clin* 41:264, 1991.

McEvoy G (ed.). *AHFS Drug Information.* Easton, MD: American Society of Hospital Pharmacists, 1992. Pp 522–661.

Pazdur R (ed.). *Medical Oncology: A Comprehensive Review.* Huntington, NY: PRR Inc., 1993.

Perry M (ed.). *The Chemotherapy Source Book.* Baltimore: Williams & Wilkins, 1992.

Portenoy R. Cancer pain management. *Semin Oncol* 20(Suppl 1):19, 1993.

Subject Index

Note: Page numbers followed by *f* indicate figures; page numbers followed by *t* indicate tabular material.